国家卫生和计划生育委员会“十三五”规划教材
全国高等学校教材
供本科护理学类专业用

Psychiatric Nursing

精神科护理学

双语

第2版

主　编　雷　慧　李小麟

副主编　杨　敏　王再超　王小琴

编者名单（以姓氏笔画为序）

王小琴 · 西安交通大学医学部护理系
王再超 · 湖北中医药大学护理学院
方　华 · 西安交通大学医学部护理系
李小麟 · 四川大学华西护理学院
杨　敏 · 中南大学湘雅护理学院
杨冰香 · 武汉大学健康学院
谷岩梅 · 河北中医学院护理学院
张　荣 · 承德医学院护理学院
张曙映 · 同济大学医学院护理系
陈　娟 · 四川大学华西医院心理卫生中心
赵　伟 · 郑州大学护理与健康学院
董方虹 · 河北大学护理学院
曾　慧 · 中南大学湘雅护理学院
雷　慧 · 承德医学院护理学院

秘　书　张　荣 · 承德医学院护理学院

人民卫生出版社

图书在版编目(CIP)数据

精神科护理学 : 英汉对照 / 雷慧，李小麟主编. —2版. —北京：人民卫生出版社，2021.2

ISBN 978-7-117-30005-6

Ⅰ. ①精… Ⅱ. ①雷… ②李… Ⅲ. ①精神病学 - 护理学 - 医学院校 - 教材 - 英、汉 Ⅳ. ①R473.74

中国版本图书馆 CIP 数据核字(2020)第 109445 号

精神科护理学（双语）
第 2 版

主　　编：雷　慧　李小麟
出版发行：人民卫生出版社（中继线 010-59780011）
地　　址：北京市朝阳区潘家园南里 19 号
邮　　编：100021
E - mail：pmph @ pmph.com
购书热线：010-59787592　010-59787584　010-65264830
印　　刷：人卫印务（北京）有限公司
经　　销：新华书店
开　　本：850 × 1168　1/16　　印张：40　　插页：1
字　　数：1075 千字
版　　次：2010 年 7 月第 1 版　2021 年 2 月第 2 版
　　　　　2021 年 2 月第 2 版第 1 次印刷（总第 3 次印刷）
标准书号：ISBN 978-7-117-30005-6
定　　价：119.00 元
打击盗版举报电话：010-59787491　E-mail：WQ @ pmph.com
质量问题联系电话：010-59787234　E-mail：zhiliang @ pmph.com

第六轮修订说明

为了在“十三五”期间，持续深化医药卫生体制改革，贯彻落实《“健康中国2030”规划纲要》，全面践行《全国护理事业发展规划（2016—2020年）》，顺应全国高等护理学类专业教育发展与改革的需要，培养能够满足人民群众多样化、多层次健康需求的护理人才。在对第五轮教材进行全面、充分调研的基础上，在国家卫生和计划生育委员会领导下，经第三届全国高等学校护理学专业教材评审委员会的审议和规划，人民卫生出版社于2016年1月进行了全国高等学校护理学类专业教材评审委员会的换届工作，同时启动全国高等学校本科护理学类专业第六轮规划教材的修订工作。

本轮教材修订得到全国百余所本科院校的积极响应和大力支持，在结合调研结果和我国护理学高等教育的特点及发展趋势的基础上，第四届全国高等学校护理学类专业教材建设指导委员会确定第六轮教材修订的指导思想为：坚持“规范化、精品化、创新化、国际化、数字化”战略，紧扣培养目标，遵循教学规律，围绕提升学生能力，创新编写模式，体现专业特色；构筑学习平台，丰富教学资源，打造一流的、核心的、经典的具有国际影响力的护理学本科教材体系。

第六轮教材的编写原则为：

1．**明确目标性与系统性** 本套教材的编写要求定位准确，符合本科教育特点与规律，满足护理学类专业本科学生的培养目标。注重多学科内容的有机融合，减少内容交叉重复，避免某些内容疏漏。在保证单本教材知识完整性的基础上，兼顾各教材之间有序衔接，有机联系，使全套教材整体优化，具有良好的系统性。

2．**坚持科学性与专业性** 本套教材编写应坚持“三基五性”的原则，教材编写内容科学、准确，名称、术语规范，体例、体系具有逻辑性。教材须符合护理学专业思想，具有鲜明的护理学专业特色，满足护理学专业学生的教学要求。同时继续加强对学生人文素质的培养。

3．**兼具传承性与创新性** 本套教材主要是修订，是在传承上一轮教材优点的基础上，结合上一轮教材调研的反馈意见，进行修改及完善，而不是对原教材进行彻底推翻，以保证教材的生命力和教学活动的延续性。教材编写中根据本学科和相关学科的发展，补充更新学科理论与实践发展的新成果，以使经典教材的传统性和精品教材的时代性完美结合。

4．体现多元性与统一性 为适应全国二百余所开办本科护理教育院校的多样化教学需要，本套教材在遵循本科教育基本标准的基础上，既包括有经典的临床学科体系教材，也有生命周期体系教材、中医特色课程教材和双语教材，以供各院校根据自身教学模式的特点选用。本套教材在编写过程中，一方面，扩大了参编院校范围，使教材编写团队更具多元性的特点；另一方面，明确要求，审慎把关，力求各章内容详略一致，整书编写风格统一。

5．注重理论性与实践性 本套教材在强化理论知识的同时注重对实践应用的思考，通过教材中的思考题、网络增值服务中的练习题，以及引入案例与问题的教材编写形式等，努力构建理论与实践联系的桥梁，以利于培养学生应用知识、分析问题、解决问题的能力。

全套教材采取新型编写模式，借助扫描二维码形式，帮助教材使用者在移动终端共享与教材配套的优质数字资源，实现纸媒教材与富媒体资源的融合。

全套教材共50种，于2017年7月前由人民卫生出版社出版，供各院校本科护理学类专业使用。

人民卫生出版社

2017年5月

获取图书网络增值服务的步骤说明

❶ 扫描封底圆形图标中的二维码，登录图书增值服务激活平台。

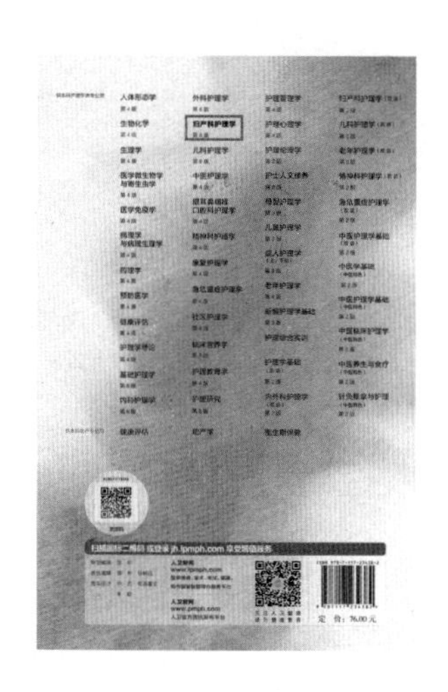

❷ 刮开并输入激活码，激活增值服务。

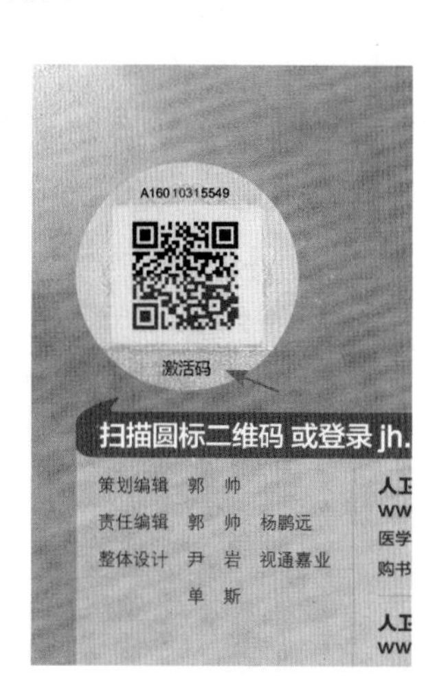

❸ 下载“人卫图书增值”客户端。

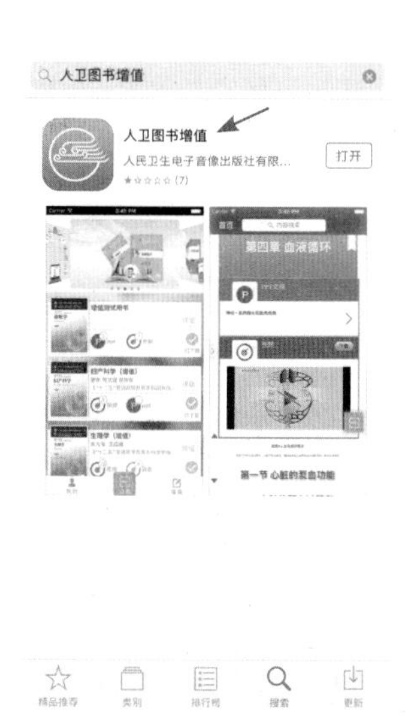

❹ 使用客户端“扫码”功能，扫描图书中二维码即可快速查看网络增值服务内容。

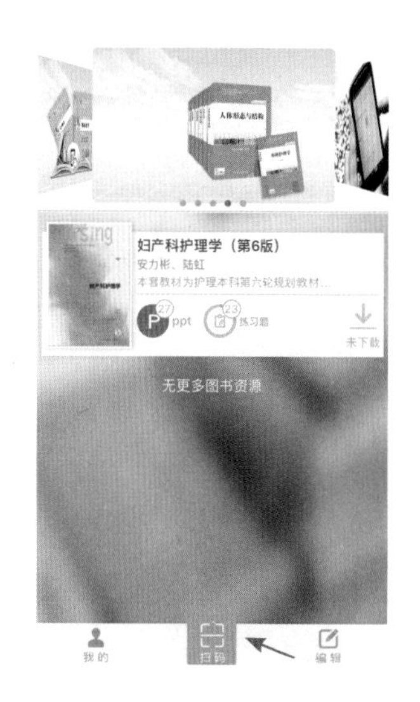

国家卫生和计划生育委员会“十三五”规划教材
全国高等学校本科护理学类专业规划教材

第六轮教材目录

1. 本科护理学类专业教材目录

序号	教材	版次	主审	主编	副主编
1	人体形态学	第4版		周瑞祥　杨桂姣	王海杰　郝立宏　周劲松
2	生物化学	第4版		高国全	解　军　方定志　刘　彬
3	生理学	第4版		唐四元	曲丽辉　张翠英　邢德刚
4	医学微生物学与寄生虫学	第4版		黄　敏　吴松泉	廖　力　王海河
5	医学免疫学	第4版	安云庆	司传平	任云青　王　炜　张　艳　胡　洁
6	病理学与病理生理学	第4版		步　宏	王　雯　李连宏
7	药理学	第4版		董　志	弥　曼　陶　剑　王金红
8	预防医学	第4版		凌文华　许能锋	袁　晶　龙鼎新　宋爱芹
9	健康评估	第4版	吕探云	孙玉梅　张立力	朱大乔　施齐芳　张彩虹　陈利群
10	护理学导论	第4版		李小妹　冯先琼	王爱敏　隋树杰
11	基础护理学	第6版		李小寒　尚少梅	王春梅　郑一宁　丁亚萍　吕冬梅
12	内科护理学	第6版		尤黎明　吴　瑛	孙国珍　王君俏　袁　丽　胡　荣
13	外科护理学	第6版		李乐之　路　潜	张美芬　汪　晖　李惠萍　许　勤
14	妇产科护理学	第6版	郑修霞	安力彬　陆　虹	顾　炜　丁　焱　罗碧如
15	儿科护理学	第6版		崔　焱　仰曙芬	张玉侠　刘晓丹　林素兰
16	中医护理学	第4版		孙秋华	段亚平　李明今　陆静波
17	眼耳鼻咽喉口腔科护理学	第4版		席淑新　赵佛容	肖惠明　李秀娥
18	精神科护理学	第4版		刘哲宁　杨芳宇	许冬梅　贾守梅
19	康复护理学	第4版		燕铁斌　尹安春	鲍秀芹　马素慧
20	急危重症护理学	第4版		张　波　桂　莉	金静芬　李文涛　黄素芳
21	社区护理学	第4版		李春玉　姜丽萍	陈长香
22	临床营养学	第4版	张爱珍	周　芸	胡　雯　赵雅宁
23	护理教育学	第4版		姜安丽　段志光	范秀珍　张　艳
24	护理研究	第5版		胡　雁　王志稳	刘均娥　颜巧元

续表

序号	教材	版次	主审	主编	副主编
25	护理管理学	第 4 版	李继平	吴欣娟　王艳梅	翟惠敏　张俊娥
26	护理心理学	第 4 版		杨艳杰　曹枫林	冯正直　周　英
27	护理伦理学	第 2 版		姜小鹰　刘俊荣	韩　琳　范宇莹
28	护士人文修养	第 2 版		史瑞芬　刘义兰	刘桂瑛　王继红
29	母婴护理学	第 3 版		王玉琼　莫洁玲	崔仁善　罗　阳
30	儿童护理学	第 3 版		范　玲	崔文香　陈　华　张　瑛
31	成人护理学（上、下册）	第 3 版		郭爱敏　周兰姝	王艳玲　陈　红　何朝珠　牟绍玉
32	老年护理学	第 4 版		化前珍　胡秀英	肖惠敏　张　静
33	新编护理学基础	第 3 版		姜安丽　钱晓路	曹梅娟　王克芳　郭瑜洁　李春卉
34	护理综合实训	第 1 版		李映兰　王爱平	李玉红　蓝宇涛　高　睿　靳永萍
35	护理学基础（双语）	第 2 版	姜安丽	王红红　沈　洁	陈晓莉　尼春萍　吕爱莉　周　洁
36	内外科护理学（双语）	第 2 版	刘华平 李　峥	李　津　张静平	李　卡　李素云　史铁英　张　清
37	妇产科护理学（双语）	第 2 版		张银萍　单伟颖	张　静　周英凤　谢日华
38	儿科护理学（双语）	第 2 版	胡　雁	蒋文慧　赵秀芳	高　燕　张　莹　蒋小平
39	老年护理学（双语）	第 2 版		郭桂芳　黄　金	谷岩梅　郭　宏
40	精神科护理学（双语）	第 2 版		雷　慧　李小麟	杨　敏　王再超　王小琴
41	急危重症护理学（双语）	第 2 版		钟清玲　许　虹	关　青　曹宝花
42	中医护理学基础（双语）	第 2 版		郝玉芳　王诗源	杨　柳　王春艳　徐冬英
43	中医学基础（中医特色）	第 2 版		陈莉军　刘兴山	高　静　裘秀月　韩新荣
44	中医护理学基础（中医特色）	第 2 版		陈佩仪	王俊杰　杨晓玮　郑方遒
45	中医临床护理学（中医特色）	第 2 版		徐桂华　张先庚	于春光　张雅丽　闫　力　马秋平
46	中医养生与食疗（中医特色）	第 2 版		于　睿　姚　新	聂　宏　宋　阳
47	针灸推拿与护理（中医特色）	第 2 版		刘明军	卢咏梅　董　博

2．本科助产学专业教材目录

序号	教材	版次	主审	主编	副主编
1	健康评估	第 1 版		罗碧如　李　宁	王　跃　邹海欧　李　玲
2	助产学	第 1 版	杨慧霞	余艳红　陈　叙	丁　焱　侯　睿　顾　炜
3	围生期保健	第 1 版		夏海鸥　徐鑫芬	蔡文智　张银萍

第四届全国高等学校护理学类专业

教材建设指导委员会名单

第四届全国高等学校护理学类专业教材建设指导委员会

本科教材评审委员会名单

指导主委	尤黎明	中山大学护理学院
主任委员	李小妹	西安交通大学护理学院
	崔 焱	南京医科大学护理学院
副主任委员	郭桂芳	北京大学护理学院
	吴 瑛	首都医科大学护理学院
	唐四元	中南大学湘雅护理学院
委 员（按姓氏拼音排序）	陈 垦	广东药科大学护理学院
	陈京立	北京协和医学院护理学院
	范 玲	中国医科大学附属盛京医院
	付菊芳	第四军医大学西京医院
	桂 莉	第二军医大学护理学院
	何朝珠	南昌大学护理学院
	何桂娟	浙江中医药大学护理学院
	胡 荣	福建医科大学护理学院
	江智霞	遵义医学院护理学院
	李 伟	潍坊医学院护理学院
	李春玉	延边大学护理学院
	李惠玲	苏州大学护理学院

第四届全国高等学校护理学类专业教材建设指导委员会

数字教材评审委员会名单

指导主委

段志光 · 山西医科大学

主任委员

孙宏玉 · 北京大学护理学院
章雅青 · 上海交通大学护理学院

副主任委员

仰曙芬 · 哈尔滨医科大学护理学院
熊云新 · 广西广播电视大学
曹枫林 · 山东大学护理学院

委　员
（按姓氏拼音排序）

柏亚妹 · 南京中医药大学护理学院
陈　嘉 · 中南大学湘雅护理学院
陈　燕 · 湖南中医药大学护理学院
陈晓莉 · 武汉大学 HOPE 护理学院
郭爱敏 · 北京协和医学院护理学院
洪芳芳 · 桂林医学院护理学院
鞠　梅 · 西南医科大学护理学院
蓝宇涛 · 广东药科大学护理学院
李　峰 · 吉林大学护理学院
李　强 · 齐齐哈尔医学院护理学院
李彩福 · 延边大学护理学院
李春卉 · 吉林医药学院

李芳芳 ‣ 第二军医大学护理学院
李文涛 ‣ 大连大学护理学院
李小萍 ‣ 四川大学护理学院
孟庆慧 ‣ 潍坊医学院护理学院
商临萍 ‣ 山西医科大学护理学院
史铁英 ‣ 大连医科大学附属第一医院
万丽红 ‣ 中山大学护理学院
王桂云 ‣ 山东协和学院护理学院
谢　晖 ‣ 蚌埠医学院护理学系
许　勤 ‣ 南京医科大学护理学院
颜巧元 ‣ 华中科技大学护理学院
张　艳 ‣ 郑州大学护理学院
周　洁 ‣ 上海中医药大学护理学院
庄嘉元 ‣ 福建医科大学护理学院

秘　书

杨　萍 ‣ 北京大学护理学院
范宇莹 ‣ 哈尔滨医科大学护理学院
吴觉敏 ‣ 上海交通大学护理学院

数字内容编者名单

主　编　王小琴　雷　慧

副主编　李小麟　王再超　杨　敏

编　委　（以姓氏笔画排序）

马明芳　西安交通大学第一附属医院精神卫生科
王小琴　西安交通大学医学部护理系
王再超　湖北中医药大学护理学院
方　华　西安交通大学医学部护理系
李小麟　四川大学华西护理学院
杨　敏　中南大学湘雅护理学院
杨冰香　武汉大学健康学院
谷岩梅　河北中医学院护理学院
张　荣　承德医学院护理学院
张曙映　同济大学医学院护理系
陈　娟　四川大学华西医院心理卫生中心
赵　伟　郑州大学护理与健康学院
董方虹　河北大学护理学院
曾　慧　中南大学湘雅护理学院
雷　慧　承德医学院护理学院

主编简介

雷慧，研究生学历，教授，硕士生导师，作为河北省优秀专家赴澳大利亚悉尼地区Bankstown Hospital学习进修，作为教育部留学基金委访问学者赴美国乔治梅森大学研究精神科护理。他的主要研究方向为精神科护理、护理英语。编写教材及参考用书20余部，其中主编规划教材《精神科护理学》等7部，《精神护理》荣获河北省第十一届社会科学优秀成果三等奖。主持省、市（厅）级科研课题十余项，发表中文核心期刊论文10余篇。先后获得河北省优秀教师、承德市专业技术拔尖人才（终身享受）、首批承德市科学技术学术带头人、承德市跨世纪学术及技术带头人、第四届金龙杯承德杰出人才贡献奖、承德医学院校级教学名师等。

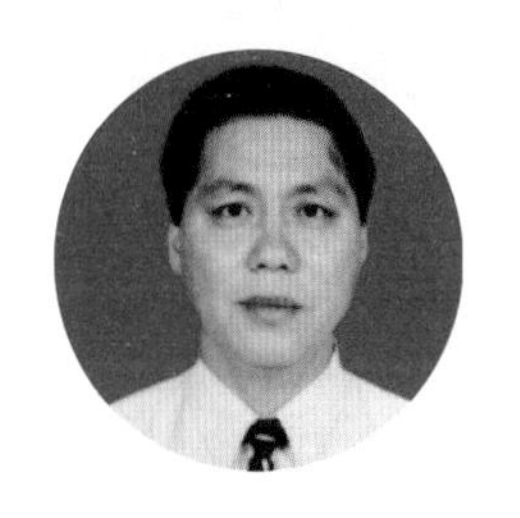

雷　慧

李小麟，硕士，毕业于泰国清迈大学，现任四川大学华西医院护理学院教授、硕士生导师，国家二级心理咨询师和心理治疗师。四川西部精神医学心身护理专委会主任委员，中国心理学会护理心理专委会委员。长期从事精神、心理临床护理与教学和临床心理咨询与治疗，有丰富的临床护理管理与教学经验，主要研究方向为精神心理护理及灾害心理救援。近年出版有关精神心理护理教材10余部，发表相关论文40余篇，负责课题10余个。

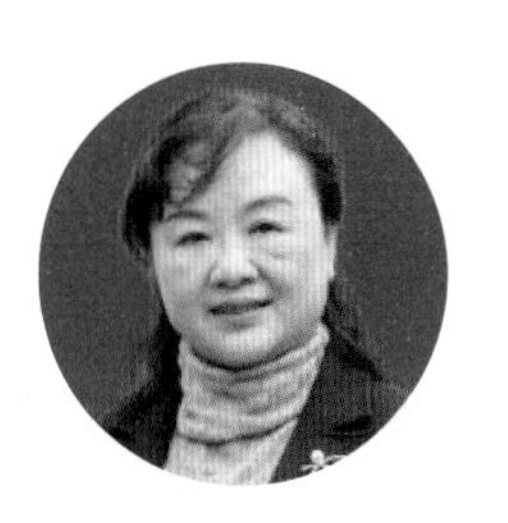

李小麟

副主编简介

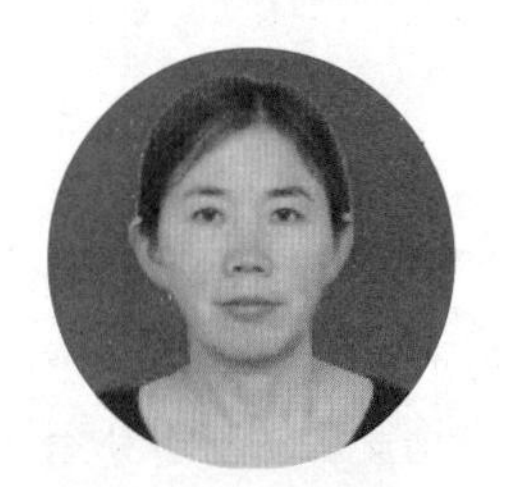

杨 敏

杨敏，生命伦理学博士，教授，硕士生导师，中南大学湘雅护理学院人文学系主任，中南大学湘雅护理学院伦理审查委员会主任，湖南省护理学会精神科护理专业委员会副主任委员。主要研究方向为精神心理护理、医学伦理。其主要承担护理专业《精神科护理》《基础护理学》《护理伦理》的课程教学；主编护理专业教材3部，副主编4部；发表学术论文20余篇。

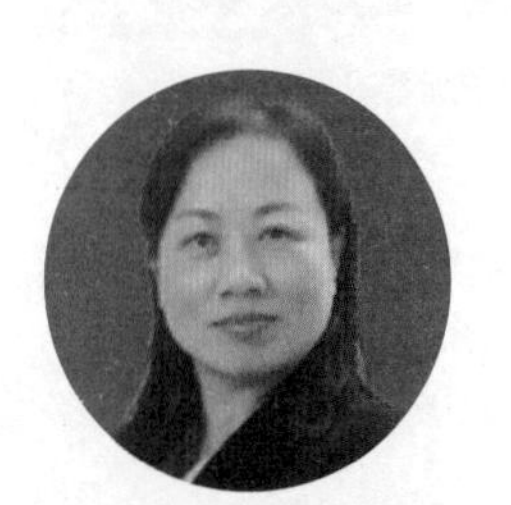

王再超

王再超，硕士，副教授，湖北中医药大学护理学院临床教研室专任教师，国家中医药管理局重点学科（中医护理学）、湖北省重点培育学科（护理学）护理标准化与信息化方向学术带头人。美国北卡罗莱纳州大学教堂山分校访问学者。兼任中国卫生信息与健康医疗大数据学会护理学分会委员，湖北省护理学会精神心理专业委员会常委。主讲《精神科护理学》《内科护理学》《护理信息学概论》等课程。研究方向为护理教育、护理标准化与信息化。近十年来，承担省级及以上课题4项，发表论文10余篇，参编人民卫生出版社规划教材6部。

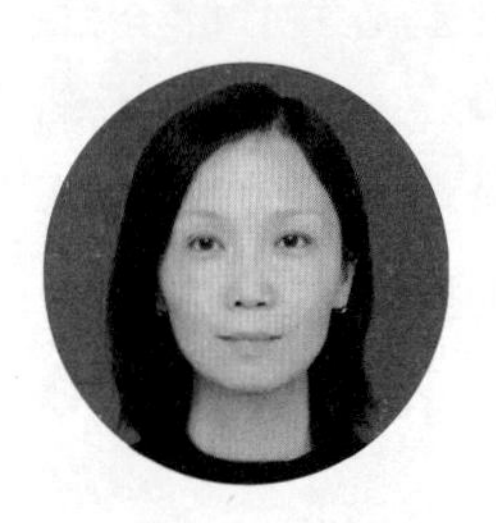

王小琴

王小琴，教授，就职于西安交通大学医学部护理系。本科毕业于西安医科大学，硕士毕业于泰国清迈大学妇幼护理学院，博士毕业于西安交通大学公共卫生学院，博士后毕业于美国阿肯色州立大学公共卫生学院。发表学术论文70余篇，其中第一作者SCI 17篇，单篇高被引112次；副主编本科教材2部，参编20余部；主持国家级和国际课题3项。其兼任《中国医学伦理学》编委和英文编辑，《中华现代医院管理杂志》常务编委，《中华现代护理杂志》核心审稿人；中华医学会医史陕西分会会员，陕西省性学会肿瘤专业委员会副主委等。研究方向为肿瘤护理学研究（胃癌的发病机制研究和营养学研究）和儿科护理学研究（营养学研究和行为研究）。

前 言

随着社会的进步、物质的丰富以及人类文明程度的提升，人们愈来愈意识到保持精神健康、防止精神疾病的重要性。我国的疾病谱发生了明显的变化，从建国初的防治传染病时代，到后来的以治疗躯体疾病为主，有专家提出目前已经到了“精神疾病时代”。因此，精神疾病已成为21世纪影响人类健康的最主要疾病之一。精神科护理学作为护理学的主要专业课程之一，既研究对精神障碍患者实施护理，也担负着帮助健康人保持精神健康、防止精神疾病发生的任务。

《精神科护理学》（双语）第2版的编写，吸收了国外发达国家精神护理的先进理念和治疗技术，并结合我国国情，以英汉对照的形式，反映当今精神科护理的最新理论及实践内容。本书的定位是培养适应国际护理服务需求的护理人才，供护理本科层次双语教学使用，亦可作为留学生护理本科专业汉语授课教材。通过对《精神科护理学》（双语）第2版的学习，不但能使学生了解对精神疾病的预防和护理知识，而且能更好地了解人的精神（心理）与行为的关系，从而提升对社会、家庭以及个人生活经历的认识。

《精神科护理学》（双语）第2版的编写，基本沿袭了第1版的主要框架，即在诊断名词的选择上，尽量采用《中国精神障碍分类与诊断标准第3版》（*Chinese Classification and Diagnostic Criteria of Mental Disorders, Third Edition*，*CCMD-3*），同时也参考并选择性地介绍了美国精神病学会的《精神障碍诊断和统计手册第5版》（*Diagnostic and Statistical Manual of Mental Disorders*，*Fifth Edition*，*DSM-IV*）和《国际疾病分类第10版》（*International Classification of Diseases*，*Tenth Revision*，*ICD-10*）的相关内容。并在如下方面做了修订：① 基于护理本科层次的需求和课时要求，对本书章节做了部分调整。首先，将第1版中的第一章和第二章合并，成为第2版的第一章。其次，将第1版的第十一章和第十二章合并为一章，成为第2版中的第十章。本书共18章，第一章至第五章是精神科护理学的总论部分，主要介绍精神科护理的基本概念和沿革、精神科护理程序、精神疾病护理中的护患关系与治疗性沟通、精神科常见的意外及防范、精神科护理中的伦理及法律问题等。第六章至第十四章是常见精神障碍患者的护理，主要介绍精神分裂症患者的护理、心境障碍患者的护理、人格障碍患者的护理、创伤与应激相关障碍患者的护理、神经症患者的护理、精神活性物质所致精神障碍患者的护理、器质性精神障碍患者的护理、心理因素所致生理障碍患者的护理，以及婴儿、儿童及青少年精神障碍患者的护理等。第三部分是具体的治疗和护理方法部分，主要介绍药物治疗及护理、躯体治疗、心理治疗及护理、精神卫生连续性护理等。② 原则上尊重第1版的编写思路、编写内容及形式，不做大的变动，但在前沿知识方面给予更新，如流行病学特点、相关护理理论和技能以及护理诊断和护理措施等内容。③ 由于本书第 1 版的篇幅较多，因此本次编写提倡压缩理论的描述，突出护理干预，特别是护士的护理技能以及处理问题和解决问题的能力等。④ 根据本次教材的统一编写要求，增设了学习目标、案例导入、思考题以及数字内容等。数字内容包括 PPT 课件、英文难点注释、相关知识拓展、图片、微视频和练习题等内容。

本教材的编写参考了国内外大量参考文献内容，在此我们对相关作者及出版单位表示诚挚的感谢。由于我们的编写能力和水平有限，书中难免会有疏漏之处，敬请使用本教材的教师、学生、其他读者以及护理界的同仁不吝指正，以不断提高本书的编写水平。

特此感谢湖北中医药大学护理学院童安港、袁锡，西安交通大学医学部惠沼沼、马梅，感谢他们在数字资源建设上给予的帮助。

雷　慧

2020 年 5 月

目 录

Chapter 1

001 **Introduction**

004 Section 1 Basic Concepts
- 004 I. Mental Health
- 008 II. Mental Illness
- 011 III. Psychiatric Nursing

013 Section 2 Historical Development of Psychiatric and Mental Health Nursing
- 013 I. History of Psychiatric and Mental Health Nursing Development in the World
- 016 II. History of Psychiatric-Mental Health Nursing Development in China
- 017 III. Challenges of Psychiatric and Mental Health Nursing

017 Section 3 Dimensions, Roles, and Functions of Psychiatric Nurses
- 018 I. Dimensions of Psychiatric Nurses
- 019 II. Continuum of Mental Health Settings
- 020 III. Roles of Psychiatric Nurses
- 023 IV. Functions of Psychiatric Nurses

第一章

001 **绪论**

004 第一节 基本概念
- 004 一、精神健康
- 008 二、精神疾病
- 011 三、精神科护理学

013 第二节 精神科护理发展史
- 013 一、国外精神科护理发展史
- 016 二、中国精神科护理发展史
- 017 三、精神科护理面临的挑战

017 第三节 精神科护士的工作范围、角色及功能
- 018 一、精神科护士的工作范围
- 019 二、精神卫生整体 - 连续性服务场所
- 020 三、精神科护士的角色
- 023 四、精神科护士的功能

Chapter 2

027 The Nursing Process in Psychiatric and Mental Health Nursing

029 Section 1 Introduction of the Nursing Process
- 029 I. Definition
- 030 II. Nursing Process in Psychiatric and Mental Health Nursing

031 Section 2 Nursing Assessment
- 032 I. Types of Assessment
- 032 II. Contents of Assessment

045 Section 3 Nursing Diagnosis
- 045 I. Definition of Nursing Diagnosis
- 046 II. Nursing Diagnosis in Psychiatric and Mental Health Nursing
- 048 III. Deriving Nursing Diagnosis

048 Section 4 Nursing Care Plan
- 049 I. Setting Nursing Objectives
- 049 II. Setting Nursing Interventions
- 051 III. General Principles of Writing Care Plans

051 Section 5 Nursing Implementation
- 052 I. Interventions during Nursing Implementing Phase
- 053 II. Evidence-Based Nursing Practice

055 Section 6 Nursing Evaluation
- 055 I. Definition of Nursing Evaluation
- 055 II. General Principles of Nursing Evaluation

056 Section 7 Documentation to the Nursing Process in Psychiatric and Mental Health Nursing

第二章

027 精神科护理程序

029 第一节 护理程序概述
- 029 一、护理程序的概念
- 030 二、精神疾病的护理程序

031 第二节 护理评估
- 032 一、评估的方式
- 032 二、评估的内容

045 第三节 护理诊断
- 045 一、护理诊断的概念
- 046 二、精神科护理中常用的护理诊断
- 048 三、护理诊断的形成

048 第四节 护理计划
- 049 一、制订护理目标
- 049 二、制订护理措施
- 051 三、书写护理计划的原则

051 第五节 护理实施
- 052 一、护理措施实施方法
- 053 二、循证护理实践

055 第六节 护理评价
- 055 一、护理评价的概念
- 055 二、护理评价的原则

056 第七节 精神科护理程序的记录方法

Chapter 3

061 **Relationship Development and Therapeutic Communication**

063 Section 1 Development of Nurse Client Relationship

064 I. Characteristics of Therapeutic Relationship in Psychiatric Settings

065 II. Conditions Essential to the Therapeutic Relationship

069 III. Development of Therapeutic Relationship in Psychiatric Settings

071 IV. Professional Characteristic Requirement for Psychiatric Nurses

072 V. Barriers of Therapeutic Relationship

075 Section 2 Therapeutic Communication

076 I. Therapeutic Communication Techniques

082 II. Barriers of Therapeutic Communication

084 III. Record of the Therapeutic Communication

第三章

061 **精神疾病护理中的护患关系与治疗性沟通**

063 第一节 精神疾病护理中的护患关系

064 一、精神疾病护理中护患关系的特征

065 二、精神疾病护理中建立治疗性护患关系的条件

069 三、精神疾病护理中护患关系的建立

071 四、精神疾病护理对专科护士的要求

072 五、精神疾病护理护患关系中常见的障碍及护理

075 第二节 治疗性沟通

076 一、治疗性沟通技巧

082 二、沟通中的常见障碍

084 三、沟通记录

Chapter 4

087 **Common Contingency and its Nursing Interventions**

089 Section 1 Nursing Care of Clients with Aggression

090 I. Introduction

090 II. Reasons of Aggressive Behavior

092 III. Application of the Nursing Assessment

103 Section 2 Nursing Care of Clients with Suicide

104 I. Classification

第四章

087 **精神科常见的意外与防范**

089 第一节 攻击行为的防范与处理

090 一、概述

090 二、攻击行为的原因

092 三、护理程序的应用

103 第二节 自杀的防范与处理

104 一、分类

105 II. Reasons of Suicide
108 III. Application of the Nursing Process
118 Section 3 Nursing Care of Clients with Spontaneous Leave
118 I. Risk Factors of Spontaneous Leave
119 II. Application of the Nursing Process
122 Section 4 Nursing Care of Clients with Other Contingencies
122 I. Choke
124 II. Eating Different Objects

Chapter 5
129 Ethical and Legal Issues in Psychiatric and Mental Health Nursing
131 Section 1 Introduction
132 I. Ethics and Related Concepts
133 II. Law and Related Concepts
137 Section 2 Common Ethical Considerations in Psychiatric Nursing
137 I. Ethical Principles of Nursing
140 II. Ethical Issues in Psychiatric and Mental Health Nursing
144 Section 3 Common Legal Considerations in Psychiatric Nursing
144 I. Types of Law
146 II. Legal Issues in Psychiatric and Mental Health Nursing
151 III. Nursing Interventions to Prevent Legal Issues

Chapter 6
157 Nursing for Clients with Schizophrenia
160 Section 1 Introduction
160 I. Definition
161 II. Epidemiology

105 二、自杀的原因
108 三、护理程序的应用
118 第三节 出走的防范与处理
118 一、与出走相关的因素
119 二、护理程序的应用
122 第四节 其他意外事件的防范与处理
122 一、噎食
124 二、吞食异物

第五章
129 精神科护理中的伦理及法律问题
131 第一节 概述
132 一、伦理及相关概念
133 二、法律及相关概念
137 第二节 精神科护理中常见的伦理问题
137 一、护理伦理的基本原则
140 二、精神科护理中常见的伦理问题
144 第三节 精神科护理中常见的法律问题
144 一、相关法律
146 二、精神科护理中常见的法律问题
151 三、预防法律问题发生的护理措施

第六章
157 精神分裂症患者的护理
160 第一节 概述
160 一、精神分裂症的定义
161 二、流行病学

161 Section 2 Etiology
162 I. Biological Factors
164 II. Psychological Factors
164 III. Environmental Factors

165 Section 3 Clinical Symptoms of Schizophrenia
165 I. Schizoid Personality Phase
165 II. Prodromal Phase
165 III. Active Phase
169 IV. Residual Phase

170 Section 4 Prognosis

171 Section 5 Treatment
172 I. Hospitalization
172 II. Somatic Treatments
176 III. Psychosocial Treatments and Rehabilitation

179 Section 6 Application of the Nursing Process
179 I. Nursing Assessment
183 II. Nursing Diagnosis and Nursing Objective
184 III. Nursing Plan and Implementation
187 IV. Nursing Intervention for Three Types of Behaviors

Chapter 7

199 **Nursing Management for Clients with Mood Disorders**

202 Section 1 Introduction
202 I. Concepts
202 II. Epidemiology

203 Section 2 Etiology
203 I. Biological Theories
204 II. Psychosocial Theories

204 Section 3 Clinical Manifestation of Mood Disorders
205 I. Manic Episode
206 II. Special Clinical Manic Situation
207 III. Depressive Episode
208 IV. Bipolar Disorder
209 V. Persistent Mood Disorder

161 第二节 病因及发病机制
162 一、生物学因素
164 二、心理社会因素
164 三、环境因素

165 第三节 精神分裂症的临床表现
165 一、精神分裂症人格期
165 二、前驱期
165 三、活跃期
169 四、残留期

170 第四节 预后

171 第五节 治疗
172 一、住院治疗
172 二、躯体治疗
176 三、心理治疗

179 第六节 护理程序的应用
179 一、护理评估
183 二、护理诊断和护理目标
184 三、护理计划和实施
187 四、针对特殊行为的护理

第七章

199 **心境障碍患者的护理**

202 第一节 概述
202 一、概念
202 二、流行病学

203 第二节 病因及发病机制
203 一、生物因素
204 二、心理社会因素

204 第三节 心境障碍患者的临床特点
205 一、躁狂发作
206 二、特殊的躁狂状态
207 三、抑郁发作
208 四、双相障碍
209 五、持续性心境障碍

209 Section 4 Treatment
209 I. Treatment Principles
209 II. Treatment of Mania
210 III. Treatment of Depression
213 Section 5 Application of the Nursing Process
213 I. Mania
218 II. Depression

Chapter 8

225 **Nursing Management for Clients with Personality Disorders**

228 Section 1 Introduction
228 I. Definition
228 II. Characteristics of Personality Disorders
229 III. Epidemiology
229 IV. Etiology and Mechanism
230 Section 2 Types and Clinical Manifestation
230 I. Paranoid Personality Disorder
231 II. Schizoid Personality Disorder
232 III. Dissocial Personality Disorder
233 IV. Emotionally Unstable Personality Disorder
234 V. Histrionic Personality Disorder
234 VI. Anankastic Personality Disorder
234 VII. Avoidant Personality Disorder
235 VIII. Dependent Personality Disorder
235 Section 3 Treatment and Prevention
236 I. Treatment
236 II. Prevention of Personality Disorders
237 Section 4 Application of the Nursing Process
237 I. Nursing Assessment
238 II. Nursing Diagnosis
239 III. Nursing Care Plan
242 IV. Nursing Evaluation

209 第四节 治疗
209 一、治疗原则
209 二、躁狂发作的治疗措施
210 三、抑郁发作的治疗措施
213 第五节 护理程序的应用
213 一、躁狂发作的护理程序
218 二、抑郁发作的护理程序

第八章

225 **人格障碍患者的护理**

228 第一节 概述
228 一、概念
228 二、人格障碍的共同特征
229 三、流行病学
229 四、病因及发病机制
230 第二节 常见类型及临床表现
230 一、偏执型人格障碍
231 二、分裂样人格障碍
232 三、社交紊乱型人格障碍
233 四、情绪不稳型人格障碍
234 五、表演型人格障碍
234 六、强迫型人格障碍
234 七、回避（焦虑）型人格障碍
235 八、依赖型人格障碍
235 第三节 治疗和预防
236 一、治疗
236 二、预防
237 第四节 护理程序的应用
237 一、护理评估
238 二、护理诊断
239 三、护理计划
242 四、护理评价

Chapter 9

245 **Nursing Care of Clients with Trauma and Stressor-Related Disorders**

247 Section 1 Introduction
247 I. Stress
248 II. Cognitive Appraisal
249 III. Stress Responses
251 IV. Coping Resources and Coping Mechanisms
252 Section 2 Trauma and Stressor-Related Disorders
252 I. Introduction
254 II. Etiology and Mechanism
254 III. Types and Clinical Manifestations
259 IV. Treatment
260 V. Application of the Nursing Process
267 Section 3 Crisis Intervention
268 I. Introduction
268 II. Types of Crisis
269 III. Phases in the Development of a Crisis
270 IV. Crisis Intervention and the Role of the Nurse

第九章

245 **创伤与应激相关障碍患者的护理**

247 第一节 概述
247 一、应激
248 二、认知评价
249 三、应激反应
251 四、应对资源及应对机制
252 第二节 创伤与应激相关障碍
252 一、概述
254 二、病因及发病机制
254 三、常见类型和临床表现
259 四、治疗
260 五、护理程序的运用
267 第三节 危机干预
268 一、概述
268 二、危机的种类
269 三、危机的发展阶段
270 四、危机干预及护士的角色

Chapter 10

281 **Nursing Management for Clients with Neurosis**

284 Section 1 Nursing Management for Clients with Anxiety Disorders
284 I. Normal Anxiety and Pathological Anxiety
286 II. Panic Disorder
289 III. Generalized Anxiety Disorder
291 IV. Application of the Nursing Process

第十章

281 **神经症患者的护理**

284 第一节 焦虑障碍患者的护理
284 一、正常焦虑与病理性焦虑
286 二、惊恐障碍
289 三、广泛性焦虑障碍
291 四、护理程序的应用

297 Section 2 Nursing Management for Clients with Phobic Anxiety Disorder
298 I. Etiology and Mechanism
299 II. Clinical Manifestation
301 III. Treatment
302 IV. Application of the Nursing Process
305 Section 3 Nursing Management for Clients with Obsessive Compulsive Disorder
306 I. Etiology and Mechanism
307 II. Clinical Manifestation
308 III. Treatment
311 IV. Application of the Nursing Process
315 Section 4 Nursing Management for Clients with Somatoform Disorders
316 I. Somatization Disorder
319 II. Hypochondriasis
320 III. Application of the Nursing Process
324 Section 5 Nursing Management for Clients with Dissociative Disorder
326 I. Etiology
327 II. Clinical Manifestation
329 III. Treatment
330 IV. Application of the Nursing Process

297 第二节 恐惧性焦虑障碍患者的护理
298 一、病因及发病机制
299 二、临床表现
301 三、治疗
302 四、护理程序的应用
305 第三节 强迫性障碍患者的护理
306 一、病因及发病机制
307 二、临床表现
308 三、治疗
311 四、护理程序的应用
315 第四节 躯体形式障碍患者的护理
316 一、躯体化障碍
319 二、疑病障碍
320 三、护理程序的应用
324 第五节 分离性障碍患者的护理
326 一、病因
327 二、临床表现
329 三、治疗
330 四、护理程序的应用

Chapter 11
337 **Nursing Management for Clients with Substance-related Disorders**
340 Section 1 Introduction
340 I. Definitions and Terms
341 II. Classification of Psychoactive Substances
342 III. Epidemiology
342 IV. Etiology and Mechanism
345 V. Diagnosis and Prognosis
346 Section 2 Alcohol-related Disorders
346 I. Clinical Manifestation

第十一章
337 **精神活性物质所致精神障碍患者的护理**
340 第一节 概述
340 一、相关概念
341 二、精神活性物质的分类
342 三、流行病学
342 四、病因及发病机制
345 五、诊断与预后
346 第二节 酒精相关障碍
346 一、临床表现

349 II. Treatment

350 Section 3 Opioid-related Disorders
350 I. Clinical Manifestation
351 II. Treatment

352 Section 4 Stimulant-related Disorders
352 I. Clinical Manifestation
352 II. Treatment

353 Section 5 Other Substance-related Disorders
353 I. Cannabis-Related Disorders
354 II. Hallucinogen-Related Disorders
354 III. Inhalant-Related Disorders
355 IV. Sedative, Hypnotic, or Anxiolytic-Related Disorders
355 V. Tobacco-Related Disorders

356 Section 6 Application of the Nursing Process
356 I. Nursing Assessment
357 II. Nursing Diagnosis
358 III. Nursing planning
363 IV. Nursing Evaluation

349 二、治疗

350 第三节 阿片类物质相关障碍
350 一、临床表现
351 二、治疗

352 第四节 兴奋剂相关障碍
352 一、临床表现
352 二、治疗

353 第五节 其他物质相关障碍
353 一、大麻相关障碍
354 二、致幻剂相关障碍
354 三、吸入剂相关障碍
355 四、镇静、催眠药及抗焦虑药相关障碍
355 五、烟草相关障碍

356 第六节 护理程序的应用
356 一、护理评估
357 二、护理诊断
358 三、护理计划
363 四、护理评价

Chapter 12

367 **Nursing Care of Clients with Organic Mental Disorders**

370 Section 1 Mental Disorder Due to Cerebral Organic Disease
370 I. Delirium
372 II. Dementia

376 Section 2 Alzheimer's Disease and Vascular Dementia
376 I. Alzheimer's Disease
379 II. Vascular Dementia

382 Section 3 Application of the Nursing Process for Clients with Cognitive Impairment
382 I. Nursing Assessment
383 II. Nursing Diagnosis
384 III. Nursing Objectives
384 IV. Nursing Intervention
386 V. Nursing Evaluation

第十二章

367 **器质性精神障碍患者的护理**

370 第一节 脑器质性精神障碍的常见综合征
370 一、谵妄
372 二、痴呆

376 第二节 阿尔茨海默病和血管性痴呆
376 一、阿尔茨海默病
379 二、血管性痴呆

382 第三节 认知功能障碍患者的护理
382 一、护理评估
383 二、护理诊断
384 三、护理目标
384 四、护理措施
386 五、护理评价

Chapter 13

第十三章

389 **Nursing Management for Children and Adolescents with Psychiatric Disorders**

389 儿童及青少年精神障碍患者的护理

392 Section 1 Nursing Management for Children and Adolescents with Mental Retardation
392 I. Introduction
392 II. Etiology and Mechanism
393 III. Types and Clinical Manifestation
394 IV. Treatment
397 V. Application of the Nursing Process

392 第一节 精神发育迟滞患者的护理
392 一、概述
392 二、病因及发病机制
393 三、常见类型与临床表现
394 四、治疗
397 五、护理程序的应用

402 Section 2 Nursing Management for Children and Adolescents with Autistic Disorder
402 I. Introduction
402 II. Etiology and Mechanism
403 III. Types and Clinical Manifestation
405 IV. Treatment
406 V. Application of the Nursing Process

402 第二节 儿童孤独症患者的护理
402 一、概述
402 二、病因及发病机制
403 三、常见类型与临床表现
405 四、治疗
406 五、护理程序的应用

409 Section 3 Nursing Management for Children and Adolescents with Attention Deficit and Hyperactivity Disorder
409 I. Introduction
410 II. Etiology and Mechanism
411 III. Types and Clinical Manifestation
411 IV. Treatment
412 V. Application of the Nursing Process

409 第三节 注意缺陷与多动障碍患者的护理
409 一、概述
410 二、病因及发病机制
411 三、常见类型与临床表现
411 四、治疗
412 五、护理程序的应用

415 Section 4 Nursing Management for Children and Adolescents with Conduct Disorder
415 I. Introduction
416 II. Etiology and Mechanism
417 III. Types and Clinical Manifestation
418 IV. Treatment
421 V. Application of the Nursing Process

415 第四节 品行障碍患者的护理
415 一、概述
416 二、病因及发病机制
417 三、常见类型与临床表现
418 四、治疗
421 五、护理程序的应用

424 Section 5 Nursing Management for Children and Adolescents with Tic Disorders
424 I. Introduction
424 II. Etiology and Mechanism
425 III. Types and Clinical Manifestation
426 IV. Treatment
426 V. Application of the Nursing Process

424 第五节 儿童抽动症患者的护理
424 一、概述
424 二、病因及发病机制
425 三、常见类型与临床表现
426 四、治疗
426 五、护理程序的应用

428 Section 6 Nursing Management for Children and Adolescents with Emotional Disorder
428 I. Introduction
429 II. Etiology and Mechanism
429 III. Types and Clinical Manifestation
430 IV. Treatment
430 V. Application of the Nursing Process

428 第六节 儿童情绪障碍患者的护理
428 一、概述
429 二、病因及发病机制
429 三、常见类型与临床表现
430 四、治疗
430 五、护理程序的应用

Chapter 14

437 Nursing Management of Clients with Physiological Disorders Related to Psychological Factors

第十四章

437 心理因素所致生理障碍患者的护理

440 Section 1 Eating Disorders
440 I. Anorexia Nervosa
444 II. Bulimia Nervosa

440 第一节 进食障碍
440 一、神经性厌食症
444 二、神经性贪食症

446 Section 2 Sleep Disorders
447 I. Primary Insomnia
450 II. Primary Hypersomnia
451 III. Circadian Rhythm Sleep Disorder
452 IV. Sleepwalking Disorder

446 第二节 睡眠障碍
447 一、失眠症
450 二、嗜睡症
451 三、睡眠的昼夜节律障碍
452 四、睡行症

453 Section 3 Application of the Nursing Process
453 I. Eating Disorders
457 II. Sleep Disorders

453 第三节 护理程序的应用
453 一、进食障碍
457 二、睡眠障碍

Chapter 15

463 **Psychopharmacology and Nursing Care**

466 Section 1 Introduction
466 I. History of Psychiatric Medication
467 II. Mechanism of Psychiatric Medication
469 Section 2 Common Medications
469 I. Antipsychotic Drugs
476 II. Drugs for treating mood disorders
493 III. Drugs for Treating Anxiety and Sleep Disorders
497 Section 3 Nursing Care of Clients with Psychiatric Medication
497 I. Nursing Assessment
498 II. Diagnosis/Outcome Identification
499 III. Nursing Intervention
500 IV. Evaluation

第十五章

463 **药物治疗及护理**

466 第一节 概述
466 一、精神药物发展概况
467 二、精神药物的作用机制
469 第二节 常用药物
469 一、抗精神病药物
476 二、治疗心境障碍的药物
493 三、治疗焦虑和睡眠障碍的药物
497 第三节 使用精神药物患者的护理
497 一、护理评估
498 二、护理诊断 / 护理目标
499 三、护理措施
500 四、护理评价

Chapter 16

503 **Somatic Therapy**

505 Section 1 Electroconvulsive Therapy
506 I. Introduction
506 II. Mechanism of Action
507 III. Indications
507 IV. Contraindications
507 V. Clinical Guidelines
511 VI. Adverse Effects
513 VII. Nursing Care in Electroconvulsive Therapy
521 VIII. Role of Nurses in Electroconvulsive Therapy
521 Section 2 Other Therapies
521 I. Transcranial Magnetic Stimulation Therapy
523 II. Light Therapy
524 III. Hypnotherapy

第十六章

503 **躯体治疗**

505 第一节 电抽搐治疗
506 一、概述
506 二、作用机制
507 三、适应证
507 四、禁忌证
507 五、治疗方法
511 六、治疗的不良反应及并发症
513 七、电抽搐治疗的护理
521 八、护士在电抽搐治疗中的角色
521 第二节 其他治疗
521 一、经颅磁刺激治疗
523 二、光感治疗
524 三、催眠疗法

Chapter 17

527 **Psychotherapy and Nursing Care**

529 Section 1 Introduction
530 I. Definition and Classification of Psychotherapy
531 II. The Role of Nurses in Psychotherapy

531 Section 2 Psychoanalysis
531 I. Mechanism of Action
532 II. Indication
532 III. Techniques of Psychoanalysis
533 IV. The Role of Nurses in Psychoanalysis

534 Section 3 Behavioral Therapy
534 I. Mechanism of Action
534 II. Indication
535 III. Techniques of Behavioral Therapy
541 IV. Role of Nurses in Behavioral Therapy

542 Section 4 Cognitive Therapy
542 I. Mechanism of Action
543 II. Indication
543 III. Techniques of Cognitive Therapy
547 IV. Role of Nurses in Cognitive Therapy

548 Section 5 Client-centered Therapy
548 I. Mechanism of Action
548 II. Indication
548 III. Techniques of Client-Centered Therapy
549 IV. Role of Nurses in Client-Centered Therapy

550 Section 6 Complementary Therapies
550 I. Introduction
550 II. Types of Complementary Therapies
553 III. The Role of Nurses in Complementary Therapies

第十七章

527 **心理治疗与护理**

529 第一节 概述
530 一、心理治疗的概念及分类
531 二、护士在心理治疗中的角色

531 第二节 精神分析法
531 一、作用机制
532 二、适应证
532 三、精神分析法的基本技术
533 四、精神分析疗法中护士角色

534 第三节 行为疗法
534 一、作用机制
534 二、适应证
535 三、行为疗法常用技术
541 四、护士在行为疗法中的角色

542 第四节 认知疗法
542 一、作用机制
543 二、适应证
543 三、认知疗法常用技术
547 四、护士在认知疗法中的角色

548 第五节 来访者中心疗法
548 一、作用机制
548 二、适应证
548 三、来访者中心疗法基本技术
549 四、以人为中心疗法中的护士角色

550 第六节 补充治疗
550 一、概述
550 二、补充疗法的种类
553 三、补充治疗中护士的角色

Chapter 18

557 Continuity of Mental Health Nursing Care

560 Section 1 Introduction
560 I. Interdisciplinary Team and the Role of Nurses
562 II. Components of Continuity of Mental Health Nursing Care
565 III. Referrals along the Continuum of Mental Health Care

568 Section 2 Psychiatric Rehabilitation
568 I. Fundamental Principles of Psychiatric Rehabilitation
569 II. Role of the Nurse in Psychiatric Rehabilitation
570 III. Program Elements in Psychiatric Rehabilitation

573 Section 3 Community Mental Health Care
573 I. Principles of Community Mental Health Care
575 II. Roles of Nurses in Community Mental Health Nursing
576 III. Program Elements in Community Mental Health Nursing

580 Section 4 Family Care
580 I. Family assessment
583 II. Family Interventions

590 英文索引

608 参考文献

第十八章

557 精神卫生连续性护理

560 第一节 概述
560 一、精神卫生连续性护理的多学科团队和护士角色
562 二、精神卫生连续性护理的内容
565 三、精神连续性护理过程中的转介机制

568 第二节 精神康复
568 一、精神康复的基本原则
569 二、护士在精神康复中的角色
570 三、精神康复项目的内容

573 第三节 社区精神卫生护理
573 一、社区精神卫生护理的原则
575 二、护士在社区精神卫生中的角色
576 三、社区精神卫生的服务内容

580 第四节 家庭护理
580 一、家庭评估
583 二、家庭干预

598 中文索引

Chapter 1 Introduction
第一章 绪 论

Learning Objectives

Memorization

1. Describe concepts of mental health and mental illness, and continuum of them.
2. Summarize the criteria of mental health and factors influencing mental health.

Comprehension

1. Explain the history of psychiatric nursing as a foundation for current mentally ill care practice with cases.
2. Identify patients' possible signs of mental illness.
3. Explain the impact of psychotherapeutic drugs on psychiatric nursing.

Application

Play effective roles of nurses in the practice of psychiatric nursing settings.

学习目标

识记

1. 能准确描述精神健康、精神疾病的概念，以及二者之间的整体连续性。
2. 能正确概述精神健康的标准及影响精神健康的因素。

理解

1. 能用实例说明精神科护理发展历史是目前精神科护理实践的基础。
2. 能识别精神病患者可能出现的征兆。
3. 能具体说明精神病治疗药物对精神科护理的作用。

运用

正确发挥护士在精神科护理实践中的作用。

Linda, a 20-year-old girl, who is a grade 3 college student, is brought into emergency room after a suicide attempt. She has been extremely depressing since her parent's death 3 months ago in a car crash driven by her. Linda has epilepsy and has had several seizures since the car accident happened. She thinks she should be punished for her carelessness, and does not care what happens to herself. She has not gone to school or shown up for her part-time job which is tutoring children in writing.

Please think about the following questions based on the case:

1. What might be the actual and potential nursing diagnoses for Linda?
2. How do psychiatric mental health nurses with either basic or advanced role cooperate together to provide effective care for Linda?

患者，琳达，女，20岁，是一名大三的学生，因有自杀倾向被送到急诊科。3个月前，琳达带着父母驾车出行，不幸出了车祸，父母双亡，从此，琳达一直精神不振，茶饭不思。患者自幼有癫痫病史，自从上次车祸后多次出现癫痫抽搐发作。她为自己因粗心大意而造成的惨痛结果而内疚，甘愿被惩罚。琳达的病情已经影响到她的社会功能，目前不能继续上学，兼职家教的写作课也停止了。

请思考：

1. 患者目前及潜在的护理诊断是什么？
2. 普通护士与临床护理专家应如何互相配合，为患者提供有效的护理措施？

In June of 2013, we were all stunned by the news of a man from Baiyun District Guangzhou City China, who was said to suffer from psychiatric and mental disorder, killing 6 people and wounding seven with an axe. A long list of similar tragic events can be generated. You may ask why these criminals did these tragic and inconceivable events. Such issues are complex and related to what you'll be studying in this text. Although most of you will not work full time in psychiatric hospitals, you can learn a lot about mental health, mental illness, yourself, and the relation between the psychiatric activity and the behavior by reading this text.

Psychiatric nursing involves the diagnosis and treatment of human responses to actual or potential mental health problems. It is a specialized area of nursing practice that uses theories of human behavior as its scientific framework and requires the purposeful use of self as its art of expression. This chapter discusses fundamental concepts of psychiatric nursing, roles and functions of psychiatric-mental health nurses, and history. When you understand the history, you understand the context. It provides a foundation for the rest of the book.

2013年6月，人们都被这样一件事情震惊了，广州市白云区一位患精神病的男子，手持利斧，砍死6人，砍伤7人。像这样惨痛的事件举不胜举。然而，究竟这些肇事者都属于什么精神（心理）问题？为什么要做出这些不可思议的事情？接下来的章节将解开你的疑惑。尽管大多数护生毕业后不一定做全职的精神科护士，但通过本书的学习，能使你懂得什么是精神健康、精神疾病，更好地了解自己，理解人的行为与精神（心理）的关系。

精神科护理学涉及诊断和处理人对现实或潜在的精神疾病的反映。它是护理学的一个分支，以人类行为学理论为科学框架，艺术地为个体提供心理健康服务。本章将讨论精神科护理的基本概念、护士的角色和功能以及精神科护理发展史。便于读者更好地理解各章间的关系。

Section 1 Basic Concepts

I. Mental Health

People struggle long for freedom of pain, for the joy that accompanies a healthy body and mind, for the opportunity to live in harmony with their environment, and for a long and productive life. The concept of health includes a sense of independence, optimism, a sense of psychological well-being, and a state of physical, emotional, social, and spiritual wellness. Mental health is a crucial part of health. A person's state of health directly influences his or her daily choices, independence, individuality and lifestyle. Therefore, health is the foundations and indicators of personal achievement, families' happiness, social stability and country's prosperity. Nurses are in a unique position to assist clients in achieving and maintaining optimal levels of health.

i. Mental Activity

Mental activity is a special phenomena of human being which is developed in the process of evolution. Mental activity reflects the complex functions of the brain, which includes the psychological process and personality. Psychological process is the reflection of a person's comprehension of the world around him, including perception, emotion and conation. Personality is the unique character of the person consisting of temperament, character and capacity. Each part of mental health functions interdependently and collaboratively as a whole maintaining the normal mental activity and functioning. The human being's mental activity is generally influenced by genetics, developmental levels, social cultures, historical background, learning and cultural tradition.

ii. Mental Health

Mental health is a multidimensional concept and must be viewed from a broader perspective. The concept of health is influenced by a person's age, educational level, physical condition, self-care competence, social class, customs and habit, value system, technology development and other factors. There is no universal definition of mental health. A number of theorists have attempted to define the concept. Many of the definitions deal with various aspects

第一节　基本概念

一、精神健康

免除痛苦，保持身心健康与幸福，人与环境和谐共处，享受长寿而有价值的生活是人类共同追求的目标。健康的意义在于独立感、乐观向上、心理上的幸福感及生理、情感、社会心理和精神方面的满足感，精神健康是健康的主要内容之一。健康直接影响着一个人的日常行为、独立自主性、个性及生活方式。因此，健康是个人成就、家庭幸福、社会安定、国家富强的基础及标志，护理的目标是使每个人达到并保持最大程度的健康。

（一）精神活动

精神又称心理，是生物进化过程中表现出的一种特殊的生命现象，精神一般通过精神活动表现出来。精神活动是人脑在反映客观事物的过程中所进行的一系列复杂的功能活动的总称。精神活动按照心理现象可以划分为心理过程及个性心理两个部分。心理过程是人在认识客观事物的过程中所表现出来的一系列心理现象，包括认识过程、情感过程及意志过程。个性心理是在心理过程中所表现出的具有一定倾向性、稳定性的心理特征总和。它包括个性心理倾向、个性心理特征及自我意识三个部分。精神活动的各个部分相互联系、精密协调，维持着精神活动的统一与完整。人的精神活动一般受遗传、发育水平、社会文化、历史背景、学习及文化传统等因素的影响。

（二）精神健康

精神健康（精神卫生）是一个复杂、多维、综合性、且不断变化的概念。其意义相当广泛，且涵盖不同的层面。对健康的理解受个人年龄、教育程度、生理状态、自我照顾能力、社会阶层、风俗习惯、价值观及科技发展等因素的影响，不同的字典、学者及

of individual functioning. For example, Abraham Maslow emphasized an individual's motivation in the continuous quest for self-actualization. Robinson has defined mental health within the framework of stress adaptation as "the successful adaptation to stressors from the internal or external environment, evidenced by thoughts, feelings, and behaviors that are age-appropriate and congruent with local and cultural norms."

机构对精神健康有不同的解释，但都包含对人体各种功能状态的描述。例如，美国人本主义心理学家马斯洛强调精神健康中自我实现的一面。美国学者Robinson从压力适应的观点将精神健康定义为"成功的适应内外环境中的压力，表现为感觉、思维及行为符合个人的身份、年龄及当地的文化风俗习惯。"

The World Health Organization defined health as "A state of complete physical, mental, and social well-being, not merely the absence of disease or infirmity." The significance of this definition is that it emphasizes the positive, and does not focus on the lack of disease or disorder. Persons are in a state of emotional well-being, or mental health, function comfortably within society and are satisfied with their lives.

世界卫生组织对健康定义："健康不但是没有疾病和身体缺陷，还要有完整的生理、心理状态和良好的社会适应能力。"此概念从积极的方面看待健康，而不是将健康仅仅看成没有疾病或身体缺陷。由此概念出发，可知精神健康指人能在社会中自如的生活，对他们所取得的成绩感到满意。

The American Psychiatric Association (APA) defines mental health as "Simultaneous success at working, loving and creating with the capacity for mature and flexible resolution of conflicts between instincts, conscience, important others and reality."

美国精神疾病学会对精神健康的定义是"精神健康是具有成熟的心态，有良好的工作及爱的能力，具有一定的创造性，并能灵活地解决本能、良心、重要人际关系及现实的冲突。"

It should be emphasized that cultural beliefs influence the determination of mental health and mental illness. For example, acceptable behavior in one culture may not be tolerant in others.

值得注意的是，文化信仰会影响人对精神健康与疾病的认识。例如一种文化认为是健康的行为，在另一种文化中可能会认为是异常行为。

iii. Components of Mental Health

（三）精神健康的组成部分

1. Self-governance The person demonstrates autonomy, a sense of detachment, independence, and a tendency to look within for guiding values and rules to live by. The person acts independently, dependently, or interdependently as the need arises, without permanently losing independence.

1. 自我管理 独立自主、不依赖，遵守社会规则及要求。能根据环境条件的不同而表现为独立、依赖或相互依赖，但永远不会失去自己的独立性。

2. Growth Orientation The person is willing to depart from the status quo to progress towards self-realization, and maximization of capacities.

2. 不断成长 不满足现状，最大程度地发挥自己的潜能，能朝着自我认识、自我完善的方向不断发展。

3. Tolerance of Uncertainty The person faces the uncertainty of living and certainty of death by means of faith and hope.

3. 能忍受生活的不确定性 能以自己的信念及希望从容面对生活的不确定性及死亡的不可避免性。

4. Self-esteem The person's self-esteem is built on self-knowledge and awareness of talents, abilities, and limitations.

4. 自尊 能意识到自己的优点、才智及不足，具有良好的自我认知能力。

5. Mastery of the Environment The person is effective, capable, competent, and creative in dealing with and influencing environment.

5. 有一定的环境控制感 能以有效、卓越、创新性的方式控制及影响环境。

6. Reality Orientation The person distinguishes fact from fantasy, the real world from the dream world, and

6. 一定的现实感 能分清现实与幻想，能区别梦境中的世界与现实世界，并在行为

acts accordingly.

7. Stress Management The person experiences appropriate depression, anxiety, and so forth in daily life, and can tolerate high levels of stress. People should know that the feeling is not going to last forever. The person is flexible and can experience failure without self-castigation. Usually the person copes with crises without needing help beyond the support of family and friends.

上表现出恰当的现实感。

7. 压力控制及应对 在日常生活中会经历和面对一定程度的抑郁、焦虑等短暂的情绪问题，能承受较高强度的压力，并能清楚地意识到这些负性的情绪是暂时的。对生活压力有一定的耐受性。能灵活处世，面对失败从容应对，面对生活危机，不过分要求家人及朋友的帮助。

Maslow investigated some historical people who represented self-actualized and moved in the direction of reaching and achieving their highest potentials. Box 1-1 shows his description of the characteristics of self-actualizing people.

马斯洛调查了许多历史上颇有成就的人物，并研究这些人是如何实现他们的最大潜能。Box 1-1 列出了马斯洛对自我实现者人格特征的描述。

BOX 1-1 Learning More

Some Characteristics of Self-actualized Persons

1. Accurate perception of reality.
2. Acceptance of themselves, others, and nature.
3. Spontaneity, simplicity, and naturalness.
4. Problem-centered rather than self-centered orientation.
5. Enjoyment of privacy and detachment.
6. Freshness of appreciation.
7. Mystical or peak experiences.
8. Active social interest.
9. An non-hostile sense of humor.
10. Democratic character structure.
11. Creativity, especially in managing their lives.
12. Resistance to conformity (enculturation).

BOX 1-1 知识拓展

自我实现者具有的特征

1. 全面和准确地感知现实。
2. 接纳自己、他人和自然。
3. 对人自发、坦率和真实。
4. 以问题为中心，而不是以自我为中心。
5. 具有超然于世和独处的需要。
6. 具有永不衰退的欣赏力。
7. 具有难以形容的高峰体验。
8. 积极的社会兴趣。
9. 处事幽默风趣。
10. 具有民主精神。
11. 富有创造性，尤其在处理自己的生活方面。
12. 在环境和文化中能保持相对的独立性。

iv. Characteristics of Mental Health

The basic characteristics provide a description of mental health. In general, a person is mentally healthy when he possesses knowledge of himself, meets his basic needs, assumes responsibility for his behavior and for self-growth, has learned to integrate thoughts, feelings and actions, and can resolve conflicts successfully. In relation to others, a mentally healthy person maintains normal relationships with others, communicates directly with others, and respects others. A mentally health person adapts to changes in his environment.

（四）精神健康的特征

精神健康的特征提供了认识精神健康的最佳方式。一般认为，精神健康具有三个方面的特征。第一，在自我认知上，精神健康表现为具有良好的自我认知，能满足个人的基本需要，对自己的行为及自我成长负责，并能融合各种思维、感觉及行为，能成功地解决生活中的各种矛盾及冲突。第二，在人际关系上，一个精神健康的人能尊重他人，直接与他人交流，能与他人保持正常的人际关系。第三，在适应内外环境上，一个精神健康的人能适应各种环境的变化。

v. Criteria of Mental Health

It is important to remember that, as people, we all share more similarities than differences. We all concern about our lives, our health, our relationship, and our well-being. As human beings, we experience happiness, anger, loneliness, and joy. Within a framework of thoughts and feelings, we function with varying degree of mental health. Mental health has been defined as the most appropriate adjustment that a person can make at a particular time based on internal and external resources. This definition implies that mental health is like physical equilibrium, it is necessary to constantly adjust it in order to cope with new situation. A mentally healthy person must meet the following criteria:

1. Self-esteem, self-respect that prevails even in the face of discouragement, failure, or frustration.

2. An open, flexible approach to life; the ability to experience a failure without beating oneself or others.

3. A spontaneous, outgoing temperament; the ability to enjoy others and the capacity of giving and receiving love, the ability to express strong feeling appropriately.

4. Minimal nervous tension; freedom from crippling worry and strain; the ability to face life in a relaxed, confident manner.

5. Appropriate depression, anxiety and anger under stress; a philosophy that facilitates the handling of frustration and pressure reasonable well.

Of course, meeting the above criteria completely and continuously is practically impossible. No one is expected to cope with, adjust or adapt perfectly to one's life stress and crisis.

vi. Factors Influencing Mental Health

1. Inherited Characteristics Some theorists believe that no one is completely normal and that the ability to maintain a mentally healthy outlook on life is partly due to one's genes. Similarly, genetic defects may predispose a person to cognitive disability, schizophrenia, or bipolar disorder. Such people have innate differences in sensitivity and temperament that prompt various responses to their environment.

2. Nurturing during Childhood Nurturing during childhood means the familial-child interactions. This also affects the development of mental health.

（五）精神健康的标准

人类既有差异，也在许多方面具有共同点。人们都关心自己的生活、健康、人际关系及福利，会经历幸福、愤怒、孤独、快乐等情感。从思维及情感上来说，人在不同的时期处于不同的精神健康水平。精神健康是人在特定时间范围内，根据内外各种环境及资源条件，适时调整自己以适应环境。这说明精神健康像躯体健康一样，是一个需不断调整以维持其相对稳定的动态过程。由此来看，精神健康的标准包括：

1. 不断维持个人的自尊及自我价值感，即使在受到挫折、失败及打击的情况下，也不丧失自我。

2. 开放而灵活的生活态度，在失意的时候不过分自责，也不指责他人。

3. 自然而积极向上的性格，能与他人快乐的相处，并能以恰当的方式给予和接受关爱，能以适当的方式表达强烈的个人情感。

4. 很少有精神紧张，没有极度的忧虑和精神疲惫，以放松而自信的方式对待人生。

5. 当有压力时，会有适度的焦虑、抑郁及愤怒。能以一定的生活宗旨及态度面对压力及挫折，处理好各种问题。

必须指出，精神健康只是一种相对状态。绝对满足以上标准只是一种理想状态，没有人能在压力及危机状态下完全应对及适应生活，也没有人能达到绝对的精神健康。

（六）影响精神健康的因素

1. 遗传 有研究表明，人不可能保持绝对的精神健康，但能否在生活中保持相对的精神健康主要受遗传基因的影响。分子遗传学揭示，遗传基因的缺陷可能与认知障碍、精神分裂症及双相情感障碍有关。遗传基因缺陷者在对人对事的敏感性及自身的脾气秉性等方面与众不同，他们对周围环境有与正常人不一样的感受与反应。

2. 童年的经历 童年的亲子关系会影响一个人的精神健康。健康的家庭养育方式包括在孩子出生时建立良好的亲子关系纽带，

Positive nurturing starts with bonding at childbirth and includes feelings of love, security, and acceptance. The child experiences positive interaction with parents, siblings and other family members. Negative nurturing includes circumstances such as maternal deprivation, parental rejection, sibling rivalry, and early communication failures. Individuals who are exposed to poor nurturing may develop poor self-esteem or poor communication skills. They may also display socially unacceptable behaviors as they seek to have their basic needs met.

使孩子感受到接纳、安全与爱。在此健康生活环境中的孩子能感受到与父母、兄弟姐妹及其他家庭成员的关爱。不健康的养育方式包括缺乏母爱、父母排斥、兄弟姐妹敌对及沟通交流障碍等。在此种不良环境中生长的人会出现自尊心差，沟通交流障碍等。这些人在寻求满足自己的基本需要时，有时会出现不能被社会所接受的行为。

3. Life Circumstances Life circumstances can influence one's mental health from birth. Individuals who experience positive circumstances are generally emotionally secure and successful in school and establish healthy interpersonal relationships. Negative circumstances, such as poor physical health, economic constrains, feelings of helpless, hopeless, or worthlessness, may place a person at risk for depression, substance abuse, or other mental health disorders.

3. **生活环境** 一个人的生活环境及生活气氛从出生时起就会影响其精神健康。一个生活在和谐美满环境中的人，感情安全稳定，学业有成，并能与他人建立健康的人际关系。而不良的生活环境，如身体健康问题、经济拮据、无助感、绝望感、无用感等会使人出现抑郁、滥用药物或其他的精神健康问题。

II. Mental Illness

二、精神疾病

i. Definition

A universal concept of mental illness is difficult since cultural factors can influence the definition. Some cultures are quite liberal in the range of behaviors that are considered acceptable, while others may have very little tolerance for behaviors that deviate from the culture norms. The American Psychiatric Association (APA) (2000) defines mental illness or disorder as "Clinical significant behavioral or psychological syndrome or pattern that occurs in an individual and that is associated with present distress (a painful symptom) or disability (impairment in one or more important areas of functioning) or with a significantly increased risk of suffering death, pain, disability, or an important loss of freedom."

（一）精神疾病的概念

目前对精神疾病仍然没有一个公认的概念，因为文化因素会影响人们对行为的看法，有些文化对行为的宽容性很大，但有些文化对是否偏离正常行为具有严格的界限。美国精神病协会于2000年对精神疾病的描述为："精神疾病是指患者在临床上出现明显的行为和心理的异常，伴有相当的痛苦和无能力，或有残疾并失去自由的危险倾向。"

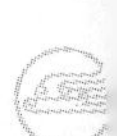

Mental illness can be caused by chemical imbalances in the brain, by transfer of drugs across the placental barrier, or by organic changes within the brain. Additionally, if a person is unsuccessful in dealing with environmental stresses because of faulty inherited characteristics, poor nurturing during childhood, or negative life circumstances, mental illness may develop.

精神疾病可由脑内的化学物质失衡、药物通过胎盘屏障或脑器质性病变所引起。同时，由于遗传、童年的不良经历或不健康的生活环境，也会使人消极应对环境压力而出现精神疾病。

ii. Possible Signs of Mental Illness

1. Marked personality change over time.

2. Confused thinking, strange or grandiose ideas.

3. Prolonged severe depression, apathy, or extreme highs and lows.

（二）精神疾病可能出现的征兆

1. 一段时间内出现明显的人格改变。

2. 思维混乱，出现怪异离奇或夸大的想法。

3. 长期且严重的抑郁、冷漠，或出现极度高峰和低谷体验。

4. Excessive anxiety, fear, or suspiciousness, blaming others.

4. 极度焦虑、恐惧、怀疑、常指责他人。

5. Withdrawal from society, friendlessness; abnormal self-centeredness.

5. 社会退缩，无友善感；异常的自我为中心。

6. Denial of obvious problems; strong resistance to help.

6. 拒绝明显的问题，强烈拒绝他人的帮助。

7. Thinking or talking about suicide.

7. 想象或谈论自杀。

8. Numerous, unexplained physical ailments; marked changes in eating or sleeping habits.

8. 出现多处解释不清的身体不适，饮食及睡眠习惯明显改变。

9. Anger or hostility out of proportion to the situation.

9. 愤怒或敌意的程度与当时所处的情景明显不符。

10. Delusions (false beliefs that are firmly maintained even though they are not shared by others), hallucinations (perceptual distortions, arising from any of the senses-hearing voices or seeing images that others do not hear or see).

10. 妄想、幻想等。

11. Abuse of alcohol or drugs.

11. 滥用酒精或其他药物。

12. Growing inability to cope with problems and daily activities such as school, job, or personal needs.

12. 持续表现为无法应对日常生活问题，如学校、工作或个人需要等方面的问题。

iii. Misconceptions about Mental Illness

（三）有关精神疾病容易出现的误区

1. Abnormal behavior is different or odd, easily recognized. Patients are irrational at times and behave in an unusual or different manner. Such behavior may occur in the privacy of one's home, at work, or even in a public place, and still may go unnoticed by other. Maladaptive behavior may not occur obviously, for instance, a person may be suspicious of everyone and avoid contact with people. Their thoughts and behavior may not be noticed unless they voice. Depressed persons who are diagnosed as mentally ill may appear quiet, sullen, or distracted but do not necessarily exhibit abnormal behavior.

1. 异常行为表现怪异，容易辨认 患者有时会出现不合逻辑或异常的行为，这些行为可能会出现在私人空间如家庭，或工作场所，甚至公共场合，但通常不被他人认为是异常。人的适应不良性行为可能表现并不明显，例如，患者会怀疑他周围的任何人，并避免与他人接触，但如果自己不直接说出来，这种行为异常就难以被他人发现。一个被诊断为精神病性抑郁症患者，可能会表现为安静、闷闷不乐或注意力不集中，但并不一定有异常行为。

2. Abnormal behavior can be predicted and evaluated. Numerous media has proven otherwise. A nice, smart and quiet person may suddenly have unpredicted abnormal behavior, which no one can explain the motivation behind the behaviors.

2. 异常行为可以被预测和评价 但事实上许多新闻媒体有相反的报道，一个和蔼、聪明、文静的人可能会突然出现难以预料的异常行为，无人能解释其行为的真正动机。

3. Internal forces are responsible for abnormal behavior. Although internal forces may cause abnormal behavior, other factors such as people, culture, environment and others may also influence one's behavior; for example, a person with marriage problems may have abnormal behaviors, such as regression, hostility, or even suicide attempts.

3. 内在力量是引起异常行为的主要原因 虽然内在力量是异常行为的主要原因，但不同的人、文化、环境或其他因素也会影响其行为，如一个有婚姻问题的人可能会出现退化、敌意、甚至有自杀企图等异常行为。

4. People who exhibit abnormal behavior are

4. 行为异常的人很危险 统计资料证明，

dangerous. According to statistics, approximately 60%-65% of individuals, who are hospitalized for psychiatric treatment, are discharged and live with their families. Many of these people function to some extent in society and are not considered dangerous. They may turn to others for help in an attempt to cope with their problems.

5. Maladaptive behavior is always inherited. Heredity plays a part in the development of some types of abnormal behavior; however, learning also influences behavior. Some people may observe specific behaviors used by others to meet their needs. As a result, they imitate behavior that they believe to be acceptable to others.

6. Mental illness is incurable. Much progress has occurred in the diagnosis and treatment of mental illness. Early diagnosis and treatment may alleviate symptoms and allow the person to function normally in society. People with a chronic mental disorder may receive maintenance doses of medication, attend various therapies, or care for themselves with minimal supervision. As a result of deinstitutionalization and implementation of managed care, clients are empowered to function as independent as possible. Resources in the community are utilized to provide education for the client and family. Ongoing supervision and support are available to minimize recidivism.

iv. Correct Views of Patients with Mental Illness

Patients with mental illness may have some absurd behaviors, which may create a feeling of danger or fear for others to avoid them. Understanding patients with mental illness correctly may help psychiatric nurses to help them professionally.

1. Patient with mental illness has unique social value. The patient has his unique personality, thinking, emotion, perceptions and needs. Whether his behaviors are strange or not, or his behaviors may has no rationale behind, nurses should help to maintain his self-esteem and value, not to discriminate, humiliate or mistreat him.

2. Patients with mental illness are partly deviate from normal. Patients with mental illness may not totally diverge from normal, most of them are partly normal and partly abnormal, and these two kinds of states may replace each other in different kind of situations.

3. Patient's behaviors have their own meaning and purpose. The mental illness patient's signs and symptoms are meaningful and purposeful for him, these behaviors for him are the attempt to cope with or adapt to environment, not as others think as no purpose.

约60%～65%的住院治疗的精神疾病患者，出院后与其他家庭成员共同生活。许多精神疾病患者能在社会生活中发挥一定的作用，并没有出现危险行为。他们有时求助别人，目的是需要别人的帮助以应对自身所面对的困难。

5. 适应不良行为具有遗传性 虽然某些异常行为具有一定的遗传性，但习得性同样影响其行为。有些人观察、模仿别人的行为来满足自己的需要，因此，他们便模仿那些自认为可被他人接受的行为。

6. 精神疾病难以治愈 目前在精神疾病的诊断及治疗方面已经取得了很大的进展。早期诊断及治疗能减轻患者的症状，并使其在社会中发挥正常的功能。慢性精神障碍的患者可能会服用维持剂量的药物，参与各种治疗活动，或在他人的监护下自我恢复。随着精神疾病治疗机构的逐渐分散化、社区化及个案管理护理的应用，患者能逐渐地独立发挥作用。人们应用社区资源为患者及家属提供健康教育。各种持续监护及支持可以减轻疾病的复发。

（四）正确认识精神病患者

精神病患者可能会出现某些怪异的行为，会使人感到恐惧和危险，从而厌恶或躲避患者。因此，正确认识精神病患者是做好护理工作的前提。

1. 精神病患者是有社会价值的人 精神疾病患者具有自己独特的人格、思维、情感、感知觉及需求，无论其行为如何怪异，或不符合逻辑，护士都应维护其做人的尊严，不能歧视、侮辱及虐待患者。

2. 精神病患者只是部分偏离了正常 精神病患者可能出现部分的异常，但也有正常的部分，一般在精神活动中正常与异常相互交织，同时存在。

3. 精神病患者的行为具有一定的目的性和意义 精神病患者表现出的症状体征对其他人看来没有什么特殊意义，但对其本人是有意义的，他们的异常行为是为了应对和适应周围环境的反应。

4. Mental illness patients are very sensitive to the environment. Because of the manifestation of mental illness, patients may feel insecure. They have high perceptions to the surroundings and take "normal" behavior to protect themselves from imaged environmental dangers.

4. 精神病患者对环境具有高度的敏感性 由于精神症状的影响，精神病患者常有不安全感，对周围环境具有高度的感知性，并采取自认为正确的方式来保护自己。

5. Mental illness behaviors are learned. Some patients' behaviors are learned to adapt to their environment, they can also learn to correct their abnormal behavior.

5. 精神病患者行为具有习得性 精神病患者的某些行为可能是为了适应环境而习得的，但他们同样可用学习的方法矫正病态行为。

6. Mental illness patients may hurt themselves and others. When patients have some mental symptoms, such as delusion, hallucinations, or mood disorders, they may have suicide behaviors, hurt themselves or others, or damage materials around them. Therefore, nurses need to take protective measures to maintain the safety of patients and others.

6. 精神病患者可能发生危害自己及他人的行为 精神病患者在出现严重的精神症状时（如幻觉、妄想或情感障碍等）会出现自杀、自伤、毁物或伤人等事件，因此精神科护士应及时采取防范措施，保证患者及他人的人身安全。

Mental health and illness are not static conditions. Rather, they are vital concepts that are subject to continuous evaluation and change. Therefore, it is helpful to image mental health and illness as a continuum, a range of well-being from excellent health through wellness and illness to death. Excellent mental health appears at one end of the continuum, death at the other end.

精神健康与精神疾病不是一成不变的绝对状态，相反，他们是不断变化的，需要持续的评估。一个人的精神健康与疾病经常处于不断动态的变化过程。因此，可以将一个人的精神健康与精神疾病想象成一个连续的过程，其中一端为非常健康，一端为病危乃至死亡，中间部分则是处于两种情况的中间状态。一个人的精神健康与精神疾病总是动态地处于这种连续状态的某种范围。

III. Psychiatric Nursing

三、精神科护理学

i. Definition

Psychiatric nursing involves the diagnosis and treatment of human responses to actual or potential mental health problems. It is a specialized area of nursing practice that uses theories of human behavior as its scientific framework and requires the purposeful use of self as its art of expression. It is concerned with promoting of optimum health of people and the society as a whole. Comprehensive nursing care focuses on prevention of mental illness, health maintenance, management of mental and physical health problems, diagnosis and treatment of mental disorders, and rehabilitation. *American Nurses' Association Scope and Standards of Psychiatric Nursing* defined it as a "specialized area of nursing practice, employing the wide range of explanatory theories of human behaviors as its science and purposeful use of self as its art" in 2000.

（一）概念

精神科护理学是护理学中一个重要的分支。它主要涉及诊断和处理人对现存的与潜在的精神障碍及精神疾病的反应。精神科护理需要护士应用行为学、护理学等相关的科学知识，艺术地为服务对象提供心理健康服务。通过促进精神健康、预防疾病、治疗及护理各种精神健康障碍患者，以及进行康复训练等各种综合性的护理服务，提高公众及整个社会的精神健康。美国护理学会在2000年出台的《精神科护理的范围及标准》中将精神科护理学定义为"精神科护理学是护理学中一个重要的分支；它以行为科学为理论基础，科学而艺术地向服务对象提供精神卫生服务。"

ii. Philosophical Beliefs of Psychiatric and Mental Health Nursing Practice

The practice of psychiatric nursing is based on a number of philosophical beliefs, which is described as the followings:

1. The individual has intrinsic worth and dignity, each person is worthy of respect solely because of each person's nature and presence.

2. The goal of the individual is growth, health, autonomy, and self-actualization.

3. Every individual has the potential to change and the desire to pursue personal goals.

4. The person functions as a holistic being that acts on, interacts with, and reacts to the environment as a whole person. Each part affects the total response, which is greater than the sum of each separate component.

5. All people have common, basic, and necessary human needs. These include physical needs, safety needs, love and belonging needs, esteem needs, and self-actualization needs.

6. All behavior of the individual is meaningful. It arises from personal needs and goals and can be understood only from the person's internal frame of reference and within the context in which it occurs.

7. Behavior consists of perceptions, thoughts, feelings, and actions. From one's perceptions, thoughts arise, emotions are felt, and actions are conceived. Disruptions may occur in any of these areas.

8. Individuals vary in their coping capacities, which depend on genetic endowment, nature of environmental influences, degree of stress, and available resources. All individuals have the potential for both health and illness.

9. Illness can be growth-producing experience for individual. The goal of nursing care is to maximize positive interactions with the individual's environment, promote wellness, and enhance self-actualization.

10. All people have a right to an equal opportunity for adequate health care regardless of gender, race, religion, ethics, sexual orientation, or cultural background. Nursing care is based on needs of individuals, families, and communities, and mutually defined goals and expectations.

11. Mental health is a critical and necessary component of comprehensive health care services.

12. The individual has the right to participate in decision-making regarding physical and mental health.

（二）精神科护理学的宗旨

精神科的护理实践必须在一定的实践原则及理念的指导下进行，精神科护理实践的哲学理念主要包括：

1. 每个人都具有自己的价值及尊严，应尊重个体独特的个性特征及生存方式。

2. 人的目标是成长、健康、自主及自我实现。

3. 每个人都具有改变的潜力及追求实现自我目标的愿望。

4. 每个人都以整体的方式发挥其功能，能以整体的方式自我行动、与环境相互作用，对环境的变化产生反应。每部分会影响其最终的功能，整体的功能大于各部分的简单组合。

5. 每个人都具有一定的基本需要，包含生理、安全、爱及归属、自尊及尊重及自我实现的需要。

6. 每个人的行为都有一定的意义，它是个体需求及目的的外在表现，护士应从患者的内心世界和所处环境来理解他 / 她的行为。

7. 行为包含感知、思维、情绪及行动。个人在感知的基础上会产生思维、感受情绪、采取行动。处于功能障碍或疾病状态，上述任何环节都可能出现问题。

8. 每个人的应对能力不同，它主要取决于遗传因素、环境影响的性质、压力的程度及可以采用的应对资源。任何人都具有向健康或疾病方向发展的潜力或可能。

9. 疾病是人成长的经历之一。护理的功能是尽可能帮助个体与环境之间产生积极的交互作用，促进人的健康及自我实现。

10. 每个人都有追求健康的平等权利，不论性别、种族、宗教、伦理、性倾向、文化背景等。护理应满足个体、家庭及社区的健康需要。护理目标必须由护患双方共同制订。

11. 精神健康是综合健康护理实践的必要组成部分。

12. 每个人都有参与制订自我生理或精神

The person has the right to make self-determination. It is the decision of the individual to pursue health or illness.

健康决策的权利。在这一方面每个人都是独立的，他们既有追求健康的权利，当患上疾病时也值得他人的尊重。

13. An interpersonal relationship has the potential for producing change and growth within the individual. It is the vehicle for the application of the nursing process and the attainment of the goal of nursing care.

13. 良好的人际关系能促进个体成长及改变，它是应用护理程序及达到护理目标的工具或媒介。

14. The goal of nursing care is to promote wellness, maximize integrated functioning, and enhance self-actualization. Nursing care is mutually determined with individuals, families, groups, and communities based on health care needs and expected treatment outcomes.

14. 护理的目标是促进个体的健康、最佳功能状态、潜能的发挥及自我实现。护理实施应根据个体的健康需求及预期的治疗结果，护士在整个过程中要经常与患者、家庭、团体及社区商量决定。

iii. The Holistic Mental Health Care

（三）精神科整体化护理

Holistic mental health care involves the whole person in the total environment. Holistic mental health care encompasses these concepts:

精神科整体化护理涉及患者内外环境的全部，包括以下观念：

1. The uniqueness of the client includs the unique life history and personal style of expression and fulfillment.

1. 每个人都是独一无二的个体，具有自己独特的人生经历，有自己的表达及行为方式。

2. The healing partnership between caregiver and client, which alters the traditional authoritarian relationship and empowers the client.

2. 在精神科护理中，应改变传统的权威型护患关系，建立平等合作的新型护患关系。

3. The healing ability of the caregiver, that is, the use of interpersonal skills and instillation of hope in the client.

3. 充分发挥照顾者的能力，应用治疗性沟通技术，帮助患者重新树立生活的信心及希望。

4. The view is that a disorder is an opportunity to grow, not just to recover, and that it is a challenge to understand and overcome, and as a result, learn new, and heal their ways of functioning.

4. 有一种观点将患病看成是个体的成长机会，而不仅仅是疾病的恢复。患病后，患者开始尝试了解疾病的特点，设法战胜疾病，最终学会了更健康的生活方式。

Section 2 Historical Development of Psychiatric and Mental Health Nursing

第二节 精神科护理发展史

The purpose of this section is to provide a brief history of the evolution of psychiatric nursing and to track the major development that led to the recognition of psychiatric and mental health nursing as an important nursing specialty in the world, as well as in China.

本节将回顾国内外精神科护理的发展历史，以更好地明确精神科护理作为一个专科的发展方向及未来趋势。

I. History of Psychiatric and Mental Health Nursing Development in the World

一、国外精神科护理发展史

Nursing has existed since the beginning of

自有人类以来，就有了各种精神活动，

civilization. The origins of psychiatric and mental health nursing is rooted in the past, paralleled the development of psychiatry.

随之出现了精神疾病及对精神疾病的治疗。精神科护理的过去、现在及未来始终伴随着精神医学及护理学的发展而存在。

Before 1860, the emphasis in psychiatric institution was on custodial care, attendants were hired to maintain control of the patients. Those attendants were little more than cell-keepers with little training, and psychiatric care was poor. The mentally ill were chained. The young and the old, women and men, the insane, criminals, and paupers were indiscriminately mixed. They often were placed on display for the amusement of the paying public. During this period, the need for special institutions for individuals with psychiatric disorders was identified, while patients were regarded as "lunatics". Soon after assuming leadership, Philippe Pinel (1745-1826) in France unchained the shackled, fed the hungry, clothed the naked, and abolished the whips and other instruments of abuse.

1860年以前，精神病患者的治疗机构主要采用囚禁的方式，条件非常差，雇佣人员没经过任何专业培训，他们的任务是负责控制患者，就像监狱的看守一样。精神病患者身负手铐脚镣，与罪犯、乞丐等关在一起。患者没有任何尊严，常被看管者取乐或被当作赚钱的工具。在此阶段，虽然人们意识到应建立特殊机构来管理，但精神病患者不被认为是受疾病困扰，而被视为疯子，即魔鬼附体、灵魂出壳。18世纪后期，法国医生菲力普·比奈尔（Philippe Pinel，1745—1826年）作为世界上第一位精神病院的院长，主张用人道主义的态度对待精神病患者，为患者提供衣服、食物，并提出要清除禁制，砸碎锁链，从而也开创了精神科护理的先河。

In US, the first school to prepare nurses to care for the mentally ill opened at McLean Hospital in Waverly, Massachusetts, in 1882. It was a two-year program. The care was mainly custodial. Nurses took care of the patients' physical needs, such as medications, nutrition, hygiene, and ward activities.

1882年，美国第一所专门培养精神科护士的学校在马萨诸塞州的McLean医院建立，规定需要两年的学习时间。当时精神科护理的主要形式仍然为看管式。护士的主要职责是满足患者的身体需要，如用药、营养、卫生及病房活动。

Nursing as a profession began to emerge in the later nineteenth century. By 1880, there were approximately 30 psychiatric hospitals in U.S. In 1872, New England Hospital for Women and Children in Boston and Women's Hospital of Philadelphia had established schools of nursing, but among them, only one psychiatric service was available. The nurse's role was to oversee the care given and to ensure the smooth operation of the ward. Housekeeping duties, dietary management, and laundry care were considered nursing responsibilities.

精神科护理真正成为一个专业是19世纪下叶，到1880年，美国已经有约30所精神病院。1872年，波士顿的新英格兰妇幼医院和费城妇科医院建立了护士学校，但只有其中一家开设了精神科护理。当时护士的主要职责是保证病房工作的正常运转，其主要角色包括病房的清洁、饮食管理及被服的清洗。

Until the end of the nineteenth century, it's little changed in the role of psychiatric nurses. They had limited training in psychiatry, and they primarily adapted in the principles of medical-surgical to the psychiatric setting. At the time psychological care consisted of kindness and tolerance toward the patients.

直到19世纪末，精神科护士的角色并没有发生明显的改变。护士所受的专科培训很少，主要应用内外科的护理技术照顾患者。当时所谓的心理护理主要体现在护士对待精神病患者的仁慈及容忍的态度。

Linda Richards, the first graduate nurse in the United States, developed better nursing care in psychiatric hospitals and organized nursing services and educational

琳达·理查兹（Linda Richards）是美国的第一位护理专科（非精神科）培养的护士，她在美国伊利诺伊州的精神病医院开展了全新的

programs in State Mental Hospitals in Illinois. Her basic care theory is "the mentally sick should be at least as well cared for as the physically sick".

护士培训及服务项目，其基本思想是按照其他专科如内外科的护理模式来护理精神疾病患者，由此奠定了精神科护理的基本模式。

In 1913 Johns Hopkins became the first school of nursing to include a fully developed course for psychiatric nursing in the curriculum. Other schools soon followed. Until the late 1930s that nursing education recognized the importance of psychiatric knowledge in general nursing care for all illnesses.

1913年，Johns Hopkins大学开设了正规的精神科护理课程。紧接着，美国其他学校也相继开展了此类课程。直到20世纪30年代后期，护士学校才逐渐认识到从事其他科专业工作的护士也需要精神心理等方面的知识。

Sigmund Feud (1856-1939) described human behavior in psychological terms. His contributions include the theory of motivation, the usefulness of talking, the importance of dream, and unlocking the hidden parts of the mind.

弗洛伊德（Sigmund Freud，1856—1939年）用心理学的术语来描述人的行为，创造了动机理论，利用梦的解析和自由联想治疗精神病患者，从而创立了精神心理分析学派，首次从心理学的角度探讨精神疾病的病因。

An important factor in the development of psychiatric nursing was the emergence of various somatic therapies including insulin shock therapy, psychosurgery, and electro-convulsive therapy. These techniques all required the medical-surgical skills of nurses. Although these therapies did not help the patient understand his or her problems, they did control behavior and make the patient more amenable to psychotherapy.

19世纪末至20世纪初，精神医学中涌现出了多种躯体治疗方法，如胰岛素休克疗法、精神外科治疗、电痉挛治疗等。而这些治疗方法同时需要护士具备内外科的护理知识及技能。虽然当时这些治疗方法还不能使患者明确自己的问题，但却很好地控制了其精神症状，从而提高了患者接受精神心理治疗的依从性。

Hildegard Peplau (1909-1999) developed the nurse-client therapeutic relationship in 1952. Her theory emphasizes that nursing is a process of relationship among people in which both nurse and client learn and grow as a result of the nurse-client interaction. It's not social but therapeutic.

1952年，佩普勒（Hildegard Peplau，1909—1999年）在前人的基础上，经过大量的临床实践，形成了精神科护理护患治疗关系理论。她认为，护理是护士与患者互相作用的过程，是有意义的、治疗性的人际关系，而不是社会关系。在此关系中，护士与患者共同学习，共同成长。护理就是进一步完善患者的人格。

The first antipsychotic drug, chlorpromazine, was discovered around 1950, and then lithium and imipramine were produced and introduced a few years later whose impact has been really powerful. Patients with mental illness such as schizophrenia, depression, and mania became less agitated and regained normal feelings. Patients' hospital stays were obviously shortened.

20世纪50年代初，随着第一位抗精神病药物氯丙嗪问世，锂剂及丙咪嗪相继出现并及时地被应用于临床实践，收到了前所未有的疗效。许多患精神分裂症、或抑郁症、躁狂症患者的症状得到了有效的控制，极大地缩短了患者的住院时间。

The Community Mental Health Center's Act was enacted in America in 1963, which a deliberate shift was made from institutional care to extra institutional care. From that time on, some advanced countries such as America and Britain established community treatment centers and community living arrangement to keep the mentally disordered individual close to the family. In

1963年美国颁布了《社区精神卫生法案》，该法案规定，大力发展社区精神卫生运动，即对精神疾病患者的治疗和护理，从当时单纯的住院治疗，开始向社区发展。英美等发达国家开始在社区建立了许多社区治疗中心及社区生活设施，使精神障碍患者能在

America, the state hospital population reached its peak in 1955, while the state hospital population had a decline of over 85% in 2007.

住所的附近接受相应的治疗。1955年，美国精神病患者住院人数达到历史高峰。然而到2007年，住院精神病患者人数与1955年相比下降85%。

The 1990s were believed as the Decade of the Brain, which a steep increase in brain research occurred. Scientists were interested in biologic explanations for mental disorders. About 100 years ago, Emil Kraeplin (1856-1926) believed that brain pathology was at the root of the serious mental disorders. It was 100 years later that people emphasized on and started working on the research of brain and biology. It seems to represent a completion of the circle, and crystallize the fact that some abnormal behaviors are caused by biologic irregularities. Now all textbooks in America provide the information about psychobiology and psychopharmacology. Nurses are able to address relatively complex topics with patients and families.

20世纪90年代是大脑研究迅速发展的10年。科学家们决心用生物学理论解释精神病现象。100年前，德国的精神病学专家克雷丕林（Emil Kraeplin，1856—1926年）通过分析大量的临床病例，率先提出重症精神疾病的根源是大脑的生物病理学的改变。100年后的今天，人们开始从生物病理学的角度研究大脑结构，这看起来像是一个百年循环，即用事实证明，异常行为的背后是有生物学基础的。目前，美国的《精神科护理学》教科书中均包含心理生物学及精神药理学等知识。从而，护士能够向患者及家属解释相对复杂的精神病现象。

II. History of Psychiatric-Mental Health Nursing Development in China

二、中国精神科护理发展史

The development of psychiatric-mental health nursing is much slower than that of the other nursing specialties in China. It has paralleled the development of psychiatry and has passed the following historical development stages.

精神科护理学在中国的发展比其他专科护理学科缓慢，它始终伴随着精神医学的发展而发展，并经过了不同的历史发展时期。

Mental disorders have existed throughout the ages and were reported in Chinese medical books and records in early times. Mental health activities were described in an ancient Chinese medical book called *Huang Di Nei Jing* in 3-2 B.C. In Qin and Han dynasties, some Chinese books like *Nan Jing, Shang Han Lun, Jin Gui Yao Lue* described symptoms of the mentally ill as "Kuang" "Zao" "Zhan Wang" "Dian" "Xian", which were extremely similar to modern medical terms as mania, delusion, schizophrenia, and epilepsy.

自古以来，中国的书籍中就有关于精神疾病的记载。公元前3～公元前2世纪，医学典籍《黄帝内经》中就提到了人的精神活动。秦汉时期，医书《难经》《伤寒论》《金贵要略》中记载的“狂”“躁”“谵妄”“癫”“痫”等与当代医学术语“mania”“delusion”“schizophrenia”“epilepsy”极为相似。

In 1898, the first psychiatric hospital was established in Guangzhou city, followed by several other cities and provinces as in Beijing, Suzhou, Shanghai, and Nanjing. Peking Union Medical University offered the first psychiatric course in 1922, but no nursing course existed at that time.

1898年，广州成立了中国第一所精神病医院，随后在北京、苏州、上海、南京等地陆续建立了多所精神病医院。1922年协和医科大学率先开始了精神病学的教学，但没有相关的护理课程。

Education of psychiatric-mental health nursing has been improved tremendously after the founding of the People's Republic of China in 1949. Institutes of psychiatric-mental health care were established in

建国以后，中国的精神科护理事业得到了迅速的发展，各地纷纷建立了精神病院，培养了一批受过专门训练的护理人员充实到

almost all parts of China. Nurses are trained to take care of the mentally ill in hospitals. With the development of undergraduate nursing program in 1980s and the higher nursing education in 1990s, "psychiatric nursing" has become a core course of nursing curriculum.

In 1990, the Chinese Nursing Association formed the Psychiatric and Mental Health Nursing Committee. The committee held meetings every two years to evaluate and oversee the quality of psychiatric nursing care.

了精神科护理工作岗位。随着20世纪80年代护理本科教育的逐步开展以及20世纪90年代更高层次的护理教育，精神科护理学已经成为护理专业的核心课程之一。

中华护理学会于1990年成立了精神科护理专业委员会，委员会每两年召开一次会议，以制订和完善相关的护理规章制度及标准。

III. Challenges of Psychiatric and Mental Health Nursing

At present, psychiatric and mental health nursing is facing challenges from:

1. The growth in scientific knowledge, which is providing new insights into the biological roots of mental illness.

2. Technological advances allowing more precise administration of the structure and function of the brain than that has been impossible in the past.

3. Changes in the delivery system of mental health care such as deinstitutionalization and the rise in outpatient treatment.

4. More and more poor, aged, ethnic people, and the chronically mentally ill who uninsured or underinsured.

5. The continuing stigmatization of mentally ill persons.

6. A changing definition of nurse's role in the evolving specialty.

三、精神科护理面临的挑战

随着各种新的精神治疗方法的不断发展及完善，精神科护理将面临更多的挑战。

1. 科学技术不断发展，为从生物病理学角度研究精神疾病的原因提供了更广阔的空间。

2. 先进技术及手段的不断完善，为大脑结构及功能的精确研究提供了前所未有的条件。

3. 精神卫生服务系统的不断发展，将逐渐加强社区及门诊对精神疾病患者的康复服务。

4. 服务对象中未得到保险或保险额不足的穷人、老人、少数种族及慢性精神障碍患者人数不断增加。

5. 长期存在对精神障碍患者的歧视。

6. 护理工作随着专业服务的具体化，护士角色的定义将进一步具体、明确。

Section 3 Dimensions, Roles, and Functions of Psychiatric Nurses

Psychiatric and mental health nurses play important roles in many areas. Psychiatric nurses must be able to make rapid and comprehensive assessments, use effective problem-solving skills in making complex clinical decisions; act autonomously as well as collaboratively with other professionals; be sensitive to issues such as ethical dilemmas, cultural diversity, and access to psychiatric care for special populations; be comfortable working in decentralized settings; and be sophisticated about the costs and benefits of providing care within fiscal constraining.

第三节 精神科护士的工作范围、角色及功能

精神科护士在许多护理岗位扮演着重要角色。他们能够应用各种解决问题的方式，快速作出综合的护理评估及临床护理决策。在保持自己专业独立性的同时，与其他专业人员密切配合。高度注意专业实践中的伦理及法律、不同文化及特殊人群的服务等问题。同时必须学会在人口分散的环境中工作，能够在资源有限的情况下为患者提供经济实用的护理服务。

I. Dimensions of Psychiatric Nurses

Psychiatric nurses may practice in settings that vary widely according to the purpose, type, location, and administration. The nurses' responsibilities in settings include health promotion, therapy, rehabilitation, and health education.

i. Health Promotion and Disease Prevention

Health promotion and disease prevention are mainly provided in the community settings, which can also be given in schools and factories as well. Knowledge from psychology, psychiatrics, sociology, public health and nursing provides a base for psychiatric-mental health nurses, which nurses are able to provide health education to community based on the total assessment of their environment, population, occupations, education and other characteristics. The fundamental of the service is to raise people's consciousness regarding mental health, to provide guidance and counseling, and to help the community to learn positive coping strategies for stress and ultimately promote people's mental health.

ii. Implementation of Treatment Interventions

One of the most important roles of psychiatric-mental health nurse is implementing treatment interventions, which is usually in the inpatient settings, and partial care settings. The nurse applies psychiatric-mental health knowledge and principles to provide a safe environment, to establish a therapeutic relationship with patients, and to meet patients' daily needs. The goals of nursing care in this dimension include reducing the hospital stay of the patients, relieving the pain of patients and their family, and prepare for discharge to the community.

iii. Rehabilitation

Rehabilitation usually takes place in communities, residences, and homes. Psychiatric-mental health nurses collaborate with therapists using a variety of rehabilitation methods to help the patients to reach their highest level of function, reintegrating them into community. A broad range of psychiatric rehabilitation programs are used by nurses to help patients adapt to community life through social, residential, vocational, educational and recreation rehabilitation services. These programs emphasize on acquiring skills such as communication skills, vocational skills, social skills and interpersonal relationship which are designed to increase the functioning of patients with psychiatric disabilities so that they are successful and satisfied in their environment of choice with the least amount of ongoing professional intervention necessary.

一、精神科护士的工作范围

精神科护士由于工作目的、性质、岗位的不同，其工作范围非常广泛，如健康促进、治疗、康复训练及健康教育等多方面服务。

（一）健康促进和预防保健

预防保健工作主要在社区进行，亦可在学校、工厂等场所进行。护士针对社区居民的生活环境、人口、职业、教育等方面的特点，应用心理学、精神医学、社会学、公共卫生、护理学等方面的知识对公众实施有关心理卫生方面的指导与咨询，并适时实施心理健康教育，指导人们关注个人及团体的心理卫生，学习适当的调节压力方法，满足个体的自尊及其他心理健康的需要，以促进公众的心理健康，预防精神障碍或疾病的发生。

（二）治疗性护理

治疗性护理主要是针对住院的精神病患者或需部分照顾的患者所提供的护理。护士按照精神疾病的治疗及护理原则，为患者提供安全舒适的治疗环境，并与其建立良好的护患关系，提供日常生活护理，满足患者日常需求。其目的是尽量缩短患者的病程及住院时间，减轻疾病给患者及家属带来的伤害及痛苦，为患者能融入社区及家庭生活做好出院计划及准备。

（三）康复训练

康复工作主要在社区及家庭进行。护士与康复治疗师等人员互相配合，采用社交技能、职业功能训练、健康教育、沟通技巧、建立人际关系以及文体娱乐活动等训练方法对患者进行康复训练。其目的是协助患者，最大程度地恢复功能水平，重返社会生活。社区康复适合慢性患者的管理。

iv. Health Education

Health education can be given to different clients in a variety of settings. In the community psychiatric and mental health care settings, nurses provide health education to the residents for preventing them from getting mental health problems and promoting their mental health. In hospitals, the nurse provides health education regarding treatment, prevention, nursing care and rehabilitation to the mentally disordered patients and their families. In community and home, the nurse provide health education to patients and their families for community rehabilitation, medication safety, prevention of relapse, and reduce re-hospitalization and help to live in the community independently. The purpose of health education is to maximize all people's potential and to help them to remain a high level of mental health.

（四）健康教育

在不同服务场所，针对不同服务对象，健康教育的形式及内容不同。在社区，护士为居民提供有关促进精神健康、防止精神疾病的知识。在医院，针对患者及家属的实际问题，提供有关精神疾病的治疗、护理、预防、康复等方面的健康指导。在社区和家庭，指导患者及家属实施有关精神疾病的社区康复、安全用药指导、预防疾病复发、减少再次入院次数，培养患者独立生活的能力。健康教育的目的是使所有服务对象能发挥自己的潜能，保持最佳的心理健康状态。

II. Continuum of Mental Health Settings

Traditional settings for psychiatric nurses include psychiatric facilities, community mental health centers, psychiatric units in general hospitals, and residential facilities, and private practice. More recently, alternative treatment settings have emerged throughout the continuum of mental health care. The hospital is being transformed into the integrated clinical system that provides inpatient care, partial hospitalization or day treatment, residential care, home care, and outpatient or ambulatory care (figure 1-1).

In addition, community based treatment settings have expanded to include foster care or group homes , hospices, visiting nurse associations, home health agencies, emergency departments, nursing homes, shelters, primary care clinics, schools, prisons, industrial settings, managed care facilities, and health maintenance organizations.

二、精神卫生整体－连续性服务场所

传统的精神科护理工作场所包括精神病医院、社区精神卫生服务中心、综合医院的精神科室、寄宿服务中心及私立机构。随着精神疾病治疗及护理的不断发展，相继出现了多种可供选择的新型服务机构，包括住院护理、部分住院或日间护理、寄宿照顾、家庭护理、门诊及流动护理等，精神疾病的治疗及护理将发展成一个整体－连续的立体网络结构（图 1–1）。

除此之外，以社区为中心的护理场所已经扩展到集体家庭护理、临终关怀中心、探访护士协会、家庭保健服务机构、急诊服务中心、老人院、庇护所、初级卫生保健所、学校、监狱、企业、各种服务管理机构以及促进及保持健康机构等。

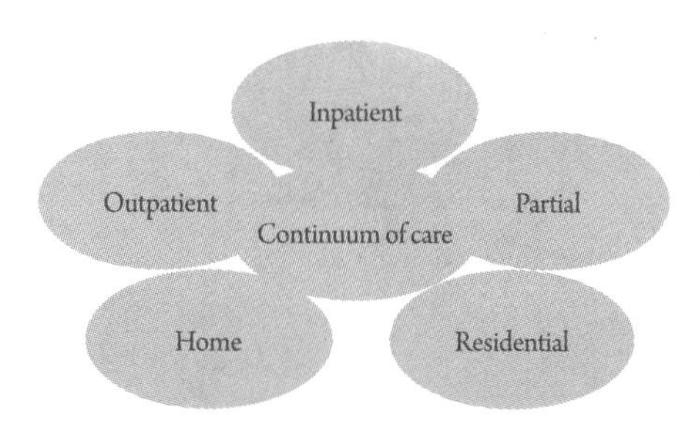

Figure 1–1　Continuum of psychiatric–mental care settings

The new opportunities for psychiatric nursing practice that are emerging throughout the continuum of mental health care are very exciting. They allow psychiatric-mental health nurses to be proactive in demonstrating their expertise in designating intervention, planning programs, implementing treatment strategies, and manage staff in a wide variety of traditional and non-traditional settings. Psychiatric nurses must also continue to demonstrate flexibility, accountability, and self-direction as they move into these expanding areas of practice.

随着精神科护理连续性服务的不断发展及完善，护士的专业服务场所将不断扩展，为护士提供了在各种传统及非传统机构展示其专业才能、知识及技能的广阔空间，包括制订护理措施、规划各种服务项目、实施治疗措施及对其他人员的管理等。当护士在不断发展自己的服务领域时，必须时刻牢记要以灵活、负责、独立的方式提供服务。

III. Roles of Psychiatric Nurses

三、精神科护士的角色

The role of a nurse is determined by the purpose, mission, organizational structure, work responsibility, and dimensions of work.

由于精神科护理工作的目的、任务、组织结构、工作责任和范围不同，精神科护士承担着如下角色。

i. Basic Roles of Psychiatric Nurses

The contemporary practice of psychiatric nursing occurs within a social and environmental context. Thus the nurse-patient relationship has evolved into a nurse-patient partnership that expands the dimension of the professional psychiatric role. These elements include clinical competence, patients and family advocacy, fiscal responsibility, interdisciplinary collaboration, social accountability, and legal-ethical responsibilities (figure 1-2).

The basic roles of the psychiatric-mental health nurses are consisted of skilled communicator, role model of adaptive behavior, director of the therapeutic milieu, advocator for a client and his family, member of health care team, primary health care nurse for a specific client, and therapist.

（一）基本角色

精神科护理工作是在一定的社会和生活环境中进行。因此当今的护患关系已发展成为新型的伙伴关系，从而形成了精神科护士的多种专业角色，具体体现在以下方面：临床工作能力、为患者及家庭代言、帮助患者筹措看病资金、与其他专业合作、社会责任、伦理与法律责任等（图 1-2）。

精神科护士的基本角色包括熟练的沟通者、适应性行为的示范者、治疗活动的指导者、患者及家庭的代言者、医疗服务团队的成员、患者的责任护士及治疗师等。

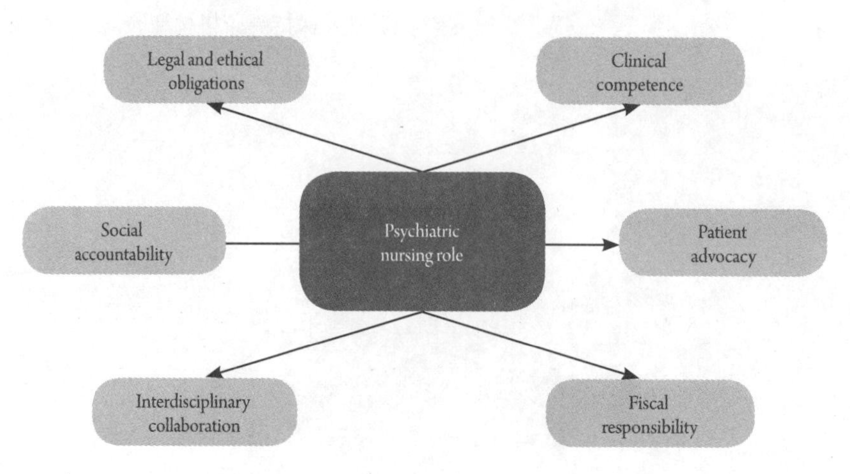

Figure 1-2 Elements of psychiatric nursing roles

ii. Advanced Roles

During the later 20th century, psychiatric nursing began to evolve as a clinical specialty. By advanced study and clinical practice in a master program in psychiatric nursing, clinical specialists and nurse practitioners gained expert knowledge in the care and prevention of psychiatric disorders. Therefore, the advanced roles are developed as nurse practitioners as well as therapist.

（二）高级角色

从20世纪后期开始，精神科护士开始由通科向专科方向发展。通过研究生或其他毕业后的继续教育，精神科护士获取了进行高级专科护理的知识与技能，开始了高级精神专科护理服务。本领域中最重要的两个角色为精神科高级执业护师及临床护理专家。

iii. Expended Roles (Clinical Specialists)

The role of nurses continues to expand with the developmental of health care system. Currently, the field of psychiatric nursing offers a variety of opportunities for specialization. These roles include nurse liaison in general hospitals, therapist in private practice, consultant, educator, expert witness in legal issues, employee assistance counselor, mental health provider in long-term care facilities, and association with a mobile psychiatric triage unit.

（三）扩展角色（临床专家）

随着社会对精神科护理需求的不断增加，精神科护士的角色功能进一步扩展，专业化的前景更加广阔，机会更多。目前，精神科护士可以发挥下列扩展的角色功能：综合医院的联系者、私立机构的治疗师、咨询者、教育者、法律问题的专业证人、雇员心理支持咨询师、长期住院的护理者、流动性精神病分类病区的护理者。

The role of nurses is also expanding in the area of tele-health. As technology becomes cheaper and more reliable, demand for this convenient delivery method grows. Experts predict more dramatic changes in the delivery of health care once technical and practical barriers are overcome.

随着先进技术的不断发明及应用，各种费用低廉、性能可靠的先进仪器设备将会逐步应用到精神疾病的治疗、康复及护理中。专家估计，随着精神疾病远程医疗护理服务的进一步完善，护士将在此领域发挥重要的角色功能。

Forensic nursing is expected to become one of the fastest growing nursing specialties of the 21st century in the western countries. Forensic nursing focuses on advocacy for and ministration to offenders and victims of violent crime and the families of both. Forensic nursing is a significant resource in forensic psychiatric practice and in the treatment of incarcerated persons.

在西方社会，法医学护理将会成为21世纪护理专业的一个快速发展的专科。法医学护士作为受害者或被告的代言人，为双方以及他们的家庭提供护理服务。

iv. Factors Determine the Roles of Psychiatric-Mental Health Nurses

The role of a nurse in any psychiatric-mental health settings depends on the followings:

1. Philosophy, mission, values and goals of the treatment settings.

2. Definition of mental health and mental illness that prevail in the setting.

3. Needs of the consumers of the mental health services.

4. Number of clinical staff available and the services they are able to provide.

5. Organizational structure and reporting relationships in the setting.

（四）影响精神科护士角色的因素

精神科护士角色影响因素如下：

1. 所在机构的服务理念、任务、价值体系及目标。

2. 所在机构对精神健康及精神疾病定义的认识。

3. 服务对象对精神健康服务的需要。

4. 医务人员的数量及所能提供的服务。

5. 组织机构及机构内部各部门之间的关系。

6. Consensus reached by the mental health care providers regarding their respective roles and responsibilities.

7. Resources and revenues available to offset the cost care needed and provided.

8. Presence of strong nursing leadership and membership.

A supportive environment for psychiatric-mental health nurses is one of which there is open and honest communication among staff, interdisciplinary respect, recognition of nurses' contribution, nursing involvement in decision making about both clinical care and the work environment, delegation of nonessential nursing tasks, opportunity to expand into new roles and responsibilities, and the encouragement of involvement in professional psychiatric-mental health nursing activities and organization.

6. 组织机构内的各种专业人员对自己的职责范围达成共识的程度。

7. 资源和收入能否满足服务需要。

8. 呈现出强有力的护理团队精神和领导协调能力。

在精神科的护理服务过程中，应采取多种方式促进护士不断发挥自己的角色功能，包括护理人员之间建立开放、诚实的沟通渠道；不同专业的人士互相尊重；对护士的工作业绩表示认可；使护士参与临床护理及管理决策；将非主要的护理工作授权给其他人员做；向护士提供不断扩展自己角色空间的机会；鼓励护士参与精神科护理的专业组织及活动。

Box 1-2 describes phenomena of concern for psychiatric mental health nurses.

Box 1-2 列出了美国精神科护理协会等所描述的精神科护士需关注的行为现象。

BOX 1-2 Learning More

Phenomena of Concern for Psychiatric-Mental Health Nurses

1. Promotion of optimal mental and physical health and well-being and prevention of mental illness.
2. Impaired ability to function related to psychiatric, emotional, and physiological distress.
3. Alterations in thinking, perceiving, and communicating due to psychiatric disorders or mental health problems.
4. Behaviors and mental states that indicate potential danger to self or others.
5. Emotional stress related to illness, pain, disability, and loss.
6. Symptom management, side effects, or toxicities associated with self-administered drugs, psychopharmacological intervention, and other treatment modalities.
7. The barriers to treatment efficacy and recovery posed by alcohol and substance abuse and dependence.
8. Self-concept and body image changes, developmental issues, life process changes, and end-of-life issues.
9. Physical symptoms that occur along with altered psychological status.
10. Psychological symptoms that occur along with altered physical status.

BOX 1-2 知识拓展

精神科护士需关注的行为现象

1. 最大限度地促进身心健康，预防精神疾病的发生。
2. 由于精神、心理及生理应激引起的社会功能受损。
3. 由于精神障碍或精神健康问题导致的思维、感知觉及沟通能力的改变。
4. 表现出对自己或对他人潜在伤害危险的异常行为及精神状态。
5. 表现出因病痛、残疾或丧失引起的情感应激。
6. 由于自服药物、服用处方精神治疗药物以及其他治疗方法所引起的药物副作用、毒性反应以及患者的症状处理方式。
7. 由酒精等滥用物质及药物依赖对治疗效果及疾病康复所造成的影响。
8. 自我概念或机体形象改变、生长发育问题、生活方式改变以及临终问题。
9. 由心理问题伴发生理疾病。
10. 由生理问题伴发心理疾病。

11. Interpersonal, organizational, sociocultural, spiritual, or environmental circumstances or events which have an effect on the mental and emotional well-being of the individual and family or community.
12. Elements of recovery, including the ability to maintain housing, employment, and social support, that help individuals re-engage in seeking meaningful lives.
13. Social factors such as violence, poverty, and substance abuse.

11. 因为人际关系、组织机构、社会文化、精神信仰、周围环境或生活事件等给个体、家庭或社区带来的影响。
12. 个体重归社会的影响因素，如住房、工作及社会支持等问题。
13. 社会因素，如社会暴力事件、贫穷及吸毒等。

IV. Functions of Psychiatric Nurses

i. Nurse's Function in Psychiatric Patients Care

1. Dealing with patients' problems of attitude, mood, and interpretation of reality.

2. Exploring disturbing and conflicting thoughts and feelings.

3.Using the patients' positive feelings toward the therapist to bring about psycho- physiological homeostasis.

4. Counseling patients in emergencies, including panic and fear.

5. Strengthening the well part of patients.

ii. Nurses' Functions in Three Levels of Prevention

The concepts of primary, secondary, and tertiary prevention provide a framework for contemporary psychiatric nursing practice. Nurses' functions in each level of the preventions are presented here.

1. Primary Prevention Primary prevention involves lowering the incidence of mental illness in a community by changing causative factors before they can do harm. It is a concept that precedes disease and is applied to a generally healthy population. It includes protection against disease, illness prevention, health maintenance, and health promotion. Primary mental health care is important because many people are not receiving the mental health care they need. Some are undiagnosed in general settings. Others are correctly diagnosed but lack a consistent care provider. Still others have problems with their prescribed treatments and have relapses that could have been prevented.

Psychiatric nurses are moving into the domain of primary care and working with other nurses and physicians to diagnose and treat psychiatric illness in patients with somatic complaints. For examples,

四、精神科护士的功能

（一）一般功能

1. 处理患者由于态度、心境及现实感悟等方面所出现的问题。

2. 了解患者思维和感受等方面是否有错乱或冲突。

3. 抓住患者对治疗师信任的机会，及时实施有效的治疗，使其达到身心衡状态。

4. 当患者处于紧急情况而出现恐惧或恐慌时，及时为其提供咨询服务。

5. 当制订护理计划时，尽可能考虑到患者的优势。

（二）三级预防模式中的功能

护士在三级预防模式的框架指导下为患者提供如下护理服务：

1. 一级预防 即通过干预可能的原因或诱因，降低精神疾病的发病率。该级预防主要针对社区的健康居民，采取各种促进健康的措施，以预防精神疾病的发生，具体包括疾病预防、健康维护、健康促进等工作。由于社区中许多人不能及时得到有关精神健康的干预，或在综合医院中漏诊，即使诊断正确，或因缺少长期的照顾者，或因未能坚持服药而复发。因此，初级卫生保健对预防社区精神疾病的发生及发展具有重要的作用。

精神科护士逐渐在初级卫生保健中发挥着重要的作用，并与医生或其他护士合作，诊断及治疗由于躯体疾病而引起的精神障碍。如评

cardiovascular, gynecological, respiratory, gastrointestinal, and family practice settings are appropriate for assessing patients for anxiety, depression, and substance abuse disorders. As health care initiates and continues to move into schools and other community settings, psychiatric nurses are assuming leadership roles in providing expertise through consultation and evaluation.

估心血管疾病，妇科疾病，呼吸系统疾病，胃肠道疾病的患者，甚至家庭成员是否有焦虑、抑郁或药物滥用等。随着精神健康护理体系进入学校等其他社区单位，精神科护士可以通过咨询及评价等方法提供专业帮助。

Nurses have many independent functions within this area. Direct nursing care functions include:

护士在一级预防保健模式中将发挥如下具体作用：

(1) Health teaching regarding principles of mental health.

（1）有关精神卫生的理念和相关的健康教育。

(2) Effective changes in improved living conditions, freedom from poverty, and better education.

（2）有效地改善居民的生存环境，脱离贫困，提高教育水平。

(3) Consumer education in such areas as normal growth and development and sex education.

（3）对服务对象进行正常人体的生长发育及性教育。

(4) Making appropriate referrals before mental disorder occurs based on assessment of potential stressors and life changes.

（4）及时评估社区居民潜在的应激及生活改变所造成的问题，并采取适宜的干预措施，以预防疾病的发生。

(5) Assisting patients in avoiding future psychiatric problems in a general hospital setting.

（5）协助综合医院工作，防止患者出现精神心理问题。

(6) Working with families to support family members and group functioning.

（6）帮助家庭及团体维持其正常功能。

(7) Be active in community activities related to mental health.

（7）及时参加社区与精神卫生有关的相关活动。

2. Secondary Prevention This level of prevention involves reducing actual illness by early detection and treatment of the problem. Direct nursing functions include:

2. 二级预防 二级预防主要涉及精神疾病的早期发现、早期治疗，减轻或控制病情。护士在二级预防中的重要角色包括：

(1) Ongoing assessment of individuals at high risk of disease exacerbation.

（1）对精神疾病易发人群要持续评估。

(2) Home visits for preadmission or treatment services.

（2）为入院前及治疗中的患者提供家庭护理。

(3) Emergency treatment and psychiatric services in the general hospital.

（3）为综合医院提供有关精神疾病的急症处理和服务。

(4) Providing a therapeutic environment.

（4）提供治疗性环境。

(5) Supervising patients receiving medication.

（5）监测患者用药情况。

(6) Suicide prevention services.

（6）提供防自杀服务。

(7) Counseling on a time-limited basis.

（7）进行限时咨询。

(8) Crisis intervention.

（8）危机干预。

(9) Psychotherapy with individuals, families, and groups of various ages ranging from children to older adults.

（9）向各年龄段的人提供个体、家庭或团体性的心理治疗。

(10) Intervention with communities and

（10）针对社区或团体所出现的（精神）

organizations based on an identified problem.

3. Tertiary Prevention This level of prevention involves reducing impairment or disability resulting from an illness. Direct nursing care functions include:

(1) Promoting vocational training and rehabilitation.

(2) Organizing after-care programs for patients discharged from psychiatric hospitals to ease their transition from the hospital to the community.

(3) Providing partial hospitalization option for patients when necessary.

In addition to direct nursing care functions, psychiatric nurses engage in indirect activities that affect all three levels of prevention. These activities include training nursing personnel in various education programs; administrating in mental health settings to help provide optimal psychiatric care; supervising nursing personnel to improve the quality of nursing services; consulting with other professionals, community care givers, local national agencies, and research agencies.

(Lei Hui Zhang Rong)

健康问题，采取相应的干预措施。

3. 三级预防 三级预防涉及如何最大限度地减轻由精神疾病引起的损伤或残障程度，恢复社会功能。护士在三级预防中的角色包括：

（1）加强职业及康复训练。

（2）为出院的精神病患者安排由医院到社区的连续康复训练项目。

（3）必要时为患者提供部分住院服务。

除上述直接角色功能，精神科护士在三级预防中也间接地发挥各种作用，包括为其他领域护理人员提供各种教育培训项目；在精神科病房做好组织管理工作并提供选择性的护理干预；指导护理人员提高护理服务水平；向其他专业人员、社区人员、当地政府机构以及科研机构提供必要的咨询。

（雷 慧 张 荣）

Key Points

1. Mental health is a positive state in which one functions well in society, is accepted within a group, and is generally satisfied with life. It includes the way a person thinks, feels, interacts, and behaves within his or her environment.

2. Mental illness is characterized by psychological or behavioral manifestations and impairment in functioning due to a social, psychological, genetic, physical/chemical or biologic disturbance. Persons with mental illness frequently have worries, distorted perceptions, fears, and may be irrational.

3. Psychiatric nursing is a specialized area of nursing practice, employing the wide range of explanatory theories of human behaviors as its science and purposeful use of self as its art.

4. Before 1860, the mentally ill was treated inhumanly. It's Philippe Pinel that unchained the shackled, and patients were treated humanely in his hospital.

内容摘要

1. 精神健康是一种良性状态，表现为个体社会功能良好，能被所在的团体及社会接纳，对生活有基本的满意度。具体体现在所处环境中个体的思维状态、感受、与他人的关系以及行为表现形式等方面。

2. 精神疾病是由社会、心理、遗传、体内的化学物质或生物失衡等原因引起，以心理行为异常及功能受损为主要临床表现的疾病。精神疾病的患者经常表现出异常的焦虑、担心、思维紊乱、恐惧及行为异常等。

3. 精神科护理学是护理学的一个分支，它以社会心理学、生物及生理学、人格发展、行为学等方面的知识为理论基础，科学地、艺术性地为服务对象提供精神卫生护理服务。

4. 1860 年以前，精神病患者面临的是非人道的对待。法国医生菲利普·比奈尔作为世界上第一位精神病院的院长，率先提出要砸碎锁链，主张人道地对待精神病患者。

5. Freud and Kraepelin studied people objectively, and their efforts led to both psychodynamic and biologic understanding of mental disorders.

5. 弗洛伊德及克雷丕林等精神心理专家客观地分析精神病患者，他们开辟了用精神动力学及生物学知识研究精神病现象的时代。

6. Antipsychotic drugs, antidepressant drugs (1950s), and other drugs were developed, which greatly contributed to the treatment of specific mental disorders.

6. 20世纪50年代，抗精神病药及抗抑郁药问世，伴随着更多治疗精神疾病的药物的出现，实现了针对不同的精神疾病采用对应的药物治疗。

7. Deinstitutionalization changed the focus of treatment of mental illness from hospitals to the community.

7. 20世纪60年代以来，越来越多的精神病患者能够在社区接受治疗及康复。

8. Challenges facing psychiatric-mental health nursing include recent biological discoveries and technological advances and changes in health care system.

8. 新形势下，精神科护理面临诸多机遇和挑战，如新的生物学发现、科学技术的进步及医疗卫生体制变化等。

9. Roles of psychiatric-mental health nurses include advocate, communicators, role model, member of health care team, and nurse therapist.

9. 精神科护士的角色功能包括代言人、沟通者、角色示范者、卫生服务组织的成员及治疗师等。

10. The psychiatric mental health nurse works to promote patients' mental health ether as a basic level nurse or as an advanced practice nurse if he or she gains additional training.

10. 精神科护士由于接受教育的层次不同，工作角色也不同。一般护士从事患者的常规护理，经过特殊训练的护士可做一些特殊的高级护理。

Exercises

思考题

1. Analyze respectively the characteristics of mental health and mental illness, and describe the continuum of them.

1. 分析精神健康与精神疾病各自的特点，并描述二者的连续性。

2. Describe the concept of psychiatric nursing and the essentials of the holistic mental health care.

2. 描述精神科护理学的概念及整体化精神科护理的精髓。

3. List people who have made contributions to mental health care and outline their theories or views in different historical stages.

3. 列举在不同历史时期对精神科护理有贡献的人物，并概述他们的主要理论或观点。

4. Describe the roles and functions of psychiatric nurses.

4. 描述精神科护士的角色和功能作用。

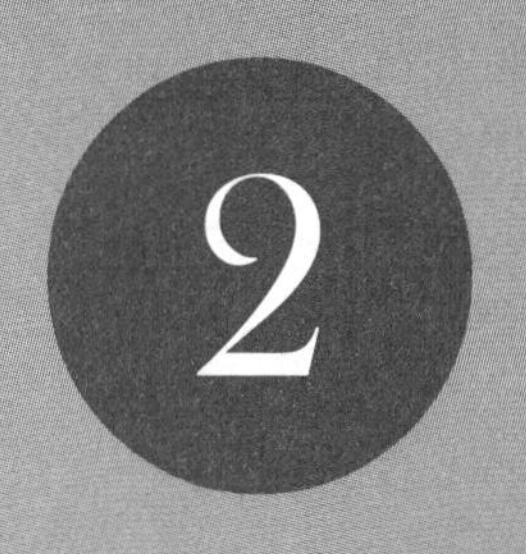

Chapter 2 The Nursing Process in Psychiatric and Mental Health Nursing

第二章 精神科护理程序

Learning Objectives

Memorization

1. Describe the concepts of nursing process.
2. Summarize the assessment contents of psychiatric and mental health nursing.
3. State the contents of mental status examination.

Comprehension

1. Explain the five consecutive steps of nursing process including assessment, diagnosis, planning, implementation, and evaluation with examples.
2. Explain the key points of evidence-based practice.

Application

1. Use nursing process to conduct nursing assessment, diagnosis, planning, implementation, and evaluation.
2. Document correctly using the method of problem-oriented recording.

学习目标

识记

1. 能准确复述护理程序的概念。
2. 能正确阐述精神科护理评估的内容。
3. 能简述精神状况检查的项目。

理解

1. 能结合实例说明护理程序中评估、诊断、计划、实施和评价的五个连续步骤。
2. 能说明循证护理实践的要点。

运用

1. 能科学地运用护理程序进行护理评估、作出护理诊断、制订护理计划、实施护理措施并评价。
2. 能正确应用以问题为中心的记录方法进行护理记录。

Susan, a 30-year-old female accountant, was hospitalized as she suspected to be hurt for two months. Two months ago, Susan argued with the boss and became insane. At present, she was always suspected that her colleagues were talking about her, speaking ill of her, and that they would conspired to murder her. She holed up at home, fidgeted, whispered and sleepless at night. Susan believed that there was eavesdropping and monitoring around her, what's more, her families persuaded invalidly. This had seriously affected Susan's social function, so she could not continue to work at present.

Please think about the following questions based on the case:

1. What might be the present and potential nursing diagnosis for Susan?
2. How do psychiatric mental health nurses provide effective care for Susan?

患者，苏珊，女，30岁，某单位会计员，因疑人害2个月余收住院。2个月前与上司争吵急起精神失常，现在总怀疑单位同事在议论她，说她坏话，觉得大家要谋害她。在家她闭门不出、坐卧不安、小声说话、夜间不眠，说有人窃听、监视她，家人劝说无效。苏珊的病情已经严重影响到她的社会功能，目前不能继续工作。

请思考：

1. 患者目前及潜在的护理诊断是什么？
2. 护理人员应如何为患者提供有效的护理措施？

The nursing process has provided a systematic framework for the delivery of nursing care for many years. It is nursing's means of fulfilling the requirement for a scientific methodology in order to be considered a profession. It is a way of thinking that allows nurses to reflect on nursing care and work in an organized and systematic manner. As a nurse, to provide care in the psychiatric and mental health setting, it is important to recognize that the nursing is a complex process of step-by-step analysis that can help one to understand and reflect on the nursing care more than it actually reflects activities as they are experienced in real life. This chapter discusses fundamental concepts of nursing process, the steps of nursing process, and nursing document. It provides a foundation for the delivery of nursing care.

护理程序是一种系统而科学地安排护理活动的工作方法，可使护理工作建立在组织化和系统化的基础之上。作为精神科护士，充分认识护理工作是根据患者的需要而进行的一系列有计划、有步骤、系统地解决问题的过程，将有助于其在护理实践中对患者进行全身心的护理。本章主要介绍护理程序的基本概念、护理程序的具体步骤以及护理记录的方法，将为护士提供护理服务提供指导。

Section 1 Introduction of the Nursing Process

第一节 护理程序概述

I. Definition

一、护理程序的概念

Nursing process is an effective method for nurses to identify and solve problems scientifically in order to achieve nursing objectives. The nursing process is a five-step problem-solving approach to nursing that also serves as an organizational framework for the practice of nursing. Nurses use nursing process to confirm the clients' response of health and disease status, design specific

护理程序是一种护士通过科学地确认问题和解决问题，以达到护理目标的有效工作方法。护士运用护理程序确认服务对象对健康和疾病状态的反应，进而设计具体措施，实施护理，并通过服务对象行为的改变确定

measures, implement, and evaluate the effectiveness through changes in the behavior of the clients. It is an ongoing process continues for as long as the nurse and client have interactions, directed toward change in the client's physical or behavioral responses (figure 2-1).

其有效性。护理程序共包括五个连续的步骤，是一种有计划、系统而科学地解决问题的工作方法，为护理实践提供了严密的组织框架。护士全面评估和分析患者身心状态、确定其需要，并根据需要制订相应的护理计划、实施计划并对护理效果作出评价，从而使患者得到全身心的护理（图 2–1）。

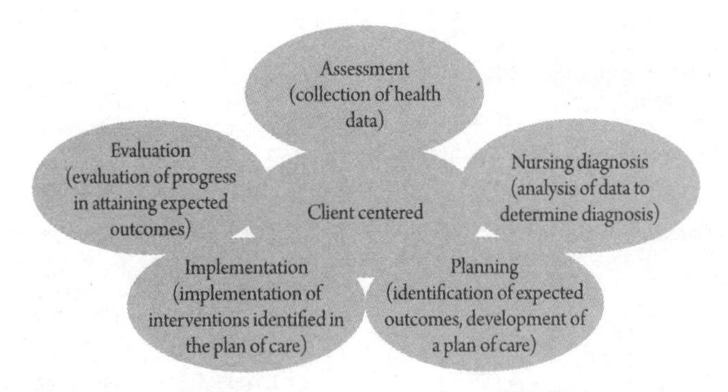

Figure 2–1 The ongoing nursing process

II. Nursing Process in Psychiatric and Mental Health Nursing

In dealing with the clients with psychiatric and mental health disorders, the nursing process can present unique challenges. Psychiatric problems may be vague and elusive, not tangible or visible like many physiological disruptions.

Geach (1974) has identified three aspects of problem-solving with psychiatric clients:

- The nurse involves the client in the process.
- The problem that the nurse and client address has immediate relevance to what is initially happening between them.
- The nurse and client form some sort of relationship so that they can solve problems within a relationship rather than in isolation.

It is essential that the nurse and the client become partners in the problem-solving process. If clients avoid or resist becoming involved, nurses may be tempted to exclude them. However, this should be avoided.

The phases of nursing process are assessment, nursing diagnosis, planning, implementation, and evaluation. Validation is part of each step, and all phases may overlap or occur simultaneously. Nurses should pay attention to the nursing conditions and nursing behaviors related to each one of these phases, in order to provide holistic nursing care.

二、精神疾病的护理程序

护理精神障碍患者常具有挑战性，因为精神问题不像躯体疾病那样明确，往往不确定或难以判断。

Geach（1974）针对精神障碍患者的护理，总结了三方面的应对策略：

① 护士应让患者参与护理过程；

② 护士应与患者共同确定护理问题；

③ 护士应与患者建立和谐的护患关系，以共同解决其存在的护理问题。

护士应充分认识到在解决问题过程中与患者的伙伴关系是对精神障碍患者进行全身心护理的关键。

护理程序由评估、诊断、计划、实施和评价五个步骤组成，这五个步骤是相互联系、互为影响的，并且可重叠或同时发生。在精神科护理中，护士应注意每一步骤的护理要求及护理行为，以便更好地为精神障碍患者提供全身心护理。

BOX 2-1 Learning More

The Core of Orlando's Nursing Process Theory

Orlando's nursing process focuses on improvement in the patient's behavior by actions that are based on a patient's needs found through effective interaction with the patient. The most important contribution of Orlando's theoretical work is the primacy of the nurse-client relationship. According to Orlando when a person is not able to meet the needs that he/she has, he/she becomes distressed and is in need of nursing care. Accordingly, the persons that are able to meet their own needs are not distressed, and do not need nursing care. Orlando highlights that it is crucial not only to meet the patient's needs but first of all find out what those needs are. If interventions are carried out before identifying if those interventions give benefits for the patient, nursing is not highly professional. Orlando explained four major dimensions in the nursing process:

- The role of the nurse is to find out and meet the patient's immediate need for help.
- The patient's presenting behavior may be a plea for help; however, the help needed may not be what it appears to be.
- Therefore, nurses need to use their perception, thoughts about the perception, or the feeling engendered from their thoughts to explore with patients the meaning of their behavior.
- This process helps nurse find out the nature of the distress and what help the patient needs.

BOX 2-1 知识拓展

Orlando 护理程序的核心

Orlando 的护理程序主要是依据患者的需求并采取相应的措施改善其行为，患者的需求是在与其互动的过程中获知的。护患关系是 Orlando 护理程序理论中很重要的一部分。Orlando 认为当一个人的需求不能得到满足时，就会处于应激状态并需要护理。与此相对，如果能满足其需求，则不需要护理。Orlando 强调满足患者的需求是至关重要的，并且首先应该评估需求。如果实施护理前护士不能确定护理措施是否有益于患者，则意味着护士的不专业。Orlando 在护理程序理论中提出：

① 护士的作用是发现和满足患者的直接需求；

② 患者行为可能是在请求帮助，但其真正的需求或许不是其表现的那样；

③ 护士需要感知并思考以探索患者行为的真正意义；

④ 护理程序则是帮助护士发现患者痛苦的本质和如何满足其需求。

Section 2 Nursing Assessment

Nursing assessment is the first step of nursing process. Effective nursing interventions are based on accurate and relevant information about the individual receiving assistance. The assessment phase of the nursing process includes the collection of health data of an individual, family, or group with the methods of observing, examining, and interviewing. Before any steps it can be taken to relieve symptoms, assist an individual with adaptation, or implement other interventions to improve the quality of life, the nurse must firstly define the difficulties experienced by the individual, understand the response to these difficulties, and identify influences from the context of the individual's life, in which these difficulties occur. This section focuses especially on the assessment of clients with psychiatric disorders.

第二节 护理评估

护理评估是护理程序关键的第一步，有效的护理干预建立在对患者准确而全面的评估上。护理评估是指护士通过观察、体格检查及访谈等方法对个体、家庭甚至群体进行全面的资料收集并对其进行整理判断的过程。护士只有全面认识患者存在的健康问题，理解这些问题所引起的社会及心理反应，并确定影响患者健康的环境因素，才能有效地实施护理措施，以帮助其适应内外环境的改变，提高其生活质量。

I. Types of Assessment

The type of assessment that occurs depends on the client's needs, presenting symptoms, and clinical setting. Three kinds of nursing assessment exist including comprehensive, focused, and screening assessment.

A comprehensive assessment includes data related to the client's biologic, psychological, cultural, spiritual, and social needs. This type of assessment is generally completed in collaboration with other health care professionals such as a physician, psychologist, and neurologist. Comprehensive assessment is helpful to judge the reasons of psychiatric disorders. A physical examination is performed to rule out any physiologic causes of disorders such as anxiety, depression, or dementia.

A focused assessment includes the collection of specific data regarding a particular problem as determined by the client, a family member, or a crisis situation such as a suicide attempt.

A screening assessment is the collection of data to identify individuals who have not as yet recognized the presence of symptoms due to a psychiatric disorder, who have risk factors for the development of a psychiatric disorder, or who may be experiencing emotional difficulties but not yet formally sought treatment. This type of assessment is usually conducted in a fairly structured census depending on the setting. For example, after a natural disaster such as an earthquake, community mental health services may establish screening clinics to recognize early symptoms, individuals at risk of developing post-traumatic stress disorder or other psychiatric disorders.

一、评估的方式

在对精神科患者进行评估时，医护人员常根据患者的需要、症状及临床环境确定采用何种评估方式。评估方式一般包括综合评估、针对性评估和筛选评估。

综合评估是指对患者生理、心理、社会、文化及精神等各方面资料的收集。这种评估方式往往需要护士和精神科医生、心理学家、神经科专科医生等人员共同合作完成。通过综合评估可以帮助判断引起患者精神障碍的原因，确定疾病诊断，如全面的体格检查可以判断患者是否存在焦虑、抑郁或痴呆等精神障碍的躯体原因。

针对性评估是指护士就患者某一具体问题所进行的相关资料的收集，如针对有自杀企图这一问题所进行相关资料的收集及整理。

筛选评估是指通过资料的收集与分析，确定那些具有精神症状但尚未认识到其属于精神疾病，或存在引起精神障碍的危险因素，或虽经历情感障碍但未寻求正规治疗的个体。此种评估方式常是根据环境而采取的有组织普查，如在一次自然灾害之后，社区精神卫生机构通过建立临床普查，早期发现并诊断创伤后应激障碍。

II. Contents of Assessment

The assessment of the human's response to emotional difficulties or mental disorders includes the collection of biologic, psychological, and social data. Individuals are inherently biopsychosocial human beings with physical, emotional, cognitive, behavioral, spiritual, and other responses that interact with the environment, including their interpersonal, economic, political, legal, and cultural context. Any single event in the individual's life may produce responses in all of these dimensions. A thorough assessment of biological, psychological, and sociocultural status contribute to judge the client's present and potential problems, and thus to conduct effective nursing interventions.

二、评估的内容

对精神障碍患者的评估主要包括对患者生理、心理及社会资料的全面收集和整理。每一个个体都不仅有生理、情感、认知、行为和精神信仰，还与周围环境相互作用，具有经济、政治、法律及文化背景。个人生活中的某一事件，往往会引起复杂的身心反应。护士全面地评估精神障碍患者生理、心理及社会文化状况将有助于判断患者现存以及潜在的问题，从而进行有效的护理干预。

i. General Information

The assessment of general information includes name, gender, age, nationality, degree of education, marital status, medical diagnosis, and so forth.

ii. Health History

The assessment of health history includes present history, past history, personal history, family history, medication history, and so forth. Present history include the cause of the onset, cardinal symptom, and duration; past history refers to the diseases that the client ever had and the therapeutic regimen in the past; personal history includes drug abuse history, allergy history, and so forth; family history refers to whether the client's three generations of two lines had mental disorders. If the client is to receive psychopharmacologic treatment, the review of systems will serve as a baseline by which the nurse may judge if new symptoms develop or are increased by the medication.

iii. Physical Examination

Once historical information has been obtained, physiologic systems should be examined to evaluate the client's current physical condition. For the psychiatric and mental health nurse, particular attention is paid to the neurologic status, such as recent head trauma, episodes of hypertension, and changes in personality, speech, or ability to handle activities of daily living.

iv. Laboratory Data

Laboratory tests can help rule out organic causes of psychiatric symptoms. For example, impaired copper metabolism in Wilson's disease and a positive result on an antinuclear antibody (ANA) test in systemic lupus erythematosus (SLE). Laboratory work is additionally used to monitor treatment, such as measuring the effects of lithium (Eskalith) on electrolytes, thyroid metabolism, and renal function. However, laboratory data serve only as an underlying support for the essential skill of clinical assessment.

v. Mental Status Examination

Mental Status Examination (MSE) is referred as an organized systematic approach to the assessment of an individual's current psychiatric condition. It provides a detailed and systematic description of the client at that time. MSE makes clues and inferences that are required for the generation of diagnostic hypotheses. The MSE, guided by the hypothetic-deductive approach to diagnosis, is an essential part of the subsequent inquiry plan. The contents of MSE include the following parts. Each of these areas is described more detailed below.

（一）一般资料

一般资料的评估主要包括患者姓名、性别、年龄、民族、受教育程度、婚姻状况、门诊或住院诊断等。

（二）健康史

健康史的评估是指对现病史、既往史、个人史、家族史、用药史等资料的收集。现病史包括患者发病的原因、主要的精神症状、持续的时间；既往史是指患者过去患过何病，治疗如何；个人史包括药物滥用史、过敏史等；家族史是指患者两系三代内有无精神疾病患者，有无自杀身亡者等。若患者接受过药物治疗，护士应详细询问其用药情况，以协助判断患者新出现的症状是否与其用药有关。

（三）体格检查

一旦详细获得患者的病史资料，护士便应对患者进行全面的体格检查，以评估患者当前的身体状况。对于精神科护士来说，尤其应注重评估患者神经系统状况，如最近的脑外伤、高血压意外，以及患者的人格、语言或日常生活能力的改变。

（四）实验室检查

实验室检查可以帮助排除器质性精神障碍。例如，威尔逊氏症有铜代谢异常，系统性红斑狼疮抗核抗体阳性。实验室检查也可用于治疗的监测，如监测抗抑郁剂的血药水平，估计锂剂（碳酸锂）对电解质、甲状腺代谢和肾功能的影响，但实验室检查结果仅是临床评估基本技术的辅助指标。

（五）精神状况检查

精神状况检查是对精神科患者进行系统观察和评估，从而提供患者目前状况全面而系统的描述。精神状况检查对得出诊断假设非常重要。通过假设－推测的方法来引导精神状况检查以形成诊断，同时它也是有次序地对患者进行全面评估的重要组成部分。检查的内容主要包括：

① 外表和行为；

- Appearance and behavior
- Affect and mood
- Cognition and memory
- Language
- Perception
- Thought
- Intelligence
- Insight and judgment

Psychiatric nurses should fully understand and master the content of mental status examination in order to evaluate patients as a whole.

1. Appearance and Behavior General appearance includes physical characteristics, physiognomy, expression of the eyes, hair, apparent age, peculiarity of dress, cleanliness, and use of cosmetics. General appearance lends clues to several aspects of mental state. For example, depressed people often neglect their personal appearance, appear disheveled, and wear drab-looking clothes that are generally dark in color, reflecting a depressed mood.

In the process of assessment, the nurse should record activity and posture generally. Abnormal action and behavior in mental disorders include psychomotor excitement and psychomotor inhibition. Psychomotor excitement is referred as the increase of action and behavior. It is called coordinated psychomotor excitement if the action and behavior increase is accorded with thought, affect, and external environment, which is more common in manic episode. In contrast, it is called non-coordinated psychomotor excitement if the increase of action is not accorded with the thought, affect and environment, which is common in catatonic schizophrenia, hebephrenic schizophrenia, and delirium. Psychomotor inhibition is the reduction of the action and speech activity. Clinically it includes stupor, the action and speech activity are totally suppressed or reduced. The client keeps a fixed posture for a long time, although it is uncomfortable. Flexibilitas cerea: it refers that the limbs are at the mercy of others, appeared on the basis of stupor. Even if it is uncomfortable posture, the client remains motionless for a long time like wax sculpture. For instance, the client maintains still for a certain time with head elevated to a pillow height position, known as "air pillow". Mutism: the client keeps silent, doesn't answer the questions, and only gives hand signals. Behavior disorders also include negativism, stereotyped act, echopraxia, and mannerism.

2. Affect and Mood Affect and mood are often used as synonyms in psychiatric and mental health

② 情感和心境；

③ 认知和记忆；

④ 语言；

⑤ 知觉；

⑥ 思维；

⑦ 智能；

⑧ 自知力和判断力。

精神科护士应全面认识和掌握精神状况检查内容，以便对患者进行整体的评估。

1. 外表和行为 外表评估主要是对患者整体外观特点的观察和评价，如患者的体格、面容、眼神、头发、外观年龄、穿着、个人清洁以及装扮。对患者进行包括面部表情在内的外表评估，有助于判断患者的精神状况。如精神抑郁者常不注重外表穿着，衣着凌乱，衣服颜色单调且灰暗。

在评估过程中，护士一般还应记录患者的活动及姿态。精神疾病患者动作与行为的异常包括精神运动性兴奋和精神运动性抑制。精神运动性兴奋是指动作和行为增加。若动作和行为的增加与思维、情感活动、外界环境协调一致，称作协调性精神运动性兴奋，多见于躁狂发作。患者的言语动作增多与思维、情感及环境不相协调，则称作不协调性精神运动性兴奋，常见于紧张型精神分裂症、青春型精神分裂症及谵妄。精神运动性抑制是指行为动作和言语活动的减少。临床上包括木僵，患者动作行为和言语活动的完全抑制或减少，长时间保持一种固定姿势，尽管这种姿势并不令人感到舒适。蜡样屈曲指在木僵的基础上出现的患者肢体任人摆布，即使是不舒服的姿势，也较长时间似蜡塑一样维持不动。如将患者头部抬高似枕着枕头的姿势，患者也纹丝不动并维持很长时间，称之为"空气枕头"。缄默症指患者缄默不语，也不回答问题，有事可以手示意。另外，行为动作障碍还包括违拗症、刻板动作、模仿动作和作态。

2. 情感和心境 情感和心境在精神医学中常作为同义词，是指个体对客观事物的主

nursing, which refers to the individual's subjective attitude towards the objective things and the corresponding inner experience. It is the conscious component of monitoring system that signals whether the individual is on track toward a personal goal, whether he or she is frustrated or prevented from achieving the goal. In contrast, mood refers to a weak and sustained emotional state.

Affective disorders include changes in the nature, stability or coordination of the emotion. Changes in the nature of the emotion often continue for a long period, such as hyperthymia, euphoria, depression, anxiety, and fear. Emotional stability disorder refers to the changes of the emotional response threshold, such as apathy, emotional numbness, emotional fragility, raptus, pathological affect, and irritability. Affective corariance disorders include parathymia, emotional infantility, ambivalence, imposed emotion, and dysphoria.

Morbid euphoria, a sense of well-being expressed in inexorable good spirits, encountered in hypomania or mania episode and less common in schizophrenia and organic brain disorder. It also happened in frontal lobe dysfunction, neurosyphilis, disseminated sclerosis and after lobotomy, may be associated with fatuous joking and lack of foresight. Depression, a pervasive lack of interest and drive (also known as anergia), may be observed in patients with preschizophrenic, schizophrenic, depressive, and organic brain disorders.

The nurse notes the presence of histrionic affect, the blatant but rather shallow expression of emotion often observed in those who exaggerate their feelings in order to avoid being ignored and who need to capture, or who fear to lose the center of the interpersonal stage. Histrionic affect is often encountered in people with histrionic, narcissistic, or borderline personality disorder.

3. Cognition and Memory The contents of cognitive functions are listed in the following. Each of these areas is described in more details below:

- Level of consciousness and awareness;
- Orientation, attention, and concentration;
- Memory;
- Information;
- Comprehension;
- Conceptualization and abstraction.

(1) Level of consciousness and awareness: Changes in level of consciousness and awareness include coma and stupor. Coma is a state of nonawareness from which the patient cannot be aroused. Diminished awareness is called semicoma or stupor, in which case the subject is temporarily aroused (e.g., by pain or noise) but reverts to

观态度和相应的内心体验。情感是监督系统的意识部分，提示人是否在向目标前进，是否在到达目标的途中被阻止或打击，或者是否妨碍成功。心境则是指一种较弱而持续的情绪状态。

情感障碍包括情感性质的改变、情感稳定性的改变以及情感协调性的改变。情感性质的改变多为持续较长时间的心境障碍，如情感高涨、欣快、情绪低落、焦虑、恐惧、抑郁。情感稳定性障碍是指情绪反应阈值发生了变化，如情感淡漠、情感麻木、情感脆弱、情感爆发、病理性激情、易激惹性。情感协调性障碍包括情感倒错、情感幼稚、矛盾情感、被强加的情感、病理性心境恶劣。

病态的欣快是一种持续精神愉快的感觉，常见于轻躁狂或躁狂发作，少见于精神分裂症和器质性脑损害，亦可出现于前额叶功能异常、神经梅毒和散发性硬化症以及前脑叶白质切除术后，表现为愚蠢的玩笑及缺乏远见。抑郁是一种悲伤感觉，常与丧失、遭拒、失败或失望等生活事件有关。

此外，护士还应记录表演性情感，即喧嚣而肤浅的情绪表达，这常在为引起注意或关注而夸张感情的个体中出现，见于表演型、自恋型或边缘型人格障碍中。

3. 认知和记忆 精神状况检查中能够评估的认知功能包括：

意识水平；

定向力；

注意力和专注力；

记忆；

知识；

理解力；

概念化和抽象能力。

（1）意识水平：意识程度的改变包括昏迷和昏睡。昏迷是指患者处于一种不能被唤醒的无意识状态。意识程度减轻称为半昏迷或

stupor when the stimulus ceases. In stupor, eye movements become purposeful when the painful stimulus is applied and wincing or miosis may occur, but the patient remains akinetic and mute. When consulting on a comatose or stuporous patient, the important thing is to clear whether a nonorganic cause hypothesized.

Disturbance of consciousness that changes mainly in the content of consciousness includes twilight state, dreamy state and delirium. In twilight or dreamy states, restricted awareness is manifested as disorientation for time and place, with reduced attention and short-term memory. In addition, the client may have the sense of being in a dream. Delirium is a common condition in medical and surgical wards. It is caused by a diffuse cerebral dysfunction of acute or subacute onset, with fluctuant or reversible course. A large amount of illusions and hallucination are characteristic of delirium. Visual hallucinations are more common than auditory hallucinations in delirium, and always horrible or threatening. They are more evident at night and can be provoked by stimulus. Affect is usually labile in delirium, but persistent blunting, anxiety, suspiciousness, hostility, depression, or euphoria may be encountered and is usually congruent with the prevailing illusions or hallucinations. In addition, delirious patients may exhibit wandering attention and concentration, with disconnected or incoherent thought and impaired memory even memory fiction.

(2) Orientation, attention and concentration: Disorders of orientation are most often involved when the sensorium is clouded, as in torpor, obtundation, dreamy state, delirium, or fugue. Orientation is usually lost in the following order: time, place, and then person. Disorientation for time and place usually indicates organic brain disorder. Disorientation for personal identity is rare and always associated with psychogenic or postictal fugue state, other dissociative disorders, and agnosia (loss of the ability to recognize sensory inputs). The psychiatric nurse assesses the client's orientation by asking him or her for the information listed in table 2-1.

Concentration refers to the capacity to maintain attention focused despite distraction. Attention is involved when a client is alerted by a significant stimulus and sustains interest in it. An inattentive patient often ignores the interviewer's question, for example, or soon loses interest in them. The distractible patient is diverted from mental work by incidental sights, sounds, and ideas. Table 2-2 describes simple clinical tests for attention and concentration.

昏睡，患者可被短暂唤醒（如通过疼痛或声音刺激），但当刺激停止后立即又转入昏睡。在昏睡状态下当有疼痛刺激时，眼运动变得有目的性，并有可能出现受刺激部位的回缩或瞳孔缩小，但患者仍保持不动、不语。对一个处于昏迷或昏睡状态的患者，首先应确定其是否为器质性原因造成。

以意识内容变化为主的意识障碍包括朦胧状态、梦样状态和谵妄状态。在朦胧或梦样状态时，患者意识范围缩窄，表现为对时间、地点的定向力障碍，可伴有注意力和短时记忆力降低。另外，患者还可能有一种在梦中的感觉。谵妄状态在内科和外科病房中均常见，由急性或亚急性起病的广泛性脑功能异常引起，病程具有波动性或可逆性。大量错幻觉是谵妄的特征性表现。其中视幻觉较听幻觉更常见，且多是恐怖或具威胁性的。谵妄状态往往昼轻夜重，在患者受到刺激时最易出现。谵妄状态时情感常不稳定，可能出现持久的迟钝、焦虑、多疑、敌对、抑郁或愉快感，且与主要的错觉或幻觉关系密切。此外，谵妄患者可出现游移的注意力和专注力，表现为思维变得不连续或不连贯及记忆力受损，甚至会出现记忆的虚构。

（2）定向力、注意力和专注力：定向障碍最多见于感觉的混浊状态，如麻钝状态、迟钝、梦样状态、谵妄或漫游。定向力受损的顺序为时间、地点、人物。时间和地点定向力障碍提示为器质性脑障碍。人物定向力障碍少见，可见于心因性或发作后漫游症、其他分离性障碍和失认症（感受性认知能力丧失）。护士可通过表2-1所列的信息询问患者，以评估其定向力。

专注力是指在有干扰时保持注意力集中的能力。当患者被刺激所警觉并对其保持兴趣时，则需要专注力的参与。例如，注意力差的患者常不注意访谈者提出的问题，并很快就对问题丧失兴趣，会由于意外的景象、声音和想法而转移注意力。表2-2描述了有关注意力和专注力的简单临床测验。

Table 2-1 Clinical tests of orientation

Time	Place	Person
Hour	Building	Name
Day	City	Address and telephone number
Date	State	Age
Month		Occupation
Year		Marital status

表 2-1 定向力的临床测验

时间	地点	人物
小时	建筑物	姓名
天	城市	地址和电话
日期	州	年龄
月		职业
年		婚姻状况

Table 2-2 Clinical tests of attention and concentration

Examples
● Subtract seven or three serially from 100 ● Reversely speak the days or months of the year ● Spell simple words backward (e.g., world) ● Repeat digits (two, three, four, or more) forward and backward ● Perform mental arithmetic (Interest on 200 CNY at 2% for 18 months?)

表 2-2 注意力和专注力的临床测验

举例
1. 从 100 连续减 7 或 3 2. 倒着说日期或一年中的月份 3. 从后向前拼写简单的单词（如世界） 4. 从前向后和从后向前重复数字（2 个，3 个，4 个或更多） 5. 心算（200 元以 2% 计息存入银行 18 个月，有多少利息？）

(3) Memory: In clinical practice, abnormal memory is manifested as amnesia (memory loss) or dysmnesia (distortion of memory). Psychogenic amnesia occurs in several forms. During and after severe anxiety, memory is likely to be defective.

Organic amnesia occurs in acute, subacute, and chronic forms. After acute head trauma, retrograde amnesia (loss of memory of past events) is likely to occur as a result of a disruption of short-term memory. However, the extent of anterograde amnesia (inability to form new memories) is an index of the severity of brain injury

（3）记忆：异常的记忆在临床上常表现为失忆症（记忆丧失）或记忆障碍（记忆损害）。严重的焦虑发生时或发生后，常出现记忆受损，称为心因性遗忘，可表现为多种形式。

器质性遗忘可为急性、亚急性或慢性。当急性头部外伤后会出现短时记忆受损，表现为逆行性遗忘（对过去事件的遗忘）。而顺行性遗忘（无形成新记忆的能力）的程度是脑损害程度的一个指标。遗忘也可在酒精中

after head trauma. Amnesia also occurs after alcoholism (e.g., blackouts), delirium, or epileptic seizures. Subacute amnesia occurs in Wernicke's encephalopathy, which is caused by thiamine deficiency, and encountered most commonly in alcoholic patients. Table 2-3 lists the clinical tests for immediate, recent, and remote memory.

(4) Information: The client's general knowledge depends on the education and current interest in contemporary affairs. Table 2-4 provides a clinical test of information. Organic disorders are suggested if the client makes 12 or more mistakes (≥60%) on this test. If administration is standardized, the reliability is high. The test is quite useful as an estimate of organic function state, although it does not assess a unitary level of information.

毒（如黑朦）后、谵妄或癫痫发作时出现。亚急性遗忘可见于韦尼克脑病，由硫胺素缺乏引起，最常见于酒精中毒者。表 2–3 列出了对瞬时、近期和远期记忆的临床测验。

（4）知识：患者的知识水平有赖于受教育程度和对事物的兴趣。表 2–4 列出了对知识的临床测验，如果患者在这个测验中错误项达到或超过 12 个（≥ 60%），则提示器质性障碍。如果操作正确的话，它的信度较高。尽管此测验不能评估患者整体的知识水平，但有助于估计其器质性功能状态。

Table 2–3 Clinical tests of memory

Items
Testing immediate recall
● Repeat digits forward and backward (present digits at 1-second intervals. The average adult performance is up to six forward and four backward)
● Repeat three unrelated words (e.g., pear, table, grass) immediately
● Repeat three three-part words (e.g., 25 Park Avenue, brown mahogany table, 18 red roses)
Testing recent memory
● Repeat the three simple phrases after 1, 3, and 5 minutes
● Repeat the three three-part phrases after 1, 3, and 5 minutes
● Recall events in the recent past (e.g., a chronological account of the present illness, the last meal, names of the physicians and nurses who are caring for the patient in the hospital)
● Repeat this sentence: One thing a country must have to become rich and great is adequate supply of wood
● Recount a story with as many details as possible
● The average patient should be able to reproduce half of the separate ideas in this paragraph.
Less adequate performance suggests defective recall of information that requires hierarchical analysis, short-term memory storage, and sequential recall
Testing remote memory
● Recall parents' or children's names, date and place of birth, graduation dates, age and year of marriage, and occupational history

表 2–3 记忆的临床测验

项目
测验瞬时记忆
1. 顺向和逆向重复数字（以 1 秒的间隔读数，一般成年人可顺向重复 6 位、逆向重复 4 位数字）
2. 立即重复 3 个无关的单词（如梨、桌子、草）
3. 重复 3 个由 3 部分组成的复合词组（如公园街 25 号、棕色的红木桌子、18 支红玫瑰）
测验近期记忆
1. 在 1 分钟、3 分钟、5 分钟后重复 3 个简单短语
2. 在 1 分钟、3 分钟、5 分钟后重复 3 个 3 部分构成的短语
3. 回忆最近发生的事件（如目前疾病病程、上次就餐的食物、医院内治疗患者的医生和护士的名字）
4. 重复这个句子：一个国家要变得富裕和强大就一定要有大量、充足的木材供应。
5. 尽可能详细地讲述一段故事：（一般的患者应能够说出一段故事里一半的单独概念，若不够，则提示存在要求层级分析、短时记忆贮存和序列回忆的信息记忆障碍）
测验远期记忆
回忆父母或子女的姓名、出生日期和地点、毕业的日期、结婚的年龄和年份及工作经历

Table 2-4 Clinical test of information

Examples
● Name the last four presidents, starting with the current president
● Name the mayor, state governor, and province governor
● Name four large United States cities
● Discuss four important current events
● Four famous people and why they are famous

表 2-4 知识的临床测验

举例
1. 最近 4 个国家领导人的名字
2. 省、市、区（县）领导人的名字
3. 4 个大城市的名字
4. 讨论当前 4 件重要的事情
5. 4 位著名人物因何而著名

(5) Comprehension: A client's comprehension is evaluated by his or her grasp of the importance of the immediate situation. For example, does the client know why he or she is where he or she is? Does the client understand the purpose of the examination? There are no tests for the client's comprehension. It is evaluated as the interview proceeds.

(6) Conceptualization and abstraction: Level of conceptualization is assessed by testing the client's capacity to discern the similarities and differences between sets of individual words. The client's capacity to abstract is tested by asking the client to discern the meaning of well-known proverbs. The tests listed in table 2-5 have poor reliability and validity. They are affected by intelligence, educational level, culture, as well as age, and have little discriminating power.

（5）理解力：临床上常常通过患者对当前处境的理解来评估其理解力。例如，患者知道自己为什么处于此地吗？患者是否理解检查的目的？临床上没有检测理解力的测验，它常在访谈过程中同时评估。

（6）概念化和抽象化：通过测试患者区分系列独立词之间异同性的能力，可评估其概念化的水平。通过要求患者解释一些众人皆知的谚语的意义，来测验患者的抽象化能力（表 2-5）。但这些测验方法信度和效度差，受智力、受教育水平、文化及年龄的影响，几乎没有鉴别力。

Table 2-5 Clinical tests of conceptualization and abstraction

Examples
1. How are the following pairs similar or alike?
A child and a dwarf
A tree and a bush
A river and a canal
A dishwasher and a stove
2. How are the following pairs different?
A lie and a mistake
Idleness and laziness
Poverty and misery
Character and reputation
3. What is the meaning of the following proverbs? (Ask the client if he or she has heard them before)
"A rolling stone gathers no moss."
"People who live in glass houses should not throw stones."
"Strike while the iron is hot."

表 2-5 概念化和抽象化的临床测验

举例
1. 下列各对词语之间的相似性是什么？ 孩子与侏儒 树与灌木 河流与水渠 洗碗机与暖炉 2. 下列各对词语之间的区别是什么？ 谎言与错误 闲散与懒惰 贫穷与不幸 身份与名誉 3. 下列谚语的意义是什么？（首先应询问患者以前是否听过） “滚石不生苔，转业不聚财” “己所不欲，勿施于人” “趁热打铁”

4. Language Language competence is assessed from the client's speech during the psychiatric interview. Any history of spoken or written language difficulty, or any observation of clumsy articulation, disordered rhythm, and difficulty in the understanding or choice of words, should be noted and identified further. The psychiatric nurse may ask the client to perform a series of actions in an arbitrary sequence to test language comprehension. Language expression can be evaluated by asking the client to repeat words, phrases, and sentences and to name a number of objects. Expression and comprehension are evaluated by asking the client to read a passage aloud and to answer several related questions about it, or asking the client to take dictation tests. Any errors and slowness in performance should be noted.

5. Perceptions Perception is the integration and reflection of different sensory stimuli, of which the process is influenced by past experience. Perception may be increased or decreased in intensity.

An illusion is sensory stimulation given an incorrect interpretation, that is, a false perception. Illusions are most likely to occur when the mind is under the sway of intensive emotion, when sensory clarity is reduced, or when both sets of circumstances are operating.

A hallucination is a visional perception without a sensory stimulus that occurs in the waking state. It is not merely a sensory distortion or misinterpretation, and it carries a subjective sense of conviction. A genuine hallucination appears to the subject to be substantial and to occur in external objective space. In contrast, a mental image is insubstantial and experienced within internal subjective space, called pseudo

4. 语言 护士在访谈过程中，通过与患者的交谈来评估其语言能力，应记录患者任何口头或书面语言障碍、发音笨拙、节律错误及理解或词语选择困难的病史，并进一步明确。访谈者可随意要求患者做一系列动作检测其语言理解力。通过让患者重复词组、短语和句子，并对物体正确命名来评估其语言表达力。亦可通过让患者朗读短文，并回答相关问题来评估其表达和理解能力。让患者听写来检测其描绘语言的能力。

5. 知觉 知觉是对不同感觉刺激进行整合而在人脑中的反映，这个过程常受既往经验的影响。知觉的强度可出现增高或降低。

错觉是对感觉刺激给予了错误的解释，是一种错误的知觉。错觉最常发生于思维受强烈情感支配、感觉清晰度降低的情况下，或以上两种情况共存时。

幻觉是在觉醒状态时，没有感觉刺激的情况下产生的虚幻知觉，它不仅是对感觉的歪曲或误解，还有判定的主观感觉。真性幻觉对患者来说是真实的，产生于外部客观世界。相反，头脑中的表象是不真实的，产生于主观世界，叫假性幻觉。幻觉可为听觉的、视觉的、嗅觉的或味觉的、触觉的或躯体化

hallucination. Hallucinations can be auditory, visual, olfactory or gustatory, tactile, or somatic, and auditory hallucination is the most common. In form, they may be amorphous, elementary, or complex. Hallucinations may be unsystematic, appearing no association with life circumstances, or systematized, related to delusions.

的，其中幻听是临床上最常见的幻觉。在形式方面，可能是无定型的、原始的或复杂的。幻觉可能表现为非系统的，看起来与生活环境没有关系；或者系统化的，并与妄想形成有关。

6. Thought Thought is the reflection of the human brain to indirect generalization of objective things. Pathology of thought may be found in the process, in the form, or in the content of thinking. The process and form of thinking may be disordered in terms of tempo, fluency (including continuity and control), logical organization, and intent.

6. 思维 思维是人脑对客观事物间接概括的反映。思维异常可表现为思维过程、思维形式和思维内容的异常。思维过程和形式可出现速度、流畅性（包括连续性和可控制性）、逻辑组织和意图方面的异常。

(1) Abnormalities of thought process and form

（1）思维过程和形式障碍

1) Tempo: The tempo of thinking is accelerated in flight of thought, which may reach such a pitch that goal direction is lost and the connection between ideas is governed not by meaning but by clang association, idiosyncratic verbal or conceptual associations. Flight of thought is the characteristic of mania, but it may also occur in excited schizophrenic patients. The tempo of thinking may be slowed in retardation of thought, especially in unipolar depression. In the extreme, retardation of thought becomes mutism or even stupor.

1）速度：思维奔逸是指思维速度加快，严重时可出现思维没有目的性，其内容之间不是根据意义连接，而是表现为音联、特殊的词语或概念间的联系。思维奔逸是躁狂的特征性表现，也可见于兴奋状态的精神分裂症患者。思维迟缓是指思维速度减慢，多见于单相抑郁症。思维迟缓严重时可出现缄默甚至木僵。

2) Fluency: In circumstantiality, although the goal direction of thinking is retained, associations meander into fruitless, overly detailed, or barely relevant byways. Circumstantiality is said to be characteristic of pedantry and perseveration happened in some epileptic patients, so called viscous quality.

2）流畅性：病理性赘述患者的思维尽管不离题，但抓不住主要问题，不厌其烦地作不必要的细节描述。病理性赘述是癫痫所致精神障碍的特征性表现，有迂腐、持续症等特点，也将这种思维称为有黏滞性。

3) Continuity: In thought blocking, the client's speech is interrupted abruptly by silences that last for from one second to several minutes. During the pause, the client often blinks his or her eyes, and sometimes the client's mind becomes blank. The client recommences on an apparently different track. Blocking is almost pathognomonic of schizophrenia but must be differentiated from the absentia of petit mal epilepsy, hesitancy of anxiety and the hesitation mental fixity of amphetamine intoxication.

3）连续性：思维中断的患者在谈话中可突然出现停顿，持续时间从1秒到数分钟不等。在停顿期间患者通常不停地眨眼，有时患者在这时感到头脑一片空白。患者在思维中断后开始谈论另一明显不同的话题。思维中断几乎可成为精神分裂症的诊断标志，但必须将它与癫痫小发作的失神、焦虑引起的迟疑及安非他明中毒的暂停性精神固定区别开。

4) Control: Akin to the subjective phenomena described in the previous section is the client's sense that speed, direction, forming, or content of thought are out of control. Complaints such as "confused" "racing thoughts" "unable to concentrate" "scatterbrained", and "doing crazy" often reflect the subjective perception of pathologically accelerated, dysfluent, or discontinuous thinking.

4）控制性：前面所述症状的共同特点是患者感到思维速度、方向、形式或内容难以控制，诸如"混乱""思维赛跑""杂乱""注意力不集中"及"变疯了"等主诉反映出有思维异常加速、不流畅或不连续的主观感觉。

5) Logical organization: Psychotic thinking may reflect disorders in thinking form or logic. Commonly

5）逻辑组织：精神病性的思维可反映出患者有思维形式或思维逻辑方面的障碍。

the schizophrenic patient uses a private logic, with over personalized concrete symbols. Within this logical framework, conceptual boundaries are blurred, and the thinking patterns are metaphorical and idiosyncratic, almost as if they emerged directly from a dreamy state.

精神分裂症患者常使用具有个体化具体象征的逻辑，这种逻辑形式使得概念界限模糊，思维形式隐喻且奇异，甚至似乎来自于梦样状态。

6) Intent of communication: The conventional purpose of discourse is to communicate, but the psychiatrist and nurse may be misled by the intentions of a schizophrenic patient. The schizophrenic patient may subtly converse in an obscure, remote, supercilious, attacking, ironic, or farcical manner to attempt to remain private or to deride the clinician.

6）交谈的意图：一般说来，谈话的目的是为了交流，但临床医务人员可能被精神分裂症患者的意图误导。精神分裂症患者有时为了保留隐私或嘲弄临床医生和护士而巧妙地采用模糊的、疏远的、傲慢的、攻击性的、讽刺的或开玩笑的方式进行谈话。

(2) Abnormalities of thought content

（2）思维内容的异常

1) Abnormal belief: A delusion is a false belief that is not susceptible to argument and that is inconsistent with the subject's sociocultural background. Bordering on delusion is the overvalued idea, a notion that may be eccentric rather than false but that becomes a governing force in the client's life. As for the content of delusions, the commonest is of persecution, jealousy, being loved, grandiosity, disease, poverty, and guile.

1）异常的信念：妄想是指不易被说服，与本人社会文化背景不相符的错误观念。超价观念位于妄想的边缘，是一种怪癖的、非错误的观念，但它是患者生活的主导力量。妄想常见的内容有迫害、嫉妒、钟情、夸大、疾病、贫穷和欺骗等。

2) Abnormal preoccupations and impulses: An obsession is a persistent idea, desire, image, phrase, or fragment of music that cuts into the stream of conscious thinking. The client recognizes the alien nature of the obsession and attempts to resist it in vain. The obsession often presses the subject to perform compulsive acts to relieve anxiety. Impulsions tend to occur in externalizing personalities, whereas compulsions are more typical of introverted and constricted persons. Impulsive acts often spring from an emotional setting of anger, anxiety, frustration, rejection, sadness, or humiliation, particularly when the subject is excited by alcohol.

2）异常的先占观念和冲动：强迫观念是指插入意识思维流中持续的想法、意愿、表象、短语或音乐片段。患者能意识到强迫观念的外来性质，并徒劳地努力抵制。强迫观念常迫使患者采取强迫行为以减轻焦虑。冲动易发生于外向人格，而强迫在内向、退缩的人格中较常见。冲动行为常发生于生气、焦虑、受挫、被拒、痛苦或蒙羞等情绪状态，尤其是当患者受酒精作用而兴奋时。

3) Abnormal self-sensation: The normal person has a sense of selfhood composed of the following elements: a sense of existing and being involved in one's own body and behavior; a sense of personal continuity in time between past, present, and future; a sense of personal integrity; and a sense of distinction between self and outside world. In psychiatric disorders, any or several of these phenomena may be disturbed. For example, the individual may feel uninvolved in his or her own body or actions, like a spectator looking at another person.

3）自我感觉的异常：正常人对自身的感觉由以下成分组成：①存在并属于自己的身体和行为的感觉；②过去、现在和将来个人连续性的感觉；③个人完整的感觉；④自身与外界有区别的感觉。精神障碍可出现这些自我感觉中的某个或数个异常。例如，人格解体患者可能感到与自己的身体或行为无关，就像一个旁观者看另外一个人一样。

7. Intelligence Intelligence is a complex and comprehensive function of mental activity, reflects the individual differences in cognition, refers to the capability to solve new problems and form new concept using previous knowledge and experience. Disturbance of intelligence can be classified with mental retardation and dementia.

7. 智能 智能是一种复杂的综合的精神活动的功能，反映的是个体在认识活动方面的差异，是指利用既往获得的知识、经验来解决新问题、形成新概念的能力。智能障碍可分为精神发育迟滞和痴呆两大类型。

(1) Mental retardation: It refers to brain dysplasia or blocked before the individual grows mature (less than 18 years old), and then the intellectual development stays at a certain stage. The intelligence level is significantly lower than the normal peers with age, and often accompanied by social dysfunction.

（1）精神发育迟滞：是指个体生长发育成熟以前（18 岁以前），大脑的发育不良或受阻，智能发育停留在一定的阶段。随着年龄增长其智能明显低于正常的同龄人智力水平；由于智力发育受阻，患者往往还伴有社会功能障碍。

(2) Dementia: It refers to a syndrome that the acquired intelligence, memory and personality are damaged due to organic lesion, without disturbance of consciousness. In clinical, the manifestations for loss of acquired knowledge and declined learning ability, or even functional dependence, come with other psychiatric symptoms, such as apathy, childish behaviors, enhanced instinctive intention, and so forth. It occurs in Alzheimer's disease and dementia paralytica. Pseudo dementia may occur after a strong mental trauma, of which the clinical manifestation is similar to dementia without organic damage of brain tissue.

（2）痴呆：是指个体由于器质性病变，虽没有意识障碍，但后天获得的智能、记忆和人格全面受损的一种综合征。临床表现为后天获得的知识丧失，工作和学习能力下降或丧失，甚至生活不能自理，并伴有其他精神症状，如情感淡漠、行为幼稚及本能意向亢进等。它可见于阿尔茨海默病和麻痹性痴呆。临床上，强烈的精神创伤后也可见一种类似于痴呆的表现，而大脑组织结构无任何器质性损害，称之为假性痴呆。

8. Insight and Judgment

8. 自知力和判断力

(1) Insight: Insight refers to the client's attitude and judgement of their own psychiatric illness. It has three aspects: understanding of disease, symptoms and treatment. For disease aspect, it means to recognize the psychiatric disease; for symptom aspect, that is, the behavior of lesions and various abnormal experiences can be correctly identified and described, and the client recognizes that the symptoms are the manifestations of the disease; for treatment aspect, the client has active desire or acceptance to the treatment, namely the treatment compliance. Insight is an indispensable index for clinical diagnosis, differential diagnosis, effect prediction, and judging prognosis. The hypomanic patients feel very well, and the schizophrenic patients do not recognize their disease and abnormal behaviors and thus refuse to treat.

（1）自知力：是指患者对自己精神疾病的态度和判断力。自知力包括三方面：对疾病的认识，即承认有病；对症状的认识，即对病变的行为表现以及各种不正常体验能正确分辨和描述，认识到它们是疾病的表现；对治疗的认识，即存在治疗依从性，有主动接受治疗的愿望或者服从治疗。自知力是临床上进行诊断、鉴别诊断、预测疗效、判断预后的一个必不可少的重要指标。轻躁狂患者常自我感觉很好，而精神分裂症患者多不承认自己有不正常的行为，更不认为自己有病，因而拒绝治疗。

(2) Judgment: The psychiatric nurse can ask the client one of the following questions to test judgment. What would you do if you found a stamped and addressed envelope in the street? Why are there laws? Why should promises be kept? Good judgment requires intact orientation, concentration, and memory.

（2）判断力：精神科护士可通过询问以下问题来检测患者的判断力：如果你在街上拣到一个贴了邮票、写了地址的信封，你怎么办？为什么有法律？为什么应遵守诺言？良好的判断力要求有定向力、专注力及记忆力的完整。

Mental status examination is always by means of interview. The purpose of the psychiatric interview is to obtain information from the client about the presenting problem and its precipitation, biopsychosocial strengths and limitations, reason for the current presentation, insight, and desire for help. Mastering the information of

精神状况检查常是通过访谈的方式实现，访谈的目的是获得患者目前的问题及其原因，了解患者的自知力和寻求帮助的愿望等方面的信息。对患者这些信息掌握，有助于精神科护士进行判断，并监测患者症状的改

the patient helps psychiatric nurses judge and monitor the patient's symptoms. A psychiatric interview may last about 50 minutes, which is long enough for a rapid survey but not so long as to exhaust the client. A concluding summary of the material points of the interview can be very helpful. It allows the client to correct or modify misinterpretations and leads naturally into the nurse's plan for what happens next-another interview.

vi. Social Dimension

The assessment of the social aspects of the client will help the nurse anticipate how the client may get along with other clients in a social setting, and also will allow the nurse to plan for any anticipated difficulties. The social assessment includes functional status, social systems, spiritual assessment, family assessment, community and support resources, and occupational and economic status.

1. Functional Status It is necessary and important for the psychiatric nurse to assess how the client functions in a social setting whether it is with family or in the community. How the client copes with strangers and those that cause problems is also important information.

2. Social Systems The social systems to be examined include the family, culture to which the client belongs, and the community in which he or she lives. Culture can profoundly affect a client's worldview. During cultural assessment, the nurse should keep in mind that the culture aspects may be a part of the current mental disorder. In addition, the nurse needs to assess what community resources are connected with the client and what the pattern of usage is.

3. Spiritual Assessment Spirituality is defined as "the unifying force of a person; the essence of being that shapes, gives meaning to, and is aware of one's self-becoming. Spirituality permeates all of life and is manifested in one's being, knowing, and doing. It is expressed and experienced uniquely by each individual through and within connection to life force, the environment, nature, other people, and self". Nurses must clear about their own spirituality to be sure it does not interfere with assessment to the client's.

4. Occupational Status The nurse should document the occupation that the client is now in as well as his or her previous job. If the client has changed jobs frequently, ask about the reasons. If the client has the problems of inability to focus on the job or get along with others, the nurse needs to explore them further.

5. Economic Status Finances are a private matter to many people, so questions about economic status must be asked carefully. What the nurse needs to ascertain is whether or not the client feels stressed by

变。一次精神状况检查约需50分钟，这一时间足以进行快速的筛查而又不至于使患者疲劳。护士在访谈过程中有必要对资料进行总结，这能使患者改正或修订错误的陈述，并能自然地进入访谈计划的下一步。

（六）社会评估

对患者进行社会方面的评估，有助于护士制订护理计划并防范患者潜在的健康问题。社会评估主要包括对患者社会功能状况、社会系统、精神信仰、家庭状况、社区及支持资源、职业和经济状况等方面资料的收集和评价。

1. 社会功能状况 精神科护士应全面评估患者在家庭或社区等环境中的社会功能状况，如患者在社会环境中如何与人相处，如何应对面临的困难等。

2. 社会系统 主要包括对患者的文化、家庭及所居住社区的评估。人的世界观会深受其文化的影响，在对患者的文化进行评估时，护士应始终认识到患者所拥有的文化可能正是其目前精神障碍的一部分。此外，护士还应评估与患者有关的社区资源以及患者使用这些资源的方式。

3. 精神信仰 人的精神信仰渗透着人生活的全部，而人的本质、思想及行为又可反映其所拥有的精神信仰。它可以通过每个人生存的动力、生存的环境、自然、周围人群和自我而体现。每一个护士都必须明确自己的精神信仰，并确保在对患者进行评估时不会受自己精神信仰的影响。

4. 职业状况 护士应询问和记录有关患者目前及从前的职业状况，若患者频繁更换工作，应进一步询问原因；若患者存在工作能力问题或与同事相处的问题，亦应做进一步评估。

5. 经济状况 对于很多人来说，其经济状况属于个人隐私，因此，护士在询问患者的经济状况时应小心谨慎。护士应着重评估

finances or whether there is enough for basic needs, rather than specific money amounts.

患者是否因为经济而感到压力或其经济收入是否满足基本需要，避免询问患者的具体收入情况。

During the assessment, the information must be included in the client's written or computerized record. This may take on several different formats. Examples are forms, checklists, and problem-oriented notes. Whatever the formats, the psychiatric and mental health nurse must be careful to describe behavior exhibited rather than interpret or judge. They must provide a brief, concise, and clear picture of the individual's symptoms, behaviors, strengths and weakness, improvements, and concerns. In either case, the standard of practice is to complete a psychiatric mental health nursing assessment and generate nursing diagnoses, identify outcomes, and plan interventions from the assessment data.

在评估过程中，精神科护士可通过应用表格、问题记录等形式对患者的资料进行收集（精神科护理评估表）。无论应用何种格式，护士应仔细和认真记录患者的行为表现，而不应对其妄加评价。护士应提供一份简明、扼要、清晰的有关患者症状、行为、优势和缺点、进步及顾虑等全面的资料，从而明确，鉴别护理结果，提出有效的护理干预措施。

Section 3 Nursing Diagnosis

第三节　护理诊断

In the second step of nursing process, data gathered during the assessment will be analyzed. Once the nurse completes an assessment of the client, appropriate nursing diagnoses are chosen. The assessment data guide the nurse in choosing nursing diagnoses. A nursing diagnosis provides the basis for selection of nursing interventions chosen to achieve outcomes for which the nurse is accountable.

根据收集到的资料作出护理诊断是护理程序的第二步。当护士全面收集了有关患者的资料，并加以综合整理、分析后，应根据患者的问题作出护理诊断。全面而准确的评估资料能够指导精神科护士作出恰当的护理诊断，而每一个护理诊断又是精神科护士选择有效的护理措施、达到预期护理目标的基础。

I. Definition of Nursing Diagnosis

一、护理诊断的概念

The nursing diagnosis is a statement of an existing problem or a potential health problem that a nurse is both competent and licensed to treat. The North American Nursing Diagnosis Association (NANDA) defines a nursing diagnosis as a clinical judgment about individual, family, or community responses to actual or potential health problems/life processes. This clinical judgment is derived through a deliberate, systematic process of data collection and analysis. The basis for providing psychiatric and mental health nursing care is the recognition and identification of patterns of response to actual or potential psychiatric illnesses and mental health problems.

护理诊断是对需要护士处理的患者现存或潜在的健康问题的阐述。目前使用的护理诊断的定义是北美护理诊断协会（NANDA）提出并通过的。护理诊断是关于个人、家庭或社区对现存的或潜在的健康问题和/或生命过程的反应的一种临床判断，这种临床判断来源于护士对患者细致而系统的资料收集和分析。而对于精神科护士来说，为患者提供有效精神护理的基础是认识和明确患者现存或潜在的对精神疾病和精神健康问题的反应。

II. Nursing Diagnosis in Psychiatric and Mental Health Nursing

二、精神科护理中常用的护理诊断

According to NANDA, a nursing diagnostic statement ideally consists of three parts: a. health problem; b. etiological or contributing factors; c. defining characteristics. The health problem identifies the behavioral disruption or threatened disruption that can be improved through nursing intervention. The etiological factors identify stressors that contribute to the problem. The defining characteristics describe the signs and symptoms that related to the identified health problem. All three components are important in formulating a nursing diagnosis. The defining characteristics are particularly helpful because they reflect the objective and subjective behaviors that is the target of nursing intervention. They also provide specific indicators for evaluation the outcomes of nursing interventions and for determining whether the expected goals of the nursing care were met.

根据 NANDA 的定义，一个完整的护理诊断应由三部分组成，即健康问题、病因或相关因素、诊断依据。健康问题是指通过护理干预可以解决和改变的问题。病因是指引起健康问题的相关或危险因素。诊断依据是指与患者健康问题相关的症状和体征，诊断依据有助于护士选择有效护理干预措施，并为评价护理干预效果、判断是否达到护理目标提供标准。

The NANDA diagnostic system is organized around nine human response patterns: exchanging, communication, relating, valuing, choosing, moving, perceiving, knowing, and feeling, whereas the psychiatric and mental health nursing diagnostic system is organized around eight human response processes: activity, cognition, ecological, emotional, interpersonal, perception, physiologic, and valuation. Indeed, the American Nurses Association Task Force continues to work on the development of a single classification system that will incorporate psychiatric nursing diagnoses. Table 2-6 lists nursing diagnoses commonly seen in the psychiatric clinical setting.

NANDA 的护理诊断系统是围绕着人的 9 种反应形态作为其概念框架的，即交换、沟通、关系、价值、选择、移动、感知、认识和感觉。而精神科护理诊断则主要是围绕人的 8 种反应形态组织的，即行动、认知、生态、情绪、人际、感知、生理及评价。事实上，美国护理学会专门工作组一直致力于发展一套适用于精神科患者的护理诊断系统，表 2-6 列出了精神科常用的护理诊断。

Table 2-6　Nursing diagnoses in psychiatric and mental health nursing

No.	Nursing Diagnoses	No.	Nursing Diagnoses
1	Acute Confusion	12	Fear
2	Grieving	13	Feeding Self-Care Deficit
3	Anxiety	14	Hopelessness
4	Decisional Conflict	15	Imbalanced Nutrition: Less Than Body Requirements
5	Bathing/Hygiene Self-Care Deficit	16	Risk for Compromised Human Dignity
6	Deficient Diversional Activity	17	Impaired Memory
7	Delayed Growth and Development	18	Impaired Parenting
8	Disturbed Body Image	19	Impaired Social Interaction
9	Disturbed Sleep Pattern	20	Impaired Verbal Communication
10	Dressing/Grooming Self-Care Deficit	21	Ineffective Coping
11	Complicated Grieving	22	Ineffective Health Maintenance

continued

No.	Nursing Diagnoses	No.	Nursing Diagnoses
23	Ineffective Sexuality Patterns	30	Risk for Loneliness
24	Interrupted Family Processes	31	Risk for Other-Directed Violence
25	Noncompliance	32	Risk for Self-Directed Violence
26	Post Trauma Syndrome	33	Social Isolation
27	Powerlessness	34	Spiritual Distress
28	Relocation Stress Syndrome	35	Toileting Self-Care Deficit
29	Risk for Injury		

表 2-6　精神科常用护理诊断

序号	护理诊断	序号	护理诊断
1	急性意识障碍	19	社会交往障碍
2	悲伤	20	语言沟通障碍
3	焦虑	21	应对无效
4	抉择冲突	22	健康维护能力低下
5	沐浴 / 卫生自理缺陷	23	性生活型态无效
6	缺乏娱乐活动	24	家庭运作过程改变
7	生长发展迟缓	25	不依从行为
8	体像紊乱	26	创伤后综合征
9	睡眠型态紊乱	27	无能为力感
10	穿着 / 卫生自理缺陷	28	迁移应激综合征
11	复杂性悲伤	29	有受伤害的危险
12	恐惧	30	有孤独的危险
13	进食自理缺陷	31	有对他人施行暴力的危险
14	无望感	32	有对自己施行暴力的危险
15	营养失调：低于机体需要量	33	社交孤立
16	有个人尊严受损的危险	34	精神困扰
17	记忆功能障碍	35	如厕自理缺陷
18	养育功能障碍		

Psychiatric nurses must continue to define and describe what they do in the psychiatric setting, and this requires the use of nursing diagnoses. Nursing diagnoses pinpoint what exactly it is that nurses treat. The priorities of nursing diagnoses are according to their life-threatening potential. Maslow's hierarchy of needs is also a good model to follow in prioritizing nursing diagnoses.

精神科护士应根据对患者资料的分析和评价，确定患者的护理诊断，并以此制订相应的护理措施。如一个患者有多个护理诊断，需按其重要性和紧迫性排出主次顺序，即把威胁患者生命的问题放在首位。亦可根据马斯洛人类基本需要层次理论为依据进行排列，将与最基本的生理需要有关的问题放在首位。

III. Deriving Nursing Diagnosis

When defining nursing diagnoses for a particular client, the nurse refers to signs and symptoms of client found during the assessment phase. It is these defining characteristics, the clues given by the signs and symptoms, which join together in the nurse's mind to form a cluster. The cluster of these characteristics leads the nurse to choose certain diagnoses over others. For example, when taking an assessment, the nurse notices that the client's responses are often self-negating and that there is an indecisiveness and lack of problem-solving ability. These defining characteristics that the nurse notices during the assessment combine with the nurse's thought process and the nurse knows that the nursing diagnosis Self-esteem disturbance is appropriate. However, the nurse also turns to related factors to further support the nursing diagnosis.

Besides defining characteristics, related factors help the nurse establish a nursing diagnosis. Related factors are those factors that have influenced the health status change. The related factors may be grouped into four categories: biologic or psychological, which are called pathophysiologic; maturational; social, which are called situational; and treatment related. To continue the assessment example above, the nurse hears the client stating the loss of three jobs within the last year and the related financial problems. These situational-related factors further strengthen the nursing diagnosis of self-esteem disturbance.

The use of nursing diagnosis affords a degree of autonomy that historically has been lacking in the practice of nursing. Nursing diagnosis describes the client's condition, facilitating the prescription of interventions and establishment of parameters for outcome criteria based upon what is uniquely nursing.

三、护理诊断的形成

在对某一患者进行护理诊断时，其症状和体征为护士提供了有效的线索。因此，护士应特别留意在评估过程中患者存在的症状和体征。例如，护士在对患者进行评估时注意到患者常存在自我否定的反应，或常常犹豫不决及缺乏处理问题的能力。这些在评估过程中所发现的患者的特征再加上护士的思考，最终可以得出患者存在“自尊紊乱”这一护理诊断，而护士还需找出相关因素来支持这一护理诊断。

除了患者现有的症状和体征可以作为诊断依据外，相关因素也有助于护士作出护理诊断。相关因素是指影响患者健康状况改变的因素，可以分为4种，即病理生理因素、成熟因素、社会因素和治疗相关性因素。以“自尊紊乱”这一护理诊断为例，相关因素为患者在一年内丢掉了3份工作及存在经济问题，这些社会因素进一步支持了患者自尊紊乱这一护理诊断。

护理诊断的应用为护理工作提供了专业自主性，是具有护理专业特色的一步。护理诊断描述了患者的状态，有助于护士制订有效的护理措施和预期的护理干预结果，从而为患者提供全身心的护理。

Section 4 Nursing Care Plan

The third phase of the nursing process is the development of nursing care plan to guide therapeutic intervention and achieve expected outcomes. The plan of care is to identify expected outcomes, effective interventions and priorities of care. These written plans aid in the continuity of care for the client and are points of information for all members of the health team.

第四节　护理计划

制订护理计划是护理程序的第三步。护理计划是对患者预期的目标，护士所要采取的护理措施的一种书面说明。这种书面护理计划有助于为患者提供连续的护理，并为所有医护人员提供患者的情况。

I. Setting Nursing Objectives

Within the context of providing nursing care, the ultimate goal is to influence outcomes and improve the client's health status. Expected outcomes serve as a record of change in the client's health status. They are client-oriented goals that must be measurable and attainment estimated in a certain time. They are derived from the diagnosis and the client's present and potential capabilities. When possible, the nurse, client, significant others, and multidisciplinary team members formulate the outcomes. As for psychiatric patients, they always cannot participate in the nursing care plan identification. Also, because the formulation of outcomes involves the client, it is important that the nurse and multidisciplinary team members understand the problems identified by the client and the outcomes the client hopes to achieve.

The client's outcomes are both short term and long term. They should be clearly stated by the nurse and should describe the expected result of care. Outcomes are the consequences of a treatment or an intervention. An example of a stated outcome for the nursing diagnosis of Risk of Injury is the following:

Risk for injury: related to extreme agitation and constant, uncontrollable motor activity as evidenced by less than 2-hours rest a night, severe skin turgor, and abrasions on hands and arms.

Possible long-term outcomes include: (a) the client will be sleeping 6 to 8 hours per night by the time of discharge; (b) the client will willingly maintain an adequate diet and fluids by the time of discharge; (c) the client will be free from infections and abrasions; (d) the client will adhere to medication regimen. The short-term goals might include: (a) the client will sleep 3 to 4 hours per night within 2 days with the aid of medication; (b) The client will drink 1500 to 2000 ml of fluid per day with the aid of nursing intervention; (c) the client's skin turgor will be within normal limits within 24 hours.

It is important for psychiatric nurses to realize that expected outcomes can be classified into three domains: cognitive, affective, and psychomotor. Table 2-7 shows the content, an example, and representative verbs of each domain.

II. Setting Nursing Interventions

Each stated goal should include nursing interventions, which are instructions for all people working with the client. A care plan is used to guide therapeutic intervention systematically and achieve the

一、制订护理目标

护理目标是指通过护理干预，护士期望患者达到的健康状态或行为。目标的主语应该是患者，并且是可以测量的，是患者在一段时间内所需要达到的程度。护理目标来源于患者的护理诊断并与患者现有或潜在的能力有关。护理目标一般是由护士、患者、患者亲属以及其他医护人员共同制订的，但对于精神障碍的患者来讲，患者本人往往无法参与护理计划的制订。由于护理目标是期望患者发生改变，医护人员尤应注意患者自己确认的问题和期望达到的结果。

护理目标可以分为长期目标和短期目标，用以描述期望患者达到的结果，即治疗或干预的效果。下面以“受伤的危险”这一护理诊断为例来陈述护理目标。如受伤的危险　与患者极度兴奋及持续的、无法自我控制的机体运动有关。诊断依据包括：① 每晚睡眠少于 2 小时；② 皮肤严重肿胀；③ 手及手臂皮肤破溃。

可能的长期目标包括：① 患者在出院前能够每晚睡眠 6～8 小时；② 患者在出院前能够摄入足够的食物和水分；③ 患者没有皮肤感染和破溃；④ 患者能够遵医嘱用药。短期目标则可能包括：① 患者在 2 天内能够在药物的帮助下每晚睡眠 3～4 小时；② 患者能够在护理干预下，每天饮水 1 500～2 000 ml；③ 患者的皮肤肿胀能够在 24 小时内恢复正常。

精神科护士应认识到，患者的预期护理结果一般包括三个方面，即认知方面、情感方面和精神运动方面。上述三方面的内容、举例和常用来描述的行为动词如表 2-7 所示。

二、制订护理措施

护理措施是护士为帮助患者达到预定目标所采取的具体活动，指导所有护士为患者提供服务。护理干预措施应针对护理目标制

Table 2-7 Three domains of expected outcomes

Domain	Example	Representative Verbs
Cognitive		
Outcomes associated with acquired knowledge or intellectual abilities	Learning the signs and symptoms of depression	Define, list, describe, discuss, explain, identify, apply, analyze, compare, contrast, examine, construct, create, design, organize, plan, assess, critique, evaluate
Affective		
Outcomes associated with changes in attitude, values, or beliefs	Describing that previous eating habits needed to be changed	Accept, realize, recognize, comply, observe, accept, believe, defend, prefer, seek, value, display, judge, weigh, express, share, internalize
Psychomotor		
Outcomes associated with development motor skills	Completing self-care activities	Place, position, prepare, imitate, inject, repeat, build, set up, coordinate, operate, change, develop, supply, construct, design, produce, demonstrate, practice, perform, administer, give

表 2-7 预期护理结果的三方面内容

项目	举例	行为动词
认知		
与所获得的知识或智力有关的结果	患者能够学习抑郁的症状和体征	定义、列出、描述、讨论、解释、确定、应用、分析、比较、对比、检测、构成、引起、设计、组织、计划、评估、批判、评价
情感		
与态度、价值或信念改变有关的结果	患者能够描述以前需要改变的进餐习惯	接受、认识、承认、遵从、观察、同意、相信、防护、更喜欢、寻求、重视、展现、判断、斟酌、表达、分享、使内在化
精神运动		
与发展运动技巧相关的结果	患者能够完成自我护理活动	放置、安置、准备、模仿、注射、重复、建造、树立、合作、操作、改变、发展、提供、创立、设计、生产、证实、实践、履行、执行、给予

expected outcomes. It is individualized to the client's mental health problems, condition, or needs and is developed in collaboration with the client, significant others, and other health professionals. If possible, for each diagnosis identified, the most appropriate interventions, based on current psychiatric and mental health nursing practice and research, are selected. Client education and necessary referrals are included.

Nursing interventions planned for meeting a specific goal need to be (a) safe: they must be safe for the client as well as for other clients, family, and staff; (b)appropriate: they must be compatible with other therapies, the client's personal goals, cultural values, as well as institutional rules; (c) effective: they should be based on scientific principles; (d) individualized: they should be realistic:

订，制订应个体化，围绕患者的精神健康问题、机体状况或需要，并与患者、患者亲属及其他医务人员共同做出决策。精神科护士在选择护理措施时，应以精神护理实践及科研为指导，并注意包括患者教育及必要的治疗安排。

为了达到护理目标，护理措施的选择应注意以下几点：① 安全。护理措施必须是对患者自身、患者的病友、患者家庭以及医务人员均安全的。② 适当。护理措施必须与其他治疗协调一致，符合患者的个人目标、文化价值及规章制度。③ 有效。护理措施的选

written within the client's age, physical strength, condition, and willingness to change; based on the number and capabilities of staff available; reflective of actual available community resources.

Prioritization of nursing care is determined by considering the urgency or seriousness of the problem or need and its impact on the client. Is there a threat to the client's life, dignity, or integrity? Are there problems or needs that negatively affect the client? Do problems that affect normal growth and development exist? Moreover, Maslow's hierarchy of needs usually is the guide for problem solving during the formulation of a care plan. For instance, the needs such as hunger and safety take precedence over self-esteem and self-actualization.

III. General Principles of Writing Care Plans

It is very important for nurses to remember the following principles when writing care plans:

- Individualize or personalize the plan of care according to the nursing diagnosis.
- State short-and long-term goals.
- Use simple, understandable language to communicate information about the client's care.
- Be specific when stating nursing interventions.
- Prioritize nursing care according to the urgency or seriousness of the problem.
- Indicate the responsible party for each nursing intervention.

Interventions selected during the planning stage are executed, taking into considerations of the nurse's ability of clinical practice, education, and certification. The care plan serves as a blueprint for delivery of safe, ethical, and appropriate interventions.

Section 5 Nursing Implementation

During the implementing phase, the psychiatric and mental health nurse uses a wide range of interventions designed to prevent mental and physical illness and promote, maintain, and restore mental and physical health. The nurses select interventions according to their level of practice.

择应建立在科学的基础上。④ 个体化。应根据现实情况，护理措施要符合患者的年龄、体力、病情及对自己健康的期望等；同时也要考虑护士的数量、能力，以及可能获得的社区资源等。

护理措施排序时应根据患者问题的轻重缓急，并考虑到其是否威胁患者的生命或尊严、是否对患者有消极影响、是否影响患者的生长与发展等。此外，亦可以根据马斯洛人类基本需要层次理论为指导来执行护理计划，如患者的饮食、安全等需要的满足应优先于自尊和自我实现需要的满足。

三、书写护理计划的原则

在书写护理计划时，护士应注意以下原则：

① 强调个体化，应根据患者的护理诊断制订护理措施。

② 陈述长期和短期护理目标。

③ 尽量使用简单、易懂的语言描述对患者的护理措施。

④ 描述护理措施时应具体和明确。

⑤ 应根据患者问题的迫切程度来排列护理措施。

⑥ 应明确每一项护理措施应由谁来负责完成。

完善的护理计划保证了安全、合乎伦理并适当地为患者实施护理措施，护士应根据自己的临床实践能力及教育水平选择护理措施，以达到期望的护理目标，恢复和促进患者的身心健康。

第五节　护理实施

在护理程序的实施阶段，精神科护士对患者进行护理措施的干预，以实现预期护理目标，促进、保持和恢复患者的身心健康。

I. Interventions during Nursing Implementing Phase

Implementation is the actions that the nursing staff takes to carry out the nursing measures identified in the care plan in order to achieve the expected outcome criteria. In implementation of the care plan, the nurses use various skills to implement the care plan. The psychiatric nurses select interventions according to their clinical practice. At the basic level, the psychiatric nurse may select counseling, milieu therapy, self-care activities, psychobiological interventions, health education, case management, health promotion and health maintenance, and a variety of other approaches to meet the mental health needs of the clients. In addition to the intervention options available to the basic-level psychiatric and mental health nurse, the nurse specialist may provide consultation and psychotherapy at the advanced level. Table 2-8 presents the interventions for psychiatric and mental health nurses.

一、护理措施实施方法

护理措施实施阶段是护士应用各种方法和技巧，将护理计划中的措施应用于患者以达到预期护理目标的过程。精神科护士往往根据其临床实践水平，选择不同的干预方法实施护理计划。在一般情况下，精神科护士会选择心理咨询、环境治疗、自护训练、心理生理干预、健康教育、个案管理、健康促进等基本护理措施来满足患者的精神健康需要。此外，精神科护理专家，还可通过专业咨询和心理治疗进一步促进患者的精神健康。精神科护士实施护理计划常用的干预方法如表 2-8 所示。

Table 2-8　Interventions for psychiatric and mental health nurses

Areas	Explanations
Basic Level	
Counseling	The psychiatric nurse uses counseling interventions to assist clients in improving or regaining their previous coping abilities, fostering mental health, and preventing mental illness and disability
Milieu Therapy	The psychiatric nurse provides, structures, and maintains a therapeutic environment in collaboration with the client and other health-care providers
Self-care Activities	The psychiatric nurse structures interventions around the client's activities of daily living to foster self-care and mental and physical well-being
Psychobiological	The psychiatric nurse uses knowledge of psychobiological interventions and applies clinical skills to restore the client's health and prevent further disability
Health Education	The psychiatric nurse assists clients in achieving satisfying, productive, and healthy patterns of living through health education
Case Management	The psychiatric nurse provides case management to coordinate comprehensive health services and ensure continuity of care
Health Promotion and Health Maintenance	The psychiatric nurse employs strategies and interventions to promote and maintain mental health and to prevent mental illness
Advanced Level	
Psychotherapy	The nurse specialist in psychiatric and mental health nursing uses individual, group, and family psychotherapy, child psychotherapy, and other therapeutic treatments to assist clients in fostering mental health, preventing mental illness and disability, and improving or regaining previous health status and functional abilities
Consultation	The nurse specialist provides consultation to health-care providers and others to influence the plans of care for clients and enhance the abilities of others to provide psychiatric and mental health care and effect change in systems

表 2-8 精神科护士实施护理计划常用干预方法

方法	解释
基本护理措施	
心理咨询	精神科护士通过心理咨询协助患者认识其以前的应对能力和精神健康状况，从而提高其应对能力和预防精神疾病
环境治疗	精神科护士通过与患者及其他医务人员的合作，提供、创造和保持一个良好的治疗环境
自护训练	精神科护士对患者的日常生活进行指导，以促进患者的自护能力和恢复其身心健康
心理生理干预	精神科护士在临床应用心理生理干预的知识来恢复患者的健康，预防患者出现身心障碍
健康教育	精神科护士通过健康教育协助患者选择满意、健康的生活方式
个案管理	精神科护士向综合健康服务机构提供有关患者的个案情况，以保证患者出院后护理和治疗的连续性
健康促进	精神科护士通过实施干预措施和技巧来促进和保持患者精神健康和预防精神疾病
高级护理措施	
心理治疗	精神科护理专家应用各种心理治疗方法协助患者恢复精神健康，预防精神障碍和疾病，促进和恢复机体功能
专业咨询	精神科护理专家为其他健康工作者提供专业咨询，以有效改变和提高这些人员在精神健康护理方面的能力

II. Evidence-Based Nursing Practice

Evidence-based nursing practice is the conscientious, explicit, and judicious use of the best evidence gained from systematic research for the purpose of making informed decision about the care of individual patients in the nursing planning. It also takes into account the patients' value, characteristics, preferences, and circumstances, as well as the skill and resources of the nurse (figure 2-2). Evidence-based nursing emphasizes to start with a specific and concrete problem in clinical practice, combine the research with clinical experience and the patient's needs, so as to facilitate the integrated application of direct experience and indirect experience in practice. This implementation can motivate the team spirit and collaborative atmosphere, reform the work procedures and methods, and improve the level of care and patient satisfaction. Only based on the synthesis of daily nursing experience, relevant research results as well as patients' own willing, the optimal care service can be offered by nurse. Finding the evidence is the key point of evidence-based nursing and may be challenging. However, advances in information technology have provided a broad platform for information retrieval (box 2-2).

二、循证护理实践

循证护理实践是指护理人员在计划其护理活动过程中，审慎地、明确地、明智地将科研结论与临床经验及患者愿望相结合，获取证据，作为临床护理决策的过程。循证护理强调以临床实践中的特定、具体化的问题为出发点，将来自科学研究的结论与临床知识和经验、患者需求进行结合，促进直接经验和间接经验在实践中的综合应用，并通过实施过程，激发团队精神和协作气氛，改革工作程序和方法，提高照护水平和患者满意度（图 2–2）。护士在护理实施过程中综合自身临床经验、相关科研结果和患者的意愿，才能为其提供最优的护理服务。实施循证护理的关键在于寻找并评价证据。然而，信息技术的进步为文献检索提供了广阔的平台（box 2–2）。

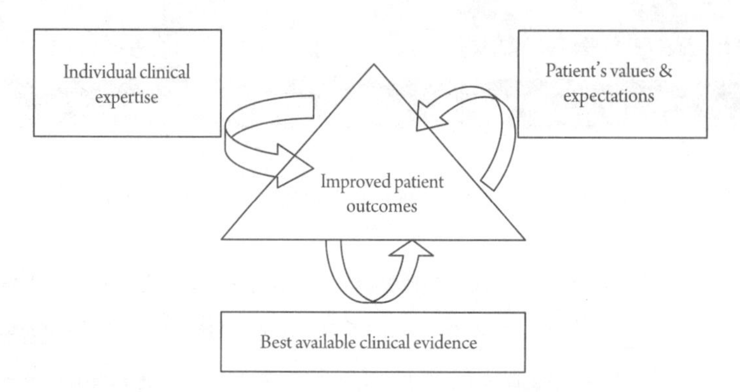

Figure 2-2 Evidence-based nursing practice

BOX 2-2 Learning More

Evidence-based Nursing Practice Resources

- **The Cochrane Collaboration** is a regularly updated electronic library available on computer disk and the Internet. It contains a unique, cumulative collection of systematic reviews that are valuable not only because they are rigorously methodological but also because they are regularly updated as new research evidence is published.
- **The National Guideline Clearinghouse**, sponsored by the U. S. government, is a database of evidence-based clinical practice guidelines and related documents.
- **The Substance Abuse and Mental Health Services Administration** (SAMHSA) and its Center for Mental Health Services (CMHS) have six Evidence-Based Practice Implementation Resource Kits to encourage the use of evidence-based practice in mental health.
- **The Joanna Briggs Institute**, based in Australia, produces best-practices information sheets and systematic reviews.
- **World Views On Evidence-Based Nursing** is a quarterly journal from the Honor Society of Nursing, which bridges knowledge and application and takes a global approach to research, policy and practice, education, and management.
- ***Evidence-Based Mental Health*** is a quarterly British journal that publishes abstracts and commentaries on research in the field.

BOX 2-2 知识拓展

循证护理实践资源

- Cochrane协作网是一个定期更新的电子图书馆，可于计算机磁盘和互联网上使用。它独家持续性地收集有价值的系统评价，不仅方法严谨，而且如若有新的研究证据发表就会定期更新。
- 国家临床指南，由美国政府资助，是一个循证临床实践指南和相关文献的数据库。
- 物质滥用和心理健康服务管理局及其心理健康服务中心有六个循证实践资源包，鼓励在心理健康中进行循证实践。
- Joana Briggs研究中心，总部设在澳大利亚，制订最佳实践信息表并发表系统综述。
- 循证护理世界观是护理荣誉学会的季刊，在知识和应用之间架起了桥梁，为研究、政策与实践、教育及管理提供了全球策略。
- 《循证心理健康》是一本英国季刊，刊登该领域的研究摘要和评论。

Nursing implementation is the process of implementing the care plan, and consummate care plan ensure the implementation to proceed smoothly. In the nursing practice, the nurse applies the scientific method and delivery a variety of nursing measures to achieve the goal of nursing, guided by the theories. At this stage, it not only needs rich professional knowledge, but also

护理实施是执行护理计划的过程，完善的护理计划能够保证实施的顺利进行。在护理实践中，护士应用科学的方法，以理论为指导，选择多种护理措施以达到护理目标。此阶段，不仅需要护士具备丰富的专业知识，还需要护士具有熟练的操作技能，良好的人

the clinical experience and interpersonal skills to ensure coordinated care plan and enable the patient to obtain optimal nursing care. Psychiatric patients often still have somatic diseases, therefore, psychiatric nurses need to use biological, psychological and social and cultural skills, and understand the development of biomedicine and social psychology to perform nursing measures, so as to restore the physical and mental health of patients.

际沟通能力，才能保证护理计划协调进行，使患者得到高质量的护理。精神科患者往往还存在躯体疾病，因此，需要精神科护士运用生物的、心理的和社会文化技巧，并了解生物医学及社会心理学的发展来执行护理措施，以恢复患者的身心健康。

Section 6 Nursing Evaluation

第六节　护理评价

Nursing care is a dynamic process involving change in the client's health status over time, giving rise to the need for new data, different nursing diagnoses, and modifications in the plan of care.

护理是帮助患者改变健康状态的动态过程，需要不断收集患者的资料，修订患者的护理诊断和护理计划，以达到护理目标。

I. Definition of Nursing Evaluation

一、护理评价的概念

The different client or the same client at the different stage of disease has various nursing problems. The phase of nursing evaluation focuses on the client's status, progress toward goal achievement, and ongoing reevaluation of the care plan. Therefore, nursing evaluation is a continuous process of appraising the effect of nursing interventions and the treatment regimen on the client's health status and expected health outcome.

不同患者或同一患者在疾病的不同时期，护理问题可能不同。因此，护士除了在患者入院时需要进行一次全面评估外，还应根据患者病情变化，连续不断地进行再评估，即护理评价。因此，护理评价是鉴定整体的护理效果，判断执行护理措施后患者的反应及预期目标是否达到的过程。通过护理评价，护士可以对执行护理措施后是否达到护理目标作出判断。

II. General Principles of Nursing Evaluation

二、护理评价的原则

When evaluating care, the nurse should review all previous phase of the nursing process and determine whether the expected outcomes for the client have been met. Four possible outcomes may occur: a. the client may respond favorably or as expected to nursing interventions, b. short-term goals may be met but long-term goals may remain unmet, c. the client may be unable to meet or achieve any goals, or d. new problems or needs may be identified. All members of multidisciplinary treatment team, as well as the client, should be encouraged to provide feedback regarding the effectiveness of the care plan. As a result of the evaluation process, the care is maintained,

在护理评价阶段，应注重执行措施后患者的反应，将其与护理目标比较，衡量目标是否达到，并复审护理计划，探讨护理目标部分实现或未实现的原因。在护理评价时，应对护理程序的前4个步骤进行全面回顾，以确定是否达到预期的护理目标。可能的护理评价结果包括：① 患者达到了预期的护理目标；② 短期目标实现了，但长期目标仍未实现；③ 患者无法达到护理目标；④ 患者有了新的问题和需要。所有医护人员及患者都应

modified, or totally revised.

对护理计划实施的效果予以反馈，以确定是否需要继续执行计划、修改护理计划或重新制订新的护理计划和措施。

Section 7 Documentation to the Nursing Process in Psychiatric and Mental Health Nursing

The written documentation is equally important as using nursing process in the delivery of care. Some contemporary nursing leaders are advocating that with solid standards of practice and procedures in place within the institution, nurses need only chart when there has been a deviation in the care as outlined by that standard. However, many legal decisions are still based on the precept that "If it was not charted, it was not done." Some health care organization accrediting agencies require that nursing process be reflected in the delivery of care. In these instances, documentation must bear written testament to the use of the nursing process.

A variety of documentation methods can be used to reflect use of the nursing process in the delivery of nursing care. Problem-oriented recording (POR) is presented here as an example, which follows the subjective, objective, assessment, plan, intervention, and evaluation (SOAPIE) format. It has its basis on a list of problems. When it is used in nursing, the problems (nursing diagnoses) are identified on a written plan of care with appropriate nursing interventions described for each. Documentation written in the SOAPIE format includes:

1. S=Subjective data Information gathered from what the client, family, or other source has said or reported.

2. O=Objective data Information gathered by direct observation of the person may include a physiological measurement such as blood pressure or a behavioral response such as affect.

3. A=Assessment The nurse's interpretation of the subjective and objective data.

4. P=Plan The treatments or nursing care to be carried out (may be omitted in daily charting if the plan is clearly explained in the written nursing care plan and no changes are expected).

5. I=Intervention Those nursing actions that were actually carried out.

6. E=Evaluation Evaluation of the problem following nursing intervention (some nursing

第七节　精神科护理程序的记录方法

在精神科护理中，文件记录与护理程序的实施同样重要。护理管理者提倡在临床实践中使用具体而统一的护理实践及程序表格，护士只需记录护理中所遇到的特殊问题。然而，这种方法有一定的法律争议，认为如果在表格中没有相应的记录，就证明护士没有做相应的工作。因此，医院及其他的健康机构要求护士认真、详细、完整地记录护理过程。

临床有很多护理程序的记录方式，在此主要讨论以问题为中心的记录，即按照主观资料（S）、客观资料（O）、评估（A）、计划（P）、干预（I）、评价（E）的格式进行记录。它以一系列问题（护理诊断）为基础，针对每一问题作出护理干预的书面计划。SOAPIE格式的记录包括以下几方面：

1. S= 主观资料　患者、家属或相关人员所提供的资料。

2. O= 客观资料　指对患者进行客观检查获得的资料，包括体格检查、行为反应等。

3. A= 评估　护士对所收集的主观和客观资料进行分析整理后的资料。

4. P= 计划　将要对患者实施的治疗和护理措施。如果每天的计划是重复的，则不必在每天的记录表格里书写。

5. I= 干预　实际执行的护理措施。

6. E= 评价　护理措施实施后，对护理效果及存在问题的评价。

interventions cannot be evaluated immediately, so this section may be optional).

Table 2-9 shows how POR corresponds to the steps of the nursing process.

In summary, the nursing process provides a methodology by which nurse may deliver care using a systematic and scientific approach. The focus is goal directed and based on a decision-making or problem-solving model, consisting of five steps: assessment, diagnosis, planning, implementation, and evaluation. The psychiatric nurse uses the nursing process to assist clients successfully adapting to stressors within the environment. Goals are directed toward change in thoughts, feelings, and behaviors that are age-appropriate and congruent with cultural norms. The nurse serves as a valuable member of the interdisciplinary treatment team, working both independently and cooperatively with other team members.

表2-9列举了如何将POR与护理程序的步骤一一对应。

总之，护理程序是一个系统性的、科学的解决问题的程序，是护士为患者提供护理服务的工作方法，包括评估、诊断、计划、实施和评价5个步骤。作为一种科学的工作方法和指导框架，精神科护士应用护理程序协助患者适应压力，改变患者的思想、情感和行为，使其认知、情感和行为与年龄和社会文化规范相符。精神科护士作为多学科治疗队伍的成员，可以独立或与其他成员配合进行护理，从而恢复和促进精神障碍患者的身心健康，使患者得到连续性和全面护理服务的保证。

Table 2-9 Validation of the nursing process with POR

Problem-Oriented Recording	What is Recoded	Nursing Process
S and O (Subjective and Objective data)	Verbal reports, and direct observation and examination by the nurse	Assessment
A (Assessment)	Nurse's interpretation of S and O	Diagnosis and outcome identification
P (Plan)	Description of appropriate nursing actions to resolve identified problem	Planning
I (Intervention)	Description of nursing actions actually carried out	Implementation
E (Evaluation)	A reassessment of the situation to determine results of nursing actions implemented	Evaluation

表2-9 以问题为中心的记录与相应的护理程序步骤

POR	记录内容	护理程序步骤
S和O(主观和客观资料)	患者等口头表述，护士直接观察及检查所获得的资料	评估
A(评估)	护士对所获得主、客观资料的分析和归纳	诊断和预期结果
P(计划)	针对问题所制订的恰当护理措施	计划
I(干预)	实际执行护理措施的描述	实施
E(评价)	对实施的护理措施重新评估，以判断目标是否达到	评价

(Wang Xiaoqin)

(王小琴)

Key Points

1. The nursing process is a five-step problem-solving approach, which also serves as an organizational framework for the practice of nursing. The five steps include nursing assessment, nursing diagnosis, planning, implementation, and evaluation.

2. Assessment is the deliberate and systematic collection of biopsychosocial information or data to determine current and past health and functional status and to evaluate present and past coping patterns.

3. The nurse determines which of the three types of assessment (comprehensive, focused, or screening) to use based on the client's needs, presenting symptoms, and clinical setting.

4. The nursing diagnosis should include the client's adaptive or maladaptive health response, defining characteristics of that response, and contributing stressors. Knowledge of NANDA diagnoses is needed by psychiatric nurses.

5. The plan of care should include expected outcomes, as well as prescribed nursing strategies to achieve those outcomes.

6. Nursing interventions should be directed toward helping the client develop insight and resolve problems through carrying out a positive plan of action. Psychiatric nursing practice includes both basic and advanced activities.

7. Evidence-based practice is the conscientious, explicit, and judicious use of the best evidence gained from systematic research for the purpose of making informed decision about the care of individual patients in the nursing planning.

8. Evaluation involves reviewing all previous phases of the nursing process and determining the degree to which expected outcomes were attained.

9. Nurses must document that the nursing process has been used in the delivery of care. Its use is mandated by the Nurse Practice Act and also required by some health care organization accrediting agencies. The method of POR is commonly used.

Exercises

(Questions 1 to 3 share the same question stem)

The patient, 43 years old, appeared unprovoked depressed for nearly 3 weeks. The symptoms were severe in the

内容摘要

1. 护理程序是一种包括护理评估、诊断、计划、实施和评价五个连续步骤的科学的解决问题的工作方法。它为护理实践提供了严密的组织框架。

2. 护理评估是全面而系统地收集患者生理、心理及社会资料，以确定患者的健康状况，并评价患者的应对方式。

3. 精神科护士应根据患者的需要、临床症状及临床环境确定采用何种评估方式。评估方式一般包括三种，即综合评估、针对性评估和筛选评估。

4. 护理诊断包括患者适应或不适应的健康反应，反应的诊断依据及相关因素。精神科护士需掌握有关 NANDA 的护理诊断知识。

5. 护理计划应包括针对护理诊断的预期护理目标和达到护理目标所应采取的护理措施。

6. 护理实施应帮助患者培养其自知力，并通过实施积极的措施解决护理问题。在精神科，护士常采用基础及高级护理措施进行护理干预。

7. 循证护理实践是指护理人员在计划其护理活动过程中，审慎地、明确地、明智地将科研结论与临床经验及患者愿望相结合，获取证据，作为临床护理决策的过程。

8. 护理评价是指对护理程序的前 4 个步骤进行全面回顾，以确定是否达到预期护理目标的过程。

9. 护士行为法及其他的健康组织授权机构要求护士认真、详细、完整地记录护理过程，常用的方法为以问题为中心的记录（POR）。

思考题

（1～3 题共用题干）

患者，女，43 岁，近 3 周无诱因出现情绪低落，晨重夜轻，兴趣丧失，易疲乏，少语，动作迟缓，自觉脑子反应慢，性欲减退，失

morning and reduced at night, which included loss of interests, fatigue, a little speaking, slow action and thought, loss of sexual interest, insomnia and early awaking. She said, "Why should I live? I am an encumbrance", and attempted to suicide several times.

1. What's the patient's thought disorder?

2. What's the optimal nursing diagnosis for the patient?

3. Aimed at the self-inflicted injury and suicide, what is the optimal measure for the nurses?

(Questions 4 to 7 share the same question stem)

The patient, 32 years old, hospitalized due to schizophrenia four years ago and the symptoms relieved after treatment. Two days ago, he took medicine and had a bed rest because of fever and headache, after several hours, the families could not arouse him and the patient kept still when he was pushed. The examinations showed no signs of pathology, but the patient was still wordless, has rigid limbs, and refused the food and medicine.

4. What's the main psychiatric symptom for the patient?

5. What's the optimal nursing diagnosis for the patient?

6. What's the most important nursing intervention for the patient?

7. What's the primary aim to arrange the patient in a single room?

(Questions 8 to 10 share the same question stem)

The patient, 18 years old, was afraid of fatness and began to go on a diet one year ago, meanwhile, she often induced vomiting. Recently, she only ate an apple one day. Her body weight decreased significantly and the menstruation ceased. Although Lee has been quite thin with the weight of 35 kilograms, she still thought that she was very fat and ugly.

8. What's the optimal nursing diagnosis for the patient?

9. What's the best measure for diet nursing?

10. The patient always said that she was very fat and ugly although she was only 35 kilograms. To solve this problem, what should the nurse firstly do?

眠、早醒，称“活着干嘛，就是个累赘”，多次想自杀。

1. 患者有什么思维障碍？

2. 患者最主要的护理诊断是什么？

3. 针对自杀自伤行为首选的护理措施是什么？

（4～7题共用题干）

患者，男，32岁。4年前曾因精神分裂症住院，治疗后病情缓解。2天前因发热头痛服感冒药后卧床休息，数小时后家人多次不能唤起患者，推之不动，送至医院做相应检查无任何病理征象，但患者仍不言不语、四肢呈僵硬状态，拒食拒药。

4. 该患者最主要的精神症状是什么？

5. 针对该患者，最主要的护理诊断是什么？

6. 对该患者的护理中最重要的是什么？

7. 将患者安置于单人房间的主要目的是什么？

（8～10题共用题干）

患者，女，18岁，1年前因担心发胖开始节食，饭后常自我催吐，最近每天只进食1个苹果，体重明显下降，月经停止。体重35kg，虽已明显消瘦，仍认为自己很胖。

8. 该患者最主要的护理诊断是什么？

9. 对患者进行饮食护理时，首要的措施是什么？

10. 患者虽只有35kg仍说：“我太胖，太难看了”。针对此，护士首先应做什么？

Chapter 3 Relationship Development and Therapeutic Communication

第三章 精神疾病护理中的护患关系与治疗性沟通

Learning Objectives

Memorization

1. Describe the terms nurse-client relationship, therapeutic relationship.
2. Describe characteristics of nurse-client relationship in psychiatric settings.
3. Explain phases of the relationship, and tasks and targets in each phase.

Comprehension

1. Explain attributes essential to the psychiatric nurse in the relationship.
2. Discuss conditions essential to the therapeutic relationship.

Application

1. Apply the therapeutic communication techniques in caring for patients with mental illness.
2. Deal with the barriers of the therapeutic relationship properly.

学习目标

识记

1. 能描述护患关系、治疗性沟通的概念。
2. 能描述精神疾病护理中护患关系的特征。
3. 能描述精神疾病护理护患关系分期，每一期的目标、任务。

理解

1. 能解释精神疾病护理护患关系的建立基本要素。
2. 能讨论精神疾病护理中治疗性护患关系建立的基本条件。

运用

1. 能在护理工作中灵活应用治疗性沟通技巧。
2. 能意识并处理沟通中的常见障碍。

03章

Jenny is a 22-year-old woman who calls the crisis hot line on a weekly basis. Tonight she is once again threatening suicide because her current boyfriend has broken up with her. Last month, Jenny took an overdose of twenty Panadol tablets in front of her boyfriend, forcing him to drive her to the emergency department where her stomach was pumped. Jenny is an attractive, bright woman who defines herself as very demanding and needy. She says that she cannot live without her boyfriend, even though he has repeatedly cheated on her and stolen some of her property.
Please think about the following questions based on the case:
1. What is Jenny's prior nursing diagnosis?
2. What might be some of the potential obstacles to establishing a therapeutic relationship with Jenny?

珍妮，22 岁，每周都会给危机干预热线打电话。今晚，她因为跟男朋友分手，打电话说要自杀。上个月时，珍妮在男朋友面前服用过量扑热息痛，被送至急诊科进行洗胃。珍妮是一个阳光有魅力的女孩，但她描述自己是一个很强势的人。虽然他的男朋友多次欺骗她，并随意拿其钱财，但她称没有男朋友就活不下去。
请思考：
1. Jenny 目前最主要的护理诊断是什么？
2. 与 Jenny 建立治疗性关系的潜在障碍有哪些？

Providing nursing care for people with a mental illness is very different to care for those with other illnesses. The foundation of mental health nursing is the nurse-client relationship.

Nurse-client relationship is a type of therapeutic relationship; it is a kind of working relationship built up by dynamic interactivities occurs in medical situation based on each other's need and, ethic, law, financial and technological disciplines. During the nursing process, this relationship is of importance on itself, and acts as part of the technology. Nurses may apply therapeutic communication skills effectively to promote patients development, mature and growing, to improve patients' coping ability. This chapter will explore the therapeutic relationships the mental health nurse initiates and utilizes as his or her "tool of trade".

精神疾病的护理与其他疾病的护理差别很大。精神科疾病的护理的基础是治疗性护患关系。本章将探讨治疗性关系的相关内容以及其在护理工作中的应用。

护患关系是治疗关系的一种，是护士与患者之间在医疗情境中基于互相间的需要和伦理、法律、经济和技术性的规范，经由互动而形成的工作关系。在精神疾病护理过程中，这种关系本身就具有治疗价值，是操作技术的一部分。护士可以有效地应用治疗性沟通技巧促进患者的成长、发展及成熟，提高患者应对能力。本章主要讨论精神疾病护理中护患关系的特点与治疗性沟通的技巧。

Section 1 Development of Nurse Client Relationship

第一节 精神疾病护理中的护患关系

The nurse-client relationship is fundamental of intervention for mental diseases. Therapeutic nurse-client relationship may help the client follow the nurse's advice and cooperate with the treatment. Nurse-client relationship in mental health nursing is characterized by professional, therapeutic and goal-oriented.

护患关系是精神疾病护理干预的基础，治疗性的护患关系能使患者自愿采纳护士的建议，配合医疗和护理工作。精神疾病护理中的护患关系具有专业性、治疗性和目的性等特征。

I. Characteristics of Therapeutic Relationship in Psychiatric Settings

1. Professional Relationship Unlike the social relationship, such as friendliness and love, the nurse-client relationship is a professional relationship. It is a kind of professional behavior and cannot be avoided. Developing a well relationship with the client is basic responsibility and obligation of the nurse, especially for the psychiatric nurse. In this relationship, the client's needs are core of interaction.

2. Therapeutic Relationship The nurse-client relationship is a therapeutic relationship. Peplau (1952) emphasized that nursing is a process of relationship developing among people; this process is not social but therapeutic and educational relationship. Evidences exist that the therapeutic alliance in the context of psychotherapy has a positive effect on client outcomes. As a helper in the relationship, the nurse's personal exhibition in nursing has significant influences on the client.

BOX 3-1 Learning More

Hildegard Peplau

Hildegard Peplau was born in Reading, Pennsylvania on September 1st, 1909. After graduating from the Pottstown, Pennsylvania Hospital School of Nursing in 1931 she worked as an operating room supervisor at Pottstown Hospital. She got her B.A. in interpersonal psychology from Bennington College, Vermont, in 1943, an M.A. in psychiatric nursing from Teachers College, Columbia, New York, in 1947, and an Ed. D in curriculum development from Columbia in 1953.

Hildegard Peplau attended World War II as a member of the Army Nurse Corps and worked in a neuropsychiatric hospital in London, England. She also served at Bellevue and Chestnut Lodge Psychiatric Facilities and was in contact with renowned psychiatrists Freida Fromm-Riechman and Harry Stack Sullivan. Hildegard Peplau holds numerous awards and positions. She retired in 1974. On March 17th, 1999, Hildegard Peplau died peacefully at her home in Sherman Oaks California after a brief illness at the age of 89.

3. Goal Oriented Relationship The therapeutic nurse-client relationship is goal oriented. Ideally, the goal of the relationship is decided together by the nurse and the client. Most often the goal is directed at learning and growth promotion, in an effort to bring about some type of change in the client's life. In psychiatric nursing, the

一、精神疾病护理中护患关系的特征

1. 专业性 精神疾病护理中的护患关系是一种专业性的人际关系。同其他的社会人际关系不同，护士与患者之间的人际关系是一种职业行为，且不可避免。建立良好的护患关系是精神科护士的一项基本职责。护士利用自身的专业素养及能力来协助患者，引导整个关系过程并维持其专业性。护士与患者交往、互动的重点是患者的需要。

2. 治疗性 护患关系也是一种治疗性的人际关系。Peplum（1952）强调，护理是人与人之间关系发展的过程，具有治疗性与教育性。证据表明，这种治疗性人际关系有利于患者病情的恢复。治疗性关系以患者为中心，医护人员无条件的积极关注患者的健康。

BOX 3-1 知识拓展

Hildegard Peplau

Hildegard Peplau 1909年9月1日出生于宾夕法尼亚州的Reading。1931年从Pottstown的Pennsylvania Hospital护校毕业后在Pottstown医院做手术室护士。1943年在佛蒙特州Bennington College拿到人际心理学学士学位。1947年拿到哥伦比亚大学护理心理学硕士，1953年获得哥伦比亚大学教育学博士学位。在二战期间，Hildegard Peplau在英国伦敦陆军护理团神经心理科工作。她曾经于Bellevue和Chestnut Lodge精神病院与著名的心理学家Freida Fromm-Riechman和Harry Stack Sullivan一起共事。Hildegard Peplau一生拥有许多荣誉和头衔。1974年退休，1999年3月17日在加利福尼亚州的家中安详的去世，享年89岁。

3. 目的性 治疗性护患关系具有明确的目的。理想状态下，目的应该由护士和患者共同确定。在精神科护理中，治疗性护患关系有以下几个目的：

general goals of the nurse-client relationship include the following:

- Self-awareness, self-acceptance, and an increased genuine self-respect of the client.
- A clear sense of personal identity and an improved level of personal integration of the client.
- An ability of the client to form an intimate, interdependent, interpersonal relationship with a capacity to give and receive love.
- Improved functioning and increased ability of the client to satisfy needs and achieve realistic personal goals.

- 使患者能够自我了解、自我接受、增强自尊；
- 能够达到个人认同和个人统合；
- 有能力去发展亲密、相互依赖的人际关系，能够接受及给予爱；
- 增加个人能力以满足自己的需要，并完成自我实现的个人目标。简而言之，就是增进患者与他人交往，提高患者自尊，加强患者解决问题的能力并使其获得满意、丰富的生活。

II. Conditions Essential to the Therapeutic Relationship

The nurse-client relationship is influenced by many aspects of factors, among which some specific core conditions are essential to develop therapeutic relationship. These conditions are illustrated as followed:

i. Trust

Trust is defined as a kind of personal desire that one can depend upon others to exchange behaviors. It is one of the decisive factors for developing the therapeutic nurse-client relationship and basis of the following work. Trust in the nurse helps the client feel secure and cared for, makes him or her express feelings, attitudes or values more bluntly.

To trust another, one must feel confidence in that person's presence, reliability, integrity, veracity, and sincere desire to provide assistance when requested. Initial interaction is important for the client to establish trust in the nurse. For the nurse, it is imperative to convey an aura of trust-worthiness, which requires that he or she possess a sense of self-confidence. Self-confidence is often derived out of knowledge gained through achievement of personal and professional goals, as well as the ability to integrate these roles and to function as a unified whole. It is through nursing interventions, which convey a sense of warmth and caring that the nurse can demonstrate the trust-worthiness of self and earn the client's trust. These interventions are initiated simply and concretely, and directed toward activities that address the client's basic needs for physiological and psychological safety and security. The interventions can include: providing a blanket when the client is cold, providing food when the client is hungry; being honest(e.g., saying "I don't know the answer to your question, but I'll try to find out" and then following through); keeping promise; explaining the policy, regulation and process precisely; being with client if he/she does not want to attend some activities;

二、精神疾病护理中建立治疗性护患关系的条件

许多外在因素可以影响精神疾病护理过程中治疗性护患关系的建立和发展，以下几方面是发展治疗性护患关系的核心要素：

（一）信任

信任是指个人感觉可以依赖他人，并愿意与他人沟通。它是发展治疗性关系的决定性因素之一，也是开展护理工作的基础。对护士的信任能使患者感觉到安全和关爱，从而使患者能够更坦率地表达情感、态度和价值观。

要信任一个人，就必须对此人的存在、可靠性、正直性、真实性充满信心，并真诚地希望在接到请求时提供帮助。最初的互动对于患者建立对护士的信任非常重要。对于护士来说，表现出值得信任的形象是必要的，这需要护士本身拥有自信。自信往往通过实现个人和职业目标而获得。护士通过护理干预，传递一种温暖和关怀的感觉，展示自我信任价值，赢得患者的信任。这些干预措施简单而具体，目的是满足患者生理和心理的安全保障和基本需求。有助于建立信任的措施，如雪中送炭，患者饥饿时给予食物、寒冷时给予毛毯；诚实，如告诉患者"我不知道答案，但可以帮你寻找"，而且言出必行；信守承诺；语言准确地解释政策、法规和流程；陪伴，患者不想参与某种活动时与他做

insisting on the organization principle; developing the individualized nursing intervention; or being confidential.

伴；言行一致，始终如一；因人而异，进行个体化护理干预；对患者信息保密等。

ii. Empathy

Empathy is the ability to enter into the life of another person and to accurately perceive his or her current feelings and their meanings. The nurse does not actually have to have the experience, but has to be able to imagine the feeling associated with the experience. Accurate empathy involves more than knowing what the client means. It also contains sensitivity to the client's current feelings and the verbal ability to communicate this understanding in a language attuned to the client. It requires that the nurses lay aside personal views and values to enter another's world without prejudice.

（二）同理心

同理心是个体理解他人的情感及其内涵的能力。具有同理心的护士能够理解患者表述的同时还能洞察其情绪，并与其沟通。护士能够公平地对待患者，而不受自身观念和价值观的影响。

The use of empathy in a therapeutic relationship is central to psychiatric mental health nursing. In the first place, empathy dissolves the client's sense of alienation by connecting the client on some level to a part of the human being. The client will not feel alone when think that "some else have the same perceptions with me, so I'm not alien..." On the other hand, it helps the client feel understood, accepted, cared for and valued. Then the client will think "maybe I'm worthwhile as what other person consider" and has confidence in himself of herself. Another benefit of empathy is that the client may learn some aspects about self of which he or she may have been unaware as the feelings are explored.

同理心是精神疾病护理中治疗性护患关系的中心环节。一方面，护士的同理心使患者感到被理解、被接受、被关怀和被尊重，从而逐步建立自信；另一方面，可以化解患者的疏远感、减轻孤独感，患者感到“别人和我感觉一样，我并不特殊”。

Empathy should not be confused with sympathy. The major difference is that with empathy the nurse "accurately perceives or understands" what the client is feeling and encourages the client to explore these feelings. While with sympathy the nurse actually "shares" what the client is feeling and experiences a need to abate distress. With empathy, when understanding the client's thoughts and feelings, the nurse is able to maintain sufficient objectivity to achieve problem resolution with minimal assistance. While with sympathy, the nurse actually feels what the client is feeling and loses objectivity, and may fall into personal distress and forget to help the client resolve the problem.

同理心不同于同情心。具有同理心的护士能够准确察觉和理解患者的想法和感受，鼓励患者探索自身情感；而具有同情心的护士分享了患者的痛苦。同理心帮助护士客观地理解患者的想法和情感，解决其问题；而同情心迫使护士体验患者的感受，陷入悲伤痛苦，无法帮助患者解决问题。

iii. Rapport

Rapport is interpersonal harmony characterized by understanding and respect. It is also an important task in developing relationship and established by the nurse through interpersonal warmth, a nonjudgmental attitude, acceptance, and friendliness. Client with mental disorders often feel alone and isolated from family and friends. A skilled nurse will be able to establish rapport that will decrease this feeling of the client and alleviate their anxiety in discussing personal problems. Developing rapport also

（三）和谐关系

和谐关系是人际关系的融洽状态，沟通双方相互理解和尊重。和谐关系使患者舒适、自由地表达个人的想法，是发展良好护患关系的重要因素之一。精神障碍患者常被家庭和朋友孤立，因此，护士应通过热情、宽容、友善及非批判性的态度与患者一起建立和谐

makes the client feel comfortable and express his or her thoughts more freely. To establish rapport is to create a sense of harmony based on knowledge and appreciation of each individual's uniqueness. It is the ability to be still and experience the other as a human being-to appreciate the unfolding of each personality one to the other. The ability to truly care for and about others is the core of rapport."

的关系。建立和谐关系就是正确认识和评价个体独特性，理解和欣赏他人的个性，从而创造一种融洽的气氛，其核心是能够真诚地关心照顾他人。

iv. Respect

Respect, also named unconditional positive regard, is to believe in the dignity and worth of the client regardless of his or her unacceptable behaviors. The nurse's attitude is nonjudgmental; it is without criticism, ridicule, or reservation. It does not mean that the nurse condone or approve of all aspects of the client's lifestyle or pattern of behaving. Nevertheless, with unconditional positive regard, the client is accepted and respected for no other reason than he or she is considered to be a worthwhile and unique human being. The inexperienced nurse may have difficulty in accepting the client without transferring feeling about the client's thoughts and actions. Acceptance means viewing the client's behavior as natural, normal, and expected, given the circumstances that will be changed as the client becomes less threatened and learns more adaptive ways.

（四）尊重

尊重即肯定和尊敬。尊重患者的护士会以不带批判性、挑剔、嘲笑或怀疑的态度来对待患者，尊重其人格，忽略一些常人难以理解和接受的行为。尊重并不意味护士完全赞同患者的生活方式或行为模式，患者的异常行为是特定情况下的自然行为，会随着病情的好转而逐步改变。

Many clients with mental disorder have very little self-respect owing to the fact that, because of their behavior, they have been rejected by others in the past. Recognition that they are being respected and accepted as unique individuals on an unconditional basis can serve to promote feelings of self-esteem and self-respect. Respect can be communicated in many different ways: by sitting silently with a client who is crying, by calling the client by name (title, if the client prefers), by active listening to the client, by accepting the client's request not to share a certain experience, by being open and honest with the client, even when the truth may be difficult to discuss, by taking the client's ideas, preferences, and opinions into considerations when planning care, by promoting an atmosphere of privacy during therapeutic interaction or when the client is undergoing physical examination or therapy, and so on.

精神障碍患者由于行为异常，被他人拒绝和疏远，因此自尊降低。专科护士应无条件地关注和尊重患者，将其看作有价值的独特个体，提高患者的自尊。一些表达尊重的方式有：① 用姓名或头衔称呼患者；② 主动倾听患者说话；③ 不追问其经历；④ 即使很难沟通也要保持坦诚；⑤ 患者哭泣时坐在其身旁陪伴；⑥ 制订护理计划时，考虑患者的意见；⑦ 体格检查或治疗时保持环境隐秘。

v. Genuineness

Genuineness refers to the nurse's ability to be open, honest, and sincere in interactions with the client. It means that the nurse's response is "real", that the nurse is not thinking and feeling one thing and saying something different. When one is genuine, there is congruence between what is felt and what is being expressed. Genuineness is the opposite of self-alienation, which occurs when many of an individual's real, spontaneous

（五）真诚

真诚是专科护士与精神疾病患者沟通交流时的坦率、诚实和真挚的态度。它表明护士的反应是个人真实的感受，表里如一。压抑对生活的自然反应时会出现自我分离，与真诚截然相反。若护士出现自我分离，则会影响患者的信任。精神疾病的护理中，真诚

reactions to life are suppressed. It is an essential quality because nurses cannot expect openness, self-acceptance, and personal freedom in clients if they lack these qualities themselves. The nurse who possesses this quality responds to the client with truth and honesty, rather than with responses he or she may consider more "professional".

的护士能够对患者做出真实的，而不是"职业化"的反应。（"职业化"的应对方式对于护士自身也是一种压抑。）

vi. Self-Disclosure

Self-disclosure is personal statements about self, intentionally revealed to another person. It may occur as the nurse shares appropriate attitudes, feelings, and beliefs with the client and serves as a role model to the client. This kind of self-disclosure is an index of the closeness of the relationship and involves a particular kind of respect for the client. It is also an expression of genuineness and honesty by the nurse and is an aspect of empathy.

Disclosure by the nurse is always for the client's benefit. It has been evidenced that nurse self-disclosure boosts the likelihood of client self-disclosure and client self-disclosure is necessary for a successful therapeutic outcome. The nurse must use self-disclosure judiciously because the number and deepness of nurse's disclosure appears to be crucial to the success of the therapy. Too few and superficial nurse self-disclosures may fail to produce client self-disclosures, whereas too many and deep may reduce the time available for client self-disclosures or may alienate the client. Therefore, when self-disclosing, the nurse should take the quality, quantity and appropriateness of the disclosures into account. The criteria of self-disclosure include to promote the development of therapeutic relationship, to act as the educational and role model of the client, to be real, and to enhance the client's self-dependency.

（六）自我暴露

自我暴露指有目的地向他人描述自己的情感和经历。护士与患者分享个人的态度、情感、信念，以及作为患者的角色榜样等都是自我暴露的表现。自我暴露可以提示护患关系的亲密程度，即护士对患者的尊重、真诚及同理心的程度。

护士的自我暴露能促进患者的自我暴露，有助于患者的有效治疗。自我暴露的深度和广度对患者的治疗很重要，护士须慎重使用。护士自我暴露过少、过肤浅，不足以促使患者的自我暴露；而护士自我暴露过多过深则会减少患者自我暴露的机会和时间。护士恰当自我暴露的评价标准有：① 促进治疗性关系发展；② 具有教育和榜样作用；③ 具有真实性；④ 能促进患者独立。

vii. Concreteness

Concreteness involves using specific terminology rather than abstractions when discussing the client's feelings, experiences, and behaviors. It occurs as the nurse maintains realistic, not theoretical response to the client's clinical expressions, and avoids vagueness and ambiguity. It has three functions, to keep the nurse's responses close to the client's feelings and experiences, to cultivate accuracy of understanding by the nurse, and to encourage the client to attend to specific problem areas.

（七）具体化

具体化是护士在探讨患者的情感、体验及行为时运用明确而非抽象的语言，从具体事件上与患者进行沟通，而非泛泛地、理论上的沟通。具体化不仅可以培养护士理解的准确度，而且帮助患者关注具体问题，使护士的反应更能接近患者的情感和体验。

viii. Immediacy

Immediacy involves focusing on the current interaction of the nurse and the client in the relationship. It is a significant dimension because the client's behavior and functioning in the relationship are indicative of functioning in other interpersonal relationship. Most clients experience difficulty in interpersonal relationship; thus the client's functioning in the nurse-

（八）即时沟通

即时沟通是指在护患关系中，护士注重与患者保持即刻沟通，是治疗性护患关系的重要方面。精神障碍患者常出现人际交往障碍，需要随时评估其社会功能状态。护士即时沟通不仅能发现潜在问题，还能让患者感

client relationship must be evaluated. The nurse has the opportunity to intervene directly with the client's problem behavior, and the client has the opportunity to learn and change behavior.

受到自己被持续关注。

III. Development of Therapeutic Relationship in Psychiatric Settings

三、精神疾病护理中护患关系的建立

Based on the creative work and study of Peplau (1952) as well as other nursing theorists, there is a framework or road map for the establishment of therapeutic relationships. The stages can be summed up as an introductory beginning phase, a middle working phase and a termination phase. The basic elements within the therapeutic relationship should include:

- Therapeutic relationships are planned in order to meet the needs of the client;
- The basic tool of the therapeutic relationship is communication;
- The mental health nurse uses his or her own personality as an integral tool;
- The mental health nurse uses involvement such as 'being there' as a tool to develop the relationship.

Peplau（1952）认为咨询者是精神科护士的首要角色。为了正确有效地发挥护患关系的治疗性作用，必须明确护患关系的发展过程及工作内容。基于Peplau等人的研究和工作，目前已有多个治疗性关系的路径，它们均包含初始阶段、中间阶段和结束阶段。这些路径包含的基本要素：

- 有计划地满足患者需求；
- 沟通是建立治疗性关系的基本工具；
- 在建立治疗性关系过程中，精神科护士要发挥自己的人格特性；
- 陪伴可以作为建立治疗性关系的条件或基础。

In terms of nursing tasks, the relationship can be divided into four phases: the pre-interaction phase, the orientation (introductory) phase, the working phase, and the termination phase. Each phase builds on the preceding one and is presented as specific and distinct from the others. There may appear some overlapping of tasks, particularly when the interaction is limited.

根据护理任务的不同，治疗性护患关系的过程可以分为四期：互动前期、开始期、工作期、结束期。每个时期都是建立在前一个时期的基础上，有具体的任务。若此过程实践较短，则各期可能相互重叠。

i. Pre-interaction Phase

The pre-interaction phase begins before the nurse's first contact with the client. Most important thing is that the nurse has to do self-analysis. All individuals bring views and emotions from prior experiences to the clinical setting. For example, the nurse may have been reared in an alcoholic family and have ambivalent feelings about caring for a client who is alcohol dependent. To be effective, nurses should have a reasonably stable self-concept and an adequate amount of self-esteem. They should engage in constructive relationship with others and face reality to help clients do likewise. If they are aware of and in control of what they convey to their clients verbally and nonverbally, nurses can function as role models.

In this period, the initial assessment about the client is begun base on the information from his or her chart, significant others, or other health members, although most of the work related to it is done with the client in the

（一）互动前期

互动前期始于护士与患者第一次接触前。主要目标是护士对自我感受的探索。本期护士最重要的任务是进行自我分析。个体都会从之前的经验中获得观点和情感并联系到临床环境。例如，护士在酗酒的家庭中长大，对照顾酒精依赖的病人可能有心理冲突。护士要想胜任，须强化自我概念，获得足够的自尊。护士应该面对现实，与他人保持良好的人际关系，这样才能帮助患者。作为角色榜样，护士要以语言或非语言的方式明确传递给患者自己的态度，控制自身的情感。

此阶段还要注意收集患者的基本信息。患者的信息来源于入院病历、与患者关系密切者

second phase of the relationship. This initial information may allow the nurse to become aware of personal responses to knowledge about the client.

或其他医务人员。这些信息可以让护士明确自己对患者的反应，做出初步评估和调整。

ii. Orientation (Introductory) Phase

（二）开始期（初期）

It is during the orientation phase that the nurse and client first meet and become acquainted. The nurse assumes responsibility for initiating and sustaining the relationship. The tasks in this phase are to establish a climate of trust, understanding, acceptance, and open communication and formulate a contract with the client. To establish trust, the nurse must demonstrate caring and consistency, keep all appointments or promises and will always follow through on any activity she said or implied she would do. Establishing the contract is a mutual process in which the client participates as fully as possible. In some cases, such as, with the psychotic or severely withdrawn client, the client may be unable to fully participate, and the nurse must take the initiative in establishing the contract. As the client's contact with reality increases, the nurse should review the elements of the contract when appropriate and strive to attain mutuality. Following are the elements of a nurse-client contract: names of individuals, roles of nurse and client, responsibilities of nurse and client, expectations of nurse and client, purpose of the relationship, meeting location and time, conditions for termination, confidentiality.

开始期是护士和患者从认识到相互熟悉的过程。护士负责建立和维持这种关系。此期的主要目标是营造信任、相互理解、接纳、开放性沟通的氛围，并与患者达成共识。为了建立信任，护士须表现出关怀且言行一致、遵守约定、落实承诺。与患者共同制订护理干预计划也是此期的一项重要任务。在某些情况下，如精神病患者或严重退化无法完全参与的患者，护士须主动订立要遵守的约定。随着与患者接触的增加，护士应在适当的时候与患者一起复核约定的内容。这种护患约定的要素有双方姓名；护士和患者的角色；护士和患者的责任；护士和患者的期望；护患关系的目标；会面地点和时间；护患关系结束的条件；保密措施。

In this period of time, more data about the client are gathered by nurse through verbal and nonverbal communication. On top of this, nursing diagnoses, specific goals and a plan of action for the client are also primarily formulated.

此期，护士通过语言和非语言交流收集了更多病例资料，初步制订护理诊断、具体目标和护理措施。

iii. Working Phase

（三）工作期

During this phase, the client begins to relax, and to trusts the nurse. The patient is able to discuss mutually goals and evaluate the results of the plan with the nurse as the assessment process continues, a plan of care develops and the plan of action is being implemented. Perceptions of reality, coping mechanisms, and support systems are identified at this time. Alternative behaviors and techniques are explored to replace those that are maladaptive. Most of the therapeutic work is carried out in this period.

患者逐渐信任护士，放松沟通时护患关系进入工作期。工作期是执行治疗性护理措施的阶段，此期的主要目标是促进患者行为改变；护士的主要任务是执行护理计划，帮助患者改变不良行为。护士与精神疾病患者共同寻找压力源，促进患者在认知、思维、情感及行为方面自知力的恢复。护士应帮助患者控制焦虑、增加独立性、明确自我职责及建立积极的应对机制。

Clients often show resistance behaviors during this phase because in the problem-solving process, he or she will focus on unpleasant, painful aspects of life. The nurse should provide supportive help to the client to avoid impasse's happening, because such behaviors is an important barrier to the progress of the therapeutic relationship.

由于工作期是帮助患者解决问题的过程，患者要面对痛苦的选择与挑战，经常会有抵抗行为。护士应该为患者提供支持性的帮助，以防止因此而阻碍护患关系。

iv. Termination Phase

The termination phase of therapeutic relationship comes when the mutually agreed-on goals are reached, the client is transferred or discharged, or the nurse has finished the clinical rotation. It is one of the most difficult but most important phases of the relationship. It's a time to exchange feelings and memories and to evaluate mutually the client's progress and goal attainment. The evaluations include the client's ability to provide self-care and maintain his or her environment, demonstrate independence and work interdependently with others, display emotional stability and recognize signs of increased stress or anxiety, and cope positively when experiencing feelings of anxiety, anger, or hostility. Levels of trust and intimacy are heightened, reflecting the quality of the relationship and the sense of loss experienced by both the nurse and the client. Some clients may attempt to prolong the relationship as clinical symptoms of separation anxiety are experienced, but termination needs to occur if a therapeutic relationship is to be a complete process. Preparation for termination actually begins during the initiating phase.

（四）结束期

护理目标实现，患者转院、出院或护士结束临床轮转时，护患关系进入结束期。此期的主要目标是评价护理目标是否达到，确保护患关系顺利结束。结束期是护患关系中最困难也是最重要的一个时期。此期护士的任务之一是与患者共同评价所取得的治疗与护理效果，护理目标达到的程度。评价内容包括患者自我照顾和适应外界的能力，情绪稳定并能认识到焦虑和应激并积极应对焦虑、愤怒。护患关系结束时会出现悲伤、失落，护士要与患者共同探索和应对这些情感，帮助患者接受和经历这一过程。分离性焦虑症的患者可能会企图延长护患关系，护士须促使其接受现实，避免拖延。

IV. Professional Characteristic Requirement for Psychiatric Nurses

The nurse's answer to these questions will largely determine the progress of the relationship.

1. Can I be in some way that will be perceived by the other person as trustworthy, as dependable, or consistent in some deep sense?
2. Do I express myself ambiguously?
3. Can I let myself experience positive attitudes toward other person-attitudes of warmth, caring, liking, interest, and respect?
4. Can I be strong enough as a person to be separate from the other?
5. Am I secure enough within myself to permit him his separateness?
6. Can I let myself enter fully into the world of his feelings and personal meaning and see these as he does?
7. Can I be acceptant of each facet of the other person that he presents to me? Can I accept him as he is?
8. Can I communicate this attitude? Or can I only receive him conditionally, acceptant of some aspects of his feelings and silently or openly disapproving of others?
9. Can I act with sufficient sensitivity in the relationship that my behavior will not be perceived as a threat?
10. Can I free him from the threat of external evaluation?

四、精神疾病护理对专科护士的要求

护士对以下问题的回答将在很大程度上决定护患关系的发展：

1. 我是否可信任、可依赖或始终如一？
2. 我的表达是否清晰？
3. 我对患者是否热情、关注，是否持尊敬的态度？
4. 我自身是否独立？
5. 我是否允许他人保持独立？
6. 我是否能真正进入他人的内心与情感世界？
7. 我是否能接受他人的个性？
8. 我是否有条件地接受他人，或只接受他人情感的某些方面，对不赞同的方面保持沉默或公开反对？
9. 我的行为是否对患者造成威胁？
10. 我是否能帮助患者不受外部评价的干扰？

11. Can I meet this other individual as a person who is in the process of becoming, or will I be bound by his past and my past?

In nurse-client relationship, nurses in mental health care are supposed to have the ability to understand herself/himself, to reflect her/his own ability, to note and control her/his feelings and the awareness and ability to set up good example.

11. 我是否可以不受他人和自己过去的影响？

在精神疾病护理的护患关系中，专科护士应具备了解自我、分析自我的能力，具有洞悉和把控情感、树立角色榜样的意识和能力。

V. Barriers of Therapeutic Relationship

五、精神疾病护理护患关系中常见的障碍及护理

There are barriers that can block the progress of the therapeutic nurse-client relationship. These barriers arise for a variety of reasons, but they all create stalls in the relationship. These barriers provoke intense feelings in both the nurse and the client that may range from anxiety and apprehension to frustration, or intense anger. Three barriers are discussed here: resistance, transference, and counter-transference.

阻碍治疗性护患关系的因素会使护士和患者产生焦虑、担心受挫、甚至震怒等强烈的情感反应。识别及克服这些障碍可以帮助护士更好地建立和维持与患者的治疗性关系。治疗性护患关系中常见的障碍包括抵抗，移情及反移情。

i. Resistance

（一）抵抗

Resistance is the client's reluctance or avoidance of verbalizing or experiencing troubling aspects of oneself. Clients usually display resistance behaviors during the working phase of the relationship, because the greater part of the problem-solving process occurs in this period. Resistance may take many forms. Some of its forms are displayed in the following (Walberg, 1988):

抵抗是指护患沟通过程中，患者不愿谈及自身的问题。较常见的抵抗反应的外在表现包括（Wolberg，1988）：

(a) Suppression and repression of pertinent information.

(b) Intensification of symptoms.

(c) Self-devaluation and a hopeless outlook on the future.

(d) Forced flight into health where there is o sudden, but short-lived recovery by the client.

(e) Intellectual inhibitions, which may be evident when the client says she has "nothing on her mind" or that she is "unable to think about her problems" or when she breaks appointments, is late for sessions, or is forgetful, silent, or sleepy.

(f) Acting out or irrational behavior.

(g) Superficial talk.

(h) Intellectual insight in which the client verbalizes self-understanding with correct use of terminology yet continues destructive behavior or uses the defense of intellectualization where there is no insight.

(i) Contempt for normality, which is evident when the client has developed insight but refuses to assume the responsibility for change on the grounds that normality "isn't so great".

① 压抑或隐瞒与疾病相关的信息。

② 精神症状变化明显。

③ 自我贬低、对未来没有希望。

④ 短暂的症状改善。

⑤ 智力下降，如称自己脑子一片空白或无法考虑问题，健忘、沉默、困倦、嗜睡等。

⑥ 喜怒无常。

⑦ 肤浅的交谈。

⑧ 言行不一致。

⑨ 鄙视常人。

(j) Transference reactions.

It is often caused by the client's unwillingness to make necessary changes. Resistance may occur as the client's reaction to a nurse, if she attempts to move to clients feeling too far or too fast, or if somewhat be irrespective whether intentionally or unintentionally in communication with clients. It may also be caused by the unskillfulness of a nurse in taking care of the clients. Another reason of resistance may be caused by secondary benefits of clients from illness, referring to beneficial changes of environment or interpersonal relationship, or even getting material or financial benefit. Types of secondary benefits include financial compensation, avoiding unpleasant situations, getting more sympathy or attention from others, escaping from work or other social responsibilities, attempting to control others, or reducing social pressures for one self. Secondary benefit can become a powerful force for some clients in perpetuating an illness because the illness makes the environment more favorable for them.

When the nurse recognizes the resistance, the first thing he or she must do is to use clarification to get a focused idea of what is happening. Then reflection can be used to help clients become aware of what has been going on in their own minds. On the basis of above works, the nurse and the client may explore and analyze the reasons for the resistance's occurrence and facilitate the relationship progress smoothly.

ii. Transference

Transference is an unconscious response in which the client experiences feelings and attitudes toward the nurse that were originally associated with other significant figures in his or her life. Two types of transference are particularly problematic in the nurse-client relationship. The first is the hostile transference. If the client internalizes anger and hostility, this resistance may be expressed as depression and discouragement. The client may ask to terminate the relationship on the grounds that there is no chance of getting well. If the hostility is externalized, the client may become critical, defiant, and irritable and may express doubts about the nurse's training, experience, or competence. Hostility also may be expressed by the client in detachment, forgetfulness, or irrelevant chatter. An extreme form of uncooperativeness and negativism is evident in prolonged silence. This is not the therapeutic silence that communicates mutuality and understanding, but the silence that seems to be hostile, oppressive, and eternal. It is particularly disturbing for the nurse in the orientation phase, before a relationship has been established. The nurse should understand the meaning of

⑩ 移情。

抵抗产生的原因有两个方面：一方面患者不愿意做出必要的改变。当护士过快或过深地进入患者的内心世界，或在与患者沟通时，有意或无意地表现出不尊重，都可能引起患者的抵抗反应。另一方面是间接性获利。间接性获利指患者患病后，所处环境、人际关系等可能发生与其有利的改变，患者从中获得物质或精神利益。间接性获利的类型包括：① 经济补偿；② 逃避不愉快的情景；③ 得到同情或关注；④ 逃避工作或其他社会责任；⑤ 控制他人；⑥ 减少社会压力。间接性获利可使患者所处的环境变得舒适，因而想持久保持患病状态。

当护士意识到抵抗存在时，应首先澄清主要问题，反思患者的真正想法，然后探讨和分析发生抵抗的原因，促进护患关系的平稳发展。

（二）移情

移情是一种无意识的反应，是患者将对亲人、朋友或其他关系密切者的态度与感情转移到护士身上。两种形式的移情会严重影响护患关系。第一种是带有敌意的移情。如果患者将愤怒和敌意内化，则表现为沮丧和气馁，患者认为好转无望，要求停止治疗。如果敌意被外化，患者则会出现挑剔、不顺从、易激惹，对护士的教育、经验和能力提出质疑，通过健忘或不相关的谈话来表达对护士的敌意。极端不合作和消极态度者表现为长时间带有敌意的沉默，要与相互理解的治疗性沉默相鉴别。在护患关系还未建立的开始期，这种沉默尤其不利于护理工作。护士应努力克服难堪或无所适从，了解患者沉默的含义，并决定如何应对。

the client's silence and decide how to deal with it despite feeling somewhat awkward and uncertain.

A second difficult type of transference is the dependent reaction transference. This resistance is characterized by clients who are submissive, subordinate, and ingratiating and who regard the nurse as a godlike figure. The client over values the nurse's characteristics and qualities, and their relationship are in jeopardy because the client views it as magical. In this reaction the nurse must live up to the client's overwhelming expectations, which is impossible because these expectations are completely unrealistic. The client continues to demand more nurses, and when these needs are not met, the client is filled with hostility and contempt.

第二种是依赖性移情。其特点是患者过高地估计护士的能力，对护士十分顺从，期待护士满足其所有要求。此时的护患关系很危险，因为患者的期待是不切实际的。患者不断向护士提出更多的需求而得不到满足时，则产生敌意和蔑视。

Transference may be triggered by a similarity in appearance, such as similar facial feature or manner of speech, or by similar personality style or trait. The most obvious manifestation of transference is the inappropriate intensity of the client's response. Transference reduces self-awareness by allowing the client to maintain an inaccurate view of the world in which all people are seen in similar terms. Thus the nurse may be viewed as an authority figure, such as parents, or as a lost loved one such as a former spouse. These reactions may become harmful to the therapeutic process; even it is a client's attempt to reduce anxiety.

移情可因为外表或行为特征的相似而引发，如容貌特征、讲话方式或性格特征等。移情最显著的表现是患者情感反应的强度不当。移情使患者根据类似特征看待所有人，降低了认知能力。护士可能被视为权威人物，如父母，或是失去的亲人，如配偶。患者试图用这种方式减轻其焦虑，但不当的移情会影响治疗过程。

Transferences coming from the client can be difficult problems for the nurse. To achieve therapeutic relationship's progress, the nurse must be prepared to be exposed to and deal with the client's powerful negative and positive emotional feelings, often on an irrational basis. Whatever the client's motivations, the analysis of the transference is geared toward the client gaining awareness of these motivations and learning about being completely responsible for all actions and behavior.

患者移情会阻碍护患关系的发展。护士必须做好准备，正确地面对和处理患者强烈的、非理性的消极或积极的情绪。与患者共同分析，使其意识到移情的内在动机，并学会对自身的言行负责。

iii. Counter-transference

（三）反向移情

Counter-transference is transference applied to the nurse. It is a therapeutic impasse caused by the nurse's specific emotional response to the qualities of the client. This response is inappropriate to the content and context of the therapeutic relationship and inappropriate in the degree of intensity of emotion. Inappropriateness is the important element, as it is with transference, because it is natural that the nurse will have a feeling of warmth toward of liking for some clients more than others. The nurse also will be genuinely angry about the actions of certain clients. But in counter-transference, the nurse's responses are not justified by reality. In this case, nurses identify the client with individuals from their past, and personal needs interfere with their therapeutic effectiveness.

反向移情是护士对患者的某些特征产生了特殊的情感。护士的护理工作和情绪具有针对性，对某些患者更加热情，或更容易动怒，对其他的患者却并非如此。护士发生反向移情时不利于治疗性护患关系的建立与发展。

Three types of reactions are contained in counter-transference: reactions of intense love or caring, reactions of intense disgust or hostility, reactions of intense anxiety often in response to resistance by the client. They are expressed by many forms, following are some examples:

1. Feelings of depression during or after the session.

2. Carelessness about implementing the contract by being late, running overtime, etc.

3. Difficulty empathizing with the client in certain problem areas.

4. Drowsiness during the sessions.

5. Feeling of anger or impatience because of the client's unwillingness to change.

6. Encouragement of the client's dependency, praise, or affection.

7. Arguments with the client or a tendency to push before the client are ready.

8. Attempts to help the client in matters not related to the identified nursing goals.

9. Personal or social involvement with the client.

10. Dreams about or preoccupation with the client.

11. Sexual or aggressive fantasies toward the client.

12. Recurrent anxiety, unease, or guilt related to the client.

13. Tendency to focus on only one aspect or way of looking at information presented by the client.

14. Need to defend nursing interventions with the client to others.

To promote therapeutic goals, the nurse should constantly use self-examination throughout the course of the relationship to look out counter-transference, becomes aware of it when it occurs, and exercises control over it. Because counter-transference can be harmful to the relationship, it should be dealt with as soon as possible. If the nurse needs help in dealing with it, individual of group supervision can be most helpful.

精神疾病护理过程中，护士常见的三种反向移情反应有强烈的爱或关怀、强烈的厌恶或敌意、因患者的抵抗产生强烈的焦虑。其具体表现为：

1. 与患者会谈时或会谈后感到沮丧。

2. 执行护理计划时粗心大意，延迟，超时等。

3. 难以体谅患者的情感。

4. 会谈时昏昏欲睡，精神不振。

5. 由于患者的不合作而感到恼火或急躁。

6. 易对患者的依赖、表扬或感情产生反应。

7. 与患者争论，或在患者还未做好准备时就催促患者。

8. 试图在与护理目标以外的问题上帮助患者。

9. 与患者有个人或社会关系的纠葛。

10. 梦到患者或对患者魂不守舍。

11. 对患者有性或攻击幻想。

12. 与患者有关的反复焦虑、不安或内疚感。

13. 只对某个患者的信息感兴趣。

14. 需要与患者辩解对他人的护理措施。

精神疾病护理过程中，专科护士应在护患关系进展过程中经常进行自我反思，评估自己是否存在反向移情，及时进行自我调节。如果护士意识到自己存在反向移情但无法解决则需寻求专业帮助。

Section 2 Therapeutic Communication

第二节　治疗性沟通

Group cannot exist without communication, nor can nurses practice without communication. Communication is process of transferring information in the various media from one point, person or device to another. It is the main vehicle for establishing a nurse-client relationship.

沟通是通过各种途径将信息从某个地方、人或设备传递给另一方，是建立护患关系的主要工具。沟通既可能有利于护患关系的建立，也可能阻碍护患关系。在精神疾病护理

It can either facilitate the development of a therapeutic relationship or serve as a barrier to it. Therapeutic communication is the purposeful use of verbal and nonverbal communication skills to bring about the client's insight, control of symptoms, and/or healing. A positive nurse-client relationship is helpful for the implement therapeutic communication. The relation of relationship and communication is reciprocal.

中，治疗性沟通是有目的地应用语言和非语言沟通技巧，使患者提高自知力、控制症状以及最大限度的康复。良性的护患关系有助于治疗性沟通，二者相辅相成。

I. Therapeutic Communication Techniques

一、治疗性沟通技巧

To interact effectively with mentally ill clients, the nurse must grasp many therapeutic communication techniques and use them appropriately. Although simple on the surface, these techniques are difficult and require practice. If they are used appropriately, they can enhance the nurse's effectiveness. If they are used as automatic responses, they will block the formation of a therapeutic relationship, negate both the nurse's the client's individuality, and divest them of their dignity. These techniques are discussed now below.

精神科专科护士必须掌握和正确运用治疗性沟通技巧，以便与精神障碍患者进行有效沟通。灵活地运用这些沟通技巧能提高护士的工作效率，而机械地使用沟通技巧，则会忽略护士与患者的个体差异，损伤其尊严，从而阻碍治疗性关系的建立与发展。

i. Listening

（一）倾听

Listening is perhaps the most important communication technique, for it involves being fully present for another while obtaining information needed to truly understand the client. There are two types of listening, passive and active. Passive listening involves sitting quietly and letting the client talk. A passive listener allows the client to ramble and does not focus or guide the thought process. Passive listening does not foster a therapeutic relationship. Body language during passive listening usually communicates boredom, indifference, or hostility.

患者的情感、思维和感知等信息，只能通过倾听其亲自描述才能获得。因此，倾听是沟通的基础，是最常用的沟通技巧。

Active listening focus on what the client is saying to be able to interpret and respond to the message in an objective manner. With active listening the nurse communicates acceptance and respect for the client, and trust is enhanced. A climate is established within the relationship that promotes openness and honest expression. While listening, the nurse concentrates only on what the client is saying and the underlying meaning. He or she should usually responds to the client and not be preoccupied. Several nonverbal behaviors have been designated as facilitative skills for active listening.

倾听有两种形式，即主动倾听和被动倾听。主动倾听指倾听过程中不仅关注患者语言表述，而且关注患者的非语言信息。在倾听过程中，护士将注意力集中于患者，注重理解其语言表述及其内在含义。主动倾听表达了护士对患者的接纳、尊重和信任，有利于在治疗性关系中形成坦诚、开放的氛围。被动倾听是倾听患者讲述，不做任何引导和干扰。护士要注意自己的肢体语言；因为对患者而言，被动倾听时的肢体语言有时会传递出负面信息。因此，有些被动倾听有碍于形成治疗性的护患关系。

BOX 3-2 Learning More

SOLER of Active Listening

Those listed as active listening can be identified by the acronym SOLER.

S—Sit squarely facing the client. This gives the message that the nurse is there to listen and is interested in what the client has to say.

O—Observe an open posture. Posture is considered "open" when arms and legs remain uncrossed. This suggests that the nurse is "open" to what the client has to say. With a "close" position, the nurse can convey a somewhat defensive stance, possibly invoking a similar response in the client.

L—Lean forward toward the client. This conveys to the client that you are involved in the interaction, interested in what is being said, and making a sincere effort to be attentive.

E—Establish eye contact. Direct eye contact is another behavior that conveys the nurse's involvement and willingness to listen to what the client has to say. The absence of eye contact, or the constant shifting of eye contact, gives the message that the nurse is not really interested in what is being said. (Note: Ensure that eye contact conveys warmth and is accompanied by smiling and intermittent nodding of the head, and that it does not come across as staring or glaring, which can create intense discomfort in the client.)

R—Relax. Whether sitting or standing during the interaction, the nurse should communicate a sense of being relaxed and comfortable with the client. Restlessness and fidgetiness communicate a lack of interest and a feeling of discomfort that are likely to be transferred to the client.

BOX 3-2 知识拓展

倾听的 SOLER 技巧

一些非语言行为可以增进主动倾听技巧，可用英文首字母表示为 SOLER。

S：呈直角坐于患者对面，表示护士专心听患者讲述对所涉及话题感兴趣。

O：保持姿势开放，即手臂和腿不交叉，表示护士对患者讲述的内容保持开放的态度。若护士若采用“封闭”姿势，则会向患者传递一种防御性的态度，使患者产生类似的反应。

L：向患者方向前倾，表示护士主动参与互动，集中精力听取信息及对谈论话题感兴趣。

E：建立眼神接触。眼神接触是另一种表达护士愿意参与及接收信息的方式。缺乏眼神接触或眼神游移，会让患者以为护士对其话题不感兴趣。（注意：眼神接触时应注意眼神的温和，同时要面带微笑，并不时地点头，避免引起患者不适的凝视或瞪视。）

R：放松。在互动过程中无论站或坐，护士都应以放松舒适的姿态与患者沟通。坐立不安或烦躁会向患者暗示护士对话题不感兴趣，而且这种不适感觉很可能会传递给患者。

ii. Silence

The nurse's silence encourages the client to feel and explore emotions. To a vocal client, silence on the part of the nurse may be welcome, as long as the client knows the nurse is listening. With a depressed client, the nurse's silence may convey support, understanding, and acceptance.

Silence can also prompt the client to talk. Some introverted people find out that they can be quiet but still be liked. Silence allows the client time to think and to gain insights and self-awareness. Finally, Silence can slow the pace of the interaction. Sometimes when the nurse is unsure how to respond to a client's comments, a safe approach is to maintain silence. If the nurse's nonverbal

（二）沉默

护士的沉默可以鼓励患者思考、反省和体验情感。在交谈时，只要患者知道自己在聆听，护士可以保持沉默。对于抑郁患者，护士的沉默意味着支持、理解和接受。

护士的沉默也会鼓励患者倾诉。有些人虽然很安静，但仍然招人喜欢。护士的沉默让患者有时间思考，获得洞察力和自我反省。最后，沉默还能放慢互动的节奏。当护士不确定如何应对患者时，保持沉默是一个安全的方法。如果护士的非语言行为传递了感兴趣和参与的信息，患者通常会进一步说明或

behavior communicates interest and involvement, the client often will elaborate or discuss a related issue.

讨论相关问题。

iii. Broad Openings

Broad openings are words that permit the client to decide the manner of the response. Comments such as "What are you thinking about?" "What shall we discuss today?" and "What's on your mind today?" are all broad openings. Such statements let the client know the nurse wants to listen and permit the client a wide range of responses. The client will choose the topic, as well as the degree to which he will open up to disclose inner feelings. The broad openings allow the nurse to get the conversation started without making demands that the client talk about one particular subject.

（三）开放式表达

开放式表达是让患者来决定回答方式的措辞。它能使护士与患者的沟通不局限于某一特定主题。例如："你在想什么？""我们今天讨论什么呢？""你今天想到了什么？"等都属开放式表达。此类陈述表明护士想了解患者，并允许患者选择谈话的主题及对内心想法的暴露程度。

iv. Restating

Restating is a technique whereby the nurse repeats the main message the client has expressed. Restating lets the client know that the nurse is truly listening and making every attempt to understand. It can also serve as reinforcement or bring attention to something important that might otherwise have been passed over. For example, the client may say "I cannot learn anything; my brain is preoccupied with other things". The nurse can restate as "do you have difficulties in concentration?"

（四）复述

复述是指护士重复患者所表达的主要信息。复述可以让患者知道护士在认真倾听，并努力理解所接收的信息，从而决定是继续讲述，还是做必要的澄清。复述也可使双方共同关注那些可能会被忽略的重要信息。例如患者说："我不能学习，我脑子一直在想其他事情"。护士可以重述："您集中注意力有困难"。

v. Clarification

Clarification is a technique whereby the nurse tries to put the client's ideas into a simple statement. It is necessary because statements about emotions and behaviors are rarely straightforward. The client's verbalizations, especially if the client is upset or overwhelmed with feelings, are not always clear and obvious. Nothing should be allowed to pass that the nurse does not hear or understand. Because of this uncertainty, clarification responses often are tentative or phrased as questions. The nurse might say, "Are you saying that..." and fill in the messages she has heard to check her understanding and to make the client's thoughts or feelings explicit.

（五）澄清

澄清是指护士用简单的陈述来概括患者的想法。因为患者很少直截了当地表达感情和行为，必须借助澄清来明确其真实的含义。当患者烦躁或处于其他不良情绪时，其语言表达也经常不清楚或不明确。澄清经常是用试探性或提问性语气，例如："我不明白您的意思，您是说……吗？"或"您能再说一遍吗？"等。

vi. Reflection

Reflection is interpreting back to the client what has been heard and understood. Reflection of content is also called validation, it lets the client know that the nurse has heard that was said and understands the content. It consists of repeating the essential ideas of the client in fewer words. Sometimes it helps to repeat a client's statement, emphasizing a key word. Different from restating, reflection allows the nurse to describe a theme that the client has not identified verbally. Therefore, reflection must be used when the nurse has a good understanding of what is important to the client.

Reflection of feelings consists of responses to the

（六）反应

反应是指护士向患者解释听到的内容和自己的理解，分为内容反应和情感反应。内容反应也称确认，指用少而精的语言描述患者的主要意思，有时仅需重复患者的部分陈述或强调一个关键词。它能让患者知道护士已经听到并理解了所讲述的内容。反应不同于复述，它允许护士说出患者没有表达的含义。因此，护士可以使用反应来表达对患者的理解。

情感反应指对患者在谈话中情感的理解

client's feelings about the content. It may be a statement such as "It sound like you got mad when your roommate left the toilet dirty." reflecting on the situation and the client's feelings. These responses let the client know that the nurse is aware of what the client is feeling. Broad openings, restatements, clarifications, and reflections of content need not represent empathic understanding. But reflection of feeling signifies understanding, empathy, interest, and respect for the client. It increases the level of involvement between the nurse and the client. The purpose of reflecting feeling is to focus on feeling rather than content to bring the client's vaguely expressed feelings into clear awareness; it helps the client accept or own those feelings. The steps in reflection of feelings are to determine what feeling the client is expressing, describe these feeling clearly, observe the effect, and judge by the client's reaction whether the reflection was correct.

vii. Focusing

Focusing is a technique in which the nurse directs the conversation to focus on a topic of particular importance or relevance to the client. For example, the nurse may say "it is worth thinking of this carefully, and we can discuss this together". Effectively used, it can help the client become more specific, move from vagueness to clarity, and focus on reality.

By avoiding abstractions and generalizations, focusing helps the client face problems and analyzes them in detail. It helps a client talk about life experiences or problem areas and accept the responsibility for improving them. Encouraging a description of the client's perceptions, encouraging comparisons, and placing events in time sequence are focusing skills that promote specificity and problem analysis.

viii. Informing

Informing, or information giving, is an essential nursing technique in which the nurse shares simple facts with the client. It is a skill used by nurses in health teaching or client education, such as informing a client when to take medication and about necessary precautions and side effects. In psychiatric nursing, the client often needs information about his or her illness, the etiology and genetic basis of his or her disease, the legal aspects of care, and alternatives for medication and treatment.

ix. Suggesting

Suggesting is often used to encourage a client to consider alternatives. As a therapeutic technique, it is a useful intervention in the working phase of the relationship when the client has analyzed the problem area and is exploring alternative coping mechanisms. At that time, suggestions by the nurse will increase the client's perceived options.

与表达。例如:“你的室友把盥洗室弄脏，你好像非常生气”，既说明了当时的情形，又反映了患者的情感，使患者知道护士能理解其感觉。开放式表达、重述、澄清、内容反应都不需要移情，而情感反应则意味着对患者的理解、移情、关心和尊重，深化了护士与患者间的互动。情感反应的目的是将患者表达较为模糊的情感阐述得更清楚，并帮助患者接受这些情感。情感反应的步骤为：① 确定患者表达的情感；② 清楚地描述这些情感；③ 观察效果；④ 最后通过患者的反应判断情感反应是否正确。

（七）集中焦点

集中焦点是指由护士引导交谈，将话题集中在对患者有意义的主题上。例如，护士可以说:“这点值得仔细研究，我们可以一起讨论一下”。有效地运用此技巧能帮助患者更明确、清晰地表达自己，逐步面向现实。

集中焦点能帮助患者面对及详细分析问题，帮助其回顾生活经历及问题，使其承担完善自我的责任。集中焦点技术包括鼓励患者描述自我感觉；鼓励对事件进行对比；按时间顺序排列事件等。

（八）提供信息

提供信息是护士将客观事实告诉患者的一种基本护理技巧。护士在进行健康指导或患者教育时经常使用它，例如护士提醒患者服药，说明服用药物的作用和副作用等。在精神科护理中，患者常需要有关疾病、疾病原因和遗传学基础、法律方面以及药物选择和治疗等方面的信息。

（九）建议

建议是向患者提供备选方案。在治疗性关系工作期，建议是一种有用的干预措施。因为此时患者已对问题进行了分析，正在探索可供选择的应对方式，护士的建议可以增加患者的选择范围。

Suggesting also is non-therapeutic if it occurs early in the relationship before the client has analyzed personal conflicts or if it is a technique the nurse uses frequently. Then it negates the possibility of mutuality and implies that the client is incapable of assuming responsibility for thoughts and actions.

The nurse's intent in using the suggesting technique should be to provide feasible alternatives and allow the client to explore his or her potential value. The nurse can then focus on helping the client explore the advantages and disadvantages and the meaning and implications of the alternatives. In this way suggestions can be offered in a non-authoritarian manner with such phrases as "Some people have tried...Do you think that would work for you?"

x. Confronting

Confronting is communication that points out inconsistencies between feelings, thoughts, and actions. As a therapeutic tool, confrontation can encourage clients to explore maladaptive behaviors and further the client's growth and progress if used correctly.

Confrontation is not limited to negative aspects of the client. It includes pointing out discrepancies involving resources and strengths that are unrecognized and unused. It requires that the nurse collect sufficient data about the client's history and accumulate sufficient perceptions and observations of verbal and nonverbal communication so that validation of reality is possible.

The nurse must have developed an understanding of the client to perceive discrepancies, inconsistencies in word and deed, distortions, defenses, and evasions. The nurse must be willing and be able to work through the crisis after confronting the client. Without this commitment the confrontation lacks therapeutic potential and can be damaging to both the nurse and the client. Without question, the effects of confrontation are challenge, are possible for growth.

It is reported that effective counselors use confrontation frequently, confronting clients with their assets more often in earlier interviews and with their limitations in later interviews. In the initial interview, these confrontations were based on attempts to clarify the relationship, eliminate misconceptions, give clients more objective information about themselves and their world, and emphasize client strengths and resources. However, inexperienced nurses often avoid confrontation for not understanding its connotation and effectiveness.

xi. Accepting

Accepting is encouraging and receiving information in a nonjudgmental and interested manner. It is used to convey an attitude of reception and regard. It can help

如果在护患关系建立初期，患者还没有分析个人冲突就提供建议，或者护士频繁地使用建议，则会阻碍治疗性关系。因为它否定了护士与患者间的互动，意味着患者没有能力为自己的思想、行为负责。

护士运用建议的目的是为患者提供切实可行的备选方案，应鼓励患者探究自身的潜能，帮助患者探讨备选方案的优点与缺点、目的与含义。提供建议时可以采用较为民主的方式，例如："一些人已经试着……你认为这样做对你有用吗"。

（十）质疑

质疑是指出对方在情感、思想和行为方面的差异。质疑作为一种治疗性工具，如果正确地使用，可以鼓励患者探究其不良行为，促进患者进一步成长与发展。

质疑并不限于患者的不良方面，还包括指出未得到识别和使用的资源与能力。护士要充分收集患者的有关资料，仔细观察患者的语言和非语言沟通行为。

护士应及时察觉出患者言语和行为中的不一致、歪曲、对抗和回避等问题。护士在质疑患者后，必须愿意并能够解决危机。否则，质疑将缺乏治疗意义，并可能对护士和患者造成不利影响。质疑具有挑战性、暴露性和危险性，并蕴藏着成长。

据报道，成功的咨询者经常使用质疑，在初期的会谈中让患者面对本身的优势，在后期的会谈中让患者面对本身的局限性。因为在起始阶段，质疑是为了与患者澄清关系、消除误解，帮助其更多地了解自己，重视自身的能力和资源。但是，经验不足的护士由于不理解质疑的内涵和效果，常常避免使用质疑。

（十一）接纳

接受是以非批判式的、感兴趣的方式表达和接受信息。它表示认可和尊敬，有助于

the client develop confidence and express more about inner feelings. It also helps the nurse to build the trust and empathy with the client. For example, the nurse may say "yes, I understand what you are saying" with eye contact and nodding at the same time.

患者树立信心，更多地表达内心的感受和想法，有利于护士建立信任和同理心。例如，护士可以对患者说："是的，我理解你所说的"，并同时给予眼神接触和点头示意。

xii. Exploring

Exploring means delving further into a subject, idea, experience, or relationship. It is especially helpful with clients who tend to remain on a superficial level of communication. However, if the client chooses not to disclose further information, the nurse should refrain from pushing or probing in an area that obviously creates discomfort. For example, "Please explain this to me in detail" or "Can we talk about the issue again?"

（十二）探索

探索指进一步探讨话题、思想、经历和深入相互关系。对那些只想把沟通保持在表面阶段的患者来说，探索尤为重要。但是，如果患者不愿透露更多的信息，护士应避免一味地追根问底，以免引起患者不适。例如，"请详细解释一下这个情况"或"能否将那件事情再谈一下"。

xiii. Humor

Humor is a basic part of the personality and a constructive coping behavior. As a planned approach to nursing intervention, humor can promote insight by making conscious repressed material. It has an important place within the therapeutic communication and relationship. A change in the expression of humor and the quality of interpersonal relationships may be indicators of significant change in the client.

The functions that humor holds in the nurse-client relationship can be positive or negative. There are no rules for determining how, when, or where humor should be used in the interaction. It depends on the nature and quality of the relationship, the client's receptivity to such themes, and the relevance of the tale or witticism. Following are some instructions of how to use humor in psychiatric settings:

1. When the client is experiencing mild to moderate levels of anxiety, humor serves as a tension reducer. It is inappropriate if a client has severe or panic anxiety level.

2. When it helps a client cope more effectively facilitates learning, puts life situations in perspective, decreases social distance, and is understood by the client for its therapeutic value. It is inappropriate when it promotes maladaptive coping responses, masks feelings, increases social distance, and helps the individual avoid dealing with difficult situations.

3. When it is consistent with the social and cultural values of the client and when it allows the client to laugh at life, the human situation, or a particular set of stressors. It is inappropriate when it violates a client's values, ridicules people, or belittles others.

（十三）幽默

幽默是人格特征的一个基本部分，属于积极的应对方式。幽默作为护理干预的方法，能通过认识被压抑的思想和情感来提高患者的自知力，在治疗性沟通和护患关系中具有重要意义。幽默和人际关系的改善，常标志着患者病情的显著好转。

在精神科护理中，运用幽默应注意以下几点：

1. 当患者有轻度到中度焦虑时，幽默是紧张的缓解剂。但对于严重焦虑患者，应慎用。

2. 恰当的幽默能帮助患者更有效地应对困难、促进学习，对生活充满希望，缩短与社会的距离，且能被患者理解。

3. 恰当的幽默与患者社会文化价值观是一致的，或能使患者笑对生活、人生境遇或特殊压力。

II. Barriers of Therapeutic Communication

It is considered that some approaches can block the nurse-client interaction and inhibit therapeutic communication. The nurse should recognize and eliminate the use of these patterns in his or her communication with clients. Avoiding these barriers will maximize the effectiveness of communication and enhance the nurse-client relationship.

i. Giving Advice

Giving advice is telling the client what need to do and how to do. Normally, the client hopes that he or she can get advice from health professionals. The nurse also believes that it is her responsibility to make the judgment for the client. However, this may increase the client's dependency and pose the responsibility to nurses. If the client takes the nurses advice with poor result, the client may blame the nurse. Seeking advice is reaction of dependence, since the client has known the answers before asking for it. Feelings of dependency and inadequacy may then impair therapeutic communication if the client receives no positive feedback during nurse-client interactions. It is much more constructive to encourage problem solving by the client.

ii. Reassurance

Reassurance such as "Everything will be OK" indicates to the client that there is no cause for anxiety, thereby devaluing the client's feelings. There are too many variables. No one can predict or guarantee the outcome of a situation. If clients who receive reassurance do not respond to treatment as predicted, they will quickly learn not to trust the nurse and become more discouraged.

iii. Agreeing/Disagreeing

Agreeing or disagreeing indicates accord with or opposition to the client's ideas or opinions implies that the nurse has the right to pass judgment on whether the client's ideas or opinions are "right" or "wrong". Agreement by the nurse denies the opportunity for the client to change or modify his or her point of view. Disagree implies inaccuracy, may result in the development of a low self-concept or provoke the need for defensiveness on the part of the client. Such expressions include "this is right, I agree" or "this is wrong, I do not agree".

iv. Giving Approval/Disapproval

Giving approval or disapproval implies that the nurse has the right to pass judgment on whether the client's

二、沟通中的常见障碍

有些沟通方式可能会阻碍护患之间的有效沟通，护士应该识别并避免使用它们，改善沟通的效果，促进良好护患关系的发展。

（一）给予意见

给予意见是指告诉患者应该做什么，或应该如何去做。一些患者希望能从专业人员处得到行动的意见。同样，护士也常觉得自身职责是提供带有判断性的意见，从而会增强患者的依赖感，并把责任留给了护士。如果患者接受了护士的意见，但结果并不理想，患者会反过来责备护士。索求意见通常是依赖性的表现，其实患者已经知道应该如何去做。在护患交流过程中，如果患者不能得到正面的反馈，则患者依赖性和未被满足的感觉会损害治疗性关系，因此，应积极鼓励患者自己解决问题。

（二）反复保证

如"一切都会好的""如果我是你，我不会担心的"之类的保证意味着患者没有什么可担心的，因而忽视了患者的情感。事物发展中有很多的不确定因素，难以预测或保证其最终结果。如果患者得到的保证与预期结果不符，则会产生悲观心理，不再信任护士，使得以后的沟通失去治疗意义。

（三）同意或不同意

同意或不同意指认可或反对患者的意见或想法，意味着护士有权利判断患者的意见或想法的"对"或"错"。护士的同意会让患者失去改变或修改自己观点的机会；而不同意则意味着患者的观点是错误的，可能造成患者的自我概念下降，或激起患者的自我防御。如"这是对的，我同意""这是错误的，我不同意"等皆属这类表达。

（四）赞成或不赞成

赞成或不赞成意味着护士有权利判断患者的想法或行为是"好"还是"坏"，而患者

ideas or behaviors are "good" or "bad" and that the client is expected to please the nurse. The nurse's acceptance of the client is then seen as conditional, depending on the client's behavior. It is not helpful to the development of the therapeutic relationship. For example, "I am very happy that you can do it in this way" or "It is not good to do it, I would rather you do not do it."

要用行为来取悦护士。患者会认为护士的判断有条件，因而不利于治疗性关系的建立。如"我很高兴你这样做""那样做不好，我宁愿你不要……"等。

v. Challenging

When the nurse considers that the client's ideas or beliefs are improper and ridiculous, he or she may challenge the client with arguments, logical thinking, or accurate theory. The purpose of the nurse may want the client to recognize the incorrectness of his or her own ideas and remodel it. But this is impossible even if the nurse win in the disputation, because challenges often hurt the client and make him or her feel being belittled. Challenging not only cannot change the client's ideas and thoughts, but also may provoke his or her hostility, and then will block the progress of the therapeutic relationship.

（五）挑衅

当护士认为患者的想法或信念不正确或荒谬，就可能会通过辩论、推理或理论向患者挑衅。虽然护士的目的是想让患者认识到其错误的想法，并改正它，但即使护士在争论中获胜，患者也不会承认错误。因为争论常会伤害患者，使其感觉受轻视、自我概念下降。挑衅不仅不能改变患者的观点与想法，还可能激起敌意，阻碍治疗性关系的发展。

vi. Rejecting

Rejecting means refusing to consider or showing contempt for the client's ideas or behavior. This may cause the client to discontinue interaction with the nurse for fear of further rejection. The nurse may tell the client as "let us not discuss this" or "I do not want to hear..."

（六）拒绝

拒绝表示不考虑患者的意见，轻视患者的思想及行为，使患者因为害怕再次遭到拒绝而停止与护士的互动。如护士对患者说"让我们不要讨论……""我不想听到……"等。

vii. Over questioning or Investigating Questions

Over questioning or investigating questions refers to keeping ask questions from a client, even he or she does not want to talk about a topic. The client may feel that the nurse is imposed or irrespective for him, which may cause emotion resistance as the result. Therefore, the nurse needs pay more attention to clients' response in the communication process. If the client feels uncomfortable, the nurse needs to stop communication or interacting with clients and avoid investigating questions. For example, "Tell me, how did your mother abuse you when you were a child?" or "Tell me, how do you think about your mother after she passed away?"

（七）过度发问或调查式的提问

过度发问或调查式的提问指对患者持续提问，对其不愿讨论的话题也要寻求答案。这会使患者感到被利用和不被尊重，而对护士产生抵触情绪。因此，护士应该注意患者的反应，在患者感到不适时及时停止互动，避免对患者采用调查式的提问，如"告诉我在你小时候，你妈妈是如何虐待你的"或"告诉我你妈妈去世以后，你是如何看待她的"等。

viii. Denial

When the nurse denies that a problem exists, he or she blocks communication with the client and avoids helping the client identify and explore areas of difficulty. For example, the client may say "It is no worth living in the world." The nurse may replies as "How could you say such despondent word?" Such answer will make the client stop further talking.

（八）否定

当护士否定患者的看法或感受时，就为自己与患者的共同讨论设立了障碍，也就不可能帮助患者识别和找出所存在的困难。护士的否定会让患者感到不被接受，因而阻碍了患者的表达。如患者说"我活着没有意思。"护士回答："你怎么能说这种丧气的话呢？"这样就会使患者不愿意继续表达。

ix. Changing Subject

Changing the subject causes the nurse to take over the direction of the discussion. This may occur in order to get to something that the nurse wants to discuss with the client or to get away from a topic that he or she would prefer not to discuss. The nurse should keep the open attitude and listen to the client's expression rather than change subjects. Otherwise, the client may feel that the nurse is not interested in what she was talking and stop the communication with the nurse.

（九）改变话题

改变话题是指护士主导了谈话的方向，多见于当护士想得到某些信息或避开某个话题时。护士应保持开放的态度，倾听患者的表述，而不要突然随意改变话题，否则会使患者感到护士对其不感兴趣而中断与护士的沟通。

III. Record of the Therapeutic Communication

Nursing records is a means by which the nurse-client relationship is analyzed and nurses can use all kinds of helpful therapeutic communication technique. Nursing records includes content of the communication, interpretation of the communication techniques and assessment of being therapeutic. Several types of records are used to communicate information about clients, including verbal and nonverbal communication. Generally records include client identification and clarification of the meaning of clients' words, key points and barriers of the communication. The communication process record is not a nursing document. However, it is a very useful tool of therapeutic communication, and it is particularly useful for beginning learners. It is also useful in situation such as communication difficulties.

The nurse-client relationship is the core of nursing, based on helpful and therapeutic communication. Psychiatric nurse should learn the therapeutic communication techniques and put them into developing therapeutic nurse-client relationship.

(Gu Yanmei)

三、沟通记录

沟通记录是逐字地记录下沟通的内容、护士对所使用的特定沟通技巧的解释，以及该沟通是否为治疗性的评估。它是分析护患互动的工具，可以帮助护士有效地使用各种治疗性的沟通技巧。过程记录格式多样，通常包括护士和患者的语言和非语言的沟通。过程记录可向护士提供许多信息，通过对它的分析可帮助护士识别和明确患者言语的内涵、关键问题，以及沟通中的障碍。过程记录本身并非文件，但应该作为专业发展的一种学习工具，特别是初次学习治疗性沟通或当沟通遇到困难的时候。

护患关系是护理工作开展的核心，建立在护士与患者治疗性沟通的基础上。因此，精神科专科护士掌握治疗性沟通技巧可使护患关系紧紧围绕着患者的治疗性目标展开。

（谷岩梅）

Key Points

1. The nurse-client relationship is a professional and therapeutic relationship. It is a mutual learning experience and a corrective emotional experience for the client. The nurse uses personal attributes and specified clinical techniques in working with the client to bring about behavioral change.

2. Conditions such as trust, empathy, rapport, respect, genuineness, self-disclosure, concreteness, and immediacy are essential to develop therapeutic relationship.

3. In terms of nursing tasks, the nurse-client relationship is divided into four continuous phases: the pre-interaction

内容摘要

1. 护患关系是一种专业性、治疗性及目的性的人际关系。在护患关系中，护士利用个人品质和沟通技巧来帮助患者改变行为，而患者也可以经历正确的情感体验。

2. 护患关系的基础为信任、同理心、和谐关系、尊重、真诚、自我暴露、具体化。

3. 治疗性护患关系可分为四个时期：互动前期、开始期、工作期、结束期。

phase, the orientation phase, the working phase, and the termination phase.

4. Therapeutic impasses such as resistance, transference, and counter-transference are roadblocks in the progress of the nurse-client relationship.

5. Helpful therapeutic communication techniques such as listening, silence, restating, clarification, and so on were presented.

6. Non therapeutic techniques that can inhibit nurse-client communication such as giving advice, reassurance, agreeing/disagreeing, and so on should be avoided.

4. 精神疾病护理中治疗性护患关系的障碍有抵抗、移情和反移情。

5. 倾听、沉默、重述、澄清等沟通技巧的使用有利于建立治疗性护患关系。

6. 给予意见、反复保证等方式会阻碍治疗性沟通，应尽量避免使用。

Exercises

(Questions 1 to 2 share the same question stem)

Li is a green hand nurse in Psychiatric Unit. When she sees patients' suffering, she shows her sympathy by saying "Everything will be fine. It's going to be OK."

1. Is there any problem with Li's communication with the patients?

2. What results may this kind of communication lead to?

(Questions 3 to 4 share the same question stem)

Zhang has been a nurse for 20 years. Her parents are suffering from sickness, her husband is unemployed and her son is in a critical period in his study. Whenever the patients talk about their life pressure and discomforts, Zhang would take herself as an example to comfort the patients.

3. What results would this kind of communication lead to?

4. What are the precautions of this kind of communication?

思考题

（1～2题共用题干）

护士小李新近入职，当他看到精神疾病患者的痛苦时非常同情，因此常常安慰患者“一切都会好起来的，会好起来的。”

1. 请问护士小李在与患者的沟通方式存在什么问题？

2. 这样的沟通方式会给护患关系带来哪些后果？

（3～4题共用题干）

高年资张护士已经工作近20年，她家里有生病的老人，爱人失业在家，孩子面临高考，因此，当她听到患者讲述患病的痛苦和生活压力时，张护士都会叙述自己的家庭情况，安慰患者。

3. 分析张护士的沟通方式和可能的效果？

4. 在与患者进行此类信息交换时应注意哪些问题？

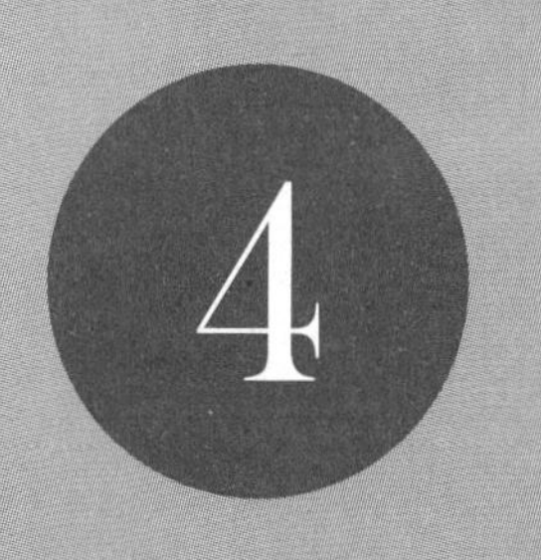

Chapter 4 Common Contingency and its Nursing Interventions

第四章　精神科常见的意外与防范

Learning Objectives

Memorization

1. Accurately summarize the common causes of aggressive behavior.
2. Correctly describe the concept and classification of suicide.

Comprehension

1. Identify the signs of aggressive behavior.
2. Correctly analyze the psychological process of suicide.

Application

1. By means of nursing assessment, work out a plan to rebuild behavior pattern together with client who has aggressive intention.
2. Use nursing procedure to assess suicide signs of client who has suicide intentions and take appropriate precautions.

学习目标

识记

1. 能准确概括攻击行为的常见原因。
2. 能正确描述自杀的概念与分类。

理解

1. 能识别攻击行为的先兆行为。
2. 能正确分析自杀行为的心理过程。

运用

1. 能运用护理评估与有攻击倾向的患者商议制订一份重建行为方式的计划。
2. 能运用护理程序评估有自杀意念患者的自杀征兆并采取相应的防范措施。

Peter, 18-year-old boy, is a student at grade 3 of senior high school. In the past three months, he felt classmates and neighbors talked about him, mocking and saying he was an adopted kid abandoned by others. He could not concentrate his minds during class time and felt difficult to study. At night he cannot sleep well and always conflicts with roommates. In the late 2 months he felt others always make comment about him in his mind and became sleepless for whole night. So he had to drop out of school and stayed at home. He was addicted to internet, reading novels and splashing money on shopping online. He asked his parents for money and assaulted or even threatened them with knife if not satisfied. Yesterday he heard several classmates' gossip that he is not his parents' own child in the neighbor's room to his home. He became furious and rushed in to overthrow the tables and beat the TV. It was out of control and the family had to send him to hospital for treatment. Admission diagnosis: Schizophrenia (paranoid).

Please think about the following questions based on the case:

1. What is the nursing diagnosis for the client at present and potentially?

2. What measures can the nurse take to help the client and prevent the assault happening again?

患者彼得，男，18岁，高三学生。近3个月来，感觉周围的同学和邻居在背后议论、嘲笑他，说他是父母领养的遗弃儿。白天上课注意力不集中，学习感觉吃力；晚上失眠，在寝室多次与同学发生冲突。近2个月来，脑海里总有人指指点点、评头论足，彻夜难眠，遂休学在家。白天沉迷网络，看网络小说，网上购物、挥霍无度，向父母要钱，如不满足，就出现攻击行为，甚则持刀威胁。昨日坐在家中听到几个同学躲在隔壁，评论他非父母亲生，大怒之下冲到邻居家掀翻桌椅、捶打电视，情况无法自控，家属无奈只好将他送医院住院治疗。入院诊断：精神分裂症（偏执型）。

请思考：

1. 患者目前及潜在的护理诊断是什么？

2. 护士可以采取哪些措施帮助患者预防攻击行为再次发生？

Psychiatric contingency indicates emergent events or conditions, which occur suddenly out of control, may endanger the client, other persons or objects and need to be intervened immediately. The most common accidents include aggression, suicide, spontaneous leaves, choke and eating different objects, etc. Contingency not only has great influence upon the health and security of the client, but also is a serious threat to other people and society. Therefore, the prevention and effective handling for contingency in psychiatric settings is a very important part of psychiatric nursing.

精神科意外事件是指由于突然失控而发生的打人、毁物事件或情境，或伤害自己，或伤害他人，对此行为需立即给予干预。常见的意外事件有攻击行为、自杀行为、出走行为、噎食和吞食异物等。这些行为不仅严重影响了患者自身的健康和安全，也会对他人和社会造成威胁。因此，意外事件的防范和有效处理已成为精神科护理的重要内容。

Section 1 Nursing Care of Clients with Aggression

第一节 攻击行为的防范与处理

Aggression is the most common contingency in psychiatric settings. In health care settings, nurses have assumed an active role in preventing and managing aggressive and violent behaviors. Nurses are more likely than physicians to be involved with clients who are aggressive or potentially violent because they spend much

攻击行为是精神科最为常见的意外事件，也是一种危机状态，对患者自己、其他患者及医务人员都具有较高的危险性。与精神科其他专业人员相比，护士与患者接触时间较长，面对攻击行为的机会也更多。因此，精

time with clients.

神科护士需要对患者的攻击行为及时预测、严加预防和及时处理。

I. Introduction

Aggressive behavior is defined as a physical act of force intended to cause harm to a person or an object based on rage, hostility, hatred, or dissatisfaction according to behavioral medicine. Its extreme form is called violence, which can result in serious physical harm or endangered life. Clients with psychiatric illness are the primary group of risk people because of their disordered mind. Clients' aggressive behaviors may happen in family, community, or hospital, and can bring serious outcome to society, families and themselves. It was reported by Rossi (1986) that about 60% clients coming to psychiatric emergency room have had aggressive behaviors; 82% clients with involuntary admission have had aggressive behavior. The forms of aggressive behavior include oral assaults such as curse, threat, deriding; physical attacks such as striking, kicking, biting, spitting; and destroying goods. Except for actual aggressive behaviors, there are some potential or possible aggressive behaviors and impulse attitudes. So accidents could be prevented if appropriate measures are taken before the aggressions occur.

一、概 述

行为医学认为，攻击行为是基于愤怒、敌意、憎恨或不满等情绪，对他人、自身和其他目标采取的破坏性行为。攻击的极端形式称为暴力行为，可造成严重伤害或危及生命。精神障碍患者因其心理活动紊乱，是发生攻击行为的主要危险人群，其攻击行为可能发生在家中、社区、医院等，给患者、家庭及社会带来危害及严重后果。据 Rossi（1986）报道，到急诊室就诊的精神障碍患者中，60% 的患者曾经出现过攻击行为，而强制入院的患者，82% 曾经有攻击行为。攻击行为可有口头攻击、身体攻击或破坏物品等，口头攻击包括谩骂、威胁、嘲笑等；身体攻击包括打人、踢人、吐口水、咬人等。除已经出现的攻击行为外，还可潜在地表现为言语性的威胁或冲动姿态，因此在攻击行为出现之前采取适当措施，可预防意外的发生。

II. Reasons of Aggressive Behavior

i. Mental Disorder

1. Schizophrenia The aggressive behaviors of clients with schizophrenia are commonly associated with delusion or hallucination. Psychic agitation, not satisfied demands, and serious side effects of meditation also contribute to clients' aggression. Some clients may feel they are abandoned by relatives and friends and therefore have grudges against them. These all can lead to the happening of aggressive behaviors.

2. Affective Disorder In acute period, manic clients may have serious violent behaviors, because clients are apt to get agitated in that time. They can fly into a fury if their requests are not met timely; ideas are denied; activities are restricted; and even they are asked to take meditation by nurse. Manic clients may also take sexual attack because of increased sexuality. Depressed clients are often connected with suicide, but some depressed clients give vent to outside in order to be punished, and ultimately

二、攻击行为的原因

（一）精神障碍

1. 精神分裂症 精神分裂症患者的攻击行为多在妄想或幻觉的支配下发生。有精神运动性兴奋、违拗症状、要求未得到满足以及药物的严重副作用也会使患者产生攻击行为；还有部分患者觉得家属或亲友嫌弃自己，从而对他们产生敌对态度，甚至攻击行为。

2. 情感性精神障碍 部分躁狂症患者在急性躁狂发作时可发生严重的暴力行为，此时患者的激惹性增高，如果要求没有得到及时满足，意见被否定，活动受到限制与约束，甚至是护士指导服药这样的常规事件就可引其暴怒，发生伤人毁物。此外，躁狂症患者可能因性欲增强而发生性攻击行为。抑郁症

put themselves to death instead of suicide.

患者虽然以自杀常见，但有些患者本意不是自杀，而是将愤怒发泄到外部，以此来寻求外部惩罚，达到结束生命的目的。

3. Alcohol and Substance Abuse Drunkenness may cause clients out of control, make their emotion unstable and judgment impaired. Temperance may make clients become fretful, agitated, or delirium. Many psychoactive substances can also bring clients to be over excited, agitated, and suspicious. These statuses will increase the occurrence of aggressive behaviors.

3. 物质滥用 醉酒可以引起攻击行为，其原因是醉酒时处于“去抑制”状态，情绪不稳定，判断能力出现障碍。戒酒亦可使患者易激惹、激动或引起谵妄状态而发生攻击行为。此外，很多精神活性物质都可使患者过度兴奋、激动和多疑，从而诱发攻击行为。

4. Personality Disorder Clients with antisocial personality disorder and borderline personality disorder are more likely to become aggressive and violent.

4. 人格障碍 人格障碍特别是反社会性人格障碍和边缘性人格障碍患者，更易发生攻击行为。

5. Others Diagnoses such as organic mental disorder, mental retardation, are also associated with all kinds of violent and destructive behaviors.

5. 其他 如脑器质性精神障碍、精神发育迟滞等都易发生各种形式的暴力和破坏行为。

ii. Biological Factors

（二）生物学因素

Current neurobiological research has focused on three areas of the brain believed to be involved in aggression: the limbic system, the frontal lobes, and the hypothalamus.

现代神经生物学研究发现，脑部的边缘系统、额叶、下丘脑三个区域可能与攻击行为有关。

1. Limbic System The limbic system is associated with the mediation of basic drives and the expression of human emotions and behaviors such as eating, aggression, and sexual response. It is also involved in the processing of information and memory. Synthesis of information to and from other areas in the brain influences emotional experience and behavior. Therefore, alterations in functioning of the limbic system may result in an increase or decrease in the potential for aggressive behavior.

1. 边缘系统 边缘系统通过整合出入大脑其他区域的信息而影响人们的情感体验与行为表达，对本能冲动（如饮食、攻击和性反应等）具有调节作用，同时也与信息的处理和记忆密切相关。因此，边缘系统功能的改变会增加或降低产生攻击行为的可能性。

2. Frontal Lobes The frontal lobes play an important role in mediating purposeful behavior and rational thinking. They are the part of the brain where reason and emotion interact. Damage to the frontal lobes can result in impaired judgment, personality changes, and problems in decision-making, inappropriate conduct, and aggressive outbursts.

2. 额叶 额叶在调节自觉行为与理性思考方面具有重要作用，是大脑理性与情感交互作用的场所。额叶的损伤可能会导致判断失误、人格改变、决策困难，并爆发不适当的行为及攻击性行为。

3. Hypothalamus The hypothalamus is the brain's alarm system. Stress raises the level of steroids, the hormones secreted by the adrenal glands. Nerve receptors for these hormones become less sensitive in an attempt to compensate, and the hypothalamus tells the pituitary gland to release more steroids. After repeated stimulation, the system may respond more vigorously to all provocations.

3. 下丘脑 下丘脑是大脑的警报系统，应激状态下会促使肾上腺所产生的激素水平升高，而神经受体则会出现代偿性敏感度降低，此时下丘脑使脑垂体释放更多的肾上腺激素进行调节。如此反复循环会使整个系统处于兴奋状态，使患者对任何刺激都易激惹。

Neurotransmitters have also been suggested as having a role in the expression or suppression of aggressive behavior. Some evidences show that low levels of the serotonin are associated with irritability, hypersensitivity to provocation, and rage.

此外，有研究表明，神经递质在攻击行为的表达或抑制上也具有一定的作用，如5-羟色胺水平的降低与患者的情绪激动、对刺激的高度敏感及愤怒等有关。

iii. Psychosocial Factors

1. Psychological Development One psychological view suggests that early psychological development or life experiences are closely associated with aggressive behavior, for they can limit one's capacity to select nonviolent coping mechanisms. Examples of these experiences are severe emotional deprivation, exposure to violence in formative years, and mental retardation. They may limit one's ability to use supportive relationships, make one become very self-centered, particularly vulnerable to injury, easily provokable. Social learning theory also proposes that aggressive behavior is a result of internal and external learning through the socialization process. Internal learning is a kind of self-reinforcement when acting aggressive behavior. External learning occurs through the observation of role models such s parents, peers, and entertainment figures.

2. Personality Psychologists consider that some special personality is closely associated with aggressive behavior. Shoham once investigated violent criminals using Cattell personality questionnaire, and found that they have some common characteristics:

(1) Suspicious, obstinate, lacking sympathy and social responsibility.

(2) Having fluctuant emotion, easy to be nervous, liking seeking for stimuli but sensitive to frustration.

(3) Lacking self-esteem and self-confidence, having poor techniques in coping with realities and interpersonal relationships.

3. Social and Environmental Factors Social and environmental factors also have impact on aggressive behavior. Influencing factors include aspects of the physical facilities, the presence of professionals and other clients, etc. For example, several studies have found that violent incidents were easy to happen when clients were over-crowded, passive, or lacked privacy. Clinicians may also intentionally or inadvertently precipitate an outbreak of clients' aggression because of the attitudes and behaviors of themselves, such as discriminating and provoking clients, inexperience in management, invading the personal space of clients, etc. In addition, involuntary admission to a psychiatric facility or closed management in psychiatric setting may constrain the development of a trusting relationship between nurse and client, and assaults may occur.

III. Application of the Nursing Assessment

i. Nursing Assessment

1. Risk Factors Predicting client's aggressive tendency is an effective method of preventing and

（三）心理社会因素

1. 心理发展 据对攻击行为的研究证明，早期的心理发展或生活经历与攻击行为密切相关，它会影响个体是否会选择非暴力应对方式的能力。例如成长期经历过严重的情感剥夺、在性格形成期接触暴力情境、智力发育迟滞等，会限制个体利用支持系统的能力，使其变得以自我为中心，对伤害异常敏感，容易产生愤怒情绪。社会学习理论认为，攻击行为在社会化过程中可自身习得，也可从外部学来。自身习得是在实施攻击时的一种自身强化，而外部学习是通过观察父母、同辈或娱乐人物的行为所获得。

2. 性格特征 心理学家认为，一些特殊的性格特征与攻击行为有密切关系。Shoham等应用Cattell个性问卷调查暴力犯罪者，发现暴力犯罪者具有下列性格特征：

（1）多疑、固执、缺少同情心与社会责任感；

（2）情绪不稳定，易紧张，喜欢寻找刺激，易产生挫折感；

（3）缺乏自尊与自信，应对现实及人际交往能力差。

3. 社会环境因素 社会环境、文化等因素会影响精神障碍患者攻击行为的发生。社会环境因素主要包括环境设施、工作人员与其他患者是否在身边等。例如：当患者聚集在一起、过分拥挤、缺乏隐私及处于被动时，容易发生暴力事件。工作人员可能由于工作态度和自身行为激惹患者（如歧视或挑逗患者），管理经验不足，与患者的人际交往距离不恰当等，有意或无意地触发了患者的攻击行为。此外，强行入院和封闭式的管理环境容易引起患者的怨恨和反感，促使攻击行为的发生。

三、护理程序的应用

（一）护理评估

1. 危险因素评估 有效预防和制止攻击

stopping aggression and violence. Many researchers have studied at this area and found that following aspects can predict these behaviors to a certain extent:

甚至暴力行为发生的关键是判断患者是否具有攻击的倾向，经研究发现下列危险因素有利于评估患者攻击行为发生的可能性。

(1) Demographic variables: Including age, gender, marital status, working conditions and environment. Young, male, single clients are more likely to catty out assaults. Unemployment, noisy and crowded environment often make the client lose his temper and attack on the people around them.

（1）一般特征：包括年龄、性别、婚姻状况、工作状态、环境等。年轻、男性、单身患者发生攻击行为的可能性较大。失业，喧闹拥挤的环境常使患者脾气不佳，容易对周围人产生攻击行为。

(2) Clinical variables

（2）临床特征

1) History of aggressive behavior: One of the best predictors of aggression appears to be a history of aggressive behavior, especially resent aggression or violence. Other important markers include previous episodes of rage and hostility, escalating irritability, intruding angry thoughts, and fear of losing control.

1）攻击行为的病史：过去尤其是最近曾有过攻击行为，很可能再次发生。此外，过去曾出现过愤怒情绪、敌对态度、激惹性的增加、侵入性的愤怒以及害怕失去控制等都可能是攻击行为的危险因素。

2) Psychotic symptoms: Some psychotic symptoms are closely associated with the aggressive behavior, such as hallucination, delusion, mania, impulsion, and unconsciousness. In general, clients with active psychotic symptoms, particularly those related to perceiving threat, such as feeling of being controlled of thoughts or being watched, can increase the risk of aggression.

2）精神症状：与攻击行为密切相关的精神症状包括幻觉、妄想、躁狂状态、冲动和意识障碍等。一般说来，活跃的精神症状，尤其是那些让患者感到有威胁的症状，如感到思想被控制、行为被监视等，会增加攻击行为发生的危险性。

3) Diagnosis: The incidence, severity, pertinence, client's age of the aggression varies greatly in different psychiatric illnesses. The incidence of schizophrenia's aggressive behavior is the highest; follows by mood disorder, alcohol and substance abuse, personality disorder and others. Thus a client's diagnosis is suggestive.

3）诊断：不同的精神障碍，攻击行为的发生率、严重性、针对性和发生年龄均不同。精神分裂症患者攻击行为的发生率最高，其次为情感性精神障碍、酒精和精神活性物质滥用，其他精神障碍如人格障碍及器质性精神障碍等亦可发生攻击行为。患者的诊断在评估时可作为参考依据之一。

2. Assessing Aggression

2. 攻击行为的征兆评估

(1) Signs of aggression: The client will show some excited behavior, some of these early behaviors before attacks, including motor agitation such as pacing, inability to sit still, clenching or pounding fists, jaw tension, breathing faster, tightening of the whole body muscle, stop the ongoing action suddenly, etc.

（1）先兆行为：患者在发生攻击行为之前会出现一些早期的兴奋行为，如踱步、不能静坐、握拳或用拳击物、下颌紧绷、呼吸增快、全身肌肉紧张，突然停止正在进行的动作等。

(2) Linguistic aspects: There also may be verbal clues such as threats to real or imagined objects or intrusive demands for attention, loud and force others to notice, or threatening postures, paranoid speech, etc.

（2）语言方面：同时还有一些语言的暗示，包括对真实或想象的对象进行威胁，或提一些无理的要求，说话声音变大，强迫他人注意，或做出威胁性的姿态，出现妄想性言语等。

(3) Emotional aspects: The affect associated with escalating behaviors, such as anger, hostility, abnormal

（3）情感方面：出现与逐步升级的兴奋行为相伴随的情感表现，如愤怒、敌意、异常

anxiety, irritability, abnormal or excessive euphoria, emotional instability, indicates that the client is about to lose control of emotions.

(4) Conscious state: Changes in the state of consciousness (such as confusion in thinking, orientation disorder, memory impairment, etc.), also suggest that aggressive behavior is about to occur.

3. Assessment Tool for Aggressive Behavior Through the specific behavior, nurses can assess the severity of the attack behavior of the clients, whether it will develop into the most serious violence(figure 4-1), suggesting that nurses need to take effective interventions for clients at once. Commonly used assessment tools are as follows:

(1) Violence risk screening-10(V-RISK-10) (table 4-1);

(2) The Broset Violence Checklist(BVC) (table 4-2);

(3) Aggressive and Violence Assessment Tool。

焦虑、易激惹、异常或过度欣快、情感不稳定，预示着患者情绪即将失去控制。

（4）意识状态评估：意识状态发生改变（如思维混乱、定向力障碍、记忆力损害等），亦提示攻击行为即将发生。

3. 攻击行为的评估工具 通过具体行为表现，评估攻击行为患者的严重程度，是否会进行性发展为最严重的暴力行为（图 4–1），提示护士是否需要立即对患者进行有效的护理干预。常用的评估工具如下：

（1）攻击风险筛查量表（表 4–1）；

（2）Broset 攻击行为评估量表（表 4–2）；

（3）攻击和暴力行为危险程度评估表。

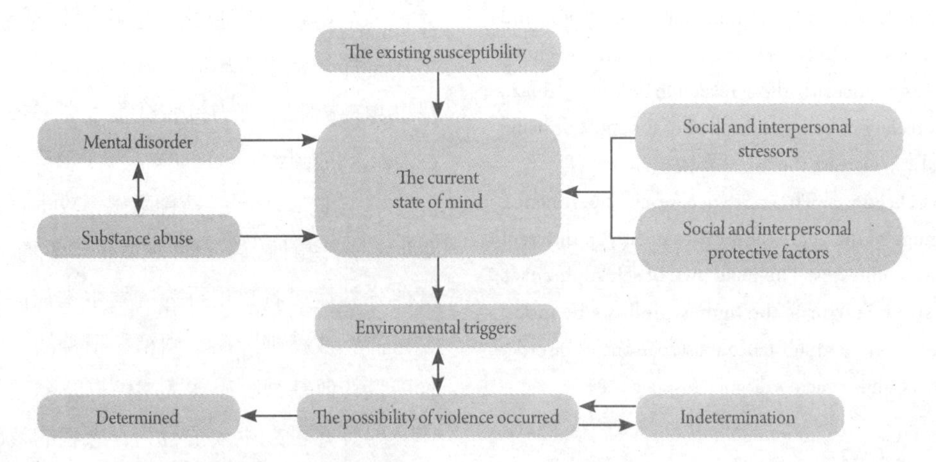

Figure 4–1 Violence risk assessment flow chart

Table 4–1 Violence risk screening–10 (V–RISK–10)

Risk Factors	No	Maybe/ Moderate	Yes	Do not Know
1. Previous and/or current violence Severe violence refers to physical attack (including with various weapons) towards another individual with intent to inflict severe physical harm. Yes: The individual in question must have committed at least 3 moderate violent aggressive acts or 1 severe violent act. Moderate or less severe aggressive acts such as kicks, blows and shoving that does not cause severe harm to the victim is rated maybe/moderate				
2. Previous and/or current threats(verbal/physical) Verbal: Statements, yelling and the like, that involve threat of inflicting other individuals physical harm Physical: Movements and gestures that warn physical attack				

continued

Risk Factors	No	Maybe/ Moderate	Yes	Do not Know
3. Previous and/or current substance abuse The client has a history of abusing alcohol, medication and/or other substances (e.g. amphetamine, heroin, cannabis). Abuse of solvents or glue should be included. To rate Yes: the client must have and/or have had extensive abuse/dependence, with reduced occupational or educational functioning, reduced health and/or reduced participation in leisure activities				
4. Previous and/or current major mental illness NB: Whether the client has or has had a psychotic disorder (e.g. schizophrenia, delusional disorder, and psychotic affective disorder)				
5. Personality disorders Of interest here are eccentric (schizoid, paranoid) and impulsive, uninhibited (emotionally unstable, antisocial) types				
6. Shows lack of insight into illness and/or behavior This refers to the degree to which the client lacks insight in his/her mental illness, with regard to for instance need of medication, social consequences or behavior related to illness or personality disorder				
7. Expresses suspicion The client expresses suspicion towards other individuals either verbally or nonverbally. The person in question appears to be "on guard" towards the environment				
8. Shows lack of empathy The client appears emotionally cold and without sensitivity towards others' thoughts or emotional situation				
9. Unrealistic planning This assesses to which degree the client him/herself has unrealistic plan for the future (inside or outside the inpatient unit). Is for instance the client himself/herself realistic with regard to what he/she can expect of support from family and of professional and social network? It is important to assess whether the client is cooperative and motivated with regard to following plans				
10. Future stress-situations This evaluates the possibility that the client may be exposed to stress and stressful situations in the future and his/her ability to cope with stress. For example (in and outside inpatient unit): reduced ability to tolerate boundaries, physical proximity to possible victims of violence, substance use, homelessness, spending time in violent environment/association with violent environment, easy access to weapons etc.				

NOTE:

Description:

1.The rater collects information about each of the ten risk factors on the V-RISK-10 checklist. Some examples of important scoring information are described under each item. Put a check in the box to indicate the degree of likelihood that the risk factor applies to the client in question.

2. No: Does not apply to this client. Maybe/moderate: Maybe applies/present to a moderately severe degree. Yes: Definitely applies to a severe degree. Do not know: Too little information to answer.

表 4-1 攻击风险筛查量表

条目	没有	可能 / 中等	有	不知道
1. 既往 / 现在的攻击行为 严重攻击是指试图对他人造成严重的身体伤害（包括性侵犯、使用各种武器）的攻击行为 有：该患者曾有过 3 次中等程度的攻击行为或 1 次严重的攻击行为 可能 / 中等：中等或轻微的攻击行为是指类似踢、打或推搡，但未对受害者造成严重影响的行为				
2. 既往 / 现在的威胁（语言 / 身体） 语言：大吼大叫或说一些威胁他人人身安全的话 身体：做出威胁他人人身安全的动作或姿势				
3. 既往 / 现在的物质滥用 患者既往有酗酒、药物和其他物质滥用（如安非他明、海洛因、大麻）或溶剂、胶体滥用史 有：是指患者有或曾有酒精、烟草等的过度滥用 / 依赖，并对其工作、学习、健康及休闲活动造成了负面影响				
4. 既往 / 现有的精神、神经疾病 患者是否患有或曾患有精神障碍（如精神分裂症、妄想性障碍、情感障碍）或癫痫、脑外伤				
5. 人格障碍 本条目是指行为古怪（精神分裂、妄想）、冲动和不能控制（情绪不稳定、反社会）				
6. 对疾病和 / 或行为缺乏认知 本条目是指患者对精神疾病认识的缺乏程度。它包括对疾病的服药必要性的认识、对疾病和人格障碍、行为改变及其造成后果的认识				
7. 猜疑的表现 患者对他人表现出语言或非语言的怀疑，对周围环境表现出“警戒”状态				
8. 情感淡漠 患者情感淡漠，对周围人的想法和感情都不敏感				
9. 不切实际地制订计划 本条目评估患者对将来（住院期间或出院后）计划不切实际的程度。如患者期望的从家庭、专业人员和社会系统中得到的帮助是否切合实际？对今后的打算是否切合实际？很重要的一点是评估患者是否能积极地去执行这些计划				
10. 将来的压力环境 本条目评估患者将来面对压力或处于压力环境的可能性及其应对压力的能力。如（住院期间或出院后）容忍度降低，接近可能的攻击对象、物质滥用、无家可归、处于充满暴力的环境中、容易获得武器或工具等				

使用说明：

1. 表格左侧列举的是影响患者伤人、自伤、自杀等攻击行为发生的 10 条危险因素（某些条目附有具体说明），请根据患者的情况选择：“没有”“可能 / 中等”“有”“不知道”，并在相应方框中划“√”做标记。

2. 没有：指该患者不存在此种情况，可能 / 中等：是指该患者存在此种情况，但不严重；有：是指该患者存在此种情况，且严重；不知道：是指信息不足，无法判断。

Table 4-2 The Broset violence checklist (BVC)

Items	day	Evening
Confused Appears obviously confused and disorientated. Maybe unaware of time, place or person		
Irritable Easily annoyed or angered. Unable to tolerate the presence of others		
Boisterous Behavior is overtly "loud: or noisy. For example slams doors, shouts out when talking etc.		
Verbally threatening A verbal outburst which is more than just a raised voice; and where there is a definite intent to intimidate or threaten another person. For example verbal attacks, abuse, name-calling, verbally neutral comments uttered in a snarling aggressive manner		
Physically threatening Where there is a definite intent to physically threaten another person. For example the taking of an aggressive stance; the grabbing of another person's clothing; the raising of an arm, leg, making of a fist or modeling of a head-butt directed at another		
Attacking objects An attack directed at an object and not an individual. For example the indiscriminate throwing of an object; banging or smashing windows; kicking, banging or head-butting an object: or the smashing of furniture		

Description: Score the client at agreed time on every shift. Absence of behavior gives a score of 0. Presence of behavior gives a score of 1. Maximum score (SUM) is 6. If behavior is normal for a well-known client, only an increase in behavior scores 1, e.g. if a well know client normally is confused (has been so for a long time) this will give a score of 0. If an increase in confusion is observed this gives a score of 1.

Interpretation of scoring:

Score=0 The risk of violence is small.

Score=1-2 The risk of violence is moderate. Preventive measures should be taken.

Score>2 The risk of violence is very high. Preventive measures should be taken. In addition, a plan should be developed to manage the potential violence.

表 4-2 Broset 攻击行为评估量表

项目	白班	中班
混乱 患者出现明显的行为、言语混乱和定向力障碍。如分不清时间、地点、人物		
易怒 患者容易生气或恼怒，极易因为小事而发火，无法容忍别人的存在		
喧闹 患者在活动时发出较大的声音或吵闹。如摔门、说话时大声喊叫		
语言威胁 患者说话声音突然提高并有恐吓和威胁他人的明确意图。如语言攻击、说粗话、谩骂，以咆哮、攻击的方式表达中立看法		
肢体威胁 患者有明显意图地用肢体威胁他人。如摆出攻击的姿势、拽别人衣服、挥动手臂、抬腿、握紧拳头或做出要用头顶人的样子		
攻击物品 患者攻击对象为物品但不是人。如乱扔物品、砰砰地敲打或砸窗户、踢、敲打或用头撞击物品、砸家具等		

使用说明：白班、中班各评估 1 次。不出现某种行为评分为 0，出现某种行为评分为 1，总分最高为 6 分。对病情熟悉的患者，行为严重程度加重时评分为 1。如患者行为总是混乱（较长一段时间来一直如此）则评分为 0，如混乱程度加重，评分为 1。

评分标准：总分为 0 攻击风险很小。

总分为 1~2 攻击风险中等，应采取预防措施。

总分 >2 攻击风险很高，应采取预防措施并制订计划以处理可能发生的攻击。

ii. Nursing Diagnosis/Goal

1. Nursing Diagnosis Risk for violence toward others: related to hallucination, delusion, anxiety, organic impairment, etc.

2. Nursing Goals There is no aggressive behavior occurred with the client. The client is able to identify the factors that caused him or her angry and agitation, can control his or her behavior, and can seek for help when feeling angry and agitation control.

iii. Nursing Interventions

1. Prevention of Aggressive Behavior Every effort should be made to carefully monitor the client who are at risk for aggressive behavior and intervene at the first possible sign of increasing agitation.

(1) Rational use of drugs to control the excitement: The judicious use of selected medications, either episodically or on a long-term basis,may be necessary. Often, haloperidol is still the drug of choice when dealing with episodes of highly agitated behavior. Selective serotonin reuptake inhibitors (SSRIs) are being increasingly used for their anti-aggressive effects as well as for their antidepressant effects. Their effect on aggressive behavior usually occurs before evidence of antidepressant action. It has been proven that lithium carbonate is effective in treating aggression resulting from mania. Some evidence also shows that lithium carbonate may be useful in decreasing aggression resulting from other disorders such as mental retardation, head injuries,and schizophrenia. Antianxiety and sedative-hypnotics (Benzodiazepines) are effective in the management of acute agitation, but these drugs are not recommended for long-term use because they can result in confusion and dependency and may worsen depressive symptoms. In addition, β blockers such as propranolol may be used for their effect in decreasing the peripheral manifestations of rage that are associated with excitement of the sympathetic nervous system. They have been shown to reduce aggressive behavior, and particularly clients with organic mental disorder.

(2) Strengthen management to remove the environmental factors: Keeping the environment quiet and orderly, and avoiding noisy and crowded can let the client feel safe. Therefore, environmental management should be strengthened, and all kinds of dangerous objects should be placed properly so as not to be used by aggressive client as tools to attack others. Units that are overly structured with too much stimulation and little regard for the privacy needs of clients may increase

（二）护理诊断 / 护理目标

1. 护理诊断有发生攻击行为的危险（针对他人） 与幻觉、妄想、焦虑、器质性损伤等因素有关。

2. 护理目标 患者没有发生攻击行为，并能确认引起自己激动、愤怒的因素，能控制自己的行为或立即寻求帮助。

（三）护理措施

1. 攻击行为的预防 若发现患者有攻击行为的先兆行为，应进行及时有效的护理干预，将攻击行为消除在萌芽状态，避免攻击行为的发生。

（1）合理用药，控制兴奋行为：长期或短期的药物治疗可有效地减少患者的攻击行为的发生。氟哌啶醇是治疗异常兴奋患者的常用药；选择性5-羟色胺再摄取抑制剂既能对抗攻击行为，又可抗抑郁，且抗攻击作用比抗抑郁效果快，使用也较为广泛；抗躁狂药碳酸锂，可有效处理由躁狂导致的攻击行为，同时对减少精神发育迟滞、脑部损伤或精神分裂症患者的攻击行为也有效。抗焦虑药与镇静催眠药（常用苯二氮䓬类药物），能有效缓冲患者的急性冲动，适合处理精神科紧急事件，但因其易致思维迟缓、药物依赖以及使抑郁症状加重等不良后果，一般不主张长期使用。此外，β受体阻滞剂，如普萘洛尔（心得安）等，可减轻由交感神经系统兴奋所致的躯体症状，尤其可减少脑器质性精神障碍患者的攻击行为。

（2）加强管理，去除环境影响因素：保持病区环境安静、整洁，避免嘈杂、拥挤，可使患者感觉到安全，因此应加强环境管理，并妥善放置好各种危险物品，以免被冲动的患者用作攻击他人的工具。如果病室的结构不合理，刺激物太多而又不注意尊重患者的隐私会使患者攻击行为增加。反之，提供多

aggressive behavior. In contrast, units that provide many productive and recreational activities can reduce the chance of inappropriate client behavior and increase adaptive social and leisure functioning. In addition, both the unit norms and the rewards associated with such activities may reduce the amount of disorganized client behavior and the number of aggressive acts.

(3) Master communication strategies to resolve the crisis: Firstly, nurses can resolve the crisis by using early language or non language communication. In order to decrease a client's agitation, nurses should pay more attention to the tone and wording during the communication, talk with them as far as possible in a calm and low voice, short and simple sentences, and avoid laughing or smiling inappropriately. Nurse may feel afraid and anxious when he or she is contacting with the aggression-prone client. The client can also perceive these responses. If the nurse can share these feelings with the client,the distance between them may be shortened. On the contrary, if these feelings are mistaken by the client, he or she will become more inclined to be furious.

Secondly, the nurse can also help reduce a rising level of agitation by acknowledging the client's feelings and reassuring the client that the staff is there to help. It may be useful to allow the client to communicate his or her concerns without interruption and engage the client's participation in treatment decisions, providing the client as much information about treatment as possible. Collaboration with clients can be enhanced, making it less likely that they will respond in an angry and aggressive manner.

Thirdly, nurses can also use appropriate nonverbal communication to enhance the outcome of intervention. The nurse's hands should be kept open and out of pockets because of crossing the arms across the chest is another posture that communicates emotional distance and an unwillingness to help; therefore, threatening, nervous, and sudden gestures should be avoided. Altering position so that the nurse's eyes are at the same level as those of the client allows the client to communicate from an equal rather than inferior position.

It is worth mentioning that the distance of communication is also a very important aspect in the treatment of communication. It has been noted that violence-prone people need four times more personal space than non-violence-prone people. So the nurse should assume a supportive stance that is at least 1 meter from the client. It is helpful if the nurse remains at an angle

种娱乐活动的病区可减少患者不适当的行为，提高患者对社会的适应能力。此外，建立与上述活动相关的病区制度和奖励办法也可减少患者的紊乱行为和攻击行为。

（3）掌握交流技巧，化解危机状态：第一，护士可以通过早期的语言或非语言的交流来化解危机状态。在沟通过程中，护士应注意语调与措词，尽量用平静低沉的声音、简短的词句与之交谈，以降低患者的激动程度，切忌发出不恰当的笑声。在与有攻击倾向的患者交流时，护士可能会有害怕或担心的感觉，而患者也会察觉到护士的异常反应。如果护士及时与患者分享自己的感受，则可缩短彼此之间的距离，也可消除自己的紧张感。反之，这种情绪一旦造成患者误解，就会使其更容易发生攻击行为。

第二，护士可向患者说明工作人员关心、理解其感受，并会尽力帮助其摆脱困境，以减轻患者的激动程度。也可通过与患者的合作来降低其敌意及攻击行为，如鼓励患者倾诉内心困扰，参与治疗决策，向患者提供治疗信息等。此外，护士还可鼓励患者控制自己的冲动，接受这种鼓励的患者会在冲动的早期就离开刺激性环境，增强对自我的控制。

第三，采用适当的非语言交流方式增强干预效果。护士可将两手分开，置于口袋外面，避免使患者感觉受到威胁、感到紧张和突然的姿势，因为两臂交叉于胸前是表达了双方在情感上的距离和不愿意提供帮助的一种肢体语言；护士还应调节身体位置，平视患者的眼睛，这样可使患者感觉交流的双方地位平等。

交往距离在治疗性沟通过程中也是一个很重要的方面。有暴力倾向的患者常需要四倍于常人的个人空间，护士与之交谈时必须保持足够的交往距离（至少1m），并与其身体之间形成一个角度。如果护士侵犯了患者的个人空间，会让其感到受到威胁，从而激发

to the client. Intrusion into a client's personal space can be perceived as a threat and provoke aggression. Finally, when approaching potentially aggressive clients and nurses should carefully observe their behavior. Clenched fists, tightening of the facial muscles, and movement away from the nurse may suggest that the client is feeling threatened. The nurse should respond by giving the client as much distance as possible.

其攻击性。因此，护士在接近具有潜在攻击性的患者时应细心观察患者的行为，紧握拳头、面部肌肉紧张或转身走开等都提示患者可能感到受到威胁，护士应立即疏远与患者的距离。

(4) Health education to improve the ability of self-control for the client: Teaching clients about communication and the appropriate way to express anger is one of the most successful interventions in preventing aggressive behavior. Many clients have difficulty in identifying their feelings, needs, and desires and even more difficulty in communicating these to others. Teaching clients that feelings are not right or wrong or good or bad can allow them to explore feelings that may have been bottled up,ignored, or repressed. The nurse can then work with clients on ways to express their feelings and evaluate whether the responses they select are adaptive or maladaptive. Providing clients with available choices in managing anger, such as physical exercise, change of environment, listen to music, etc., may be effective in reducing more restrictive interventions.

（4）健康宣教，提高自控能力：通过沟通性咨询及健康教育，教会患者人际沟通的方法和表达愤怒情绪的适宜方式是一项有效预防攻击行为的措施。许多患者很难识别自己的情绪、需求与愿望，更难将这些与他人进行交流。因此，要告诉患者情绪没有对与错或好与坏之分，鼓励他们探讨自己被尘封、忽视或压抑的情感。护士可以与患者一起探讨情绪的表达方式，不适宜的行为，如攻击他人或伤害自己等，并评估患者所选择的方式是否恰当。向患者提供处理愤怒情绪的一些实用方法，如进行体育锻炼、改变环境、听音乐等，以减少限制性措施的使用，有效控制患者的攻击行为。

2. Management of Aggressive Behavior There are times when attempts at early intervention are unsuccessful and more active intervention is necessary. Emergency treatment must follow the "SAFETY FIRST, to persuade, to minimize the damage limit" principle, which should first consider the safety of clients himself, other clients and staff. This can be accomplished by assigning a staff member to remove the other clients from the area. Effective crisis management must be organized and should be directed by one clearly identified crisis leader. In general, there is a corresponding crisis treatment group which designated specialized personnel to deal with the crisis. The leader may be the nurse manager, the charge nurse, or a staff nurse, other staff members, including physicians, nurses, and tenders, can be used for support. All members of the crisis team should be trained in crisis management and have experience working as a cohesive group. The staff should be prepared to intervene under the direction of the crisis leader. In addition, a room without furniture should always be readily available for an emergency.

2. 攻击行为的处理 当早期干预不能有效预防患者的攻击行为时，就需要采取进一步的措施来处理已经发生的攻击行为或危机状态。紧急处理遵循“安全第一，劝诱为主，将危害降到最低限度”的原则，即应首先考虑暴力行为者自身、其他患者及工作人员的安全，可指定一位工作人员将其他患者转移，离开现场。有效的危机处理必须是有组织的，并且要有组织者或危机处理的领导者。一般情况下精神科病房都有相应的危机处理小组，指定专门的人员来处理危机事件。组织者可以是护士长、责任护士或值班护士，其他小组成员（包括医生、护士和护工等）可以进行协助。所有参与危机处理的成员都应该接受过此方面的训练，在组织者的统一指导下对患者实施干预。此外，应该经常准备一间没有家具的房间，以供处理危机时使用。

(1) Verbal persuasion: During this time it is critically important that the leader relate to the client in a calm, steady voice and tone, the direct, simple and clear words should be used to remind the consequences of violence

（1）言语劝诱：在处理危机时，组织者必须用平静、平和的声音和语气与患者交流，用直接、简单、清晰的语言提醒患者暴力行

for the client. Particular attention should be paid to maintaining appropriate communication distance. As the group approach about 2 meters from the client,the staff should express concern for the client's safety and the behavior demonstrated that has caused such concern. The nurse should take good words to comfort the client, meet his or her demands, so that it is becoming possible to close to the client gradually. Any anxiety, impatient or ambivalence will be conveyed to the client and contribute to a feeling of insecurity. A leader who is anxious will be unable to make right judgment to the whole situation. Many clients are afraid of being out of control,and they become assaultive not because they want to frighten people but because they themselves are frightened. If the staff controls the situation, the client's agitation will be defused gradually. When the crisis team is overwhelmed by their own fears of the client, they cannot be effective in reducing the client's fear. Consistency is also important so that the client cannot bargain with or manipulate staff members.

为的后果。特别要注意保持适当的交往距离，当工作人员离患者2m左右时，即可向患者表达对其安全及行为的关心，好言劝慰，满足患者合理要求，逐步接近患者，切忌快速、正面冲突。任何焦虑、急躁与矛盾情绪都会传递给患者，加重其不安全感。组织者如果焦虑不安，就不能对全局作出正确的判断。许多患者都害怕失去控制，他们动武并非为了恐吓别人，而是发泄其恐惧情绪。如果工作人员能控制局面，患者一般不会长时间处于激动不安的状态。工作人员如果自己表现出恐惧、不安，就无法减轻患者的恐惧。此外，还应注意保持语言及行为的前后一致性，这样患者就不会与工作人员讨价还价或操纵工作人员了。

(2) Seclusion and restraint: When the nurse's verbal persuasion was invalid, the client's aggression cannot be controlled, the staff can take some appropriate measure to subdue the client and make he or she isolated and restricted. The isolation and restriction are used to protect the client from injury to self or others, to help the client reestablish behavioral control, and to minimize disruption of unit treatment regimens.

（2）隔离与约束：当言语劝诱无效，不能控制患者的攻击行为时，可采用适当的形式制服患者，然后将其隔离与约束。隔离与约束的目的是为了保护患者，使其不会伤害自己或他人，帮助患者重建对行为控制的能力，并减少对整个病房治疗体系的破坏。

1) Subduing the client: If a client holds a weapon in his hand, the intervention can be taken under the help of security personnel or the police instead of acting hastily. If the client has no arms, staff members involved in the intervention should be assigned to secure one of the client's extremities, escort the client to the appropriate room and inform him or her of the necessary intervention. It should be emphasized that the intervention is not a punishment but is being implanted to help ensure the safety of the client.

1）制服患者：若患者手中持有武器，不可贸然行事，可由保安人员或警察出面制服。若患者手上没有武器，则由4人行动，每人保护患者的一个肢体，陪同患者至适当的房间，同时告诉患者这是必要的处理措施，是减少损害而不是惩罚。

2) Seclusion: The rationale for the use of seclusion is based on three therapeutic principles including containment, isolation, and decrease in sensory input. Using the principle of containment, clients are restricted to a place where they are free from harming themselves and other clients. Isolation addresses the need for clients to distance themselves from relationships that can make them anxious. The third principle is that seclusion provides a decrease in sensory input for clients whose illness results in a heightened sensitivity to external stimulation. The quiet atmosphere and monotony of a seclusion room may provide some relief from the sensory overload.

2）隔离：隔离的应用基于三项治疗性原则，即封闭、孤立及减少感官刺激。封闭是指将患者限制在一个相对独立、安静、安全的地方，以防伤害自己和其他患者。孤立是指让患者暂时脱离使其不安的人际关系或环境。对外界刺激高度敏感的患者，单调而安静的隔离环境可以减轻其感官负荷，使情绪逐渐稳定。

3) Restraint involves the use of mechanical or manual devices to limit the physical mobility of the client. Such an intervention may be indicated to protect the client or others from injury, particularly if less restrictive interventions have failed. If restraints are to be used, the client should be asked to lie on the bed with arms at his or her side. Restraint should be applied efficiently and with care not to injure a combative client. Adequate personnel must be assured before the client is approached. Each staff member should be assigned to be responsible for controlling specific body parts. Padding of cuff restraints helps to protect the skin. For the same reason, the client should be positioned in anatomical alignment (figure 4-2).

During the constraint, physical needs must be included in nursing care. Vital signs should be checked,and regular observation of circulation in the extremities is necessary. Fluids should be offered regularly and opportunities for elimination should be provided. Skin care is also essential. If visitors are allowed, the nurse should explain the reason for restraints or seclusion before they see the client. This may help them accept the situation. The client in restraint may be confused or delirious and will probably be frightened at the limitation of movement. The nurse should not assume that the client understands the need for restraint. Sometimes despite explanations of the therapeutic purpose of the intervention, it is not uncommon for clients to perceive the use of restraints as a punishment. Thus providing support and reassurance is essential. Every effort must also be made to maintain a therapeutic alliance with the client in restraints. Reviewing the behavior that precipitated the intervention and the client's current capacity to exercise control over his or her behavior are key factors. The decision to terminate the use of seclusion or restraints should be well planned.

Clients are initially reintegrated by reducing restraints from four points to three points and then to two points as soon as they begin to regain control. Before the end of constraint, clients should be told which behaviors are reasonable and which behaviors or impulses need to be controlled before the intervention can be discontinued. Communication and careful documentation are critical in making an accurate assessment of a client's level of control.

(3) Medication: Effective medication can be used both in place of isolation and restriction, and at the same time. Commonly used drugs contain Haloperidol, chlorpromazine and diazepam (Valium), Haloperidol is the most popular one. These drugs are generally taken by muscle injection. It is necessary that observing the client's vital signs, medication response and emotion control after treatment.

3）约束：如果以上措施仍无法控制患者的行为，就需要对患者进行约束，以保护患者自己与他人的安全。约束前，使患者仰卧于床上，手臂放于身体两侧。约束方法包括使用机械约束或人工装置限制患者的身体行动。约束时，效率要高，不要伤害正在反抗的患者，在接近患者前，要保证有足够的工作人员，每人应该负责身体的一部分。约束后，在腕部、踝部等处塞填充物（图 4-2），以免损伤皮肤，并使其肢体处于功能位。

约束期间，需加强对约束患者的基础护理，观察其生命体征和末梢循环情况，定时给予足够的营养和液体，帮助其进行排泄，并对患者进行皮肤护理。如果有人来探视患者，护士应向其解释对其进行隔离或约束的原因。被约束的患者可能会烦躁不安或对行动受限制感到害怕。护士不应该认为患者能够理解约束的必要性。有时尽管已向患者反复解释干预措施的目的，患者仍将约束视为一种惩罚。因此仍要给予患者解释和支持，努力与其保持一种治疗性关系。护士需回顾导致隔离或约束的患者行为，适时观察患者对自己行为的控制能力，合理计划结束隔离或约束的时间。

随着患者自控能力的逐渐恢复，可将其约束部位从四个变为三个，然后再变成两个，直至解除约束。在结束前，应该告诉患者哪些行为是合理的，哪些行为或冲动是需要进行控制的。与患者的交流和详细的病史记录都可以帮助护士了解患者的自我控制水平。

（3）药物治疗：有效的药物治疗既可代替隔离约束患者，也可同时使用。常用的药物有氟哌啶醇、氯丙嗪、地西泮（安定）等，以氟哌啶醇最为常用，一般采取肌内注射方式。用药后注意观察患者生命体征、用药反应及情绪控制情况。

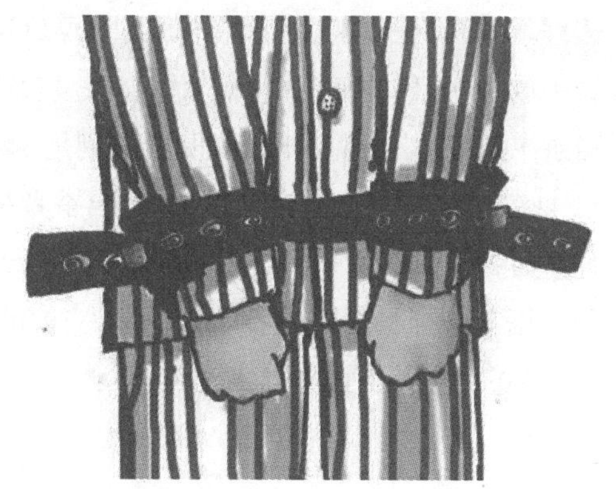

A. Arms-restraint strap

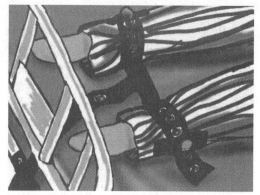

B. Legs-restraint strap

Figure 4-2 Protective constraint tools

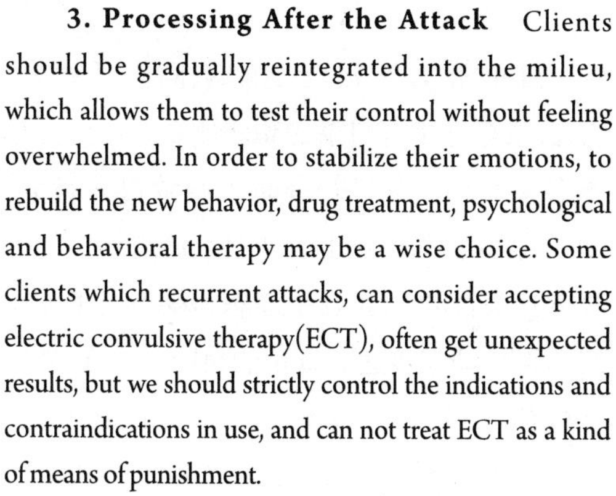

3. Processing After the Attack Clients should be gradually reintegrated into the milieu, which allows them to test their control without feeling overwhelmed. In order to stabilize their emotions, to rebuild the new behavior, drug treatment, psychological and behavioral therapy may be a wise choice. Some clients which recurrent attacks, can consider accepting electric convulsive therapy(ECT), often get unexpected results, but we should strictly control the indications and contraindications in use, and can not treat ECT as a kind of means of punishment.

iv. Evaluation

Evaluation includes the following aspects:

1. Whether the client behaves aggressively, if he or she has harmed himself or herself, or others.

2. Whether the client can recognize the aura of losing control and seek for help immediately.

3. Whether the client can deal with raging feelings in constructive ways.

3. **攻击行为发生后的处理** 被约束过后的患者应逐步使其回归到原来环境，这样可以帮助他们在不感到崩溃的情况下检验自己的控制力。为了稳定其情绪，重建新的行为方式，可适当给予药物治疗、心理行为治疗。部分反复发生攻击行为的患者，尚可考虑接受电抽搐治疗，往往会获得意想不到的效果，但使用时应严格掌握适应证和禁忌证，切忌将电抽搐治疗当作惩罚手段。

（四）护理评价

对患者的护理评价应从以下几个方面来进行：① 患者是否发生了攻击行为，有无伤害自己或他人；② 患者能否识别失去自制力前的征兆，并立即寻求帮助；③ 患者是否能以建设性的方式处理自己的愤怒情绪。

Section 2 Nursing Care of Clients with Suicide

Suicide is also a common Psychiatric contingency and one of the riskiest behaviors of clients with mental illness. It is one of the leading ten causes for the death of the disease and the leading killer of the psychotic. The definition provided by WHO is "one hurt himself or herself consciously in order to end his or her life". Some scholars also regard smoking, drinking, taking drugs, and other behaviors that can endanger one's health as chronic suicide, or indirect self-destructive behaviors.

The suicide rate was significantly higher in the clients

第二节 自杀的防范与处理

自杀是精神科较为常见的意外事件，是精神科患者最危险的行为之一，也是精神障碍患者死亡的最常见原因。世界卫生组织将自杀定义为："一个人有意识的企图伤害自己的身体，以达到结束自己生命的目的。"也有学者把诸如吸烟、酗酒、吸毒等危害健康的行为称为慢性自杀，或间接性自我毁灭行为。

精神障碍患者中，自杀率明显高于普通

with mental disorder than in the general population. Data provided by the China/WHO Mental Health Forum (1999) indicates that clients with psychiatric disorder account for 64% and 42% in China among those who commit completed suicide and attempted suicide. It was assumed by Black (1990) that more than 90% of the suicides are psychiatrically ill at the time of suicide. The data of America and Europe show that the rate of suicide of in client is range from 50 per 1 000 000 to 600 per 1 000 000 one year, which is higher than that of the common population. Most experts believe that the rate of suicide is increasing yearly.

人群。中国/世界卫生组织精神卫生高层研讨会（1999）提供的资料显示，我国自杀成功及自杀未遂者中，患精神障碍的比例分别是64%和42%。Black等（1990）认为90%的自杀者在自杀时都有精神障碍。美国和欧洲的数据表明，每年精神科住院患者的自杀率为50/100万～600/100万，明显高于普通人群。

I. Classification

Suicidal behavior is classified into five kinds according to the degree of suicide:

1. Suicidal ideation indicates having thoughts of wanting to die, but don't have specific plan and action. Strong ideation can lead to actual suicidal behavior.

2. Suicidal threat is the oral expression of a client's desire to end his or her life without specific plan and action.

3. Suicidal gesture is intentional self-destructive behavior that is clearly not life-threatening but does resemble an attempted suicide.

4. Suicidal attempt has suicidal ideation and put suicidal plan into practice, but doesn't arrive at predicted goal due to various reasons such as rescued by others, soft handed, regretting and stopping.

5. Completed suicide has suicidal ideation, takes actual suicidal action, and achieves suicide.

一、分　类

自杀行为按照程度的不同，可分为：①自杀意念指有自杀的想法或意向，但无具体自杀行动。意念较强时可导致自杀行为。②自杀威胁指口头上表达自杀的愿望，但无具体自杀行动。③自杀姿态指以不至于死亡的自杀行动来表达其真正的目的。④自杀未遂指有自杀的念头或想法，并有相应的行为，但由于各种原因（如被救、手段不坚决或懊悔而自动终止等），未造成死亡。⑤自杀死亡，又称完成自杀或成功自杀，指有自杀的念头或想法，并付诸于行为，最终造成死亡。

BOX 4-1 Learning More

World Suicide Prevention Day

According to the World Health Organization statistics (2000), there were about 1 million people died of suicide, and suicide attempts is 10 to 20 times for this data, which means on average that one person commits suicide every 40 seconds and one person suicide attempt happens every 3 seconds on average. Suicide has evolved from personal behavior into a threat against humanity development. In order to help the public to understand the risk factors of induced suicide, enhance people's ability to cope with adverse life events and prevent suicidal behavior, WHO and the International Association for Suicide Prevention（IASP）has celebrated World Suicide Prevention Day on September 10th since 2003. The theme of the first World Suicide Prevention Day is "Suicide one too many".

BOX 4-1 知识拓展

世界预防自杀日

据世界卫生组织2000年的统计数据，全球约有100万人自杀死亡，自杀未遂者则为此数字的10至20倍，这意味着平均每40秒就有一人自杀身亡、每3秒就有一人企图自杀。自杀，已从个人行为演变成威胁人类发展的一大隐患。为预防自杀和降低自杀率，自2003年开始，世界卫生组织和国际自杀预防协会将每年9月10日确定为"世界预防自杀日"，以帮助公众了解诱发自杀行为的危险因素，增强人们对不良生活事件的应对能力，预防自杀行为。首个世界预防自杀日的宣传主题是"自杀一个都太多"。

II. Reasons of Suicide

i. Genetic Factors

A family history of suicide is a significant risk factor for self-destructive behavior. Explanations for this association include identification with and imitation of a family member who has committed suicide,family stress,and transmission of genetic factors. Families of suicide victims have a significantly higher rate of suicide than families of clients who are nonsuicidal but mentally ill. In addition, monozygotic twins have a higher concordance rate for suicide than dizygotic twins.

ii. Biochemical Factors

There is growing evidence of an association between suicide or suicidal tendencies and a low level of the brain neurotransmitter serotonin, or 5-hydroxytryptamine (5-HT). 5-HT is an important monoamine brain neurotransmitter, and it is readily metabolized to 5-hydroxyindoleacetic acid (5-HIAA), which circulates in blood and cerebrospinal fluid. In general, 5-HIAA levels in assayable body fluids are thought to reflect levels of brain 5-HT(which can not be directly measured). Multiple studies suggest that a subset of suicide attempters and completers, especially those who use violent means of self-destruction,have very low 5-HIAA levels in the cerebrospinal fluid.

iii. Psychological Factors

Personality and psychological diathesis are also connected with suicide. In general,the client with following traits are likely to commit suicide under the psychological stress.

1. Having profound hostility towards the society, especially surrounding people, being accustomed to think things from the negative side. The association between hostility and suicide stems from the notion proposed by Freud that the suicidal person turns rage inward against the self.

2. Lacking of decisiveness and his or her own view, less trusting of others, expecting bad things to happen to them.

3. Isolating himself or herself from the society from thoughts and emotions, reducing social activity, regarding his or her self-value is low.

4. Being narrow-minded and extreme in treating matters, having not objective assessment of himself or herself and the environment, feeling powerless over their lives, not realizing the various ways to solve problems and just thinking of suicide.

5. Having impulsive behaviors, fluctuant emotions, nervousness.

二、自杀的原因

（一）遗传因素

自杀行为的家族史是自杀的重要危险因素。这可能与家庭成员对自杀的认同和模仿、家庭压力大以及遗传物质的传递有关。自杀者的亲属比有精神障碍但未自杀的患者亲属有更高的自杀可能性。此外，单卵双生子的自杀一致性比双卵双生子要高。

（二）生化因素

研究表明，自杀或自杀倾向可能与中枢神经系统中5-羟色胺水平下降有关。5-羟色胺是一种重要的中枢神经递质，不能直接检测其浓度。其代谢产物为5-羟吲哚醋酸，血液及脑脊液中5-羟吲哚醋酸的浓度可反映脑中5-羟色胺的水平。许多研究发现，自杀未遂者和自杀者（特别是使用暴力方式自杀者）脑脊液中5-羟吲哚醋酸的浓度很低。

（三）心理因素

不良的心理素质和个性特征与自杀有一定的关系，一般说来，具有下列心理特征者在心理应激状态下自杀的可能性比较大：

1. 对社会，特别是对周围人群抱有深刻的敌意，喜欢从负面看问题。敌意与自杀的关系源自弗洛伊德提出的“自杀者是将愤怒转向自我”的学说。

2. 缺乏判断力，表现为没有主见，遇事犹豫不决，不相信他人，总是相信坏事会发生。

3. 从思想上、感情上把自己与社会隔离开来，社会交往减少，自我价值降低。

4. 认识范围狭窄，看问题喜欢以偏概全，走极端。看不到解决问题的多种途径，在挫折和困难面前不能对自己和周围环境做出客观的评价，只是围绕着自杀而无法转向其他方法。

5. 行为冲动，情绪不稳定，神经质。

iv. Social Factors

Although suicide is a personal behavior, but it is affected by various social factors. Through the researches between social integration and the incidence rate of suicide, sociologists consider the following factors have effect on the behavior of suicide:

1. Social Support Social supports have valuable effect on the origin of mental disorder and the compliance and sensibility to the therapy. Isolating from the society will increase the client's loneliness; make him or her become fragile and vulnerable to commit suicide. People who are active in social affairs are more likely to suffer from stress; on the contrary, people who seldom participate in social activities have a higher tendency to commit suicide. In the interpersonal relationship theory, Sullivan also emphasized the association between suicide and the interpersonal relationship. He believed that the suicidal behavior is often a result of failure in dealing with interpersonal relationship problems.

2. Living Events Malign life events are likely to cause the suicidal behavior, these events include confliction with relatives, divorce, death of family members, unemployment, deterioration in economic status, being assaulted and threatened, crime, etc.

v. Psychiatric Disorder

Suicide is closely connected with the psychiatric disorder. All kinds of psychoses can increase the risk of suicide. Mental disorders with high rate of suicide are depression(unipolar or bipolar), schizophrenia, alcohol and drug abuse, and personality disorder.

1. Depression Depression is a common reason of committing suicide. It is reported that about 50% of the depressive clients have claimed that they have suicidal ideation,the rate of suicide is 50 times higher than that of common population. About 15% of the depression clients die of suicide finally. Losing confidence,feelings of uselessness, guilt, and desperation are the usual symptoms leading to suicide. Most of depressive clients who commit suicide have delusion.

2. Schizophrenia Schizophrenia has a high rate of suicide. It is one of the reasons that cause premature death of schizophrenia clients. It is reported that about 40% clients with schizophrenia have had suicidal ideation, 20%-40% clients have attempted to commit suicide,and 9%-13% clients died of suicide finally. The psychological symptoms such as hallucination and delusion are often factors leading to client's suicide. Domestic data shows that 65% suicide of the schizophrenia clients is due to delusion and hallucination. Other reasons include clients' desperation to the disease, frustration in work

（四）社会因素

虽然自杀是由个人决定的行为，但是要受多种社会因素影响。社会学家通过研究社会整合与自杀率的关系认为，对自杀行为产生影响的社会因素包括：

1. 社会支持 社会支持对精神障碍的起因、患者对治疗的依从性、敏感性都有重要的影响。社会隔离会使孤独感增加，使患者更加脆弱，容易导致自杀。研究证明，积极融入社会的人更能忍受压力。相反，很少参加社会活动的人自杀的倾向性较高。护理学家Sullivan在其人际关系理论中亦强调了人的自杀行为与人际关系的相关性，认为自杀行为是一种处理人际关系失败的方式。

2. 生活事件 不良的生活事件容易使人产生自杀行为。如与亲友间的矛盾、离婚、亲人去世、失业、经济状况恶化、被侮辱、受威胁或恐吓、犯罪等。

（五）精神障碍

自杀与精神障碍密切相关，所有精神障碍都会增加自杀的危险性。自杀率较高的精神障碍包括抑郁症（单相或双相）、精神分裂症、酒精和药物滥用以及人格障碍。

1. 抑郁症 抑郁症是自杀的一个常见原因。据报道，约有50%的抑郁症患者有过企图自杀的行为，自杀率高于普通人群50倍，约15%的抑郁症患者最终死于自杀。对生活失去信心、无用感、自罪感及绝望是导致自杀的常见症状。抑郁症自杀者中，有妄想者多于无妄想者。

2. 精神分裂症 精神分裂症的自杀率较高，是精神分裂患者过早死亡的原因之一。约40%患者有自杀意念，20%～40%患者有过自杀企图，9%～13%的患者最终以自杀结束了生命。精神分裂症患者常因幻觉、妄想等精神症状的影响而自杀。国内资料表明，引起精神分裂症患者自杀的原因中幻觉和妄想约占65%；其次是缓解期患者对疾病感到悲观，工作或婚姻受挫，社会歧视等增加了患者的

and marriage, social discrimination, and so on in the convalescence, for these factors can deepen the social isolation, and feeling of helplessness of the clients. In addition, large dose of the antipsychotics can cause serious effects such as inability to sit still, inflexible limbs, and tremble; a combination of large dose of the antipsychotics and long period usage can lead to tardive dyskinesia(TD). All these effects can cause obvious anxiety, depression, and suicide of clients.

社会隔离和无助感；此外，大剂量的抗精神病药物可引起严重的坐立不安、肢体僵硬、震颤，长期大量用药可出现迟发性运动障碍，这些原因均可使患者产生明显的焦虑、抑郁情绪，严重者会导致患者自杀。

3. Alcohol and Drug Abuse Long period of alcohol and drug abuse are the primary reason of suicide in the countries of north Europe. There are various reasons of committing suicide for these clients: most clients of alcohol and drug abuse also have symptoms of depression, and drinking can help them get rid of worry and timidity and make a strong will to suicide; excessive use of alcohol and drug can cause toxic hallucination and delusion; the withdrawal syndromes of alcohol and drug use can also lead to clients' suicide; clients who addict to drinking usually have personality disorder,which will have impulse to commit suicide under inducement.

3. 酒精中毒和药物滥用 在北欧的许多国家，长期嗜酒和药物滥用是由精神障碍引起自杀的主要原因。导致这类患者自杀的因素多种多样：酒精中毒和药物依赖患者大多伴发抑郁症，饮酒后可消除顾虑和胆怯，易于出现自杀行为；过量的酒精和药物会使患者产生中毒性幻觉或妄想；药物滥用患者产生的戒断综合征等可以引起自杀；嗜酒者常有人格障碍，在一定诱因下可出现自杀冲动。

4. Personality Disorder and Neurosis Personality disorder also has a close relationship with suicide. The research among the youth suicidal clients showed that more than 20% of them have personality problems. Clients with antisocial personality disorder and borderline personality disorder are more likely to commit suicide. The combination of antisocial personality disorder and depression is deadly to both the youth and the elderly. Furthermore,clients with histrionic and narcissistic personality disorder are also likely to commit suicide when they are aggressive and impulsive.

4. 人格障碍与神经症 人格障碍与自杀的关系也较密切。对年轻自杀者的调查显示，20% 以上有人格问题，其中边缘性人格障碍和反社会性人格障碍患者的自杀行为较多见。反社会性人格障碍和抑郁症状的同时存在对年轻人和老年人具有较高的致死性。表演性和自恋性人格伴有冲动和攻击性时也易发生自杀行为。

Long course of neurosis will also increase the danger of suicide. For example, the clients with stubborn obsession are more likely to commit suicide because they cannot get rid of obsessive idea or behavior, or have an obsessive suicidal idea; hysteric clients may perform suicidal gestures, and many of them die of suicide behaviors; hypochondriac neurosis accompanied with depression will increase the risk of suicide.

神经症病程持久会增加自杀的危险。如患有顽固强迫症的患者，因不能摆脱强迫性观念和行为的困扰，或出现强迫性自杀观念者自杀危险大；癔症患者会表现出自杀姿态，但也有不少最终自杀；疑病症患者在伴有抑郁时自杀危险性增加。

vi. Physical Disease

（六）躯体疾病

Chronic and consumptive diseases are also associated with the client's suicide. It is estimated that about 20%-70% of the suicidal clients have physical diseases. Malignancy and AIDS are common diseases of this kind. Clients with malignancy are likely to commit suicide after knowing diagnosis or within first two years of the course of disease. The rapid deterioration and acute pain are the important factors leading to suicide. Clients with HIV infection or AIDS have a high rate of suicide.

慢性消耗性的躯体疾病会让患者心生绝望，从而产生自杀意念。约有 20%～70% 自杀者患有躯体疾病。常见的疾病有：① 恶性肿瘤，此类患者容易产生自杀行为，尤其在得知诊断后及病后 2 年内。病情迅速恶化和剧烈疼痛是导致自杀的重要因素。② 艾滋病，HIV 感染者的自杀率较高，特别是明确诊断后和

The period after the diagnosis is definitely made and the primary stage of the disease are the riskiest time. Poor prognosis and disgrace often make them feel despair of life and hope to get released through suicide.

病程的初级阶段。预后差和耻辱感易使患者感到绝望，通过自杀来进行解脱。

III. Application of the Nursing Process

三、护理程序的应用

i. Nursing Assessment

（一）护理评估

Assessing the risk of suicide is the key element of preventing suicide. Nurses can do assessment to the client who is suicidal through close observational and listening skills to detect any suicide clues, the specificity of the plan,and its degree of lethality. Assessment of suicide risk is an ongoing process, not a single event. Data may be valid for only a day or two because a client's degree of suicidality is fluctuating quickly and unpredictably. Assessing individual suicidal risk factors generally requires in-depth knowledge of a client. It also may be necessary to obtain information from other sources before the degree of suicidal risk can be determined. Clearly, the more accurately risk can be predicted, the more effective prevention are the interventions. While false judgment may result in serious consequence, make the suicidal client lose chances of receiving timely treatment. It is imperative that nurses develop an awareness of suicide and predict risk for suicide of all clients in all clinical settings.

对患者自杀危险性的评估，是预防自杀的重要环节和组成部分。要评估患者自杀的危险性，必须通过严密观察和倾听来取得患者自杀的线索、自杀的计划和致死程度。对自杀的评估是一个连续的过程，因为患者自杀意愿的强烈程度不是一成不变的，而是随时可能出现预料之外的变化，患者自杀的信息有效性或许只有一两天。评估患者自杀的危险性不但需要护士对患者进行深入了解，还需要从与其相关的人那里了解信息。对自杀的危险性推测的越准确，预防的措施就越有的放矢。而错误的判断可能会导致严重的后果，使自杀者失去治疗和抢救的机会。因此，精神科护士必须了解自杀的相关知识，并对临床上所有患者的自杀危险性做出评估。

1. Methods of Assessment Psychiatric nurse can use direct conversation, observation, and other ways to estimate whether the client has suicidal idea, whether he or she will take suicidal action,and the risk degree of the client.

1. 评估的方法 判断患者是否有自杀意念，是否会出现自杀行为，通过交谈和观察的方法发现问题，并由此评价其危险程度。

(1) Conversation: Conversation can help nurse understand the client's feelings, thought, find the suicidal ideation. The encouragement of verbalization of negative feelings is essential, as well as the direct questioning about suicide ideation, such as asking if he or she feels meaningless to life, if he or she has the idea of ending his or her life. There is a wrong view that discussing such topic with the client will induce him or her to suicide. In fact, analyzing and discussing with the client about suicide will reduce the risk to suicide of him or her. Through communication with the client, the nurse begins to establish a therapeutic relationship based on trust by displaying an attitude of acceptance, empathy, and support, which is supportive to clients who experience feelings of worthlessness, helplessness, and hopelessness.

（1）交谈：交谈可以帮助护士及时了解患者的情绪、想法，发现患者的自杀意念并对其危险性作出判断。护士可以鼓励患者表达消极的情绪或直接询问患者一些关于自杀意念方面的问题。如是否觉得活着没有意义，是否有轻生的想法，是否采取过自杀行为等。有人认为与患者讨论与自杀有关的话题会诱导患者的自杀，这种观点是错误的。事实上，与患者公开坦率地交谈和分析不会促成自杀，反而会降低自杀的危险性。并且在交谈的过程中，护士通过运用接纳、同理心及支持，与患者建立起治疗性的信赖关系，以减轻患者的无用感、绝望感和无助感。

(2) Observation: Once the client has suicidal

（2）观察：自杀意念出现之后，患者的

ideation, his or her sensibilities, behaviors, and attitudes often change to a certain extent. For instance, the client may feel more anxious and fretful because of inner conflicts between living and dying; if the client has made up his or her mind to suicide, he or she will feel very calm and sedate, express regret and guilt to the relatives and friends, avoid discussing suicide with others and make specific preparation for suicide. Some clients may feel desperate at first and become hostile and aggressive to others. All these phenomena may suggest the possibility of suicide, so nurses in psychiatric setting should observe carefully the responses and changes of every client.

情感、行为及态度常会发生不同程度的变化。例如：患者一般对自杀引起的内心冲突感到更加焦虑和紧张；决意自杀后如释重负，情绪迅速平静下来，对以往的问题不再追究和抱怨；向亲友表示歉意和内疚；回避讨论自杀话题并为自杀做一些具体的准备等。此外，一些人在绝望后还会表现出明显的敌意及较强的攻击性。以上情况都预示着自杀的可能性，因此，精神科护士要注意观察患者的各种反应和行为的变化。

(3) Other clues: Nurses may communicate with the relatives and friends of the client, and they are often able to provide important information about the client. Some scales or questionnaires are also helpful.

（3）其他线索评估：应注意向家属、亲友及其他相关者了解情况，他们常常能提供较重要的信息；也可采用相应的量表或问卷，以帮助护士了解患者的自杀倾向。

2. Contents of Assessment Approximately 80% of all potential suicide victims give some clues before exhibiting self-destructive behavior. All behaviors and comments about suicide should be taken seriously. The nurse should be aware the clues that may indicate a client's suicidal intent and the intensity of the suicidal ideation intent.

2. 评估的内容 约80%有自杀倾向的患者在实施自杀行为前都曾表现过一定的自杀征兆。因此，应充分重视患者所有的关于自杀的语言和行为。具体来说，护士应该了解预示着患者自杀意图的一些征兆和自杀意图的强烈程度。

(1) Suicidal clues

（1）自杀的征兆

1) Has a history of suicide attempts.

1）有企图自杀的历史。

2) Is depressed, nervous, helpless, hopeless and cries frequently.

2）情绪低落，表现为紧张、无助、无望、经常哭泣。

3) It is unable to sleep, loses weight and fears the night.

3）失眠，体重减轻，害怕黑夜。

4) Keeps away from others due to self-imposed isolation, especially in secluded areas or behind locked doors.

4）将自己与他人隔离，特别是将自己关在隐蔽的地方或反锁于室中。

5) Listening to voices (The voices may tell the person to try to take his or her life).

5）存在命令性幻听。

6) Feels very guilty about something real or imaginary, feels that she or he is not worthy to live.

6）对现实的或想象中的事物有负罪感，觉得自己不配生活在世界上。

7) Talks or thinks about punishment, torture, and being persecuted.

7）存在被害妄想。

8) Suddenly seems very happy, without any apparent reason, after being very depressed for some time.

8）有抑郁情绪的患者，无明显原因突然出现情绪好转。

9) It is very aggressive or very impulsive, acting suddenly and unexpectedly.

9）显得非常冲动、易激惹，行为突然，出乎意料。

10) Ask suspicious questions such as "How often do the night personnel make rounds?" "How many of these pills would it take to kill a person?" "How high is

10）问一些可疑的问题。如“值夜班的人员多长时间巡视一次”“这种药要吃多少才会

this window from the ground?" "How long does it take to bleed to death?"

11) Talk about death, suicide, and want to be dead, and appear to be in deep thought. Examples of statements include "I want to die." "I don't have anything worth living for anymore." or "This is the last time you'll see me."

12) Show an unusual amount of interest in getting his or her affairs in order. Give away personal belongings.

13) Collect and hoard strings, pieces of glass, a knife, or anything else sharp that might be used for self-harm.

(2) Intensity of the suicidal intent: Intensity of the suicidal intent is determined by the frequency and degree of suicidal ideation, whether the individual has a specific plan and, if so, whether he or she has the means to carry out that plan. If pills are planned, what kind of pills? Are they accessible? In general, a client who has a suicidal plan, and has the means to carry out the plan is at very high risk. Most suicides are well planned, although they may ultimately be carried out impulsively.

(3) Suicide risk assessment tools: The psychiatric nurse may also find it helpful to use assessment tools to explore self-protective responses such as the one for inpatient settings. E.g., suicide probability scale, inpatient suicide assessment yool, nurses' global assessment of suicide risk (NGASR) (table 4-3).

死？”“这窗户离地面有多高？”或“流血死亡需要多长时间？”

11）谈论死亡与自杀，表示想死的意念，常常发呆。如患者可能会说“我不想活了”“没什么值得我活下去了”或“这是你最后一次见到我”。

12）将自己的事情处理得有条不紊，并开始分发自己的财产。

13）收集和储藏绳子、玻璃片、刀具或其他可用来自杀的物品。

（2）自杀意愿的强烈程度：自杀意愿的强烈程度取决于自杀意念出现的频率和程度以及是否有明确的自杀计划。如果有自杀计划，再看是否具备相应的条件和方法去实行此计划。如计划服药自杀，那么药物的种类和是否能够得到药物就决定了自杀的危险程度。一般来说，患者若有一个周密的自杀计划和计划实行的具体方式，其自杀的危险性就非常高。尽管患者的自杀都表现得较为突然，但大多数自杀是有精心的计划的。

（3）自杀危险程度的评估工具：临床上可采用一些评估工具来分析住院患者自杀的危险程度。如：自杀可能性量表、住院患者自杀行为评估表、护士用自杀风险评估量表（表4-3）等。

Table 4-3 Nurses' global assessment of suicide risk (NGASR)

Assessment Items	Score Key	Result	
		Yes	No
1. Feeling of despair	3		
2. Recent negative life events	1		
3. Delusion of persecution or have murdered content of auditory hallucination	1		
4. Depression/lose interest or lack of happy feeling	3		
5. Interpersonal competence and social function withdrawal	1		
6. Words with suicide attempts	1		
7. Suicide action plan	3		
8. Family history of suicide	1		
9. Death of loved ones or lose of Intimate Relationships	3		
10. History of mental illness	1		
11. The widower/widow	1		

continued

Assessment Items	Score Key	Result	
		Yes	No
12. History of suicide attempts	3		
13. Low socio-economic status	1		
14. History of drinking or alcohol abuse	1		
15. Suffering from terminal illness	1		

Scoring Key: In accordance with the above 15 items of scale, we concluded that the total sum, the higher the score, the higher the risk of suicide.

≤5 Low risk of suicide　6-8 Moderate risk of suicide

9-11High risk of suicide　12 extremely high risk of suicide.

表 4-3　护士用自杀风险评估量表

评估项目	评分标准	评估结果	
		有	无
1. 绝望感	3		
2. 近期负性生活事件	1		
3. 被害妄想或有被害内容的幻听	1		
4. 情绪低落 / 兴趣丧失或愉快感缺乏	3		
5. 人际和社会功能退缩	1		
6. 言语流露自杀意图	1		
7. 计划采取自杀行动	3		
8. 自杀家族史	1		
9. 亲人死亡或重要的亲密关系丧失	3		
10. 精神病史	1		
11. 鳏夫 / 寡妇	1		
12. 自杀未遂史	3		
13. 社会－经济地位低下	1		
14. 饮酒史或酒精滥用	1		
15. 罹患晚期疾病	1		

评分标准：上述 15 个条目量表根据加分规则得出总分，分数越高代表自杀的风险越高。

≤5 分为低自杀风险，6～8 分为中自杀风险，9～11 分为高自杀风险，

12 分为极高自杀风险。

ii. Nursing Diagnosis/Outcome Identification

1. Nursing Diagnoses Related to Suicide Include Several Aspects as Followings

(1) Risk for violence toward oneself related to hopelessness, auditory hallucination, etc.

(2) Desperation related to lacking supportive system and feeling worthless about oneself.

(3) Invalid coping related lacking adequate social support and skills of dealing with varied kinds of problems.

（二）护理诊断 / 护理目标

1. 与自杀有关的护理诊断　① 有指向自己的暴力行为的危险：与绝望的情绪、幻听等有关；② 绝望：与支持系统缺乏及感觉没有价值有关；③ 无效应对：与社会支持不足、缺乏应对技巧有关。

2. Nursing goals Include Several Aspects as Followings

(1) The client has experienced no physical harm to self.

(2) The client can identify and express painful inner experiences, has positive self-awareness, expresses some optimism and hope for the future.

(3) The client can cope with problems effectively.

iii. Nursing Intervention

1. Prevention of Suicide Suicide is considered more preventable than any other cause of death. This statement is based on the assumption that all suicidal persons are ambivalent about life and therefore are never 100% suicidal. Colvin (1980) suggested that the most important aspect of care for the suicidal person is the provision of a caring, therapeutic environment. She stated that the nurse may provide this type of environment by instituting the following plan:

(1) Communicate the potential for suicide to team members: This is an around-the-clock team effort. Any clues of potential suicide, no matter how insignificant they may seem, should be reported to all team members, including the physician. Subtle clues may well reveal intent, and after-the-fact is too late to make the determination that the client was indeed serious about suicide.

(2) Restrict lethal access: Suicidal clients should return to environments that have been made as safe as possible. Objects such as sharp items, belts, ties, and smoking materials that could be proved dangerous to the client are removed by searching the client's clothing, carry-in-items, and body in a dignified and professional manner. But do not completely isolate this person from others and strip him or her or all personal possessions unless the suicide potential is extremely acute. This only serves to intensify feelings of worthlessness. Medication stockpiles should be assessed and placed under other's supervision. Family and house-hold members will likely need education to ensure their willingness to act on a potential victim's interests.

People who seem very intent, have a specific plan for action should be hospitalized for their own protection,because hospitalization affords a safe environment in which lethal access is well restricted. Many clients will recognize that their own interests are best served by protective hospitalization, but for others, short-term involuntary commitment will be necessary.

(3) Observe the person: Clients at risk for suicide need either constant(one-to-one visual supervision) or close observation (visual check every 15 minutes)

2. 护理目标 ① 患者没有自我伤害行为；② 患者能够确认及表达自己痛苦的内心体验，并对自己有积极的认识，对将来抱有希望；③ 患者能够有效地应对问题。

（三）护理措施

1. 自杀的预防 与其他原因所致死亡相比，自杀是可以预防的，因为所有自杀者对于生命的取舍都是矛盾的。Colvin 建议在护理自杀者时，最重要的是给患者提供一个充满关怀的、治疗性的环境。一般可以通过以下的措施来预防患者的自杀行为：

（1）通知其他小组人员患者自杀的征兆：因为预防自杀需要全体医护小组成员夜以继日的共同努力。任何自杀的征兆，不管看起来是多么微不足道，都应该向其他小组人员和医生汇报。一些细微的征兆可能反映了患者自杀的真正意图，如果忽视这些细节，可能就会错过了挽救患者的最佳时机。

（2）保证环境安全：将有自杀意念的患者置于安全的环境中。用专业的方式检查患者的衣物、所带物品及身体，将危险物品如刀、剪、玻璃、绳、火种等拿走，在此过程中要注意维护患者的尊严。除非其病情非常严重，否则不要将患者与他人彻底隔离或拿走患者所有的个人物品，因为这样会加重患者的无用感。此外，药品也应放置于工作人员的视野范围内。

那些自杀意图明显且有明确计划的患者应该接受住院治疗，因为医院的环境较为安全，患者不太容易接触到危险物品。许多患者能够意识到住院治疗对于保护自身的重要性，但也有部分患者可能需要强制入院。

（3）密切观察：对于有自杀危险的患者，需要在安全的环境中对其进行持续观察（一

in a safe, secure environment. The level of observation varies according to the client's intention of suicide and established protocol of the facility or agency providing care. This observation should be carried out sensitively, with the nurse neither hovering over nor remaining aloof from the client. Constant or close monitoring of the client's behavior is important because a suicidal client's mental state often fluctuates. Watchful observation and care also give the person a sense of assurance that control will be provided until he or she can regain self-control.

对一的监护）或密切观察（大约15分钟巡视一次）。观察水平根据患者自杀意图程度和医院的规章制度来确定。护士在观察时应该认真仔细，既不应走马观花，也不应对患者表现得十分冷漠。持续地或密切性地观察患者的行为十分必要，因为患者的精神状态经常会发生波动。密切的观察及护理也会带给患者这样一种感觉：在患者能重新获得自我控制之前，外界会帮助其控制自己的行为。

Suicidal clients may appear to be feeling much better immediately before making an attempt. This is due to the feeling of relief experienced when the decision has been made and the plans finalized. Nurses have been fooled by this behavior pattern, relaxing their vigilance, only to have clients kill themselves when they are allowed to be alone for a moment. Therefore, it is important to remain alert until the mental health team and the client agree that the self-destructive crisis is over.

自杀者在采取行动之前，可能会出现情绪好转。因为当自杀的决心已定，计划都安排好时，患者会有一种情绪得到释放的感觉。若护士被患者的一时表现所迷惑而放松警惕，让患者独处，只会给患者自杀创造时机。因此，护士应在治疗小组及患者都确定自杀危机过去之前，保持高度警惕。

(4) Establish a therapeutic relationship: A therapeutic relationship conveys acceptance of the individual aside from the unacceptable act of suicide. If even one person is able to establish rapport with the client, this may well be the best protection against suicide.

（4）与患者建立治疗性关系：建立在信任基础上的治疗性关系表达了一种对患者接纳、理解、支持的态度，但其中不包括接受自杀行为的态度。这对经历着无用、无助及无希望感觉的患者来说，具有支持作用。能与患者建立一种融洽的关系，是一种最有效的预防自杀的措施。

(5) Listen to the person: The nurse's listening will convey support for the suicidal person throughout the current crisis. After the client comes to realize that the nurse is interested in and accepts him or her, the nurse should encourage the client to identify, examine, and share the source of the current emotional pain. The suicide risk may decrease if the individual feels that someone hears and understands what he or she is feeling. Explore with others who might be available to provide comfort. Perhaps communication patterns with significant others may need improvement.

（5）倾听患者诉说：护士的倾听显示了对患者的安慰及支持，在帮助患者渡过自杀危机中具有重要作用。当护士观察到患者能感受到并接受其关怀时，应抓住时机，与患者一起分析导致痛苦或自杀企图的原因，探讨可以提供帮助的潜在力量，如亲人或朋友等。如果患者感受有人能理解自己，会降低自杀的危险性。

(6) Contract for safety: Since 1973, nurses, psychologists, and psychiatrists have endorsed the use of no-harm or no-suicide contracts, believing them helpful in the treatment of suicidal clients. In such a contract, the client is asked to agree (verbally or in writing) not to attempt suicide for a specified length of time, to contact the clinician if he or she is tempted to act on self-destructive impulses. Most therapists agree that when clients readily agree to not harm themselves during a prescribed period, risk is decreased. When that time has

（6）安全契约：自1973年，护士、心理专家、精神科专家都开始赞成使用不伤害或不自杀契约，认为这种方法对治疗自杀患者非常有帮助。在此契约中，患者要同意（口头上或书面上）在一定时间内不会采取自杀行为，如果有自杀冲动应及时与工作人员联系。大多数治疗者认为当患者乐意接受在规定的时间内不伤害自己的条件时，自杀的危

elapsed,secure another promise. This gives the nurse and other professionals some time to help the client. This may also offer the client a sense of relief for getting the idea of suicide out in the open and discussing it in a nonjudgmental environment with a trusted individual. Finally, supportive others should be involved in the contracting process. Families and friends are important allies in caring for a suicidal client.

险会降低。当这个时间段过去时，再重新商定另一个条件。这种做法使得工作人员能有一段时间来帮助患者。而且，当患者在一种开放、无偏见的氛围中与所信任的人将自杀的想法说出时，会有一种解脱的感觉。患者的亲友也应该参与制订契约，因为他们都将参与到对患者的护理中。

(7) Give the person a message of hope: The suicidal person views life as hopeless,without any possibility for improvement. He or she undoubtedly has many ambivalent feelings regarding living or dying, but without hope for betterment, sees life as not worth living. After listening to the client's expression of emotional pain, encourage him or her to accept a message of optimism that life can be better. Discuss possible alternatives available to solve painful issues, and convey to the client that although the process may be very difficult, a measure of hope does exist.

（7）提供希望：想自杀的人都认为活着毫无希望，也没有改善的可能。他们无疑对生死持矛盾态度，因看不到好转的希望，才觉得活着没有意义。在倾听了患者对痛苦情感的表述后，护士应鼓励其接受一些乐观的信息，告诉患者生活会好起来的，不会总有像现在这样的感觉。应与患者讨论解决困难或矛盾的方法，告诉患者尽管解决问题的过程可能比较困难，但是问题最后总会解决的。

(8) Increase the person's self-esteem: Suicidal individuals have low self-esteem. The nurse may intervene by treating the client as someone deserving attention and concern. Positive attributes of the client should be recognized with genuine praise. An attempt to make up reasons to praise the client is usually recognized as artificial and lowers the client's self-esteem. The message is that the client is so bad that one has to search for positive characteristics. When getting to know the client, the nurse should be alert to strengths that can be built on to provide the client with positive experiences. It is also important to reinforce reasons for living and promote the client's realistic expectation.

（8）提高患者自尊：企图自杀者一般自尊都较低，护士应将其看作值得关注的人来对待。为此，护士应留意患者的优点，并真诚地给予表扬，以帮助患者建立正向的感觉和自信。但应避免凭空称赞，它会让患者觉得虚伪，自身并无可取之处，从而使其自尊下降，此外，向患者强调生活的意义，帮助其建立对现实的期望也可提高患者的自尊。

(9) Give the person something to do: Meaningful activities that release tension and anger can benefit the individual by allowing a medium for expression of hostility and aggression in a constructive manner. Activities such as washing clothes, repairing, bsanding,and refinishing furniture are best for this. It is also important that the individual resume independent participation in activities of daily living. Activities like those that promote achievement and a sense of belonging, ultimately, increase feelings of self-worth, as the individual once again becomes involved in the interactions of living.

（9）参加有益活动：一些有意义的活动可帮助患者释放紧张和愤怒的情绪，如洗衣服、打扫卫生、修理家具等。让患者独立参与日常活动也很重要，因为这些活动可以促进患者对生活的参与，增加其成就感、归属感及自我价值感。

(10) Mobilize social support: Self-destructive behavior often reflects a lack of internal and external resources. Mobilization of social support systems is an important aspect of nursing intervention. Significant others probably have many feelings about the client's self-destructive behavior. They need an opportunity to express

（10）动员家庭、社会支持：自杀行为常常反映了内在与外在资源的缺乏。动员社会支持系统是护理干预的一个重要方面。患者的亲友或许对患者的自杀行为有诸多感受，他们也需要一个机会来表达自己的感受，并

their feelings and make realistic plans for the future.

Families of suicidal client may be frightened of future suicidal activity. They need to be aware of behavioral clues to suicide and of community resources that can help with crisis. Suicidal behavior often recurs. False reassurance should be avoided. A better approach is to foster improved communication and an ability to cope in the family.

Community resources may also be important for the long-term care of the self-destructive person. There are many special institutions to provide services to the suicidal person in the USA, such as Suicide Prevention Center or Crisis Management of America. Nowadays, many professional crisis management institutions and hot lines have been developed in China to prevent the suicidal events. The nurse may be active in explaining resources to the client and initiating referrals to other agencies. Education of the public and health-care providers is needed to increase knowledge about the early warning signs of self-destructive behavior and implement effective treatment strategies.

All possible efforts must be made to protect clients and to motivate them to choose life. Nurses should align themselves with the clients' wish to live and then help them to be responsible for their own behavior. However, nurses must also understand that some clients will choose death despite their best efforts to intervene. Nurse must develop a realistic understanding of the client's responsibility for his or her own life and accept the possibility of losing a suicidal client even with the best nursing care.

2. Emergency Management It was reported that taking poison, hanging oneself, falling from high, striking, knifing wrist, getting an electrical shock,and turning on coal gas are usually used by clients with mental disorder to commit suicide. When suicidal behaviors happened,nurses should help doctors to rescue the clients immediately.

(1) Taking poison: The psychotropic medications are often used by psychiatric clients to kill themselves.

1) First, make assessment of client's consciousness, pupil, and color of skin, secretion and vomit.

2) Make a primary judgment of the quantity and the kind of the poison. If the client is conscious, try best to induce him or her to describe the quality of the poison and the process of committing suicide.

3) If the client has consciousness, first stimulate his or her throat to make him or her spew out the poison, and then clean his or her stomach. To those who are not sensitive to the stimulation can first make him or her drink

对未来作一些现实的计划。

家属可能害怕患者会再次自杀，因此，他们需要了解自杀的行为征兆和可以求助的社会资源。自杀行为经常会再次发生，所以不要做出错误的保证，而要促进家庭内的交流，以提高家庭的应对能力。

社会资源对于自杀患者的长期护理也非常重要。在许多国家和地区设立有专门的服务机构，如：美国的自杀预防中心或危机干预中心。我国在这方面的工作起步较晚，近年来部分地区已建立起了专业性危机干预机构，许多城市设立了热线电话、危机干预或心理咨询门诊，这对预防自杀起着非常积极的作用。护士可以将这些社会资源介绍给患者及其家庭。此外，还可以对公众及卫生保健提供者进行健康教育，使其了解自杀的早期征兆，并采取有效的治疗措施来进行干预。

护士应采取各种可能的措施来激发患者的生活热情，帮助患者对自己的行为负责，预防其自杀。护士应该明确，尽管他们已进行了最好的干预，有些患者还是会选择死亡。因此，护士必须认识到患者的生命掌握在自己的手中，只有患者自己才能对其生命负责。接受即使护士尽了最大努力，患者还是可能自杀死亡的现实。

2. 对常见自杀的紧急处理 根据国内外资料显示，精神障碍患者多采用服毒、自缢、坠楼、撞墙、割腕、触电、煤气中毒等方式进行自杀。当自杀行为发生时，护士应立即和医生一起对患者进行抢救。

（1）服毒：以精神药物最常见。

1）首先检查患者的意识、瞳孔、肤色、分泌物、呕吐物等。

2）初步判断所服毒物的性质及种类。对意识清醒的患者，应尽量诱导患者说出所服毒物的种类和服药的过程。

3）对意识清醒的患者，应先通过刺激咽喉部促使其呕吐，然后进行洗胃。对咽、喉部刺激不敏感者，可先口服适量洗胃液后，

some stomach washing liquid and then make him vomit.

4) According to the information, choose a suitable stomach washing liquid. For clients taking psychotropic medications or sedative-hypnotics, the best choice is 1:15 000-20 000 potassium permanganate solution. When the quality of poison is unknown, pure water is the best choice.

5) Whether time is long or short after taking poison, the client should also be made a thorough stomach washing.

6) If the poison that the client had taken is unknown, liquid washed out from client's stomach must be sent to further testing.

7) After stomach washing,use sodium sulfate solution to make him effuse.

8) If the client is unconscious or shock, cooperate with doctors to implement corresponding treatment.

(2) Hanging oneself: It is a common method adopted by psychotic to commit suicide. The main reason is that carotid is pressed by the gravity of the body, and the brain is in a condition of ischemia and hypoxia. Stimulation to the carotid sinus and causing sudden stop of the heart beating also contribute to the death. Nursing interventions are as follows:

1) Untie the rope immediately, using a knife or scissors. If the client is hung on the high, when untying the rope, we should clasp the client in order to prevent him from hurts caused by falling.

2) Lay the client on the floor, loose his collar and carotid. If the client still has heartbeat, we can put up his mandible, make him breath unobstructed, and give oxygen at the same time.

3) If the client's heartbeat and respiration have stopped, we should give heart massage and artificial respiration.

4) At the sustaining period of resuscitation, we should correct acidosis and prevent hydrocephalus caused by hypoxia, and provide some other supporting treatment.

(3) Getting an electrical shock: It is also called electric injury, caused by directly contact with electricity. The major effect of electricity to human being is burns of electric heat and muscle convulsion, which can cause the sudden stop of heartbeat. The treatments are as follows:

1) Cut off electrical source immediately.

2) If the client has consciousness, the nurse should lay him or her on the floor, loose his clothes and light up his mandible to keep him unobstructed breath.

3) If the client's heartbeat and respiration have stopped, we should give cardiopulmonary resuscitation immediately.

再进行催吐治疗。

4）根据所了解的情况，正确选择洗胃液，对服用抗精神病药物和镇静安眠药物者，可首选 1 : 15 000 ~ 20 000 高锰酸钾溶液，对毒物性质不明者，首选纯净水。

5）对服毒的患者，无论服毒时间长短均应彻底洗胃。

6）对所服毒物种类不明确者，应留取胃内容物标本送去检验。

7）洗胃后，可用硫酸钠溶液导泻。

8）对意识不清或休克的患者，应配合医生进行急救处理。

（2）自缢：自缢是精神障碍患者常用的一种自杀方法。引起死亡的主要原因是由于身体的重力压迫颈动脉使大脑缺血缺氧。此外，刺激颈动脉窦反射性地引起心脏骤停，也可能导致死亡。处理方法如下：

1）立即解脱自缢的绳带套，解套要快，可用刀切断或用剪刀剪断。如患者悬吊于高处，解套的同时要抱住患者，防止坠地跌伤。

2）将患者就地放平，松开衣领和腰带。如患者心跳尚存，可将患者的下颌抬起，保持呼吸道通畅，并给予氧气吸入。

3）如心跳和呼吸已经停止，应立即进行心肺复苏术。

4）复苏后期要纠正酸中毒和防止因缺氧所致的脑水肿，并给予其他支持治疗。

（3）触电：又称电击伤，是人体直接接触电源，电流通过人体而造成的伤害。电流对人体的损伤，主要是电热所致的烧伤和强烈的肌肉痉挛，可引起心搏骤停。处理如下：

1）立即切断电源。

2）意识清醒者就地平卧休息，松开衣服，抬起下颌，保持呼吸道通畅。

3）心跳和呼吸停止者，应立即行心肺复苏术。

4) At the sustaining period of resuscitation, we should keep the client's blood pressure stable, correct disorder of acid-base balance, prevent hydrocephalus caused by hypoxia, clear up the wound thoroughly, provide antitoxin of lockjaw and adequate antibiotics.

(4) Striking: When we find the client is striking against the wall, we should stop him immediately and distract his attention. For those who can't be persuaded and controlled, restraints can be used. Then we should observe the client's consciousness, pupil, respiration, blood pressure, pulse, and vomit immediately, cooperate with doctors to make examinations and deal with the client. If the wound is opening, we should clear up it thoroughly, and suture it immediately if necessary.

(5) Falling from high: If the client has fallen from high place, we should check if the client has consciousness, headache, and vomit, if there is liquid flowing from auricle, whether he or she has fracture and opening wounds, etc. For opening wounds, we should ligate limbs closing to heart to stop bleeding; for the client who has fracture, we only remove the client when necessary, use rigid board to fix his body and check if the client has viscera injury; if the shock has emerged, we should rescue the client on the spot. After primary treatment, we can send the client to the corresponding unit for further treatment.

(6) Self-harming: Stop bleeding of the incised wound caused by sharp instrument immediately, and ligate the limbs closing to heart. Observe client's consciousness, complexion, lip, and the quantity of urine,blood pressure,and impulse. Estimate the quantity of blood having been lost, judge whether the client is shock,and decide if it is necessary to rescue and give surgical treatment on the spot.

Because suicide is closely associated with the psychiatric disorder, and most of the suicidal clients have different degrees of mental disorder,we should give them psychotropic drug after first aid. Electric convulsive therapy (ECT) is also a good method for clients with strong intention to commit suicide. In addition, psychological treatment and crisis intervention can help clients deal with many problems and conflicts, enable changes in thoughts and behaviors of the clients so that they will increase their adaptability to the society.

iv. Evaluation

Evaluation of the suicidal client is an ongoing process accomplished through continuous reassessment of the client, and the goal achievement as well. Once the immediate crisis has been resolved, further psychotherapy may be necessary. The long-term goals of individual or group psychotherapy for the suicidal client would be to:

4）复苏后期要维持血压的稳定，纠正酸碱平衡失调，防治因缺氧所致的脑水肿，彻底清创（电灼伤面），肌注破伤风抗毒素并应用足够的广谱抗生素。

（4）撞墙：当发现患者撞墙时，应立即阻止患者，转移其注意力。对于不听劝告，又无法控制自己的患者，应将其约束。医护人员应迅速检查患者的伤情，观察患者的意识、瞳孔、呼吸、脉搏、血压及有无呕吐等。如有开放性伤口，立即进行清创、缝合。配合医生对患者进行各项检查和紧急处理。

（5）坠楼：如果发现患者自高处坠落，应立即检查有无开放性伤口、患者意识是否清醒、有无头痛或呕吐、外耳道有无液体流出、肢体有无骨折等，对开放性伤口，应立即用布带结扎肢体近心端止血。如果发现骨折，应减少搬动患者，搬运时应使用硬板，并观察有无内脏损伤。如果患者休克应就地进行抢救，对患者进行初步处理后，转入相应的科室进行进一步治疗。

（6）自伤：对于由锐器引起的切割伤，应迅速止血，用布带结扎近心端。观察患者的面色、口唇、神志、尿量，测量血压、脉搏，并根据受伤部位、时间估计失血量，判断是否存在休克，决定是否需要就地抢救和外科治疗。

由于自杀与精神障碍的关系非常密切，多数自杀者患有不同程度的精神障碍。因此，在急救之后常需要使用精神科药物进行治疗。对自杀观念非常强烈者，采用电抽搐治疗常能取得较好疗效。此外，心理治疗或危机干预可帮助患者解决存在的问题和矛盾，改变原有的思维和行为方式，提高适应能力。

（四）护理评价

对自杀患者的评价是一个持续的过程，需要不断地重新评价和判断目标是否达到。一旦自杀的危机解除，就可能需要进一步的心理治疗。自杀者长期心理治疗的目标为：① 建立和保持一个更为积极的自我概念；

1. Develop and maintain a more positive self-concept.

2. Achieve successful interpersonal relationships.

3. Learn more effective ways to express feelings to others.

4. Feel accepted by others and achieves a sense of belonging.

② 建立良好的人际关系；③ 学会更多有效地向他人表达情感的方法；④ 感觉能被他人接受，有归属感。

Section 3 Nursing Care of Clients with Spontaneous Leave

第三节 出走的防范与处理

Spontaneous leave as one of main contingencies in psychiatric settings indicates that clients leave hospital without permission of doctors. When clients run away, their treatment is interrupted. Clients without restriction and treatment may endanger themselves or other people in community and society, and may cause some other accidents. So if this behavior can't be prevented and dealt with effectively, they may cause serious consequence. So psychiatric nurses should know how to prevent and deal with spontaneous leave.

出走是精神科的重要意外事件之一，是指患者在住院期间，没有得到医生的同意而私自离开医院的行为。患者的出走会使治疗中断，可能造成自己受伤或伤害他人，还可能因走失而导致各种意外。如果不能及时有效地预防和处理精神障碍患者的出走行为，将可能给患者和他人造成严重的后果。因此，精神科护士必须了解如何对精神障碍患者的出走行为进行防范和护理。

I. Risk Factors of Spontaneous Leave

一、与出走相关的因素

In order to prevent it effectively, attributes to the spontaneous leave should be explored, and the signs should be perceived as early as possible. These attributes are psychiatric disorders and psychosocial factors.

只有了解与精神障碍患者出走相关的因素，及早地发现其出走的征兆，才能做到有目的的预防出走的发生。导致患者出走的主要因素包括精神障碍因素及社会心理因素：

i. Psychiatric Disorders

Different psychiatric disorder has various reasons for leave. Mental disorders that have relationship with leave are stated as follows:

1. Schizophrenia Some clients with schizophrenia have delusion and hallucination of persecution, so they leave hospital to avoid being persecuted. Some clients haven't insight and don't believe they are mentally ill, so that they think it unnecessary for them to receive treatment, and seek for opportunities to leave the hospital. And some clients can get lost when they are roaming about without purpose because of the reduced will and decreased responsibility.

2. Mood Disorder In order to choose a place to end their life, some depressive clients will make attempt to

（一）精神障碍因素

患有不同精神障碍的患者，出走原因是各不相同的。引起出走的常见精神障碍因素如下：

1. 精神分裂症 一些精神分裂症患者存在迫害性内容的幻觉和妄想，为了躲避迫害，患者会突然离开医院。也有一些精神分裂症患者没有自知力，认为自己没有疾病，无须治疗而选择出走来躲避就医。另外，还有一些精神分裂症患者由于意志活动的减弱及责任心的降低，会无目的地到处漫游而走失。

2. 情感障碍 有些抑郁症患者可因采取自杀行动而寻找机会离开医院，选择一个特

leave the hospital. Some manic clients try to leave hospital secretly to carry out a great plan, because they fear that their purposes would be prohibited or they can't wait to ask for permission.

3. Acute Stress Disorder Some clients may be in a condition of a hazy consciousness after exposure to acute stress and roam about without purpose. These clients can escape from dangers and do some complicated activities,but their expressions are dull. The can recover after several hours or several days, but most of them can't remember what has happened after they leave the hospital.

4. Epilepsy The spontaneous leave of the clients with epilepsy is actually a kind of automatism lasting for several hours or several days. Clients have some sensation to the surroundings and can also do complicated and harmonious activities, such as, shopping, talking, and traveling. If we make a careful observation, we can find that they are absentminded. Most of these clients will forget what they have done after seizures.

5. Mental Retardation and Dementia Clients with serious mental retardation and dementia may get lost when they go out or stroll without purpose in the hospital.

ii. Psychosocial Factors

1. Because of closed environment in hospital, clients feel boring, being constrained and want to escape as quickly as possible.

2. Some clients may feel that they have recovered and be anxious to return to work. And a few clients want to leave because of missing family members.

3. Some clients are fearful of being in hospital or some therapies, such as seclusion, restraints and the treatment of ECT.

4. The clients are unsatisfied with the indifference and impatience of the professional and want to leave the hospital.

II. Application of the Nursing Process

i. Nursing Assessment

After assessing the risk and the method of the spontaneous leave, the nurse can take correspondent measures to prevent its happening.

1. Methods of Leave Clients with clear consciousness will choose to leave in a covert way. They often search for and create opportunities to leave the hospital actively and secretly. If the client has the ideation of leaving, he or she will approach the staff, establish good

殊的地方来结束自己的生命。躁狂症患者则可能突然做出决定要实行一个宏伟的计划，常因来不及等到允许出院或怕受到阻拦而寻机离开医院。

3. 急性应激障碍 患者在精神因素刺激之后会出现意识朦胧状态，并无目的地出走。这类患者在外出时可以躲避危险，也可进行一些较复杂的活动，但患者的表情茫然。患者在几小时或几天后可以突然意识恢复，清醒后对出走的过程多不能完全回忆。

4. 癫痫 癫痫患者的出走实际上是一种持续几小时或几日的自动症。患者对周围环境有一定的感知能力，可进行复杂的协调的活动，如购物、交谈，甚至旅行。如果仔细观察，可发现患者心不在焉，绝大多数患者于发作后完全遗忘。

5. 精神发育迟滞和痴呆 严重精神发育迟滞患者和严重痴呆患者，可能外出时或到处乱走时走失。

（二）社会心理因素

精神障碍患者出走的常见社会心理因素有：① 住院患者由于处于封闭的环境中，感到生活单调、受拘束和限制，想尽快脱离此环境；② 一些病情好转的患者，因思念亲人，想早日回家，或急于完成某项工作而出走；③ 患者对住院和治疗存在着恐惧心理，如害怕被约束、对电抽搐治疗有误解等；④ 工作人员态度生硬，对患者不耐心等都会使患者产生不满情绪而想离开医院。

二、护理程序的应用

（一）护理评估

通过对患者出走方式及出走危险性的评估，护士可预先采取相应的措施，预防患者出走行为的发生。

1. 出走的方式 意识清楚的患者多采用隐蔽的方法，平时积极地创造条件，遇到有机会时便会出走。例如：与工作人员建立良好关系，取得工作人员的信任；常在门口附

relationship with them in order to gain trust and distract their attention; he or she may move around the gate to get out when guards are loose; look around all kinds of facilities in the ward, seeking possible passage to leave, such as unsolidified doors and windows. Anxiety, fidget and insomnia are usually accompanied with these behaviors.

Client with unclear consciousness always leave without purpose, plan and don not care about the method of leaving. They will leave through the gate as if there are no guards there. Once they get success, they are more dangerous to themselves and others.

2. Risk of Leave Following items can help the nurse assess the risk of leave of the client, and discover the client's intent of leave timely.

(1) Whether the client has history of leave?

(2) Whether the client has obvious hallucination and delusion?

(3) Whether the client has insight into his or her disease, and whether he or she is forced by others to the hospital.

(4) Whether the client feels fear of being in hospital and therapy, whether he or she is adaptive to the environment of the hospital?

(5) Whether the client misses relatives seriously and wants to go home?

(6) Whether the client has the signs of seeking opportunity to leave?

ii. Nursing Diagnosis/Outcome Identification

1. Nursing Diagnoses

(1) Risk of leave related to psychiatric symptoms, missing relatives, conscious disorders, etc.

(2) Risk of being injured related to psychiatric symptoms, conscious disorders, etc.

2. The Outcome of Nursing Interventions

(1) The client has correct knowledge of his or her disease and feels at ease in hospital. There is no behavior of leave when the client is in hospital.

(2) There is no accident happened to the client.

iii. Nursing Interventions

1. Prevention of Leave The nurse in psychiatric settings should increase communication with the clients and develop a therapeutic relationship with them. Close observation is also essential to know what the clients feel and need. For the clients who have the ideation of leave, the nurse should analyze the reasons with them, help them deal with problems and comfort them so as to remove their ideas of leave.

(1) Keep the environment safe. The nurse should often check the risk factors in the environment, repair the damaged doors or windows in the units at once,

近活动，窥探情况，乘工作人员没有防备时出走；观察病房的各项设施，观察可以出走的途径，如不结实的门窗等。与这些活动相伴随的是患者经常会有焦虑、坐卧不安、失眠等表现。

意识不清的患者，出走时无目的、无计划，也不讲究方式。他们会不知避讳、旁若无人地从门口出去。一旦出走成功，危险性较大。

2. 出走的危险性 下列项目可以帮助护士评估精神障碍患者出走的危险性，及时发现患者出走的意图：① 病史中是否有出走历史；② 患者是否有明显的幻觉、妄想；③ 患者是否对疾病缺乏认识，不愿住院或强迫入院；④ 患者对住院及治疗是否感到恐惧，不能适应住院环境；⑤ 患者是否强烈思念亲人，急于回家；⑥ 患者是否有寻找出走机会的表现。

（二）护理诊断 / 护理目标

1. 护理诊断 ① 有走失的危险：与精神症状，思念亲人，意识障碍等有关；② 有受伤的危险：与精神症状，意识障碍等有关。

2. 护理目标 ① 患者能对自身疾病和住院有正确的认识，表示能安心住院；住院期间没有发生出走行为；② 患者没有发生受伤等意外。

（三）护理措施

1. 预防出走 护士应加强与患者的交流，密切观察患者病情变化，了解患者的心理需求，并尽量满足。对有出走想法的患者，应了解原因，给予解释与安慰，力求消除患者的出走念头。

（1）加强安全管理。对病室及活动室损坏的门窗应及时维修，严格保管各类危险品，经常检查患者身边有无危险品。工作人员要

and remove all kinds of dangerous objects from the clients, such as knife, barrette, rope, etc. Make sure that the key of the ward are well kept by the staff, and not lend it to the clients. Once the key lost, the staff must search immediately. If the clients go out for activities or examinations, they should be accompanied by professionals. For the clients who have the intent to leave, the nurse should strengthen observation and inspection, and restrict the activities of them properly.

保管好钥匙，不可随意乱放或借给患者，如果丢失应立即寻找。患者外出活动或检查要有专人陪同。对出走危险性较高的患者，应加强对患者的观察与巡视，适当限制其活动范围。

(2) Enrich the clients' life. Carrying out indoor entertainment and productive activities regularly can make the clients feel at ease, and it is helpful to improve clients' mental activities and social functioning. If it is allowed,the nurse can organize some outdoor activities.

（2）丰富住院患者的生活。经常开展室内的娱乐活动，充实患者的住院生活，使其安心住院，而且能促进其精神活动及社会功能的恢复。如果有条件，可组织患者到户外活动。

(3) Strengthen the connection with the clients' family and colleagues, and encourage them to visit the clients,which can help the clients alleviate the feeling of being isolated and abandoned.

（3）加强与患者家属或单位的联系，鼓励他们来医院探视患者，以减轻患者的被遗弃感和社会隔离感。

At last, for the clients with mental retardation and dementia, close watch is the best manner of preventing accidents and clients' leave.

对于精神发育迟滞、痴呆患者以及处于谵妄状态的患者，应加强监护，以防止出现意外和出走。

2. Management of Spontaneous Leave When the nurse discovers the client is lost, he or she should inform other members of the unit immediately. All members must analyze and judge the time, manner and direction of spontaneous leave of the client. At the same time, some members of the unit should be assigned to search for the client.

2. 出走的处理 发现患者出走后，应立即通知其他人员，分析与判断患者出走的时间、方式、去向，并立即组织人员追踪。

For the client who wants to commit suicide, special attention should be paid whether he or she is at high place. If the client is on the top of the building, the searchers should try to calm him or her down and persuade him or her to give up the idea of suicide. At the same time, other assistance also should be provided, such as soft carpet, to prevent client's falling caused by nervousness and fear.

对有自杀企图的患者，应注意患者是否攀高，如果患者登上高层建筑的顶端，一定要稳住患者，劝说患者放弃自杀念头，引导患者自己下来。与此同时，组织救援力量，如搭建松软地铺等，预防患者因紧张、恐惧而下跌。

For the client who is wandering along the river or sea, some of the searchers should persuade them patiently, help them to realize that he or she is cared and regarded. The statement may make the client realize the serious consequence of their behavior, and give up the idea of suicide. During the course of explanation, the other searchers should get close to the client cleverly and restrict him or her so as to prevent his or her sudden jumping.

对徘徊在河边、海边等地方的患者，要耐心劝说，帮助患者感到自己受到关怀和重视，认识到自己行为的偏差，进而放弃自杀意念。同时，机智地接近患者，乘其不备，迅速将其约束，以防患者突然跳下。

If the client returns to home to escape the treatment, the searchers should cooperate with his family members to persuade and encourage him or her to return to the hospital.

如果患者因逃避治疗或不想住院而回到家里，医护人员应与家属一起做好患者的思想工作，使其返院，继续治疗。

iv. Evaluation

The evaluation can be carried out from the following aspects:

1. Whether the client has right recognition of his or her disease, whether he or she feels at ease in hospital?

2. Whether the client has an idea and plan of leave?

3. Whether the client's leave has caused injury to himself or herself or others?

（四）护理评价

护理评价可从以下方面来进行：① 患者是否对自身疾病有正确的认识，是否表示要安心住院；② 患者有无出走的想法和计划；③ 患者有无因出走而受到伤害或伤害他人。

Section 4 Nursing Care of Clients with Other Contingencies

第四节 其他意外事件的防范与处理

Besides aggressive behavior, suicide and spontaneous leave, there are other contingencies in psychiatric settings such as choke, eating different objects and falling. Psychiatric nurses must be familiar with the causes of these contingencies and the interventions to prevent and deal with them.

除攻击、自杀及出走外，精神障碍患者还可能会发生各种各样的意外事件，如噎食、吞食异物、跌倒等。为了切实保护患者的安全，护士必须熟悉各项意外的发生原因、预防及处理措施。

I. Choke

一、噎 食

Choke indicates that foods block the throat or the first narrow section of the esophagus, or enter the trachea and cause asphyxia. The rate of choke is higher in the clients with mental disorders than that in the normal persons. The symptoms of choke include acute cough and dyspnea when the client is taking foods, accompanied by the pale or violet complexion. If choke can't be relieved promptly, the client may die of it.

噎食是指食物堵塞咽喉部或卡在食道的第一狭窄部，甚至误入气管，引起窒息。精神障碍患者发生噎食以及因此而致窒息者较正常人多。患者表现为在进食中突然发生严重的呛咳和呼吸困难，出现面色苍白或青紫，甚至会窒息死亡。

i. Risk Factors of Choke

1. Antipsychotics often have the side effect of extrapyramidal symptoms (ESP), which may cause the movement of the swallow muscles becoming unharmonious, and restrain the swallow reflection.

2. Some clients with organic mental disorder such as Parkinson's syndrome, are likely to choke when eating too quickly because the swallow reflection is very slow. If a client with epilepsy seizure abruptly when eating, he or she may be choked by foods. In addition,clients eating at unconscious condition will likely to choke.

（一）危险因素

1. 精神障碍患者因服用抗精神病药出现锥体外系不良反应，引起吞咽肌肉运动不协调，抑制吞咽反射。长期服用抗精神病药容易出现噎食。

2. 患有脑器质性疾病如帕金森综合征的患者，吞咽反射迟钝，如果抢食或进食过急会发生噎食。癫痫患者在进食时抽搐发作也可能导致噎食。此外，患者在意识不清醒的状态下进食也可引起噎食。

ii. Application of Nursing Process

1. Nursing Assessment The choke of the psychotics often occurs suddenly, so it is very important for

（二）护理程序的应用

1. 护理评估 精神障碍患者噎食出现较突然，及时的发现及抢救非常重要。护理上

the nurse to detect and rescue them immediately. Nursing assessment can be processed based on the expression of the client. At prophase of the choke, the client may have cough and dyspnea with black and blue complexion, eyes open straightly, hands grabbing,and limbs convulsed. Serious symptoms include losing consciousness, body becoming soft, limbs being cold, incontinence of stool and urine, and ultimately, ceasing of respiration and heartbeat.

应从以下表现进行评估：噎食的程度较轻者会表现呛咳、呼吸困难、面色青紫、双眼直瞪、双手乱抓、四肢抽搐；严重者则意识丧失、全身瘫软、四肢发凉、大小便失禁、呼吸停止，心跳变弱进而停止。

2. Nursing Diagnosis/Outcome Identification

(1) Nursing diagnosis is the risk of choke related to the side effect of antipsychotics, organic mental disorder, etc; asphyxia related to obstruction of respiratory tract caused by choke.

(2) The outcomes include that the client knows how to prevent choke, choke or asphyxia doesn't happen.

2. 护理诊断 / 护理目标

（1）与噎食有关的护理诊断包括：① 有噎食的危险：与抗精神病药物不良反应有关，与脑器质性疾病等有关；② 窒息：进食过急而致。

（2）护理目标：① 患者知道如何防止噎食；② 患者未发生噎食或窒息。

3. Nursing Interventions

(1) Prevention of choke: Prevention is the most important treatment of the choke. Following measures can be used to prevent choke effectively.

1) The nurse should pay attention to the client's responses to the medications. If the client is taking antipsychotic,nurses should be sensitive to whether he or she has difficulty in swallowing.

2) If the client has the symptoms of side effect of medications and the swallow reflection is slow, the nurse should provide the client with soft food,semifluid or fluid when necessary. Make sure not give them foods with bone or thorn.

3) Assign special person to feed the clients having difficulties in swallowing. To those having the bad habit of crapulence or snatching foods, the nurse should control the quantity of foods, let him or her taking foods alone, and help him or her change the bad behaviors.

(2) The first aid of choke

1) If the client is choked, the rescue must be made on the spot. Clean out the foods in the mouth and pharynx to make the respiratory tract unobstructed. If the client's teeth are locked tightly, the nurse can prize up his or her mouth with chopsticks to take out the foods.

2) If the client still can't alleviate after these interventions, the staff should clasp around his or her waist with his or her head towards the floor and beat the back. Another way is making the client prostrating with the abdomen on a desk, upper part of body hung in the air, and then press the abdomen and waist in a rush to make the midriff move up. The pressure to the lung will force gases to dash out, so the food in the trachea will come out with the gases.

3) If above interventions have failed, it is essential

3. 护理措施

（1）预防：对噎食的护理应以预防为主，以下措施可以有效防止噎食的发生。

1）严密观察患者的病情和药物的不良反应，对服用抗精神病药物治疗者，要注意观察患者有无吞咽困难。

2）如果患者有药物不良反应，吞咽反射迟钝，护士应给予软食，必要时给予半流质或流质，避免带骨、带刺的食物。

3）加强饮食护理，对吞咽困难的患者，应专人守护进食或喂食；对抢食及暴饮暴食的患者，应单独进食，适当控制其进食量，并帮助患者改变不良的进食习惯。

（2）噎食的急救处理

1）如果患者发生噎食，应就地进行抢救。立即清除口咽部食物，疏通呼吸道。如果患者牙关紧闭，可用筷子等撬开口腔取出食物。

2）如果清除口咽部食物后患者仍无缓解，应立即将患者拦腰抱住，头朝下并拍背。或将患者腹部俯于凳子上，让其上半身悬空，猛压其腰腹部迫使膈肌突然上移，压迫肺部，使肺内气体外冲，从而将气管内的食物冲出。

3）上述措施无效，则要立即在环状软骨

to use a thick pinhead to stab into the trachea or cut off the trachea. It is an urgent way to keep respiration tract unclogged temporarily.

4) The client's dyspnea can be alleviated through treatment cited above. If the foods are also in the trachea, doctors of department of ENT can be asked to determine which way can be used to get the food out: bronchoscope, trachea intubations or trachea dissection.

5) When the foods are taken out, further interventions must be implemented to prevent inspiratory pneumonia.

4. Evaluation We can evaluate the effect of nursing intervention from following aspects:

(1) Whether the preventive measures are effective? Whether the client is choked?

(2) Whether the client recognizes the importance of eating slowly? Whether the client can choose what kind of foods to eat?

(3) Whether the staff provide timely and right rescue when the client is choked? Whether the treatment is effective? Whether there are complications happened?

下刺入一粗针头或行紧急气管切开，暂时恢复通气。

4）经上述处理后，呼吸困难可暂时缓解，如果食物仍滞留在气管内者，可请五官科医生会诊，决定采用气管镜、气管插管还是采用气管切开取出食物。

5）当取出食物后应及时采取护理措施防治吸入性肺炎。

4. 护理评价 ① 各种预防措施是否有效，患者有无噎食发生；② 患者是否认识到缓慢进食、细嚼慢咽的重要性，是否能对所摄食物进行选择；③ 发生噎食的患者有没有得到及时正确的抢救，急救措施是否有效，是否有并发症发生。

II. Eating Different Objects

i. Introduction

Eating different objects refers to swallow down other objects except for foods. It is a common contingency among clients with mental disorders. This behavior can be a result of thought disorder in clients with schizophrenia,or a manner of aggressive behavior or committing suicide. Clients with personality disorder may take eating different objects as a suicidal gesture. The objects the clients eat are various, including rings, pins and razor blades, thermometer, chopsticks, scissors and so on. Sometimes the client may swallow down plastics, cloth and cotton wool. Eating different objects can lead to serious outcome, so the nurse must prevent strictly, discover and deal with it in time.

ii. Application of Nursing Process

1. Nursing Assessment

(1) Assess the client's risk of eating different objects. The nurse should acknowledge whether the client likes to collect some strange objects, and whether he or she has a history of eating different objects. All these can help the nurse to judge if the client has intent to eat strange objects.

(2) If the client has swallowed down the different objects, the nurse should assess the kinds of objects and when this behavior happens, and makes a primary judgment of how dangerous the client is. The degree of danger is connected with the kind of objects. Metal or

二、吞食异物

（一）概述

吞食异物是指患者吞下了食物以外的其他物品，在精神障碍患者中常见，精神分裂症患者吞食异物可能由思维障碍引起，也可能是一种冲动行为或者想以此作为自杀的方法。人格障碍患者可采用吞食异物作为一种自杀姿态。吞食的异物种类各异，小的如戒指、别针、刀片，大的如体温表、筷子、剪刀等。除金属外，可以是塑料、布片或棉絮等。吞食异物可导致十分严重的后果，需严加防范，及时发现和正确处理。

（二）护理程序的应用

1. 护理评估

（1）评估患者有无吞食异物的倾向：了解患者的病情特点，是否有收集各种物品的嗜好，以前有无吞食异物的历史等。这些可以帮助护士预测患者吞食异物的可能性。

（2）如果患者已经吞食了异物，护士应立即评估患者吞食的异物的种类及吞食的时间，从而判断危险程度。吞食异物的危险性视吞食异物的性质不同，有锋口的金属或玻璃片

glass with a sharp edge is easy to hurt important organ or blood vessel and cause gastric or enteric perforation or massive hemorrhage. The plastics can cause poisoning,and too much fiber will cause intestinal obstruction.

2. Nursing Diagnosis/Outcome Identification

(1) Nursing diagnoses related to eating different objects include risk of being hurt, risk of poisoning,and constipation.

(2) Nursing goals.

1) The client realizes the consequence of eating different objects and changes his or her behaviors.

2) The client hasn't taken different objects.

3) The client has experienced no physical hurt.

3. Nursing Interventions

(1) Prevention: For the client with a tendency of eating other objects but foods, the nurse should analyze the reason,and not blame him or her for it. Explain the serious result of this behavior to the client and help him or her develop adaptive behaviors. In addition,strengthening the management of all kinds of objects is very important, especially the dangerous objects. The client should use scissors, needle, and nail clippers under the supervision of the nurse.

(2) Crisis management: When the client has the symptoms of intestinal obstruction or shock without other reasons, the staff should think about whether the client has taken different objects and ask the eating history. Examinations such as X-ray are also useful.

If the client is identified having taken different objects, appropriate treatment should be given to him or her according to the kinds of the objects, and treat with corresponding complications:

1) Small object can be excreted from alimentary tract naturally.

2) If the object is small and with sharp edge or needle-point, the client should be asked to rest on the bed and eat plenty of foods containing fibers such as leek. Give some evacuants to the client to facilitate his or her excretion. At the same time the nurse should pay closely attention to the abdominal symptoms and the blood pressure of the client.

3) If the object is metal, X-ray is essential to identify the place of the object, whether the mucous membrane of alimentary tract is hurt, and whether the object can be excreted from alimentary tract successfully.

4) If the mucous membrane has been hurt and is bleeding, or the object is too large to be excreted from alimentary tract, a surgery will be necessary.

5) If the client had crunched the thermometer and swallowed it down, the nurse should let him or her drink egg white or milk immediately.

可损伤重要器官或血管，因而引起胃肠穿孔或大出血，吞食塑料等可引起中毒，吞下较多的纤维织物可引起肠梗阻。

2. 护理诊断 / 护理目标

（1）常见的护理诊断：有受伤的危险，有中毒的危险及便秘等。

（2）护理目标：患者能认识到吞食异物的后果；患者没有吞食异物；患者没有发生中毒、内脏受伤等。

3. 护理措施

（1）预防：对有吞食异物倾向的患者要了解原因，不要斥责患者。耐心地向其说明吞食异物会导致的不良后果，并帮助患者改变行为方式。此外，要加强对各类物品尤其是危险物品的管理，患者如果使用剪刀、针线、指甲钳等应该在护士的监护下进行。

（2）患者吞食异物后的处理：当患者出现肠梗阻、急腹症或内出血（表现为休克）时，医护人员应想到患者有无吞食异物的可能，并追问病史，同时进行 X 线或 B 超检查，积极地予以处理。如果已确定患者吞食了异物，应根据异物性质或大小，采取不同的措施，并处理相应的并发症：① 较小的异物多可自行从肠道排出。② 若异物较小，但有锐利的刀口或尖锋，可让患者卧床休息，并进食含较多纤维素的食物如韭菜、给予缓泻剂，以利异物的排出；同时进行严密的观察，尤其注意患者腹部情况和血压的变化。③ 若异物属于重金属，应进行 X 线检查，以确定异物所在位置，胃肠道黏膜是否受损，确定异物能否自行排出。④ 若异物较大，不可能从肠道排出，或胃肠道黏膜受到损伤，出现内出血，应采用外科手术取出异物。⑤ 若患者咬碎了体温表并吞食了水银，应让患者立即吞食蛋清或牛奶。

4. Evaluation Nursing evaluation should emphasize whether the client has realized the danger of eating different objects, whether he or she has eaten different objects and experienced physical hurt.

The prevention and management of contingencies would help nurses resolve the clinical crisis in psychiatric settings, so that other nursing interventions can be conducted effectively and the harm to patients can be reduced or eliminated.

(Wang Zaichao)

4. 护理评价 护理评价应着重于患者是否认识到吞食异物的危险性，有没有吞食异物，以及是否发生了内出血、中毒等危险。

对意外事件的预防和处理可帮助护士化解精神科临床上的危机状态，更有效地实施其他护理措施；使患者免于或减少受伤，早日恢复身心健康。

（王再超）

Key Points

1. Aggressive behavior is the most common contingency in psychiatric settings. Reasons of aggressive behavior include psychiatric disorder, biological factors, and psychosocial factors.
2. Nurses need to assess risk factors and potential aggression of the client with mental illness. A screening tool may be useful in this process.
3. Many nursing interventions such as communication strategies, taking medications, seclusion, restraint, etc., may be helpful in preventing and dealing with aggressive behavior.
4. Suicide is one of the leading ten causes for the death of the disease and the leading killer of the psychotic.
5. The reasons of suicide include genetic factors, biochemical factors, psychological factors, social factors, psychiatric disorder, physical disease.
6. Conversation and observation can help nurse assess the suicidal clues and intent.
7. Nursing interventions such as establishing a therapeutic relationship, listening to the person, contract for safety, and so on can be used to preventing suicide. Once a suicidal behavior has occurred, nurses should help doctors to rescue the clients immediately.
8. Spontaneous leave as one of main contingencies in psychiatric settings indicates that clients leave hospital without permission of doctors. Psychiatric disorders and psychosocial factors are associated with the spontaneous leave.
9. The measures, including strengthen safety management, enrich the patient's life in hospital, strengthen contact with family members or units, and can effectively prevent the occurrence of the spontaneous leave.

内容摘要

1. 攻击行为是最常见的精神科意外事件，其原因有精神障碍、生物学因素及心理社会因素。
2. 护士应该评估精神障碍患者攻击行为的危险因素和前兆，以预防攻击行为的发生。此过程可利用评估工具进行评估。
3. 对患者的教育、交流技巧、服用药物、隔离、约束等措施可有效地帮助护士预防和处理攻击行为。
4. 自杀为疾病死亡的十大原因之一，是精神疾病的第一位死因。
5. 自杀原因包括遗传因素、生物化学因素、心理因素、社会因素、精神障碍因素和躯体疾病因素。
6. 谈话和观察可帮助护士发现患者的自杀征兆和意图。
7. 与患者建立良好的治疗性关系、倾听患者诉说、签订安全契约等措施可帮助预防患者的自杀。一旦患者发生自杀行为，应立即配合医生对其进行抢救。
8. 出走也是精神科的重要意外事件之一，其相关因素与患精神障碍与一些心理社会因素有关。
9. 加强安全管理、丰富患者的住院生活、加强与患者家属或单位的联系可有效预防出走的发生。

10. Other contingencies include choke, eating different objects, etc.

11. Choke indicates that foods block the throat or the first narrow section of the esophagus, or enter the trachea and cause asphyxia.

12. Eating different objects refers to swallow down other objects except for foods. For the client with a tendency of eating other objects but foods, the nurse should analyze the reason, and strengthen the management of all kinds of the dangerous objects.

10. 其他的精神科意外，还包括噎食、吞食异物等。

11. 噎食是指食物堵塞咽喉部或卡在食道的第一狭窄部，甚至误入气管，极易引起窒息。

12. 吞食异物是指患者吞下了食物以外的其他物品，对有吞食异物倾向的患者要了解原因，并加强对各类危险物品的管理。

Exercises

(Questions 1 to 2 share the same question stem)

A 21-year-old man suffered from schizophrenia and had delusion of persecution, saying someone was monitoring him outside the window across his ward and intending to harm him. So he rushed to the doctor's office, pounded the desk and shouted: "Let me out, or I'll start hitting others."

1. What is the main nursing diagnosis for the young client?

2. What kinds of the interventions should be taken by medical personnel?

(Questions 3 to 4 share the same question stem)

A 32-year-old woman committed suicide in ward by cutting neck with broken glass. She was found, treated with debridement&suturing and bound to bed. Then she said she need use the toilet and was released for a while. Consequently she opened the wound inside the toilet and committed suicide again.

3. What is the assessment method of the suicide severity?

4. What measures can the nurse take to prevent her from committing suicide again?

(Questions 5 to 6 share the same question stem)

A 19-year-old man has been hospitalized for more than 1 year since "talking to himself from and laughing himself, acting strangely, and parabulia". He was diagnosed with schizophrenia (hebephtenic type). After admission he was treated with modified electric convulsive therapy. One hour after the second treatment, he was in ambiguous sense condition, ran to the pantry, suddenly grabbed 2 cold steamed buns and swallowed him in one mouthful. The buns got stuck in the throat and caused choking. His face appeared purple with eyes fixed and hands scratching.

5. What are the primary actions which the nurses should take at this time?

6. What are the measures which can be taken to prevent the client from choking?

思考题

（1～2 题共用题干）

患者，男，21 岁，患精神分裂症，有被害妄想，说病室对面的窗外有人在监控他，想害他，于是冲到医生办公室拍桌子、大声叫嚷：“放我出去，不然我就要开始打人”。

1. 该患者的主要护理诊断是什么？

2. 此时医务人员应该采取的干预措施是什么？

（3～4 题共用题干）

患者，女，32 岁。在病室内用碎玻璃片割颈自杀被发现，经医生清创缝合处理，约束保护在病床上，期间患者称要如厕，便解除约束，结果患者在厕所内撕开伤口欲再次自杀。

3. 该患者自杀的严重程度评估方法是什么？

4. 预防患者再次自杀的主要措施是什么？

（5～6 题共用题干）

患者，男，19 岁，因“自语自笑、行为怪异、意向倒错 1 年余”收住入院，诊断为精神分裂症（青春型）。入院后给予改良电抽搐治疗，在第 2 次治疗结束后 1 小时，患者意识处于朦胧状态，跑到配餐间突然抓起 2 个冷馒头一口吞下，致使馒头卡在咽喉部而发生噎食，出现面色青紫，两眼发直，双手乱抓。

5. 此时护士首要采取的措施是什么？

6. 预防患者噎食的其他措施是什么？

Chapter 5 Ethical and Legal Issues in Psychiatric and Mental Health Nursing

第五章 精神科护理中的伦理及法律问题

Learning Objectives

Memorization

1. Describe related concepts of ethics and nursing ethnics.
2. Summarize laws related to psychiatric nursing.

Comprehension

1. Specify the rights and obligations of patients and nurses.
2. Identify ethical and legal issues arising in psychiatric nursing.

Application

Prevent or solve relevant ethical and legal issues in psychiatric nursing work.

学习目标

识记

1. 能准确描述伦理、护理伦理学及相关概念。
2. 能正确概述与精神科护理相关的法律。

理解

1. 能具体说明患者和护士的权利以及义务。
2. 能识别精神科护理中出现的伦理和法律问题。

运用

在精神科的护理工作中能够预防以及及时恰当的解决相关伦理和法律问题。

05章

Sally is the only child in her family. After graduation from university, her parents wished her to find a job in her hometown, so that they could stay closer with her. But finally Sally found a job in a big city which was far from her hometown. Her parents never stopped persuading her to go back to hometown. One year ago, Sally fell in love with a man in the big city, and planned to marry him. Her parents were very angry at her decision; they thought Sally was selfish without concerning about their feeling. And they had many unhappy disputes in the last year. Sally was very sad, and she refused to contact with her parents recently. Her parents felt despair and out of anger. So they visited Sally' house without notifying her and they had a very frustrated conversation. Sally felt helpless, crying and shouting to her parents. Her parents called the policeman and told the policeman that Sally was in a psychotic state. Sally was forced to the mental disorder center and hospitalized.

Please think about the following questions based on the case:

1. What ethical/legal problems exist in this case?
2. How would you help Sally as her primary nurse?

莎莉是独生女，大学毕业后父母想让她留在身边回家乡工作，但是不遂愿，女儿在大城市找到工作。一年前，莎莉在其工作地交了男朋友并计划结婚，父母得知消息后非常生气，觉得女儿非常自私不顾及他们的感受。去年为了这件事发生了很多次争吵，莎莉很伤心，最近她不再联系父母，父母非常生气并且感到绝望。他们在没有告知女儿的情况下找到女儿并和女儿发生了很激烈的冲突，莎莉感到无助，对父母大吼大叫，于是父母报警称她有精神方面的问题，莎莉被强制送进精神疾病中心住院。

请思考：

1. 本案例中存在哪些伦理问题？
2. 假如你是莎莉的责任护士，你会怎样帮助她？

Nursing work is embodied in moral content of providing service for patients and society, because of the strong professionalism and specialty of psychiatric nursing, ethical and legal issues arise in practice. It puts forward higher requirements to psychiatric nurses correspondingly, they should master not only basic theoretical knowledge of psychiatry and general medical professional, also knowledge about psychology, sociology etal. In this chapter we will learn the related concepts and theories of ethics and law and their application in psychiatric care. The aim is to strengthen the ethical and legal consciousness of psychiatric nurses, provide some additional tools for them to analyze situations and make considered and defensible judgments and provide better service for patients.

护理工作本身体现了为患者、为社会服务的道德内容。对于精神科护理工作而言，其本身具有极强的专业性和特殊性，因此必然会出现相关的法律及道德问题，相应的也对精神科护士提出了更高的要求。她们不仅要具备精神病学和一般医学专业基础理论知识，还要具备心理学，社会学等方面的知识。因此，本章将讨论伦理及法律的相关概念和理论及其在精神科护理中的体现，提出问题并阐述处理过程中的原则及方法，以加强精神科护士的伦理和法律意识，从而在临床上更好地为患者提供服务。

Section 1 Introduction

第一节 概 述

There exist a large number of ethical/legal issues in psychiatric nursing. It is extremely important and necessary for nurses to know the knowledge of legal and

在临床护理工作中，护士每天要向各种患者提供服务，满足其各种各样的需要，在

ethical issues, which will enhance the quality of care they provide in psychiatric and mental health nursing practice and also protect themselves within the parameters of legal accountability.

此过程中，就出现了大量的伦理和法律问题。因此，对于精神科护士，了解有关伦理和法律的相关知识非常重要而且必要。这将有助于提高精神科护理质量，并护士能在法律允许的范围内保护自己。

I. Ethics and Related Concepts

一、伦理及相关概念

i. Morals, Ethics and Ethnics

The term "ethics" derives from the Greek word "ethos" which refers to "customs, habitual usages, conduct, and character." The term "morals" derives from the Latin word "mores" for custom or habit. So the derivations of "ethics" and "morals" in West are totally the same. Thus, morals are the ethical customs of a society or ethical habits of a person. Both terms also imply goodness, worthiness, or desirability. An action or motive described as good, worthy or desirable is termed moral or ethical, whereas an action or motive described as bad, unworthy, or undesirable is considered immoral or unethical. But in China ethics and moral are different. They are the relationship between whole and part. Ethics is the whole, including two parts: the regular pattern of behavior and behavioral criteria that people should obey. Moral is the part which means how to regulate the behavior

Ethnic, a branch of philosophy science, is to deal with morals. It is a science on good moral and moral value. Ethnic is a system or code of and the behavioral rules that people indeed comply with in normal life. Moral only refers to one part: behavioral crite morals and is a discipline that seeks to formulate and systematically justify responses to moral dilemmas. Ethics can be classified into normative ethics and non-normative ethics. Normative ethics can be subclassified into general normative ethics and applied normative ethics, while non-normative ethics can be subclassified into descriptive ethics and pure ethics.

（一）道德、伦理和伦理学

伦理源于希腊文"ethos"，意为品行与气质以及风俗与习惯。道德源于拉丁文"mores"，也指风俗或习惯。所以，伦理与道德在西方的词源涵义完全相同。道德是一个社会或个人的伦理风俗或伦理习惯。两个词都意指正义、有价值或一种愿望。如果一种行为或动机是好的、有价值的、所希求的，那么它就符合道德伦理；反之，就不道德或不符合伦理。但是，在中国，伦理和道德的含义不同，它们是整体与部分的关系。伦理是整体，其涵义有二：人际行为事实如何的规律及其应该如何的规范；道德是部分，其涵义有一：人际行为应该如何的规范。

伦理学是哲学的一个分支，是研究道德的科学。它是关于优良道德的科学，是关于道德价值的科学。伦理学是一套道德准则或道德系统，以寻求道德判断确证的学科。伦理学可以分为规范伦理学和非规范伦理学两大类。规范性伦理学分为普通规范伦理学和应用规范伦理学。非规范伦理学又分为描述性伦理学和纯伦理学。

ii. Nursing Ethnics

Nursing ethnics was viewed as a subset of medical ethnics. In the 1980s, however, ethicists began to acknowledge the unique domain of nursing ethics, that is, the ethical issues and analysis used by nurses to make ethical judgments. Nursing ethnics is a science on nursing moral, which can direct nursing practice by using the ethical principles, theories and criteria, regulate the relationship within the nursing field and analyze, discuss, resolve the ethical problems in the nursing practice.

（二）护理伦理学

护理伦理学曾经被认为是医学伦理学的一个分支，自20世纪80年代以来，伦理学家逐步承认护理伦理学的学术地位，即护士作伦理判断时所运用的伦理法则。护理伦理学是研究护理道德的学科，用伦理学的原则、理论和规范来指导护理实践，协调护理领域中的人际关系，对护理实践中的伦理问题进行分析、讨论并提出解决方案。

II. Law and Related Concepts

i. Law

The term "law" derives from the Latin word "Jurisprudentia", which refers to social rules regulating human behavior. Law has a narrow sense and a broad sense definition. On the narrow sense, law is exclusively standardized documents established by the national legislature. On the broad sense, law is a standard or rule of conduct established and enforced by the government of a society. Except the standardized documents established by the national legislature, it also includes rules of conduct established and ratified by other national institutes, such as administrative statutes established by national administrative departments and local statutes established by the local departments.

ii. Rights and Responsibilities

Generally, rights are power and benefit defended by ethics or ratified by law. Responsibilities are special role claims, which are the duties that individuals must or should commit. A right is a claim one person has to a responsibility or duty on the part of another person. A responsibility is a duty or obligation of one person with the respect to another person.

1. Patients' Rights and Responsibilities Patients' rights are a complex concept related to legal, moral and ethic. It describes the legal and rational power and benefit after the individual suffering from disease. Protecting patients' right has been paid more and more attention in our country, for example, the research and legislative proposals of this aspect have being strengthened. Nowadays, special laws on patients' rights and responsibilities have not been enacted in China. However, many laws and regulations have clearly defined rights protection for patients. For example, *Constitution of the People's Republic of China* [45(1)] clearly states that citizens of the People's Republic of China have the right to get material assistance from the state and society when they are old, ill or disabled. *General Principle of the civil law of the People's Republic of China* [98] states citizens shall enjoy the rights of life and health. According to the situation of China, the patient rights include:

(1) The right to have medical, nursing, health, and rehabilitation service.

(2) The right of disease perception and informed consent.

(3) Free choice right.

(4) Privacy right.

(5) The right to exempt from some responsibilities and obligations.

(6) The right to disposite body tissue and body.

二、法律及相关概念

（一）法律

法律一词来源于拉丁语Jurisprudentia，意为调整人类行为的社会规范。法律有狭义及广义之分，从狭义上讲专指国家立法机关制定的规范性文件；从广义上讲泛指由国家制定或认可并由国家强制力保证实施的行为规范的总和。它除了国家立法机关制定的规范性文件以外，还包括其他国家机关制定或认可的行为规则，如国家行政机关制定的行政法规、地方国家权力机关制定的地方性法规等。

（二）权利和义务

从一般意义上说，权利是指法律上认可或伦理上可得到辩护的权利和利益。义务是指特定的角色要求，即主体必须或应当承担的职责。权利是一个人（权利人）从他人（义务人）那里得到某种东西的资格。义务是为满足权利人的要求应该或必需的作为或不作为。

1. 患者的权利和义务 患者权利是一个复杂的法律、道德或伦理概念，是指患者患病后应享有的合法、合理的权力和利益。在我国，对患者的权利保护也日益受到重视，医学伦理学和法学界加强了患者权利保障的相关研究以及法律保障机制的构建，虽然中国目前没有颁布关于患者权利的专门法规，但在许多法律、法规中对患者的权利保护有明确规定。如我国《宪法》第45条第1款规定"中华人民共和国公民在年老、疾病或者丧失劳动能力的情况下，有从国家和社会获得物质帮助的权利。"《民法通则》第98条规定"公民享有生命健康权。"从中国的国情出发，患者的权利应包括：

(1) 有医疗、护理、保健、康复的享有权；

(2) 疾病认知权和知情同意权；

(3) 自由选择权；

(4) 隐私权；

(5) 免除部分社会责任和义务的权利；

(6) 患者身体组织及遗体处分权；

(7) The right of indemnity.

(8) The right to supervise the realization of one's medical right.

In addition, *The Mental Health Law of the People's Republic of China* that took effect on May 1, 2013 also makes some specific rules and regulations to protect the rights of psychiatric patients including the rights of getting rescue, rehabilitation, accepting education and employment, applying for relief and getting informed consent. The rights and the responsibilities are corresponding. So the patients must assume the following responsibilities while having the rights. The patients' responsibilities include:

(1) The responsibility of self-health care.

(2) The responsibility to search for medical services and cooperate with the doctors and nurses actively.

(3) The responsibility to promote the development of medical science.

(7) 要求赔偿权；

(8) 监督自己的医疗权利实现的权利。

另外，2013年5月1日起施行的《中华人民共和国精神卫生法》还对保障精神病患者权利作了一些具体规定。它主要包括保障患者获得救助、康复的权利，保障患者接受教育和就业的权利，保障患者知情同意的权利以及保障患者申请救济的权利。义务与权利是相对应的，患者在享有权利的同时，也应履行相应的义务：

(1) 自我保健义务；

(2) 主动求医、积极配合治疗和护理的义务；

(3) 支持医学科学发展的义务。

BOX 5-1 Learning More

Declarations and Guidelines to Protect the Rights of Persons with Mental Disorders

A large number of declarations and guidelines which regulate the work in psychiatric sanitary area have been issued to protect the rights of patients with mental health disorder by various international organization including World Medical Association and World Psychiatric Association. Those declarations and guidelines contain *Declaration on the Rights of Mentally Retarded Persons* (the United Nations, 1971), *Declaration on the Rights of Disabled Persons* (the United Nations, 1975), *the Declaration of Hawaii* (World Psychiatric Association, 1977), *Mental Health Declaration of Human Rights* (World Federation for Mental Health, 1989), *Principles for the Protection of Persons with Mental Illness and the Improvement of Mental Health Care* (also called MI Principles, WHO, 1991), *Madrid Declaration* (World Psychiatric Association, 1996), *Mental Health Law: Ten Basic Principles* (WHO, 1996), *Guidelines for the Promotion of Human Rights of Persons with Mental Disorders* (WHO, 1996). Among them, the *Declaration of Hawaii* and *Madrid Declaration* are the most important ethical guidelines.

BOX 5-1 知识拓展

保护精神障碍患者权利的宣言和指南

从世界医学会的成立到世界精神病学会的组织与运作，诸多国际机构制定了不少有关的国际伦理原则、准则、规范，先后发表了大量规范精神卫生工作的宣言和指南来保护精神障碍患者的权利。这些宣言和声明包括《精神发育迟滞者权利宣言》(联合国，1971)、《残疾人权利宣言》(联合国，1975)、《夏威夷宣言》(世界精神病学协会，1977)、《精神患者人权宣言》(世界精神卫生联盟，1989)、《关于保护精神疾病患者和改善精神卫生保健的原则》(又称MI原则，世界卫生组织，1991)、《马德里宣言》(世界精神病学协会。1996)、《精神卫生保健法：十项基本原则》(世界卫生组织，1996) 和《促进精神障碍者人权的指南》等。其中《夏威夷宣言》和《马德里宣言》是最重要的伦理学指南。

2. Nurses' Rights and Responsibilities Nurses' rights and responsibilities have some specialities as well as the common characteristics of rights and responsibilities. Because of the special role relationship between nurses and patients, nurses' rights are emphasized more than responsibilities. In 1984, the report from WHO indicated that related nursing law had been enacted in more than

2. 护士的权利和义务 护士的权利和义务除了具有权利和义务的一般特点外，更具有其特殊性，即由于护士和患者的特殊角色关系，使护士一切以患者为中心，表现为更加注重护士的义务，而非权利。1984年世界卫生组织的调查报告就显示有70多个国家已经制定了相

70 countries, in which nurses' rights and responsibilities were embodied. *Nurses' Regulations* is the first regulation of protecting rights and interests of nurse in China, which passed on January 23, 2008 and provides legal basis of safeguarding nurse's legal rights. In the third chapter it points out the rights and obligations of the nurses, the details are as follows:

(1) The right to obtain remuneration, and attend social insurance.

(2) The right to obtain health protection and medical care service.

(3) The right to obtain the corresponding professional technical position, the title, to participate in professional training, academic research and exchange, to participate in industry associations and professional academic organizations.

(4) The right to obtain information related to performing nursing duty such as disease diagnosis and treatment, to give comments and suggestions on medical and health institutions.

The corresponding responsibilities include:

(1) The responsibility to comply with the laws, regulations, rules, the diagnosis and treatment norms.

(2) The responsibility to inform doctor immediately when patient is in critical condition, to implement the necessary emergency rescue first to rescue critically ill patients in emergency situations.

(3) The responsibility to respect and care for the patients, to protect the privacy of patients.

(4) The responsibility to participate in the work of public health and disease prevention and control.

iii. Legal Competence

Legal competence refers to the individual's qualification to have legal rights and commit legal responsibilities within the law system depending on his own conducts. In the psychiatric clinical practice the main legal competences include criminal responsibilities, civil capacity, trial competence, ability to serve on sentence, witness competence and self-defense ability.

1. Criminal Responsibilities　Criminal responsibilities, also called competence of responsibilities, refer to the abilities to identify and control behavior of individual. It also means that an individual has the abilities to understand the nature, meaning and consequences of the behavior and to control them. According to Chinese crime law, "anyone over 16-year-old takes criminal responsibility

应的护理法规，规定了护士的权利和义务。我国于2008年1月23日国务院第206次常务会议通过了《护士条例》，这是我国首部保护护士劳动者劳动权益的法规，为保障护士劳动者的合法权益筑起了强有力的法律保证，让护士劳动者维权做到有法可依。在第三章中明确指出了护士的权利与义务。护士的权利包括：

(1) 按照国家有关规定获取工资报酬、享受福利待遇、参加社会保险。

(2) 获得与其所从事的护理工作相适应的卫生防护、医疗保健服务。

(3) 按照国家有关规定获得与本人业务能力和学术水平相应的专业技术职务、职称；参加专业培训、从事学术研究和交流、参加行业协会和专业学术团体。

(4) 获得疾病诊疗、护理相关信息的权利和其他与履行护理职责相关的权利，可以对医疗卫生机构和卫生主管部门的工作提出意见和建议。

相应的义务：

(1) 遵守法律、法规、规章和诊疗技术规范的规定。

(2) 发现患者病情危急，应当立即通知医师；在紧急情况下为抢救垂危患者生命，应当先行实施必要的紧急救护。

(3) 尊重、关心、爱护患者，保护患者的隐私。

(4) 参与公共卫生和疾病预防控制工作。

（三）法律能力

法律能力是指行为人作为所参加的法律关系中的法律主体，以自己的行为独立地在法律关系中享有法定权利和承担法定义务与责任的资格，也称法律行为能力。在精神病学实践中主要涉及的法律能力包括刑事责任能力、民事行为能力、受审能力、服刑能力、作证能力、自我防卫能力等。

1. 刑事责任能力　又称责任能力，是行为人辨认和控制自己行为的能力，也就是行为人辨认自己行为的性质、意义和后果并自觉控制自己行为的能力。我国刑法规定："已满

when she or he is convicted for crime" and "psychiatric patients take no criminal responsibility when the harm happened on the condition that an individual couldn't discriminate or control one' behaviors under forensic evaluation".

2. Civil Capacity　Civil capacity, also called competence to behave, refers to whether an individual has the competence to stand trial when he or she deals with civilian problems such as marriage, property, testament, and contract.

iv. Forensic Psychiatry

1. Definition　Forensic psychiatry is a cross discipline based on the psychiatry and law. It is the medical subspecialty that involves the use of psychiatry expertise to assist in the resolution of legal disputes. As psychiatric knowledge and practice have developed, courts increasingly have called on psychiatrists to help solve legal problems.

2. Components　According to R. Rosner, there are seven components of forensic psychiatry as follows.

(1) Civil forensic psychiatry: It mainly includes child custody, parental competency, terminal of parental competency, child abuse, child negligence, psychotic determination, testament ability, demerits of psychiatric patient, breach of duty, lawsuit on individual trauma, etc.

(2) Criminal forensic psychiatry: It mainly includes trail competence, responsibilities competence, demurring competences, diminished capacity, ability to serve on sentence, the defense of delirium, and the release of innocent person because of delirium, etc.

(3) Legal regulation of psychiatry: It usually refers to the aspects such as right of privacy and confidentiality, right of therapy, right to refuse treatment, voluntary commitment, involuntary commitment, professional liability, and ethical codes, etc.

(4) Special issues of forensic psychiatry: Special issues of forensic psychiatry include risk appraisal of psychiatric patients, hypnotism, and the application of the anaesthesia analysis in court, responsibilities and roles of forensic psychiatrists, etc.

(5) Psychiatry in prisons: It refers to the treatment of criminals, and the psychology of criminals and the corresponding ethical codes.

(6) The essential issues of law: It mainly includes the essence of the law, the forensic system, the basic procedure of criminal law and civil law, the theory and practice of trail and punishment, etc.

(7) The representative cases: No examples.

16周岁的人犯罪，应当负刑事责任。""精神患者在不能辨认或不能控制自己行为时造成伤害结果，经法定程序鉴定确认的，不负刑事责任……"

2. 民事行为能力　又称行为能力，是当事人在处理民事法律关系，如婚姻问题、处理财产、遗嘱、订立合同时有无取得权利和承担义务的能力。

（四）司法精神病学

1. 定义　司法精神病学是建立在精神病学和法学两大基础科学上的一个交叉学科，是以涉及刑法、民法及诉讼法的精神疾病课题为研究对象，主要对专家的精神病学鉴定，对各种精神疾病的鉴定案例的临床特点、诊断、治疗，以及涉及法律问题的有关精神疾病问题进行研究的一门学科。

2. 内容　司法精神病学的内容十分广泛，美国Rosner（1982）将司法精神病学分为以下七个方面：

（1）民事司法精神病学：包括儿童监护、双亲能力、中止双亲权利、儿童虐待、儿童忽视、精神病性残疾判决、遗嘱能力、精神患者的过失、失职行为、个人外伤诉讼问题等。

（2）刑事司法精神病学：包括受审能力、责任能力、抗辩能力、限定责任能力、服刑能力、精神错乱辩护、由于精神错乱而被裁决为无罪的患者释放等问题。

（3）精神病学的法律规定：主要包括隐私保密性、治疗权利、拒绝治疗权利、自愿住院、非自愿住院、专业法律责任、伦理学准则等。

（4）司法精神病学中的特殊问题：主要包括精神患者的危险性评价、催眠术、麻醉分析等的法庭上的应用，司法精神病学鉴定中的医师的责任和作用等。

（5）监狱精神病学：主要包括拘禁患者的治疗计划、治疗安排，拘禁状态的心理学、伦理学问题等。

（6）法律的根本性问题：主要包括法律的本质，司法系统结构，刑法、民法的基本程序，审判、处罚等理论和实践等。

（7）典型案例：不再举例。

Section 2 Common Ethical Considerations in Psychiatric Nursing

第二节 精神科护理中常见的伦理问题

Psychiatric nurses may frequently confront many moral or ethical dilemmas while providing care for patients. Learning related knowledge of moral and ethics can help nurses to take effective interventions while facing moral dilemmas to prevent unnecessary disputes.

由于精神科护士在工作中面对的是患有精神疾病的个体，经常会面临许多伦理问题。通过学习有关道德及伦理的相关知识，使得护士在面对相关伦理问题时，能及时采取正确的处理措施，预防相关问题的发生，减少不必要的纠纷。

I. Ethical Principles of Nursing

一、护理伦理的基本原则

Ethical principles are fundamental guidelines that influence decision-making. Ethical principles themselves do not form a comprehensive ethical theory. Each may be used in resolving ethical dilemmas in relation to discussion of duties, rights, and goals. In ethical dilemmas, these principles can be in conflict with each other. The ethical principles of autonomy, beneficence, nonmaleficence, justice are helpful and used frequently by health care providers to understand ethical problems in health care and assist with ethical decision-making.

伦理原则为伦理决策提供基本的指导原则，但伦理原则本身并不能形成完整的理论。每一个伦理原则在解决特定的伦理问题时都起一定的作用，但是在解决伦理问题时，这些原则之间可能会有冲突。护士在伦理决策时广泛应用的伦理原则包括自主原则、无害原则、有利原则和公正原则。

i. Autonomy

（一）自主原则

Autonomy emphasizes that the persons have the right to make their own decisions free of external control even if it might conflict with medical advice. Health care providers should respect the rights and behaviors of patients with self-choice, freedom of action , self-management and self-decision-making. The principle of autonomy has been the most emphasized moral principle in modern health care ethics. Health care workers should apply the principle of autonomy flexibly in the clinical practice to make their behavior accord with the ethical code.

自主原则强调每个人都有不受外界干扰、自由选择自己行为的权利，即使有时候他们的决定会和医疗建议产生冲突。医护人员应当尊重有自主能力的患者的自我选择、自由行动或者按照个人意愿自我管理和自我决策的权利和行为。在现代健康照护伦理方面的所有道德原则中，自主原则被赋予了高度的关注。护士在临床上应灵活应用自主原则，最大限度地尊重患者的自主权，使自己的行为更符合道德规范。

1. Respect for Patients The principle of autonomy not only ensures that the autonomous decisions of patients are followed but also acknowledges the individual dignity of patients as persons able to form their own life paths. Nurses should respect personality and right of patients. Some psychiatric patients usually present childish, foolish, crude or weird behavior because of the characteristics of psychiatry. The nurse should treat them as general patients rather than sneer at or trick them. Nurses should try their best to satisfy the patients' need. If the patients have some illogical needs, the nurse should refuse euphemistically

1. 尊重原则 自主原则的实质是对人的尊重，对患者的尊重就是承认患者有作为一个人去选择自己生活方式的权利，护士应尊重患者的人格和权利。由于精神疾病的特殊性，有些精神患者常会出现幼稚、愚蠢、粗鲁或怪异的动作。护士应像对待普通患者一样尊重他们，而不是嘲笑和愚弄。对于患者提出的问题和合理要求，护士应尽量满足；对于不合理的要求，护士应婉言拒绝，而不

rather than ignore or deceit the patients. Patients should not be leashed except for special health care needs, which cannot be used for revenge, menace or terror.

2. Informed Consent Informed consent is a client's permission granted to the nurse to perform a nursing procedure, prior to which information about the procedure has been presented to the client with adequate time given for consideration about the pros and cons. Every client have the right to decide whether or nor to accept the treatment or nursing procedure and know the details about the procedure. Children, comatose patients, and the seriously mentally ill are examples of clients who are incapable of making informed choices. In these instances, a representative of the individual is usually asked to intervene with consent. The practice of informed consent has wide acceptance and approval. Its practice represents a clear effort to respect individual volition and values of patients and in this way also provide a fundamental resolution to the paternalism that was more common earlier in this century.

3. Confidentiality Medical documents may involve some secrets and privacy of patients because of the demands of diagnosis, treatment and nursing. Patients usually tell or expose to the medical personnel some private information, action or body part, which they don't want others to know for the benefit of therapy. Doctors and nurses should keep the information of patient confidential and shouldn't reveal it to others without the permission of the patient. On the other hand, information about medical professionals, such as addresses and hospital issues, also cannot be released to patients to avoid some unnecessary troubles.

ii. Beneficence

The principle of beneficence requires positive action, doing something good, preventing what is bad, and preventing what is harmful. In other words, beneficence removes what is bad, what is harmful, and promotes what is good and beneficial. This is positive in that it benefits the patient. As the theoretical basis, Utilitarianism is one of the broad ethical theories, which thinks the value of behaviors depends on the goals and consequences. Mill believed that "an ethical decision served to produce the greatest good for the greatest number of persons involved". To Mill, the basis of utilitarianism is "the greatest-happiness principle", ethical theorists of utilitarianism think that the aim of conduct is to weigh the positive and negative value of the behavior so as to alleviate pains and produce the greatest good for the greatest people. Health care workers

是不予理睬或哄骗患者。除非病情需要，否则不应约束患者，更不能以此对患者进行报复、威胁和恐吓。

2. 知情同意原则 知情同意原则强调所有护理措施都应得到患者及家属的同意，但同意的前提是患者必须完全了解有关护理措施的全部内容及信息。每个人有权决定自己是否接受某项治疗或护理措施，而且必须对该治疗或护理措施十分知情。在临床护理工作中，有些患者可能无自主能力，如婴幼儿、失去知觉者及精神疾病患者。这种情况下，通常由其代理人来代表患者行使自主权。知情同意已经得到广泛的接受和认可。它的实施不但保护了患者的自主权，而且也为20世纪初医务界的一种普遍现象——家长式作风提供了一种基本的解决方法。

3. 保密原则 出于诊断、治疗和护理等方面的需要，病历中有些内容会涉及患者的秘密和隐私。为了方便诊断与治疗，患者可能会将自己的隐私、不愿让他人知道的个人信息、私人活动或私人领域暴露给医护人员，医护人员应为患者保守秘密，未经患者本人同意，不得向他人泄露其秘密。另一方面，医护人员的有关资料如家庭住址和医院的内部事宜，也应对患者保密，防止出现不必要的麻烦。

（二）有利原则

有利原则强调一切为患者的利益和健康着想、尽量做对患者有益的事情，而不仅仅是不伤害患者。也就是说，护理人员为患者提供的所有指导和护理不仅仅是做到避免伤害，而是要对患者有积极的作用。其理论基础是被大众所接受的伦理理论之一——功利论，功利论者认为行为的价值取决于目的和结果。Mill认为行为的目的是“为最多的人带来最大的幸福”，他所提出的“最大幸福原则”是功利论的基础。功利论认为个人行为的目的就是权衡其正面和负面价值，以尽量减轻痛苦和不安，带来幸福和快乐。为患者

who act in their clients' interests are beneficent provided their actions really do serve the clients best interests. Doing good, preventing harm and removing harm are the essence of the nursing obligation to clients. However, nurses should keep in mind that an exaggerated form of beneficence that achieves good is not appropriate at the expense of autonomy. For example, the nurse might inform a postoperative patient who is in pain that a particular postoperative complication will occur if the client does not walk. Thus the nurse violates the principle of autonomy in order to obey beneficence. So in this case the nurse should explain the benefits of walking and the risk of remaining sedentary rather than tell a client that a complication will occur.

iii. Nonmaleficence

Nonmaleficence is the requirement that health care providers do no harm to their clients, either intentionally or unintentionally and also they should be empathetic, merciful and affable. For example, the nurse is responsible for not abandoning a client when the nurse disagrees with the client's ethical choices. Some nurses, for example, do not wish to care for criminals. If no other nurse is present to provide care, the nurse must stay with the clients. Some philosophers suggest that this principle is more important than beneficence. An example of this conflict might occur when administering chemotherapy to a cancer patient, knowing it will prolong his or her life, but creating "harm" (side effects) in the short term. In addition, it is challenging to obey the principle of nonmaleficence in Emergency Department since triage may strengthen the physical (long waiting times, increasing pain, and deteriorating condition et.al.) and psychological (stress, terror, feeling of being neglected et.al.) harms that come with the underlying pathological conditions). So the nurse should make the ethical decisions carefully.

iv. Justice

The principle of justice "refers to people getting what is fair or what is their due". Justice is the right of individuals to be treated equally regardless of race, gender, age, occupation, marital status, medical diagnosis, social economic level or religious belief. The term "justice" is the notion of equality. It is often used during the discussion of medical resources. When applied to health care, this principle suggests that all resources within the society ought to be distributed evenly without respect to socioeconomic status. Medical resources should be allocated to clients according to "first help with first come and urgency". The allocation should be benefit to improve the life quality, relieve the disease and prolong lifetime and also take the discrepancy between the nurses'

的利益着想、避免或消除对患者的伤害是护士最主要的职责之一。但护士在工作中应注意，不要过分的以有利原则为前提，而损害患者的自主权。如一个手术后的患者疼痛非常明显，护士却告诉患者如果不活动会产生并发症，这样，这位护士虽然是在遵循有益原则为患者利益着想，但却违反了自主原则。因此，在这种情况下护士应向患者说明术后活动的好处及不活动有可能产生的后果，而不应用并发症来威胁患者。

（三）无害原则

无害原则强调不要做有害患者的事，并要求护士做到有同情心、仁慈、和蔼。在某些情况下，虽然护士不赞成或反对患者的伦理观或行为，但从无害原则出发，不能拒绝护理患者。例如，当护士面对一个罪犯时，从无害原则出发，在没有其他护士在场的情况下，应该继续给患者提供必需的护理，而不能拒绝或停止患者的护理。有学者认为无害原则比有益原则更重要。例如，化疗可以帮助癌症患者延长生命，但短期内会对患者产生"损害"。另外，在急诊中有时候很难去遵守无害原则，因为在验伤分诊时，伴随的潜在病理状况有可能会增加患者生理（长时间等待，疼痛增加，病情恶化等）和心理（恐惧，紧张，被忽视的感觉等）方面的危害。这就需要权衡利弊，做出最合理的决策。

（四）公正原则

公正原则指的是"人们得到自己应得的或者受到公平的对待"，公正原则要求护士面对各种不同种族、肤色、年龄、职业、婚姻状况、医疗诊断、社会经济水平、宗教信仰的人，给予公正的护理。公正的实质是平等。公正原则常涉及医疗资源的分配问题。一般来说，医疗资源的公正合理分配首先应考虑根据需要来对待每个人。同时，医疗资源的分配应满足生命质量不断优化和提高的需要。再者，资源的公正分配应考虑到护患之间认识上的差距，使资源的分配有利于疾病的缓解和患者康

and clients' cognition into consideration. This principle is particularly important in Emergency Department(ED); it's really critical to maintain balance between being fair to all patients and the efficient use of medical resources in ED.

复、长寿。公正原则在急诊中的应用显得尤为重要，一方面要公平的对待每一位患者；另一方面，要保证医疗资源的有效使用，医护人员应该尽力做到平衡这两个方面。

BOX 5-2 History Corridor

Development of *The Code of Ethics* for Nurses in America

The Code of Ethics for Nurses was developed as a guide for carrying out nursing responsibilities in a manner consistent with quality in nursing care and the ethical obligations of the profession. In 1896, one of the initial goals of the newly established American Nurses Association (ANA) was to write a code of ethics, urgent issues such as nurse registration, the welfare of nurses, and accreditation processes for nursing schools took precedence. For many years, nurses had no formalized code of ethics and used Gretter's Nightingale Pledge, akin to medicine's Hippocratic Oath, to guide their practice. The first formal Code for Professional Nurses was adopted in 1950 and was edited slightly before being revised in 1960. *The Code* has been revised over time to introduce obligations to advance the profession and build and maintain a healthy work environment. ANA released the latest version of *the Code of Ethics for Nurses* in 2015, today's Code is a result of the ANA's long-standing commitment to support nurses in their daily life and practice. This code continues to provide all nurses with a firm foundation for ethical practice, it's the promise that nurses are doing their best to provide care for their patients and their communities and are supporting each other in the process so that all nurses can fulfill their ethical and professional obligations. It is important tool that can be used now as leverage to a better future for nurses, patients and health care.

BOX 5-2 历史长廊

美国护理发展之《护士伦理守则》

《护士伦理守则》在指导护士在护理工作中将专业知识和道德规范相结合中扮演着重要的角色。在1896年美国护士协会[American Nurses Association (ANA)]成立之初，就将制订关于伦理、一些重要事务（比如护士注册、护士的福利、护理学校的认证程序等的守则）作为一个目标。正如医生的希波克拉底誓言，多年来，护士一直使用南丁格尔宣言，而没有形成正式的书面伦理守则指导护理实践。1950年第1版正式的《护士伦理守则》获得通过并在1960年修订之前做了一些校正。为了使它能协助发展专业学科，让护士明白自己的职责以及建立和维护良好健康的工作环境，反复修改成了不可缺少的一步。2015年，ANA发布了最新版的《护士伦理守则》，新版守则是ANA在日常生活以及护理实践方面对护士做出的的长期承诺，一如既往的在伦理实践中为护士提供坚实的基础。它指出尽最大努力为患者、社区提供护理和相互支持，体现护士在工作中应履行的职业道德义务，同时也指出了护士应享有的权利，可为护士、患者、卫生保健服务的未来提供有效的保障。

II. Ethical Issues in Psychiatric and Mental Health Nursing

Ethical dilemma often arises when nurses are confronted with two or more choices neither of which is the perfect, especially when the reasons supporting each side of the argument for action are logical and appropriate. For example, ethical dilemma can arise from the conflicts among individual value systems, the conflicts among the clients, relatives and health care workers, the conflicts among the policies morals and laws. Nurses usually

二、精神科护理中常见的伦理问题

在面对两种或两种以上的选择，但没有一种决定完美的情况下，会产生伦理问题。伦理问题的产生可能是由于个人内在价值系统的冲突，患者、家属或医务人员的道德价值体系的冲突，或者政策、道德和法律的冲突。由于精神科护理工作的特殊性，精神科护士在工作中常会陷入道德或伦理两难的困

drop into ethical dilemmas because of the speciality of psychiatric nursing practice. Ethical problems can cause distress and confusion for both patients and nurses. Controversy is the very nature of ethical dilemmas and few people like conflict. To overcome controversy and determine a course of action, ethical issues should be processed carefully and deliberately.

境。伦理问题带给护士和患者痛苦和烦恼，争议是伦理问题的关键。为了解决争议，寻求合理的解决方法，护士和患者需要谨慎认真地来处理伦理问题。

i. Action Control

Action control is one of the biomedical ethical issues. It is also defined as that what one controlled do must be in harmony with requirement of controller. Action control is usually applied in neurotic, psychiatric and psychological therapy. It can be classified into message control and coercive control. Message control means to control individual's actions by regulating the messages inputted, for example psychological therapy. Coercive control means to change the individual's response to the stimulus by direct intervention on the body, then to influence the behavior, for example the medication.

The purpose of action control is to give the autonomy to the one controlled. But only if the autonomy is violated, action control takes effect. In psychiatric nursing, action control may violate the benefit and autonomy of the patient inevitably to cause ethical dilemmas. So the nurse must obey some moral principles while giving action control. Firstly, action control should promote patients' behavior to become normal. Secondly, action control should try to avoid the impairment on patients' body and mind. Thirdly, action control should not change the patients' personality. Finally, before action control informed consent must be involved.

（一）行为控制

通过一定的手段或方法使受控者的行为达到控制者的要求。它多应用于对神经科、精神科及有心理问题患者的治疗。行为控制可分为信息控制和强制控制。信息控制是控制者通过调节信息输入来刺激受控者并影响其行为，如心理治疗。强制控制是控制者通过直接操作和干预身体过程来改变受控者对刺激的反应，影响其行为，如精神药物治疗。

行为控制的目的是把自主性还给受控者，但只有首先在治疗中侵犯受控者的自主性这种控制才能奏效。在精神科治疗中，行为控制不可避免会侵犯患者的利益和自主权，产生了伦理学上的争议。因此，医护人员在实施行为控制时，应遵循一定的道德原则。首先，行为控制应促使患者的行为趋于正常。第二，应尽量避免对患者身体和理智能力的侵害。第三，应避免使用从根本上改变患者个性的方法。第四，应实行多种形式的知情同意，不能在隐瞒和欺骗的情况下实施行为控制技术。

ii. Self-determinism

Self-determinism can be defined as being empowered or having the free will to make moral judgment. The individual chooses a course of action without being restrained by others' expectation. A self-determined individual has intrinsic motivation to make choices based on personal goals, not to please others or to be reward. That is, a person engages in activities that are interesting, challenging, pleasing, exciting or fun requiring no "reward" other than the positive feeling that accompany them. Self-determinism is a basic and fundamental psychological need.

（二）自主决策

自主决策是指个体有权对伦理道德问题自由做出判断。个体在内在动机驱使下，达到个人目的而非取悦他人，自主决策。个体参与某项活动是因为活动本身有趣，有挑战性，而非参与活动带来的情感。自主决策是人的一项基本心理需求。

In psychiatric nursing, self-determinism is the right to choose one's health-related behaviors, which, at times, differ from those recommended by health professionals. For example, a twenty-year-old psychiatric male patient took medication regularly. He chose not to take the

在精神科护理中，自主决策是指患者自主选择与健康相关行为的权利。患者的自主决策有时可能会与医护人员的建议不相符合。例如：一个20岁的男性精神病患者，因病情

medication because of its side effects. However, the doctor insisted that the medication be helpful to the patient. If the nurse respected the patient's self-determinism only, the patient may stop the medication to make the illness worse, which violates the principle of nonmaleficence. On the other hand, it will be an offence of autonomy if client is coerced to take the medication. Confronted such dilemma, nurses should take the patient feeling into account objectively and communicate with both the doctor and the patient to try to achieve the consistence between the self-determinism and the medication. That is to say, nurse should try their best to promote the rehabilitation of the patient while respecting self-determination.

需要，定期到门诊接受抗精神病药物治疗。患者因为药物的副作用要求换药。而医生认为这个治疗方案对病情最有效。患者行使了自主决策权，但同时与疾病的治疗方案发生了冲突。这种情况下，若单一地尊重患者的自主决策，可能会导致病情恶化，违背无害原则。若强迫患者继续治疗则违背了自主原则。面对这种困境，护士需要客观地体会患者的感受，作为医患之间的桥梁与双方沟通，使患者的自主决策与医生的治疗方案尽量达成一致。也就是说，护士必须想方设法在尊重患者自主决策的同时，促进患者的康复。患者的自主决策有时无章可循。例如：患者要求给予安乐死，但没有相关法律政策可循。

iii. Informed Consent

Informed consent means that client has the right to be given adequate information about his or her disease and determine what should be done with his or her own body and mind. In psychiatric nursing, informed consent is important because of the potential side effects of many of the treatments including medication and electroconvulsive therapy. Once consent is given, nursing and medical personnel are absolved from legal liability for actions that they provide and practice according to discipline standards. Informed consent is complicated in psychiatric nursing. A patient must be competent to give consent, but the individual's decision-making ability is often compromised by the mental illness. A patient who is informed of the medication side effects refuses treatment, not because of the potential negative impact of the medication, but because of he or she denies the illness outright. The patient who is competent to give informed consent should be able to: communicate with others; understand relevant information; appreciate the situation and its consequence; use a logical thought process to compare the risks and benefits of treatment options.

In order to evaluate the psychiatric patients' competence to give informed consent objectively, many scales have been developed both at home and abroad, such as MacArthur competence assessment tool for clinical research (MacCAT-CR), Hopkins competency assessment test (HCAT), semi-structured inventory of competence assessment (SSICA), et al.

Under some circumstances, informed consent may do harm to patient, which deviates from the principle of nonmaleficence. Sometimes, informed consent may be

（三）知情同意

知情同意是指患者有权知晓自己的病情，并对医护人员采取的防治措施有决定取舍的自主权。在精神科护理中，知情同意非常重要，因为有很多治疗和护理措施，如药物治疗、电休克治疗等副作用很大。只有获得知情同意，医护人员根据相关原则所实施的治疗护理措施的法律责任才能免除。在精神科护理中，知情同意比较复杂。行使知情同意权时，患者必须有自知力、有决策能力。精神病患者的决策能力经常受到疾病的影响。患者被告知治疗的副作用后，拒绝治疗可能并非因为治疗的副作用，而是对疾病本身的否认。所以患者行使知情同意权时，护士必须充分评估患者的决策能力，主要含以下组成部分：① 能够与他人进行沟通交流；② 能够理解相关的信息；③ 能够评价有关的情景及后果；④ 能够比较各种治疗方案的优缺点。

为了客观评定精神障碍患者知情同意能力，国内外都开发了很多量化的评定工具，这其中包括麦克阿瑟临床研究知情同意能力评估工具、霍普金斯知情能力评估工具、半定式知情同意能力评估问卷等。

在某些情况下，知情可能对患者造成伤害，违背无害原则；但也可能有利于患者的健康和安全，与保密原则相符。这时护士会

beneficial to patient, which accords with beneficence. The terminal goal is to benefit patient most with the cooperation of patient, relatives and medical staff. Based on this, necessary disposal is directly introduced to patient on conditions as follows: the client's life and health would be threatened in emergency; emergency accidents defined; patients are incompetent and agents cannot be contacted with; to obtain written consent from client.

陷入两难的困境。通过与家属、患者和其他医护人员的合作，维护患者的最大利益是解决这一问题的最佳途径。基于这一点，建议在下列情况中可直接对患者实施必要的处理：① 对生命和健康有紧急威胁时；② 被认可是紧急事件时；③ 患者无行为能力，又无法联系其代理人时；④ 患者自动委托时。

iv. Protection of Privacy

The right of privacy means that the private information about the patient should be protected by law and should not be violated, collected, used illegally, and opened to the public. The private information includes the body part, physiological characteristic, psychological activities and some "demerit" behavior without harm to public. All of this information is that the patient tells the health care providers for the sake of the treatment needs. Nurse should try to protect privacy of patient. Medical record of psychiatric patient, such as personal information, primary therapeutic and prescription drugs should not be revealed without the permission of the patient. Also there are some exceptions for the protection of privacy. Psychiatric nurses usually make decisions considering the patient privacy, the health and security of patient or others. Because psychiatric patients usually have no deep knowledge of illness, it is necessary for nurse to communicate with others about the patients' condition. This may deviate the client's will, but do help to diagnosis and therapy. Also, the protection of Privacy is limited by the public health, that is, cannot do harm to others and the society.

（四）维护隐私

隐私权是患者享有的私人信息依法受到保护，不被他人非法侵犯、知晓、搜集、利用和公开的一种人格权。患者隐私主要包括患者为诊治疾病而告知医护人员的某些不愿让他人观察和接触的身体部位、生理特征、心理活动以及对公众无害的"过失"行为。护士应该尽量维护患者的隐私权，对于精神患者的个人情况、病史和治疗过程，未经本人允许不能对外公开。但是维护隐私不是绝对的。护士往往要在维护患者隐私与维护患者或第三者的健康和安全中做出决策。精神患者对自身的疾病缺乏认识，护士需要与家属、其他护士等人员一起沟通相关信息。这可能违背了患者的意愿，却有利于疾病的诊断和治疗。另外，隐私权的保护范围受公共利益的限制，即对他人和社会不能造成伤害。

Ethical decision-making in nursing practice requires determining facts, identifying the ethical problem, analyzing options by applying ethical theories and principles, and making choices. Because health care is ideally delivered by a team, ethical decisions should be team based. Many factors can affect ethical decision-making, including values, ethical theories, outer circumstance and law. It should be emphasized that nurses must take into national law and the rules and moral requirements of organization consideration to which they belong while making ethical decisions. For example, the Supreme Court in California prescribes that psychiatric medical personnel have the responsibility to protect others from the harm of psychiatric patients, which may influence the protection of Privacy. In addition, some legal right does not accord with ethical codes, which results in conflicts between legal rights and ethical codes. For example, euthanasia is legal in some countries, but it is

护理实践中伦理决策是一个复杂的过程，包括确定事实，认清伦理问题，依据伦理原则进行分析选择，最终做出决策。护理工作是团队工作，因此，伦理决策也以团队为基础。有很多因素影响伦理决策过程，包括价值观、伦理理论、外在环境、法律等。需要特别强调的是，护士在对上述问题进行决策的过程中，必须考虑到国家的法律规定和所在组织、机构的规章制度及道德要求。如美国加州最高法院规定精神科医务人员有保护第三者免于受精神患者伤害的责任。这就对维护隐私问题的决策产生了重要影响。另外，法律所规定的某些权利不符合伦理规范，法律权利和伦理规范有时会发生冲突。例如，安乐死在许多国家不合法，但有人认为是合

illegal in others. Abortion is legal in many countries, which deviates from ethical codes for religions. Nurses must obey the law rules rather than break the law in order to satisfy the patients' needs while making ethical decisions.

理的。堕胎在很多国家是合法的，但对于某些教徒来说却不合伦理。护士在处理伦理问题时，必须遵守法律规定，不能为了满足患者的要求而做出违法的事情。

Section 3 Common Legal Considerations in Psychiatric Nursing

第三节 精神科护理中常见的法律问题

Laws are the primary factor affecting the level of nursing practice. Each country has its own nursing practice act, which regulates entry into the profession and defines the legal limits of nursing practice that must be adhered to by all nurses. Nurse practice acts also address aspects of advanced practice, including prescriptive authority. Nurses must be familiar with the nursing practice act of their countries and define and limit their practice accordingly.

精神科护理常会涉及一些法律问题。作为一个特殊的群体，当精神科患者的行为涉及某种法律关系时，需要对他们的行为做出与法律相关的评定。护理法还涉及包括处方权在内的高级护理实践。而护士更应明确自己的权利和责任，减少法律问题的发生。

I. Types of Law

一、相关法律

The system of law varies from one county to another. In order to make right decision and avoid illegality, nurses should be acquainted with related regulations of law. Some related laws that nurses in China should know are as follows.

i. *Constitutional Law*

Constitutional Law, which is the basic law of nation, stands at the highest position in legal system and is the legislation basis of other laws. It is the rule of managing the national affairs. *Chinese Constitutional Law* prescribes the primary rights and responsibilities of citizens, which is one of the foundations for legal issues of psychiatric nursing.

ii. *Criminal Law*

Criminal Law includes the rules of crime and penalty. If psychiatric patients present the prohibited behavior by criminal law, the criminal legal competence at that time must be identified. The criminal legal competence refers to psychiatric patient, who reaches the legal responsibility age, has the obligation to assume the legal responsibility of his behavior in the criminal litigation. It mainly includes responsibility competence, trial competence, ability to serve on sentence, witness competence and self-defense ability.

不同的国家有不同的法律体系。为了能够合理决策并且避免违法行为的发生，护士必须要了解相关的法律法规。以下主要介绍在中国的护理工作中可能会涉及的相关法律：

（一）《宪法》

《宪法》是国家的根本法，具有最高的法律效力，是一切法律的立法基础，治国安邦的总章程，对国家生活起根本准则的作用。我国的《宪法》规定了公民的基本权利和义务，是处理精神科相关法律问题的基本依据之一。

（二）《刑法》

《刑法》是关于犯罪和刑罚的法律规范的总和。精神患者实施了我国《刑法》所禁止的行为后，必须对其在实施该行为时的刑事法律能力做出鉴定。精神患者的刑事法律能力是指达到法定责任年龄的精神障碍者，在刑事诉讼中对自己行为承担法律责任的刑事诉讼主体资格。它主要包括责任能力、受审能力、服刑能力、自卫能力和作证能力等。

iii. *Civil Law*

Civil Law is the rules to regulate the property and personal relationship between citizens, juridical persons, citizen and juridical person. If the psychiatric patient is involved in Civil Law, the civil legal competence at that time must be identified. The civil legal competence of psychiatric patient includes competence to act, marry, contract and make testament.

（三）《民法》

《民法》是调整平等主体的公民之间、法人之间及公民与法人之间的财产关系和人身关系的法律规范的总称。精神患者的行为涉及民事法律问题时，需要对其在实施该行为时的民事法律能力做出鉴定。精神患者的民事法律能力包括行为能力、婚姻能力、合同能力和遗嘱能力等。

iv. *Health Legislation*

Health Legislation is a standard or rule of conduct on medical care established and enforced by the government of a society. The aim is to protect the human health and regulate the relationship within medical activities. There are many kinds of *Health Legislation*, which include special laws, regulations, rules and relevant guidelines. Nursing law and medical malpractice law in our country, which both belong to the system of health legislation, play an important role in the psychiatric law issues.

（四）《卫生法》

《卫生法》是由国家制定或认可的，并由国家强制力保证实施的关于医疗卫生方面的法律规范的综合。它的宗旨是保护人体健康，调整人们在与卫生有关的活动中形成的各种社会关系。《卫生法》形式多样，包括专门的法律、法规和规章以及其他法律规范中的相关条款。我国的护理法、医疗事故法等都隶属于卫生法规系统，在精神科法律问题的处理中起着重要的作用。

v. *Mental Health Legislation*

Psychiatric Sanitary Legislation is various in different decades and countries. In 1800, the *Lunatics Act* was enacted in British, according to which psychiatric patients were housed and surveiled. The first law named *Psychiatric Sanitary Legislation* in the world was born in France in 1938. Other countries enacted Psychiatric sanitary legislation as follows.

The Action of Psychiatric Patients Protecting and Health Care Enhancement, which was passed in 75 session of 46 Union Congress in 1991, prescribed 25 primary principles. In 1995, they were generalized to 10 aspects by WHO, which include procurement of psychiatric health protection; medical evaluation in line with universal international standards; the provision of psychiatric health care in appropriate quality; health protection in least restrictive circumstances; self decision; the right to have others' help during self decision; the procedure to reexamine, eligible decision maker; automatic periodic reexamination procedure; respect to legal procedure.

Psychiatric sanitary legislation in Asia fell behind that in Westerns. Related mental health legislations were enacted at the end of 1980s in China. *Mental health Law of People's Republic of China* standardizes the treatment for patients with mental disorder, safeguards the rights and interests of them and promotes their rehabilitation. The law was adopted in 2012 and includes contents such as mental

（五）《精神卫生法》

《精神卫生法》在不同时代、不同国家有不同的要求。早在1800年，英国就制定了精神卫生条例，以法律形式收容或监视精神患者。世界上第一部正式命名的《精神卫生法》，于1938年诞生于法国，随后各国相继制定了各自的精神卫生法。1991年46界联大75次全体会议通过的“保护精神病患者和促进精神保健的原则”中，制定了25条原则，1995年WHO将此概括为10个内容：① 精神保健的获得；② 与国际通用原则一致的医学评定；③ 提供恰当质量的精神保健；④ 在最少限制的环境中提供保健；⑤ 自我决策；⑥ 在实施自我决策时有得到帮助的权利；⑦ 有复查程序；⑧ 合格的决策者；⑨ 自动定期复查程序；⑩ 尊重法律程序。

亚洲国家的精神卫生法方面较为落后。我国于20世纪80年代末，先后制定了多种精神卫生相关法规。历经十余年的反复审议，2012年10月26日第十一届全国人民代表大会常务委员会第二十九次会议通过了《中华人民共和国精神卫生法》，并在2013年5月1日

health promotion, prevention, diagnosis, treatment and rehabilitation. The birth of this law is definitely a good news for health care provider working in psychiatry department, they can notice potential legal issues more acutely. This law also can improve the quality of nursing service and safeguard the legitimate rights and interests of patients in a better way.

正式实施。这是首次由精神卫生人员参与起草的一部规范精神障碍患者治疗、保障精神障碍患者权益和促进精神障碍者康复的法律，其中包括心理健康促进和精神障碍预防、精神障碍的诊断和治疗、精神障碍的康复、保障措施、法律责任等多项内容。这对于在精神科工作的医务人员来说是一个好消息，让他们更加敏锐的观察到工作中所遇到的潜在的法律问题，并提出了相关的防护措施，进而提高护理服务的质量，更好地维护患者的合法权益。

II. Legal Issues in Psychiatric and Mental Health Nursing

Nurse may be involved in many legal issues in psychiatric and mental health nursing, including the admission and treatment, rights and responsibilities etal. They must be familiar with and abide by the local regulations and practice according to the laws.

i. Types of Admission

When psychiatric patients are hospitalized, the type of admission is vitally important. Various admission statutes reflect differing patient rights as well as staff treatment responsibilities. There are specific statutory regulations pertaining to each admission status that mandate procedures for admission, discharge, and commitment for treatment.

1. Voluntary Admission Patients, who present themselves at psychiatric facilities and request hospitalization, are considered voluntary admission patients. Likewise, patients were evaluated as being of danger to themselves or to others or being so seriously mentally ill that they cannot adequately meet their own needs in the community but who are willing to submit to treatment and are competent to do so have voluntary admission status. Voluntary patients have certain rights that differ from the rights of other hospitalized patients. They have the absolute right to refuse treatment, including psychotropic medication, unless they are dangerous to themselves or others, as in a violent destructive episode within the treatment unit. Voluntary patients do not have an absolute right to discharge at any time but may be required to request discharge.

2. Involuntary Admission The admission form of psychiatric patients must be different from those in general hospital because of the patients' specialty. Some

二、精神科护理中常见的法律问题

在精神科护理中常会遇到一些法律问题，内容可能涉及患者的住院和治疗、患者的权利和义务等多个方面。护士必须熟悉和遵守其工作地的相关法律规定，依法行事。

（一）患者的入院形式

精神科患者住院时，其入院形式非常重要。患者的权利和医务人员的治疗责任，也因入院形式而有所不同。每一种入院形式都对入院、出院和治疗有特定的法律规定。

1. 自愿入院 患者因自己的精神病状态而自愿要求住院时即称为自愿入院。当患者可能会对自己或他人造成危险，或者严重的精神病状态生活不能自理，但是愿意并且能够入院接受治疗时，也称为自愿入院。自愿入院患者有不同于其他形式入院患者的特定的权利。自愿入院患者如果在治疗过程中因暴力倾向可能伤害自己或他人时，也没有拒绝接受治疗的权利。自愿入院患者虽然没有任何时候都可以要求自动出院的权利，但有申请出院的权利。

2. 非自愿入院 由于精神病患者的特殊性，其入院方式与综合医院的患者必然存在差异，有时需要违背患者意志让其住院，因此会

legal issues may arise when it is necessary to hospitalize patients against their will. Patients are considered to have involuntary admission status when they would dangerous to self or others, in mentally illness and indeed of treatment, or is gravely disabled. Because involuntary admission results in substantial restrictions of the rights of an individual, the individual seeking the involuntary admission must show probable cause why the patient should be hospitalized against his or her own wishes.

(1) Coercive admission: Coercive admission usually refers to the patients who are unable to take care of basic personal needs and judge potential harm to others because of mental illness. Inability to care for oneself cannot be established by showing that the patient lacks the resources to provide the necessities of life. Rather, it is the inability to make use of available resources. Usually, the patients come to hospital accompanied by their relatives or guardian. Sometimes, police sent them to hospital if they refuse treatment.

(2) Judiciary-identified admission: Judiciary-identified admission refers to the psychiatric patients, who are convicted of crime, need hospitalization and judiciary identification. Committed institution manages the admission and discharge of the patients. Without its permission, no one has right to visit them.

Generally, the admissions to psychiatric hospitals are voluntary. However, some psychiatric patients refuse to treatment because of the mental disorder. Coercive admission may take place for the benefits of clients after the permission of related law institution. According to the citizens' right of personal freedom prescribed in constitution law and criminal law in China, patients and relatives may think that coercive admission is the "restraint of freedom" of "illegal detention", which results in law issues. Psychiatric patients, who are considered as involuntary admission patients, must meet the following two criteria.

Firstly, the patient is gravely disabled. That is, he or she has seriously violent behavior, which is dangerous to others, obvious inclination to injure self or suicide, inability to take care of basic personal needs, or the serious disturbance of social order. Secondly, if the patient is really gravely disabled, the relatives, guardian or legal attorney can apply for the admission instead of the patient. After the doctor diagnoses the illness as psychiatry and permits the admission, the patient can carry out the admission procedure.

In few cases, not only the clients but also the relatives refuse hospitalization. For example, paranoid

产生相关的法律问题。非自愿入院通常包括以下几种情况：患者可能会对自己或他人造成伤害、病情需要治疗、丧失生活能力。非自愿入院会在很大程度上限制患者的权利，因此，对于非自愿入院患者必须有明确的原因。

（1）强制入院：强制入院患者通常是指因精神病症状，患者生活不能自理，或者有潜在的对自己或他人造成伤害的可能性。生活不能自理并不是指患者缺乏日常生活资源，而是无法利用现有的资源来维持生活。此类患者一般由亲属或监护人送医院治疗。拒不接受诊治者，可以由当地公安机关强制入院。

（2）司法鉴定入院：对象是出现危害或犯罪行为，但需要住院观察，进行司法精神鉴定的人。入院和出院均由委托单位办理手续。未经委托单位同意，其他人员不能探望。

精神病患者住院，一般以自愿为原则。但是，有些精神病患者常常由于自知力障碍，不承认有病，拒绝住院治疗。在这种情况下，需要从患者的根本利益出发，在经过相关的法律程序后，违背其意愿而强制性入院。根据我国宪法和刑法关于保护公民人身自由权利的规定，强制患者入院易被患者或家属认为是“限制人身自由”或“非法拘禁”，从而引发法律纠纷。所以对非自愿入院的精神患者强迫入院时，必须具备两方面的条件：① 病情必须达到一定的严重程度。一般对重症精神患者有严重危害他人人身安全的暴力行为，或有明显的自伤、自杀行为，或生活不能自理；或严重扰乱社会秩序的，可以采取强制入院。② 符合病情严重程度的患者，可以由其亲属、监护人或法定代理人提出要求或申请，经医师检查认为确实患有精神病并签发住院证后，才能办理入院手续。

在少数情况下，会出现不但患者拒绝住院，而且家属也坚决反对的情况。如：某些

schizophrenia patients can do harm to self, others or the society if they don't take any treatment. Under these circumstances, patients must be hospitalized involuntarily after the identification of more than two experience doctors and the permission of government, police or judiciary.

Most countries have established laws about involuntary treatment of psychiatric patients, which protect the medical right of psychiatric patients. However, there are no related laws about involuntary admission in China at present. Nurses must practice according to related prescription of constitution law, criminal law and civil law.

ii. Issues on Informed Consent

Patients have the right of informed consent according to related laws. Medical institutions should be assured that the patients have right to be informed of the diagnosis and therapy and be given explicit explanation about especial examinations, surgery and therapy. Sometimes when performing the protective medical procedure, which is not suitable for the patient to know, the health care workers should tell the relatives about it.

It is difficult to obtain informed content from a mentally ill person due to the lack self-awareness, unwillingness to comply with the treatment. Furthermore, closed management mode in psychiatric ward determines that there are no family members around in most of the time. So the implementation of informed consent for the mentally ill person without capacity for civil conduct may be in dilemma. Therefore signatures by the guardian at the time of patient's admission will be required for some files such as hospitalization agreement, consent form for mandatory medical service, consent form of hospitalized patients, etal.

The doctor should establish possible therapy plans for psychiatric patients regardless of involuntary or voluntary. Before performing therapy, doctor had better obtain the consent from the client or relatives, especially written consent from the contract on "consent with the necessary therapy and protection in hospital" or other informed consent documents. For example, before the electroconvulsive treatment or adopting a new treatment, the doctor must inform the patient of the effect and side effect and obtain the consent.

Nurses may not mainly be responsible during the process of informed consent. However they have the

偏执性精神患者，如不强制入院会对患者、别人或社会造成危害。这时需要经过 2 名以上的有经验的医生鉴定同意，同时经过政府或公安、司法部门的批准，强制其入院。

在许多国家的法律中，明确规定了对精神患者的强制医疗措施，从而有效保障了精神患者应享有的疾病治疗的权利，维护了社会的安定。目前，我国对此还没有明确的立法，护士在处理相关问题时，可以依照我国宪法、刑法、民法等法律的有关规定执行。

（二）治疗中知情同意的问题

根据我国相关法律规定，知情同意权是患者享有的权利之一。医疗机构应当尊重患者对自己的病情诊断、治疗的知情权利。在实施手术、特殊检查、特殊治疗时，应当向患者做必要的解释。由于实施保护性医疗措施不宜向患者说明情况的，应当将有关情况通知患者家属。

由于精神患者的特殊性，因疾病原因会出现自知力缺乏，不愿配合治疗，从而无法履行告知义务并取得同意。再者，封闭管理模式的精神科病房决定了患者身边常常没有陪护人，因此对于无行为能力的精神患者实施知情同意权就会出现盲点。因此在精神患者入院时都会由监护人签署《住院协议》《强制性医疗行为同意书》《住院患者知情同意书》《特殊治疗知情同意书》《开放疗区住院患者及监护人知情同意书》。

对精神科患者，无论自愿或非自愿入院，入院后医生都要为其制订切实可行的治疗方案。医生在决定患者的治疗时，应取得患者或其家属的同意，最好在有“同意医院的一切必要的治疗与保护措施”内容的住院合同上签字或签署其他的知情同意文件，作为依据。例如：需要对患者进行电休克治疗或采用新的治疗方法时，必须对患者解释其疗效和副作用，在取得同意的情况下，才能执行。

在某些精神患者的知情同意过程中，护士可能不负主要责任，但有义务对护理方面

obligation to explain the details of nursing intervention to the patient. The information the nurses give to the patient should accord with the doctor's in order to avoid the misunderstanding of the patients and relatives. When the patients or relatives change their ideas, nurses should tell related staffs immediately.

According to the related law in the United State, in obtaining the patients' informed consent, nurses' main responsibilities include three aspects. Firstly, it is whether the patient has achieved adequate information before the decision-making. The second is whether the patient has the competence to make a decision. The last one is whether the patient's decision is out of his own will, without others' pressure.

The right of informed consent is a basic right of patients and the foundation of other rights. Legally, it is not appropriate to confine the patients or deprive the right of patients for ethical reasons during the period of conservative therapy. Rather, nurses should improve the level of psychological nursing and the skill of informing. Of course, the right of informed consent is not absolute. In some cases, the obligation of medical personnel to inform can be exempt. For example, nurses can constrain patient behavior in the rescue of emergency or serious patients or when the patients may do harm to self or others. But careful consideration should be taken for exempt. According to the *Shanghai Mental Health Act* [46], it should be decided by psychiatrist whether temporary protective safety measures are necessary for hospitalized patients with mental disorders to prevent accidents or to meet specific medical needs. The purpose of protective constrain is to guarantee the patient's safety, the relevant standards and norms must be followed and patients and guardians should be informed after constrain.

的服务向患者做出解释，包括护理活动执行的原因和方式。在提供有关资料时，应注意与医生保持一致，防止患者或家属产生误解；并在患者或家属改变看法时，及时通知相关人员。

在美国，相关的法律要求在获得患者的知情同意时，护士需要确认以下几点：① 患者在做出决定前，是否获得了足够的相关知识；② 患者是否具有做出决定的能力；③ 决定是否按照患者的自由意志，即没有受到他人的强迫。

知情权是患者的一项基本权利，是享有其他权利的基础。从法律角度讲，以伦理学为由在保守治疗中限制和剥夺患者的知情权是不恰当的。解决问题的思路应放在提高心理护理水平和告知技巧上。当然，知情权也不是绝对的，在客观上不能履行告知义务时，医疗机构的告知义务可以免除。例如：在急、危重症患者的抢救中或当精神患者可能危害自身或他人的时候，可以由护士使用保护性约束。对此，护士要在医疗文书中记录使用原因和使用经过，并及时向医生反映情况，争取适当的治疗，尽早出院。但是免除告知义务的情况必须谨慎对待，根据《上海市精神卫生条例》第四十六条规定，因医疗需要或者为防止发生意外，必须对住院治疗的精神疾病患者暂时采取保护性安全措施的，应当由精神科医师决定。实行约束性保护是为了保障患者的人身安全而采取的强制性措施，必须遵循相关标准及规范，并且在行约束性保护后告知患者或其家属。

iii. Issues on Privacy

There are some opinions that the obligation of the medical personnel to protect the patient's privacy belongs to moral scope rather than legal issues. According to the law in China, privacy is the right of patients and confidentiality is the responsibility of the medical personnel. In medical practice, the protection of patients' privacy and avoidance of spirit or psychological harm refer to both moral and legal issues.

The patients may confide the secret to nurses out

（三）隐私权的法律问题

有人认为，医疗人员履行对患者隐私保密的义务，属于道德范畴，而非法律问题。我国有关法律规定，维护隐私是患者的权利，也是医务人员的义务。在医疗实践中，保护患者的隐私，避免患者精神、心理受各种有害因素的侵害和刺激，不仅是道德问题，也涉及法律问题。

基于对医护人员的信任，患者在治疗中

of confidence, which may play an important role in diagnosis and therapy. Medical professionals have an obligation to keep confidentiality whether it is related to illness. Otherwise it will do harm to the reputation of the patient and the family happiness. Based on *Mental Health Law of the People's Republic of China*, members of medical staff have the obligation to keep confidential for psychiatric patients' identifiable information such as name, image, address, working unit, medical records etal. They should not violate the patients' privacy by disclosing their information or laughing at them in clinical practice.

向其倾吐心中的秘密。对于精神患者，这种倾诉行为，有时对疾病的诊断和治疗能起到重要的作用。作为医护人员，不论患者的隐私是否与病情有关，都应保守秘密，否则可能会损害患者的名誉和家庭幸福。根据《中华人民共和国精神卫生法》的相关要求，对于精神科患者的姓名、肖像、住址、工作单位、病历资料以及其他可能推断出其身份的信息，医护人员负有保密的义务。在检查中应该做好隐私保护，医护人员不得在临床上谈笑、泄露患者隐私，避免对患者的隐私权构成侵犯。

iv. Issues on Freedom of Person

Freedom of person is a basic right of citizens according to the constitution law in China. According to the *Constitution of the People's Republic of China* [37], the personal freedom of citizens in the People's Republic of China is inviolable. No citizen may be arrested except with the approval or by decision of a people's procuratorate or by decision of a people's court, and arrests must be made by a public security organ. Illegal detention or deprivation or restriction of personal freedom is prohibited. Anyone including the medical professionals has no right to imprison the patients illegally or deprive patients' freedom of person because of their weird behavior, search the patients' body illegally, invade patients' dignity, or trick, ridicule or defame patients because of the mental disorder. But there are exceptions. For example, in psychiatric setting, if the patients may hurt themselves or people around them due to their psychotic symptoms, they will be constrained which limits their personal freedom. And for safety, it is necessary to check the patient's pockets, bed, and diary, and so on to know if there are adverse events happening to the patient. But appropriate ways should be suggested to avoid violating the patient's human rights.

（四）人身自由的法律问题

人身自由权利是我国公民最基本的权利之一。我国《宪法》第37条规定：中华人民共和国公民人身自由不受侵犯，任何公民非经人民检察院批准或者决定，或者人民法院决定，并由公安机关执行，不受逮捕；禁止非法拘禁和以其他方法非法剥夺或者限制人身自由。任何人包括医务人员，对精神患者不能因为其行为乖张而非法拘禁，或以其他方法进行非法剥夺、限制其人身自由，不能非法搜身；其人格尊严也不能受侵犯，不能因其丧失理智而进行侮辱取乐、歧视或诽谤。但是由于精神科病房的特点就是封闭式管理，期间会限制一些发作期患者的自由。对于可能发生自伤、伤人、毁物等行为的患者，应及时给予暂时的保护性约束，遵医嘱给予对症治疗。但约束应适当并且注意方式手法，避免给患者造成伤害。另外出于对患者安全的考虑，应常规检查患者衣袋、床铺等防止危险物品的藏匿，服药时检查口腔防止藏药，以及检查患者信件、日记等以了解病情，制订更好的治疗方案并防止意外发生，同时也应注意方式方法，以免涉及侵犯人权。

v. Issues on Female Sex Protection

Chinese laws pay much attention to the protection of female mental health. Sexual relationship related to patients usually refers to sexual relationship between the doctor and female patients in therapy. Anyone, including the doctors who have sex with female psychiatric patients, who have no ability of sex defense or be in sexual

（五）女患者的性保护问题

我国对保护妇女的身心健康和人身权利极为重视。涉及患者的性关系，一般指医务人员对其治疗的女患者所发生的性关系。有关法律规定，任何人如果对患有精神病或重度精神发育迟滞的妇女，利用其丧失自我防

abnormality, whether volunteer or not, will be accused of rape.

卫能力或性的反常行为而与之发生性关系的，不论其自愿与否，都将作为强奸罪论处。医护人员也不例外。

Sexual relationship with patients is defined as medical malpractice by many courts in Unite State. It also can be considered as abuse of "emotion shift" on female patients. Sexual liaisons between doctors and patients are prohibited by statute in a number of states. Despite this widespread prohibition, such sexual relationships do occur. Violation of such statutes may result in loss or suspension of one's professional license and the doctor may be convicted to take the responsibility of compensation.

美国的许多法院将这种性关系宣判为医疗失责。认为是医护人员不守职责，或是对女患者所产生一种“移情”关系的滥用。美国很多州的法律都禁止医患之间发生性关系，尽管如此，这种性关系还会时常发生。其结果是，被控诉的医护人员承担医疗失责的赔偿责任，还可能根据情节吊销其执照或以刑事犯罪论处。

vi. Illegal Behavior of Mental Disorder

Illegal behavior of mental disorder refers to legal issues related to psychiatric, mental retardation or personality disorder, such as ruining property under mental disorder, murdering at the mercy of illusion. How to deal with such problems refers to criminal responsibility, which is judged by court.

（六）精神障碍者的违法行为问题

精神障碍者违法行为是指患有精神病、精神发育迟滞或人格障碍等精神障碍的人产生的相关的法律问题。如：在意识障碍状态下破坏财产的行为；在幻觉或妄想支配下的杀人行为等。对这种问题的处理主要涉及患者的刑事责任能力，可参阅司法精神鉴定的有关内容。

III. Nursing Interventions to Prevent Legal Issues

三、预防法律问题发生的护理措施

Nurses have many roles in social life, such as citizen, medical professional nurses and assume special legal responsibility and duty. In order to prevent legal problems, nurses should be acquainted with and abide by law. Acquaintance with law means that nurse should learn related knowledge of law and improve the legal consciousness. To abide by law, nurses must define and limit their practice accordingly during professional practice. When law conflicts with other codes, nurses should abide by the legal codes. As conflicts arise between inferior and superior laws, nurses should obey the superior one.

在社会生活中，护士会扮演多种角色。不论作为公民还是作为医疗卫生工作者来讲，都承担着一定的法律责任和义务。要在护理工作中杜绝法律问题的发生，护士就必须做到懂法和守法。懂法要求护士学习相关的法律知识，提高自己的法律意识。守法要求护士能用相关的法律法规规范自己的行为，遵守法律的规定。特别注意的是当法规与其他行为规范不一致时，应首先服从法律规范；低级法律规范与高级法律规范相抵触时，服从高级法律规范的规定。

i. Tort and Crime

Tort refers to violation against the right of individual or crowd. Crime means all behaviors, which disaccord with criminal laws. Tort is not equal to crime, but crime must include the violation of legal right of victims. In psychiatric nursing, nurses will offend the right of patients' privacy if they talk about the individual illness and secrets. If the patient commits a suicide as a result, nurses will be

（一）防止侵权与犯罪的发生

侵权行为指对某人或许多人的人身权利不应有的侵犯。犯罪是指一切触犯国家刑法的行为。侵权不一定是犯罪，但犯罪必定包含对被害者合法权益的侵犯。如在精神科中，护士随意议论患者的病情和隐私，则侵犯了患者的隐私权；如果因此使患者精神受到刺

convicted of crime.

Tort and crime should be avoided in mental health nursing. Most nurses won't commit tort or commit deliberately. But some legal issues on privacy, informed consent and person freedom may cause the occurrence of tort and crime potentially. For example, the following violations may occur during the process of constrain:

1. Violation of the life and health right of patients with mental disorders. As a result of patient' aggressive behavior and resistance behavior, constraint may do harm to patients both physically and psychologically, some patients may even commit suicide.

2. Violation of the right of informed consent of patients with mental disorders. Informed consent and the explanation of the constraint process are not provided for patients or their family members before the implementation of constrain.

3. Violation of the right of personal freedom of patients with mental disorders. Nursing staff may seclude the patients with aggressive behaviors without communicating with patients and doctors, and even reduce the patient's visiting hours..

4. Violation of the right of respecting the personality of patients with mental disorders. Nursing staff may tease or make fun of patients' strange behaviors during the onset of mental illness.

So nurses should be fully familiar with the related right and responsibility, respect the patients and practice according to the prescription of the law.

ii. Negligence

Negligence is defined as that the negligent conduct of a person occurring within his or her professional capacity. Usually this kind of negligence violates the legal right of others, which can be foreseen and prevented. Negligence in nursing practice may do no harm to patients, which only can cause tort. Sometimes, negligence in nursing practice may lead to serious consequences, such as death, which would be convicted of crime.

In psychiatric health care, negligence results from different kinds of wrong nursing practices, such as without observing patients on time, checking during therapy wrongly, and drug conserving. Nurses would be convicted of crime if nursing negligence results in serious medical accident. There are two important aspects to prevent negligence. One is to enhance nursing responsibility; the other is to practice under the regulation.

激而自杀身亡，则构成了犯罪。

护士在护理活动中必须防止侵权和犯罪的发生。大多数护士都不会故意实施侵权和犯罪行为，但在工作中会有导致这种行为的危机存在，如前面提到的涉及隐私权、知情同意权、人身自由权等的法律问题。举个例子，在对精神病患者进行约束时，可能会发生以下侵权行为：

1. 侵犯精神病患者的生命健康权。进行约束的过程中可能由于患者过激行为以及反抗，造成患者身体和心理方面的伤害，甚至会导致患者自杀等不良事件的发生。

2. 侵犯精神病患者的知情同意权。在实施约束前没有征得患者或者家属的同意，也未将具体流程给患者解释。

3. 侵犯精神病患者的人身自由权。在实施约束过程中，护理人员未与患者及医生沟通，私自对行为过激的患者进行隔离，甚至减少患者见访客的次数。

4. 侵犯精神病患者的人格受尊重权。在精神病患者发病期间，护理人员对其怪异的行为进行嘲笑和戏弄。

这就需要护士充分了解患者应有的权利和自己应尽的义务，尊重、爱护患者，尽职尽责，随时对工作进行评估。

（二）防止出现护理过失行为

过失是指行为人应当预见自己的行为可能危害他人的合法权益，但因为疏忽大意而没有预见，或已经预见但轻信能够避免。护理上的过失如果没有对患者造成严重的损害，只是构成了侵权；但造成恶果，如患者致死，这就构成了犯罪。

精神科护理工作中，有很多情况会导致过失行为。例如：没有及时观察病情；治疗时没有按规定查对；没有妥善保管药品等，涉及护理工作的各个方面。如果护士的过失行为造成了严重的医疗事故，就构成犯罪。而防止这种行为的出现，最重要的是两条：一是增加工作责任心，二是严格按照规章制度办事。

iii. Legality of Performing Prescription

Prescription is the foundation of nursing practices. Nurses should perform the prescription strictly rather than incorrectly or blindly. Faults on performing prescription may include four aspects as follows: performing wrong, for example, mistaking of drug quantity; changing prescription without permission, for example, changing the therapy from twice a day to once a day; not performing without any reason, for example, not using bedrails for patients; performing without prescription, for example, permitting patients to take part in entertainment. Nurses have the responsibility to check the prescription and ask the doctor to correct the faults in prescription. So the nurses must have good professional quality and plenty of working experience.

（三）执行医嘱的合法性

医嘱是护士对患者实施护理措施的依据。一般来讲，护士应严格执行医生的医嘱，不能执行错误，也不能盲目执行。执行医嘱错误可以表现为4种情况：一是执行失误，如药物计量错误；二是擅自改变医嘱，如将治疗由1天2次改为1天1次；三是无故不执行医嘱，如应为患者使用床挡，但没有使用；四是没有医嘱自行实施，如擅自让患者参加工娱治疗活动等。当医生医嘱错误时，护士有责任在执行前的查对中发现错误，并请医生纠正，而不能盲目的执行。否则，护士要对因此而发生的不良后果负责。这就需要护士具有良好的专业素质和丰富的工作经验。

iv. Other Preventing Intervention

Besides aspects mentioned above, nurses should pay much attention to the management of drugs and other items in wards. When performing medication, nurses should prevent the patients from spitting out, storing, grabbing bills or taking the wrong medicine. Nurses should record the nursing intervention accurately and timely. Obvious deficiencies in nursing records, such as obscure details, lack of continuum, no individual health education, inconsistency of the former and the latter, negligence of physical syndrome, inaccuracy of nursing diagnosis, may result in unnecessary legal troubles. The psychiatric patients may respond abnormally to the medication because of the mental disorder. For example, some patients may feel no uncomfortable even when they have temperature of 39° centigrade with heart rate over 120 times one minute. So the nurse should observe patients carefully to avoid accidents.

On the whole, nurses should know that every nursing intervention is complex, especially in mental health nursing. So nurses must obey the nursing practice act and be familiar with related law and regulations to prevent the occurrence of blunder.

(Yang Min)

（四）其他的防范措施

精神科的护士应注意对病房药物及其他物品的管理。在药疗时，要防止患者吐药、藏药、抢药、吃错药。护士要及时、真实、准确地书写护理记录。一项调查表明，在精神科护理记录中如有明显的缺陷，可能导致不必要的法律纠纷，其中包括内容不具体、缺乏连贯性、无卫生宣教个体化、前后不一致、忽视躯体状况、护理诊断不确切等。由于精神科患者感知障碍、行为紊乱，在服用抗精神药物后会出现反应迟钝，可能会掩盖某些症状。如一位患者发热超过39℃，心率高于120次/min，但没有不适的主诉，护士有可能忽视其疾病。因此，需要护士严密观察病情，及时发现和处理问题，防止意外的发生。

总之，护士应明确，每一项护理工作都不是一个简单的过程，包含有许多环节，对精神科患者的护理更是如此。精神科护士必须认真遵守护理常规和操作规程，熟悉相关的法律、法规，否则稍有疏忽，就可能酿成大错。

（杨　敏）

Key Points

1. Ethnic, a branch of philosophy science, is to deal with morals. It is a science on good moral and moral value. Ethnic is a system or code of morals and is a discipline that

内容摘要

1. 伦理学是哲学的一个分支，是研究道德的科学。它是关于优良道德的科学，是关于道

seeks to formulate and systematically justify responses to moral dilemmas.

德价值的科学。伦理学是一套道德准则或道德系统，以寻求道德判断确证的学科。

2. Nursing ethnics is a science on nursing moral, which can direct nursing practice by using the ethical principles, theories and criteria, regulate the relationship within the nursing field and analyze, discuss, resolve the ethical problems in the nursing practice.

2. 护理伦理学是研究护理道德的学科，它用伦理学的原则、理论和规范来指导护理实践，协调护理领域中的人际关系，对护理实践中的伦理问题进行分析、讨论并提出解决方案。

3. Law has a narrow sense and a broad sense definition. On the narrow sense, law is exclusively standardized documents established by the national legislature. On the broad sense, law is a standard or rule of conduct established and enforced by the government of a society.

3. 法律有狭义及广义之分，从狭义上讲专指国家立法机关制定的规范性文件；从广义上讲泛指由国家制定或认可并由国家强制力保证实施的行为规范的总和。

4. Ethical issues in psychiatric nursing refer to action control, self-determinism, informed consent and protection of privacy.

4. 精神科护理中常见的伦理问题主要涉及行为控制、自主决策、知情同意和维护隐私等。

5. Legal issues in psychiatric nursing refer to admission and treatment, patients' rights and responsibilities etal.

5. 精神科护理中常见的法律问题主要涉及患者的住院和治疗，患者的权利和义务等。

Exercises

思考题

(Questions 1 to 2 share the same question stem)

A patient hospitalized with auditory hallucinations, suspected harm, and extreme agitation. The doctor told the family that they may need to implement constraints on the patient according to the patient's condition on admission and the family signed. Later, the patient had a left radial fracture as a result of strong resistance in the process of restraint. The nurse who implement restraint and the ward were taken to court and been requested compensation by the family of the patient.

1. What evidence should be prepared if you want to prove that the nurse is not wrong in the above case?

2. Describe the related ethical issues in the above case.

（1～2题共用题干）

某患者以幻听、疑人害自己，极度兴奋躁动而收住院。入院时医生告诉患者家属，根据患者的病情，可能需要对患者实行约束，并让家属签了字。后来因患者强烈反抗，在约束过程中患者左手桡骨骨折。患者家属将实施约束的护士及其病房告上法庭，请求赔偿。

1. 上述案例中如果要证明护士没有过错，需要准备什么证据？

2. 请描述上述案例中的伦理问题。

(Questions 3 to 4 share the same question stem)

The patient is 25 years old; she is on the schizophrenia rehabilitation period and adheres to medication treatment at home. A psychiatric hospital called his family to inform that the hospital ward is undergoing a clinical drug trial of a new drug now, if the patient is involved in the case can they be provided with drugs for free. The family member made decision for the patient that the patient will participate in this experiment considering the economic conditions.

3. Weather there exist violations of the rights of patient in the above case? Make explanation If the answer is yes.

4. Weather this hospital did the right thing? Use the ethical principles to analyze.

（3～4题共用题干）

患者，女，25岁，精神分裂症康复期，在家坚持服药治疗。某精神病医院打电话给其家属告知现在病房正在进行某新药的临床药物试验，如果患者参与的话则可以免费为患者提供药物。其家属考虑到家里的经济条件，替患者决定参与此项实验。

3. 上述案例中是否存在侵犯患者权利的情况？如果有，请说明。

4. 上述案例中医院的做法是否恰当，请用伦理原则进行分析。

(Questions 5 to 6 share the same question stem)

A patient with severe depression and psychotic symptoms was forced to be hospitalized. He is not willing to eat because his intestine has become "a jelly like". The patient convinced that it is a punishment for his sins. He asked to leave the hospital, but the nurse refused. Because the doctor has carried out a ban on patients in the hospital.

5. What is the basis of banning the patient?

6. Is the action of the nurse right in this case? Give some reasons.

(5～6题共用题干)

一名重度抑郁症和有精神病症状的患者被强制送进医院。他不愿吃饭，因为他的"肠已经变成果冻状"。患者坚信这是对他的罪恶的惩罚。他要求出院，但护士拒绝同意。因为医生已经对患者进行了委托院禁。

5. 请思考，法律允许可以将患者委托院禁的依据是什么？

6. 本案例中护士的做法对吗？分析原因。

Chapter 6 Nursing for Clients with Schizophrenia

第六章 精神分裂症患者的护理

Learning Objectives

Memorization

1. Define the term of "schizophrenia".
2. Describe the clinical symptoms of schizophrenia.
3. Describe a nursing assessment of mental status for a client with schizophrenia.

Comprehension

1. Discuss various theories of the etiology of schizophrenia.
2. Identify the major pharmacological strategies in the treatment of schizophrenia, their target symptoms and their major adverse effects.
3. Describe the mental treatment and rehabilitative needs of clients with schizophrenia.

Application

1. Apply the nursing process to the care of a client with schizophrenia.
2. Provide teaching to clients, families, caregivers, and community members to increase knowledge and understanding of schizophrenia.

学习目标

识记

1. 描述精神分裂症的定义。
2. 描述精神分裂症患者的临床表现。
3. 描述精神分裂症患者的护理评估。

理解

1. 讨论精神分裂症的病因学。
2. 识别精神分裂症药物治疗的主要策略、抗精神病药物的主要作用及不良反应。
3. 描述精神分裂症患者心理治疗及康复方法。

运用

1. 运用护理程序护理精神分裂症患者。
2. 向患者、家属、照顾者和社区成员提供精神分裂症的健康教育指导。

06章

Lihua, a 25-year-old man, was staying with his father for a few weeks on a visit. His father knew Lihua couldn't sleep well at night, and he could hear Lihua talking to himself in the next room. One day when his father was at work, Lihua began to hear some voices outside the apartment. The voices grew louder, saying, "You're not good; you can't do anything right. You can't take care of yourself or protect your dad. We're going to get you both." Lihua grew more frightened and went to the closet place where his dad kept his tools. He grabbed a hammer and ran outside. One day, when his father came home from work early, Lihua wasn't in the apartment though his coat and wallet were still there. Lihua's father called a neighbor, and they drove around the apartment complex looking for Lihua. They finally found Lihua crouched behind some bushes. Although it was 7℃, he was wearing only a T-shirt and shorts without shoes. Lihua's neighbor called emergency services. Meanwhile Lihua's father tried to coax Lihua into the car, but Lihua wouldn't come. Some voices told Lihua to use the hammer and to destroy the car. He began to swing the hammer into the windshield, but someone held him back. Emergency services staff arrived and spoke quietly and firmly as they removed the hammer from Lihua's hands. They told Lihua they were taking him to the hospital where he and his father would be safe. They gently put him on a stretcher with restraints, and his father rode in the emergency van with him to the hospital.

Please think about the following questions based on the case:

1. What are the symptoms of Lihua in this case?
2. What might be the potential nursing diagnoses for Lihua? What might be the effective nursing interventions?

李华，25岁，回家探望父亲。父亲知道李华晚上睡眠不好，能听到他在隔壁和自己说话。有一天父亲在忙的时候，李华听到公寓外面有些声音，并且声音越来越大，说："你真没用，什么事都做不好。你既不能照顾自己，也不能保护父亲。我们要来整你们俩。"李华越来越害怕，跑到父亲放工具的橱柜边，拿起一个锤子就往外跑。有一次他父亲提早下班回家，发现李华衣服和钱包在公寓，但是人不在。李华父亲和邻居在公寓附近四处寻找，最终在灌木丛后面发现了蜷成一团的李华。当时温度只有7℃，但李华只穿了一件T恤和短裤，连鞋子都没有穿。这时李华又听到一个声音叫他自己用锤子去砸车的挡风玻璃。急救中心的工作人员及时赶到并阻止了他，并将锤子拿开。他们告诉李华，他们将把他送到医院，在那里他和父亲会很安全。他们用约束带将李华固定在担架上把他送到了医院。

请思考：

1. 在本案例中，李华的症状有哪些？
2. 请提出李华潜在的护理诊断和有效的护理措施。

Schizophrenia is one of the severe and common mental illnesses, which usually begins during adolescence or young adulthood and has a deteriorating course. In schizophrenia, the person is overwhelmed by an onslaught of bizarre thoughts and hallucinations, resulting in inappropriate or bizarre ways and general disorganization in daily functioning and behavior. Psychiatric nurses often are most challenged when providing nursing care to patient with schizophrenia, because the behaviors of patient with schizophrenia are difficult to be understood and sometimes frightening. They are usually unable to form close interpersonal relationships because of the demands of the illness for their attention and energy. Caring nurses must strive to make contact with schizophrenia patients and assist them to overcome or adapt to the effects of the illness.

精神分裂症是一种严重的慢性精神疾病，常见于青壮年。其病程迁延，有反复加重或恶化的过程。精神分裂症患者受其奇异想法或幻觉的影响，表现出一些不适当的或奇怪的行为，严重影响了患者的日常生活和社会功能。由于患者的行为有时难以理解并有一定的危险性，同时因受疾病的影响，患者通常难与他人形成良好的人际关系，因此护理精神分裂症患者对护士来说是一个挑战。护士应努力与患者建立良好的治疗性关系，帮助患者战胜疾病和适应疾病对其造成的影响。本章将介绍精神分裂症流行病学、病因及发病机制、主要临床表现、诊断与治疗和护理。

Section 1 Introduction

第一节 概 述

Schizophrenia is defined as a mental disorder characterized by disordered thoughts, hallucinations, and delusions and usually happens in young people. Approximately 1% of the general population will have schizophrenia during their lifetime. Schizophrenia probably caused more lengthy hospitalization, more chaos in family life, more exorbitant costs to individuals and governments, and more fears than any other diseases.

精神分裂症是一类常见的严重的精神疾病，表现为思维障碍、幻觉和妄想等，该病多见于青壮年。在一般人群中，大约1%的人有患精神分裂症的危险。该病可导致冗长的住院治疗，对个人、家庭、社会和政府等带来的影响较其他精神疾病更为严重。

I. Definition

一、精神分裂症的定义

The term schizophrenia was coined in 1908 by the Swiss psychiatrist Eugen Bleuler. The word was derived from the Greek "skihiz" (split) and "phren" (mind). Over the years, there were many debates surrounding the concept of schizophrenia. Various definitions of the disorder have evolved, and numerous treatment strategies have been proposed, but none of them has been proven to be uniformly effective or sufficient. Schizophrenia is often described as a group of psychiatric diseases with unknown etiology. Most of them start from a young age, mostly chronic or subacute. The main clinical manifestations are mental, emotional, behavioral and other disorders and mental activities. Patients are generally conscious, and most patients may experience cognitive impairment during the course of the disease and lack awareness of their own diseases.

精神分裂症最早由瑞士精神病学家Eugen Bleuler于1908年提出。他指出情感、联想和意志障碍是本病的原发性症状，而中心问题是人格的分裂，故提出了"精神分裂"的概念。"分裂"来源于希腊语"skihiz"（劈开）和"phren"（思想）。很多年以来，围绕精神分裂症的概念进行的辩论有很多。该病的定义已经历了多次演变，并提出了许多相应的治疗方法，但没有一个定义或治疗方法被大家完全认同。精神分裂症常常被描述为一组病因未明的精神病，多在青壮年起病，多为慢性或亚急性，临床主要表现为思维、情感、行为等多方面的障碍及精神活动的不协调。患者一般意识清楚，大部分患者在疾病过程中可出现认知功能的损害，对自身疾病缺乏认识能力。

Although the controversy lingers, two general concepts appear to be accepted among clinicians. The first is that schizophrenia is probably not a homogeneous disease entity with a single cause but results from the combination of genetic predisposition, biochemical dysfunction, physiological factors, and psychosocial stress. The second is that there is no single treatment that cures the disorder. Instead, effective treatment requires a comprehensive, multidisciplinary effort, including pharmacotherapy and various forms of psychosocial care, such as behavior therapy, living skills, social skills training, rehabilitation, and family therapy.

虽然临床医生对精神分裂症的概念争论不休，但有两个基本观点被大家所接受。一是精神分裂症可能不是由单一因素引起的疾病，而是由多种因素包括遗传、生物化学、生理及心理社会因素等引起。二是没有一种单一的、特效的治疗精神分裂症的方法。实际上精神分裂症有效的治疗方法常常是多种治疗方法的综合使用，包括药物治疗和各种类型的心理治疗，如行为治疗、生活技能训练、社会职业技能训练、康复治疗和家庭治疗等。

II. Epidemiology

World Health Organization estimates that the lifetime prevalence of schizophrenia is 0.3%-0.7%. In the United States, approximately 1.3% of the general population will have schizophrenia during their lifetime. In China, according to the investigation of seven areas in 1994, the lifetime prevalence of schizophrenia is 0.655%.

Schizophrenia is equally prevalent in men and women. However, some studies have indicated that symptoms occur earlier in men than in women. The onset of schizophrenia usually occurs in late adolescence or early adulthood, and sometimes occurs after age 50, though less frequently. The incidence is higher in the lower socioeconomic classes, which may be due in part to the multiple psychosocial stressors that prevail in this group. The risk of children becoming schizophrenia increases significantly when one or both parents have the disorder.

The mortality rate related to both natural causes and suicide is higher for individuals with the disorder than for normal individuals. Approximately 5%-6% of individuals with schizophrenia die by suicide, about 20% attempt suicide on one or more occasions, and many more have significant suicidal ideation. Suicidal behavior is sometimes in response to command hallucinations to harm oneself or others. Suicide risk remains high over the whole lifespan for males and females, although it may be especially high for younger males with comorbid substance use. Other risk factors include having depressive symptoms or feelings of hopelessness and being unemployed and the risk is higher, also, in the period after a psychotic episode or hospital discharge. Schizophrenia is one of the costliest mental disorders in terms of loss of productivity. From the global disease burden, schizophrenia is in the top 10 of the total burden of disease.

二、流行病学

不同国家和地区报道的精神分裂症的患病率差异性较大。世界卫生组织估计精神分裂症的终身患病率在0.3%～0.7%左右。在美国，大约有1.3%的普通人群患有精神分裂症。中国于1994年在7个地区进行的流行病学调查中发现，精神分裂症的终生患病率为0.655%。

精神分裂症的患病率在男女性别间没有显著性差异。然而有报道男性的发病年龄较女性早。经调查发现，精神分裂症的发病年龄一般在15～45岁，偶尔也有在50岁之后发病。社会经济地位较低的阶层的患病率较高，可能由多种社会心理应激源造成。父母中一方或双方患有精神分裂症，其孩子的患病危险性将升高。

精神分裂症患者因自然原因及自杀的死亡率较一般人群高，大约5%～6%的精神分裂症个体死于自杀，约20%的患者有一次以上的自杀企图，有自杀观念的比例更高。自杀行为有时是对伤害自己或他人的命令式的幻觉反应。对男性和女性来说，自杀风险在整个生命周期都较高，对于合并物质使用的年轻男性来说自杀风险尤其高。其风险因素包括有抑郁症状或感觉无望和失业。在精神病性发作或出院后的一段时间内，自杀风险也很高。另外，精神分裂症是一类疾病负担较重的疾病。从全球看，精神分裂症的疾病负担居于所有疾病负担的前10位。

Section 2 Etiology

The cause of schizophrenia is still uncertain. Many authorities suggest that multiple factors must cause schizophrenia, because no single theory satisfactorily explains the disorder. The disease probably results from a combination of influences including biological, psychological, and environmental factors (figure 6-1).

第二节　病因及发病机制

精神分裂症的病因和发病机制不是很清楚，许多学者认为该病与多种因素有关，主要包括生物学的、心理学的和环境的因素等（图6-1）。

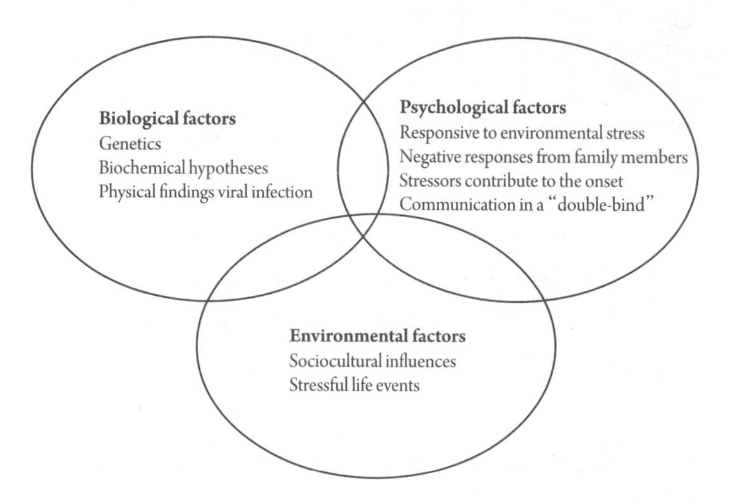

Figure 6-1 Biopsychosocial etiologies for patients with schizophrenia

I. Biological Factors

i. Genetics

The body of evidence for genetic vulnerability to schizophrenia is growing. Studies show that relatives of individual with schizophrenia have a much higher probability of developing the disease than general population. Whereas the lifetime risk for developing schizophrenia is about 0.3%-0.7%. In most population studied, the first-degree relatives of an identified client have a 5 to 10 percent risk of developing schizophrenia.

The studies of twin show that rate of schizophrenia among monozygotic (identical) twins is four times that of dizygotic (fraternal) twins, and approximately 50 times that of the general population.

The adoption studies find that children born in schizophrenic families, but adopted and reared by nonschizophrenic families, were more likely to develop the illness than the control group. From the same studies, children born of nonschizophrenic parents, but reared by schizophrenic parents, did not suffer more often from schizophrenia than those of the control group. These findings provide additional evidence for the genetic basis of schizophrenia.

ii. Biochemical Hypotheses

1. The Dopamine Hypotheses This theory suggests that schizophrenia be caused by an excess of dopamine-dependent neuronal activity in the brain. This excess activity may be related to receptor sensitivity, or reduced activity of dopamine antagonists.

2. 5-hydroxytrypatamine Hypotheses Some studies viewed that atypical antipsychotics have potent serotonin-related activities (for example, clozapine). Type

一、生物学因素

（一）遗传因素

有证据显示精神分裂症与遗传因素有关。家系研究发现精神分裂症亲属患同病的危险性明显高于一般人群。虽然精神分裂症的终生患病率在一般人群中为0.3%～0.7%，而在精神分裂症亲属中则高达5%～10%。

双胞胎研究显示在同卵双胞胎中，同时发生精神分裂症的几率是异卵双胞胎的4倍，大约是一般人群的50倍。

在寄养研究中发现，精神分裂症家庭出生的孩子寄养在无精神分裂症的家庭，其发病率较对照组高。与此同样的研究，将非精神分裂症患者的孩子寄养在精神分裂症的家庭，其发生精神分裂症的几率仍然没有对照组高，这些研究结果都提示了精神分裂症与遗传有关。

（二）生物化学因素

1. 多巴胺功能亢进假说 该假说提出，精神分裂症可能与多巴胺功能亢进有关。多巴胺活动的亢进可能与多巴胺受体的敏感性增加或拮抗多巴胺的能力降低有关。

2. 5-羟色胺（5-HT）受体假说 研究发现非典型抗精神病药物如氯氮平对 $5\text{-}HT_2$

2 (5-HT_2) receptor has been emphasized as important in reducing psychotic symptoms and in mitigating against the development of D_2 antagonism-related movement disorder.

有较强的抑制作用，能够有效地缓解精神分裂症的症状。

3. Other Biochemical Hypotheses Various other biochemical hypotheses have been implicated in the predisposition to schizophrenia. Abnormalities in the neurotransmitters norepinephrine, serotonin, acetylcholine, and gamma-aminobutyric acid, and the neuroregulators, such as prostaglandins and endorphins, have been suggested. The body may manufacture a hallucinogen or psychotomimetic that usurps the usual neurotransmitter or neuroregulator pathways in the brains of individuals with schizophrenia.

3. 其他生物化学的假说 许多学者和理论提出多种神经化学递质的代谢障碍与精神分裂症有关。如去甲肾上腺素、血清素、乙酰胆碱、γ- 氨基丁酸，以及前列腺素和内啡肽等神经调节剂。幻觉等精神病性症状与精神分裂症患者体内神经递质紊乱或神经调节通路异常有关。

iii. Physical Findings Viral Infection

（三）生理学因素

1. In postmortem studies Stevens reported observations of degenerative change within the neurons and an increase in the supporting glial cells of schizophrenic brains. These structural changes are similar to those characteristically reported in infectious inflammatory diseases such as viral encephalitis. Stevens considered these changes in the brain of individuals with schizophrenia to be consistent with a "healed inflammatory" process.

1. 病毒感染 学者 Stevens 在对精神分裂症患者的尸体研究中发现，在精神分裂症患者的大脑中有神经元的退行性变化和胶质细胞数量的增加。这些结构的变化与病毒感染相似，比如病毒性脑炎。

2. Anatomical Abnormalities Some studies have shown a significant enlargement in cerebral ventricular size in the brains of individuals with schizophrenia. One study reported 53% of those with chronic schizophrenia have ventricular size more than two standard deviations larger than the mean of controls.

2. 脑结构异常 有研究发现精神分裂症患者有明显的脑室扩大，据报道，有 53% 的慢性精神分裂症患者脑室的大小要比正常平均值大两个标准差。

3. Histological Changes Scheibel and his associates (1991) have studied the cerebral changes at the microscopic level. In studying brains of clients with schizophrenia, they found a "disordering" or disarray of the pyramidal cells in the area of the hippocampus. They compared this to the normal alignment of the cells in the brains of clients without the disorder. They have hypothesized that this alteration in hippocampal cells occurs during the second trimester of pregnancy and may be related to an influenza virus encountered by the mother during this period.

3. 组织学的改变 Scheibel（1991）报道，在显微镜下发现精神分裂症患者海马区域的锥体细胞排列紊乱。他们推测海马区锥体细胞的改变可能发生在怀孕的 4 至 6 个月，可能与母亲在此期间感染病毒有关。

4. Physical Conditions Some studies reported a well-established, positive link between schizophrenia and the following conditions: epilepsy (particularly temporal lobe), Huntington's chorea, birth trauma, head injury in adulthood, alcohol abuse, cerebral tumor (particularly in the limbic system), cerebrovascular accidents, systemic lupus erythematosus, myxedema, parkinsonism, and Wilson's disease.

4. 身体状况 一些研究报告提出，精神分裂症和下列情况有一定的联系，如癫痫（特别是颞叶）、亨廷顿舞蹈症、产伤、成年人的头部外伤、酒精滥用、脑肿瘤（特别是大脑边缘系统）、脑意外事件、全身性红斑狼疮、黏液性水肿、帕金森病和威尔逊氏症。

II. Psychological Factors

Although genetic and neurologic factors are believed to play major roles in the development of schizophrenia, researchers have also found that the prefrontal lobes of the brain are extremely responsive to environmental stress. Individuals with schizophrenia experience negative responses from family members and acquaintances that can intensify the already vulnerable neurologic state, and possibly trigger and exacerbate existing symptoms. Stressors that have been thought to contribute to the onset of schizophrenia include poor mother-child relationships, deeply disturbed family interpersonal relationships, impaired sexual identity and body image, rigid concept of reality, and repeated exposure to double-bind situations.

Communication between parents and offspring was described as frequently contradictory and placed the child in a "double-bind". This incompatible communication may interfere with ego development, thereby causing the individual to generate false ideas and exhibit extreme mistrust of all communications. Double-bind communication gives mixed messages and creates confusion in the receiver.

二、心理社会因素

虽然遗传和生物化学因素在精神分裂症的起病中扮演着主要角色，但许多研究发现精神分裂症患者脑额前叶皮质对环境压力的反应极为敏感。患者常常从其家人或他人中获得一些负性的反应，这可能引起并加重已存在的症状。应激源被认为对精神分裂症的发病起着"扳机"作用。这些应激源包括母亲与孩子之间关系的紧张、家庭成员之间关系的紧张、对性和身体的认识障碍、固执的观念及经常处于两难的情形中。

有研究发现精神分裂症患者家庭成员的沟通模式普遍存在问题。孩子常常处于"两难处境"，这种不相容的沟通可能影响自我发展，引起个人产生错误的观念，或表现出偏激和不信任等。

III. Environmental Factors

i. Sociocultural Influences

Many studies have been directed that have attempted to link schizophrenia to social class. Certainly epidemiological statistics have shown that greater numbers of individuals from the lower socioeconomic classes experience symptoms associated with schizophrenia than those from the higher socioeconomic groups. Explanations for this occurrence include the conditions associated with living in poverty, inadequate nutrition, absence of parents, care, few resources for dealing with stressful situations, and feelings of hopelessness for changing one' s lifestyle of poverty.

Some studies refute this hypothesis and view the link between low socioeconomic status and schizophrenia as merely a shift downward because of the client's difficulty in maintaining stable employment and relationships.

ii. Stressful Life Events

Many studies have been conducted that psychotic episodes may be precipitated by stressful life events. In the study of Brown and Birley, they found that stressful events were most likely to have occurred in the 3-week period just before the onset of symptoms. Other investigators of Goldstein (1987) and Liberman (1984) have supported

三、环境因素

（一）社会文化因素

许多研究提示精神分裂症的发生与社会阶层有关。流行病学研究发现处于社会阶层较低的人群比社会阶层较高的人群发生精神分裂症的几率高。这可能与社会阶层较低的人群居住贫穷、营养不足、父母关爱不足、缺乏应对压力的资源和感到改变生活环境无助等有关。

另外一些研究对该假设提出异议，认为精神分裂症患者与低阶层之间的关系是与患者很难维持稳定的职业和人际关系有关。

（二）应激性生活事件

有许多研究提出精神分裂症的发病与应激性生活事件有关。Brown 和 Birley 的研究发现患者在出现症状的前 3 个星期，多数存在明显的生活压力事件。Goldstein（1987）和 Liberman（1984）的相关研究也支持该结论。

the hypothesis that stressful life events can precipitate schizophrenic symptoms in a genetically predisposed individual.

Section 3 Clinical Symptoms of Schizophrenia

第三节 精神分裂症的临床表现

The clinical signs and symptoms of schizophrenia are complex and various. The patient's symptoms change with time. Symptoms seen in schizophrenia may also be seen in the other mental disorder. The development of schizophrenia can be viewed in four phases as following.

精神分裂症的症状复杂多样，并随时间而改变，这些症状也可见于其他精神障碍中。患者的症状与类型有关，而且随着时间可能发生变化。精神分裂症的发展过程可分为四个阶段：精神分裂症人格期、前驱期、活跃期和残留期。

I. Schizoid Personality Phase

一、精神分裂症人格期

The typical but not invariable premorbid history of schizophrenic patients is one of schizoid personality. Such a personality may be characterized as quiet, passive, and introverted. A preschizophrenic adolescent may have had no close friends and no dates, and may have avoided team sports. Such an adolescent may enjoy watching movies and television or listening to music to the exclusion of social activities. Not all individuals who demonstrate the characteristics of schizoid personality will progress to schizophrenia. However, most individuals with schizophrenia show evidence of having had these characteristics in the premorbid condition.

大多数精神分裂症患者在发病前都有精神分裂症人格史，表现为安静、消极和内向的人格特征，没有亲密的朋友，没有约会，避免参加群体活动等。他们更喜欢独处，如一个人看电视、听音乐。虽然不是所有具有这些人格特征的人都会发展为精神分裂症，但大多数精神分裂症患者在发病前都会表现出这些人格特征。

II. Prodromal Phase

二、前驱期

Characteristics of this phase include social withdrawal; impairment in role functioning; behavior that is peculiar or eccentric; neglect of personal hygiene and grooming; blunted or inappropriate affect; disturbances in communication; bizarre ideas; unusual perceptual experiences and lack of initiative, interests, or energy. The length of this phase is highly variable, and may last for many years before deteriorating to the schizophrenic state.

精神分裂症患者在此期表现为社会退缩行为，角色功能损害，行为古怪，不注意个人卫生和修饰，情感淡漠或不协调，沟通障碍，想法奇怪，有不寻常的知觉体验以及缺乏主动性、兴趣和精力。不同患者此期的差异性很大，有的患者持续多年后，病情才进一步恶化。

III. Active Phase

三、活跃期

The active phase is characterized by delusions,

活跃期患者表现出典型的幻觉、妄想、

hallucinations, disorganized speech, grossly disorganized or catatonic behavior, and negative symptoms. When onset is acute, this phase is often the first sign that others observe.

i. Thought Disturbance

Disturbed thoughts are a major characteristic of schizophrenia. It may be manifested in three major areas: content, form, and process.

1. Content Disturbance Content refers to dysfunctional beliefs, ideas, and interpretations of actual internal and external stimuli. Delusions are examples of disturbed thought content. There are some examples of delusions as follows:

The client believes that stereo speakers, TV, or computers are controlling his or her thoughts.

Intergalactic electrical waves are beaming on the world, ready to destroy the client.

The client has the power to change the seasons.

The client has a demon in the stomach that causes sounds.

Common delusions include victimized delusion, relationship delusion, controlled delusion, influence delusion, exaggerated delusion, sinful delusion, hypochondriac delusion, loving delusion, thinking by insight delusion.

2. Thinking Logic Disorder Mainly in the formation of concepts and judgment, reasoning obstacles, such as symbolic thinking, new words and phrases, etc. Clients abstract abstract concepts or specific concepts. There are some examples as follows:

The client reversed the clothes and said that they were same outside and inside.

The client wore a red cap and walking on the road paved with red brick means to take the "socialist-minded and professionally qualified" road.

The client held the oxygen cylinder tightly, indicating that it was closely integrated with the working class because the oxygen cylinder was made by the workers.

The difference between symbolic thinking of clients and normal symbolic thinking is that the purpose and meaning of pathological symbolic thinking is not clear, and its content is not accepted by the group.

3. Form Disturbance Form refers to incoherence, loose associations, tangentiality, circumstantiality, neologisms, word salad, echolalia, perseveration, verbigeration, and autistic and dereistic thinking, all of which are observable by staff as the client speaks or writes.

4. Process Disturbance Process includes

言语紊乱、紧张行为和一些阴性症状等。急性期症状容易被他人发现。常见的急性期症状有：

（一）思维障碍

思维障碍是精神分裂症的特征性症状，其主要表现在思维内容、逻辑、形式和过程的障碍。

1. 思维内容障碍 主要表现为病理性信念、想法和对内外刺激的病理性解释。妄想是最常见的一个思维内容障碍，示例如下：

“患者认为音响、电视或计算机正在控制他或她的想法。”

“星系间的电波正照耀着整个世界，准备摧毁患者。”

“患者拥有改变季节的能力。”

“患者认为在其胃中有一个恶魔发出声音。”

常见的妄想包括被害妄想、关系妄想、被控制妄想、影响妄想、夸大妄想、罪恶妄想、嫉妒妄想、疑病妄想、钟情妄想、思维被洞悉妄想等。

2. 思维逻辑障碍 主要表现在对概念的形成以及判断、推理方面的障碍，如象征性思维、语词新作等。患者将抽象概念具体化或具体概念抽象化。示例如下：

“患者将衣服反穿表示表里如一。”

“戴着红帽，并在用红砖铺的路上行走表示走‘又红又专’的道路。”

“患者紧紧抱着氧气瓶不放，表示与工人阶级紧密结合，因为氧气瓶是工人制造。”

患者的这种象征性思维与正常的象征性思维的区别在于病理性象征性思维的目的和意义不明确，其内容不被群体所接受。

3. 思维形式障碍 主要表现为语无伦次、联想松弛、答非所问、说话绕圈、语词新作、词语乱拼、语言模仿、言语反复、内向性思维、孤僻性思维等。

4. 思维过程障碍 表现在思维中断、记

thought blocking; poor memory; symbolic or idiosyncratic association; illogical flow of ideas; vagueness; poverty of speech; and impaired ability to abstract (concrete thinking), reason, calculate, and use judgment.

忆力差、象征性的或特异性的联想、思维云集、茫然、言语贫乏，抽象、概括、推理、运算和判断能力受损。

ii. Affective Disturbance

（二）情感障碍

Affective disturbance maybe characteristically evidenced by flat (blunted) or inappropriate affect. The person with flat affect demonstrates little or no emotional responsively. Facial expression is immobile, voice is monotonous, and the client describes not being able to feel as intensely as he or she once did, or not being able to feel at all. Inappropriate affect means emotional response does not match cognitive behavior or situation. For example, the individual may describe the death of a parent and laugh. Other affective manifestations may appear as sudden, unprovoked demonstrations of angry or overly anxious behavior. The person may be responding to internal stimuli such as hallucinations.

精神分裂症急性期情感障碍主要表现为情感的淡漠、不协调。情感淡漠的患者表现为情感很淡或没有情感反应、面无表情、声音平淡以及对很多事情都无情感反应。情感不协调主要是指患者的情感反应与自身认知活动和行为的不协调，以及与外界环境的不协调。例如某患者笑着说他母亲死了。

其他情感障碍可表现为在突然、未受刺激的情况下生气，或过度的焦虑等。这可能是患者对内在刺激（如幻觉）的一种反应。

Persons with schizophrenia may demonstrate or express a wide range of emotions, and say that they feel terrified, perplexed, ambivalent, ecstatic, omnipotent, or overwhelmingly alone, or that they don' t feel anything at all. These clients are frequently not in touch with their feelings or have difficulty expressing them.

iii. Perceptual Disturbance

（三）知觉障碍

Perceptual disturbance may include hallucinations, illusions, and boundary and identity problems.

知觉障碍包括幻觉、错觉、自我界限和自我认定障碍、行为障碍。

1. Hallucinations A common perceptual dysfunction in schizophrenia is the occurrence of hallucinations. Hallucination is a sensory perception by an individual that is not associated with actual external stimuli. Although hallucinations may occur in any of the senses (hearing, sight, taste, touch, and smell), the most common are auditory hallucinations. The voices that clients hear carry various types of message, but are usually derogatory, accusatory, obscene, or threatening. It is important for staff to thoroughly assess auditory hallucinations, and assess whether they harm self or others, so that staff can initiate protective interventions. In some instances clients will describe their auditory hallucinations as thoughts or sounds in their brain rather than voices outsides.

Visual, gustatory, tactile, and olfactory hallucinations are less common than auditory types but do occur. Delusions may or may not accompany hallucinations; if they do, the delusional content usually parallels the hallucination, as if the clients are attempting to "make sense" of the hallucination.

1. 幻觉 是精神分裂症最常见的知觉障碍，指在没有客观刺激作用于感觉器官的情况下，所出现的知觉体验。虽然幻觉可出现在任何感觉器官（听觉、视觉、味觉、触觉、嗅觉），但最多见的是听幻觉。患者可听到各种不同类型的声音，但常见的是听见别人议论自己，说自己的不是，或命令自己做某事等。对护士来说，最重要的是评估和判断患者幻听的性质、对患者及其他人的危险性，并及时给予保护性措施。另外，有的患者描述"声音"或"印象"来自大脑，而不是通过感觉器官感觉的。虽然视幻觉、味幻觉、触幻觉和嗅幻觉没有听幻觉常见，但也时常发生。妄想也可伴有幻觉的存在，妄想的内容与幻觉相一致，就像患者试图去解释幻觉存在的意义。

2. Illusions Occasionally the client may experience illusions that are misinterpretations of actual

2. 错觉 偶尔患者可能出现对现实环境或客观事物的错误知觉。如当太阳正在下沉

external environmental or sensory stimuli. For example, as the sun is setting, the patient looks out of the window and tells staff that his grandfather is standing behind the bush. Differentiation by staff of illusions and hallucinations is often difficult and requires keen assessment. Illusions may also occur in any of the senses.

的时候，患者指着窗外告诉护士他看见他祖父站在矮树丛后面。区分患者的错觉和幻觉常比较困难，需要护士仔细地评估。错觉也可能在任何感觉器官出现。

3. Boundary and Identity Problems The schizophrenic client may seem confused and lack a clear sense of self-awareness, in which the client is not sure of his or her own boundaries and sometimes cannot differentiate self from others or from inanimate objects in the environment. This is often frightening for the client. The client may also describe depersonalization or derealization phenomena. In depersonalization, individuals have the sense that their own bodies are unreal, as if they are estranged and unattached to the world or the situation at hand, while derealization is the experience that external environmental objects are strange or unreal. Some clients with schizophrenia may perceive a loss of sexual identity and doubt his or her own sex or sexual orientation. This may be frightening for the client and should not be interpreted as homosexuality by the staff.

3. 自我界限和自我认定障碍 精神分裂症患者可能出现自我认定的障碍。患者表现为缺乏自我意识，不能区分自己和周围环境以及自己和他人。因此，患者非常害怕，感到不真实。有些患者还可出现人格解体或现实感丧失。人格解体感觉自己身体不真实，与周围的环境不相容。非真实感是患者对周围事物和环境感到发生了变化，变得不真实。有的精神分裂症患者还可出现对自己性别的认识障碍，不知道自己究竟属于男性还是女性或对自己的性取向产生疑惑。在这种情况下，不应该将患者看成是同性恋患者。

4. Behavioral Disturbance Behavioral disturbance may be demonstrated by impaired interpersonal relationships, because the client has difficulties in communication and interaction. The individual is frequently emotionally detached, socially inept, withdrawn, and has difficulty in relating to others. Forming a therapeutic relationship with schizophrenic clients is a challenge because of the detached affective responses, illogical thinking, and egocentrism, along with many problems described previously. A concerted effort must be made to engage with the schizophrenic client because the usual encouraging cues for continue interaction is often absent. The nurse must be aware that during acute episodes the client may be more restricted in thought and speech production, so initiation of contacts by the nurse is imperative.

4. 行为障碍 精神分裂症患者常存在行为障碍，患者因语言沟通困难、行为退缩等很难与他人建立关系，影响了患者与他人之间的交往。因此，护士与精神分裂症患者建立信任性治疗关系非常重要且充满挑战。在急性发作期，患者的思维和语言能力受到严重损害，所以护士开始时需主动接触，并保持持续性互动是非常重要的。

A variety of psychomotor disturbance may be present. On one hand the patient may display symptoms of psychomotor overactivity, such as grimacing, bizarre posturing, unpredictable and unprovoked wild activity, odd mannerisms, and compulsive stereotypical or ritualistic behavior. On the other hand, the patient may display symptoms of psychomotor retardation. He may stare into space, seem totally out of touch with the external surroundings or persons in it, and show little or no emotional response, spontaneous speech, or movement. Clients may appear stiff or clumsy and be socially unaware of their appearance and habits and may fail to

精神分裂症患者的行为障碍主要表现为精神运动性兴奋。患者整个精神活动，包括感知觉、思维、情感、意志和行为等方面的活动均高出一般水平，表现为言语动作增多、情感活跃、亢奋易激惹，刻板动作（反复做单一的、无目的动作），模仿行为（无目的和意义地模仿别人的言语和动作），作态（毫无目的和意义地做出古怪、愚蠢、幼稚的动作、姿势、步态或表情）等。也可能表现为精神运动性抑制，包括木僵（精神活动全面抑制，不吃不喝、呼之不应、推之不动，肌张力增高，对外界刺激缺乏反应），缄默（在意识清楚情况下，不能用口头语言进行交流，而只能用书面言语进行交流），违拗（对外界的任

bathe or wash their clothes. They may spit on the floor and in the extreme case they may regressively play with or smear feces. Clients frequently demonstrate anxious, agitated, fearful, or aggressive behavior. Once again, staff's knowledge of the effects of antipsychotic medications is essential to distinguish between symptoms of the disorder and behavioral response to the drugs.

何指令均坚决地拒绝执行，甚至采取相反的行动加以对抗）。

One of the most difficult aspects of schizophrenia is clients' lack of awareness of symptoms or outright denial that anything is unusual or amiss. Termed "poor insight", this characteristic seriously limits the nurse's opportunity to obtain an accurate history and assessment of current and previous functioning.

精神分裂症最大的问题是患者缺乏对症状的认识，完全否认这些症状是错误的或不恰当的，而患者缺乏自知力，可影响护士准确地获得患者的病史、评估患者当前的和过去的功能状况。

IV. Residual Phase

四、残留期

Symptoms occurring before an acute episode (prodromal phase) or after an acute episode (residual phase) are similar. Following an acute episode, clients almost always lack energy and initiative to engage in goal-directed activity. Interest and drive seem absent. He or she may complain of multiple physical symptoms, such as back pain, headache, gastrointestinal problems. The individual may seem confused, perplexed, or have unusual perceptual experiences. Ideas and beliefs become odd or eccentric, and self-care and personal hygiene deteriorate. Affect is blunted or inappropriate, and anxious or angry behaviors may be vague, digressive, and lack words to express his or her point, or may be over elaborative and circumstantial. These symptoms may occur in the prodromal and residual phases.

精神分裂症患者在急性期前的症状和急性期后的症状是相似的。在急性期后，患者常常缺乏精力和主动性去从事有目的的活动，缺乏兴趣和动机。患者可表现为抱怨多种躯体不适，如背痛、头痛、胃肠不适等；显示出困惑、茫然或有一些不寻常的知觉体验；一些想法和观念非常奇怪或偏离正常；自我照顾能力和个人卫生下降；情感淡漠和不协调等。这些症状在前期和残留期都可出现。

BOX 6-1 Learning More

DSM-IV-TR: Positive and Negative Symptoms of Schizophrenia

Positive or hard symptoms

Hallucinations: False sensory perceptions or perceptual experiences that do not exist in reality.

Delusions: Fixed false beliefs that have no basis in reality.

Formal thought disorder: Disordered thinking or use of language.

Odd or bizarre behavior: Behaviors that are inappropriate to usual social convention; odd mannerisms or gestures.

Negative or soft symptoms

Flat affect: Absence of any facial expression that would indicate emotions or mood.

BOX 6-1 知识拓展

DSM-IV-TR：精神分裂症的阳性和阴性症状

阳性症状

幻觉：没有客观刺激作用于感觉器官而在相应器官出现了知觉体验。

妄想：没有事实根据的顽固错误信念。

思维形式障碍：思维或者语言使用的障碍。

行为怪异：不适于通常的社会惯例的行为；奇怪的习惯或手势。

阴性症状

情感淡漠：对外界可引起情感变化的各种刺激所做出的面部表情变化减少或完全没有变化。

Alogia: Tendency to speak very little or to convey little substance of meaning (poverty of content).
Anhedonia: Feeling no joy or pleasure from life or any activities or relationships.
Avolition: Lack of motivation; apathy; impaired ability to initiate activity.
Inattention: Observable impairment in attention.

思维贫乏：联想数量减少，概念与词汇贫乏。
兴趣缺失：感觉生活中的活动和关系都缺乏乐趣。
意志缺乏：缺乏意志、抱负和采取行动或完成任务的动力。
注意力障碍：可观察到的注意力障碍，如涣散。

Section 4 Prognosis

第四节　预后

Several studies have found that over the 5 to 10 year period after the first psychiatric for schizophrenia, only about 10% to 20% of the patients can be described as having a good outcome. More than 50% of the patients can be described as having a poor outcome, with repeated hospitalizations, exacerbations of symptoms, episodes of major mood disorder, and suicide attempts. In spite of those glum figures, schizophrenia does not always run a deteriorating course, and a number of factors have been associated with good prognosis. Table 6-1 shows those factors that relate to the outcome of schizophrenia.

研究发现在精神分裂症发病5～10年后，只有约10%～20%的患者预后较好，超过50%的患者预后较差，表现为反复住院治疗、症状恶化、出现片段的情绪障碍和自杀企图。尽管上述数字显示精神分裂症的预后不是很好，但并不表明精神分裂症的病程总是进行性恶化的。其预后与多种因素有关（表6-1）。

Table 6-1　Factors that relate to the outcome of schizophrenia

Favorable course and prognosis	Unfavorable course and prognosis
1. Late age of onset	1. Early age of onset
2. Acute onset	2. Insidious onset
3. Good premorbid social, sexual, and work/school history	3. Poor premorbid history of socialization
4. Preceded by definable major psychosocial stressors	4. No clear precipitating factors
5. Adequate support systems	5. Few if any supports
6. Paranoid or catatonic features	6. Undifferentiated and disorganized features
7. Family history of mood disorders	7. Withdrawn and isolative behaviors
	8. Chronic course with relapses and few remissions
	9. Perinatal brain injury
	10. Poor response to medications
	11. Inappropriate affective response
	12. Substance abuse

表6-1　与精神分裂症预后相关的因素

有利于预后的因素	不利于预后的因素
1. 起病年龄较晚	1. 起病年龄较早
2. 急性起病	2. 缓慢起病
3. 发病前社会、性关系、工作或学习方面功能较好	3. 发病前社会、性关系、工作或学习方面的功能状态不好
4. 有明显的生活压力事件	4. 无明确的影响因素
5. 有较强的支持系统	5. 支持系统弱

续表

有利于预后的因素	不利于预后的因素
6. 偏执型和紧张型特征	6. 未分化型和瓦解型特征
7. 有心境障碍的家族史	7. 有退缩和孤僻行为
	8. 慢性反复发作的病程，并且很少缓解
	9. 出生前后有大脑受伤的历史
	10. 对药物治疗不敏感
	11. 不协调的情感反应
	12. 物质滥用

The range of recovery rates reported in the literature is from 10% to 60%, and a reasonable estimate is that 20% to 30% of all schizophrenic patients are able to lead somewhat normal lives. About 20% to 30% of patients continue to experience moderate symptoms, and 40% to 60% of patients remain significantly impaired by their disorders for their entire lives. Schizophrenic patients do much less well than do patients with mood disorders, although 20% to 25% of mood disorders patients are also severely disturbed at long-term follow-up.

在不同的研究报告中，精神分裂症康复率为10%~60%。据合理估计有20%~30%的精神分裂症患者能够过正常人的生活。大约有20%~30%的患者可能继续保持中等程度的症状。大约40%~60%的患者可能因疾病而出现社会功能和生活学习能力的明显损害。精神分裂症患者的预后较心境障碍患者的预后差，在长期随访中发现后者有20%~25%存在严重的社会功能损害。

Section 5 Treatment

第五节 治 疗

Schizophrenia is a complex disorder. The cause of schizophrenia is still uncertain. Many authorities suggest that multiple factors cause schizophrenia. Probably specific environmental and psychological factors have contributed to development of the disorder. Schizophrenia occurs in a person who has unique individual, familial, and social psychological profile. The treatment approach must be tailored to how the particular patient has been affected by the disorder and how the particular patient will be helped by the treatment. Thus, just as pharmacological agents are used to address presumed chemical imbalances, nonpharmacological strategies must address nonbiological issues, and any single therapeutic approach is rarely sufficient to address the multifaceted disorder satisfactorily.

精神分裂症是一个复杂的疾病，其病因至今未完全清楚。许多学者都认为与多种因素有关，特定环境和心理社会因素对疾病的发生有影响。每个精神分裂症患者都有其独特的个人、家庭、社会、心理的背景，应根据不同的个体和背景来制订适合于患者的治疗方案。因此，正如其发病与多种因素有关一样，精神分裂症的治疗也根据其特点，多采用综合性治疗，任何单一的治疗方法都不能满意地解决患者的问题。

Although antipsychotic medications are the mainstay of the treatment of schizophrenia, research has found that psychosocial interventions can augment the clinical improvement. Psychosocial modalities should be carefully integrated into the drug treatment regimen and should support it.

虽然抗精神病药物是精神分裂症治疗的主要方法，但有研究发现心理社会干预能促进患者的临床康复。因此，临床上常常在药物治疗过程中进行适当的心理社会干预。

I. Hospitalization

Because of suicidal or homicidal ideation, the client may display grossly disorganized or inappropriate behavior, including the inability to take care of basic needs, such as food, clothing, and shelter. The primary indications for hospitalization are for diagnostic purposes, stabilization on medications, patient safety, and to establish an effective link between the patient and community support system.

Hospitalization decreases stress on patients and helps them structure their daily activities. The length of hospitalizations depends on the severity of the patient's illness and the availability of outpatient treatment facilities. Research has shown that shout hospitalizations (four or six weeks) are just as effective as long-term hospitalizations.

The hospital treatment plan should have a practical orientation toward issues of living, self-care, quality of life, employment, and social relationships. Hospitalization should be directed toward aligning patients with aftercare facilities, including their family homes, foster families, board-and-care homes, and halfway houses.

II. Somatic Treatments

i. Antipsychotics

1. Principles of Antipsychotics Antipsychotic medications, also called neuroleptics, are the mainstay of pharmacologic treatment. Although these drugs have the potential to treat some of the most disturbing psychotic symptoms, they may lead to adverse effects and potentially life-threatening reactions. Many psychiatrists viewed the use of antipsychotic medications in schizophrenia should follow five major principles:

(1) The clinician should carefully define the target symptoms to be treated.

(2) An antipsychotic that has worked well in the past for the patient should be used again.

(3) The minimum length of an antipsychotic trial is four to six weeks at adequate dosages.

(4) In general, the use of more than one antipsychotic medication at a time is rarely.

(5) Patients should be maintained on the lowest possible effective dosage of medication. The dosage is often lower than the dosage that was needed to achieve symptom control during the psychotic episode.

一、住院治疗

精神分裂症患者因受精神症状的影响，可能出现杀人或自杀等危险行为，并且患者自我照顾能力下降，无能力照顾自己的个人卫生、饮食、睡眠、活动等。住院治疗的主要目的是确定诊断、保证药物治疗的稳定和患者的安全，同时建立患者和社区支持系统之间的有效联系。

住院治疗可减少患者的压力和帮助患者建立日常生活的规律。住院治疗时间的长短有赖于患者疾病严重程度和院外治疗服务的有效性。研究显示，一般患者住院治疗四或六个星期能取得与长期住院治疗同等的治疗效果。长期住院可能导致患者社会功能的退缩和适应困难，不利于患者的康复和重返社会。

医院治疗计划还应关注患者居住、生活照料、生活质量、职业技能训练和社会关系建立、住院治疗后的连续性服务（家庭护理、日间护理、家庭访视）等。

二、躯体治疗

（一）抗精神病药物治疗

1. 抗精神病药物治疗原则 精神分裂症的治疗以药物治疗为主。虽然抗精神病药物能治疗和缓解精神病症状，但对人体也有副作用，甚至能威胁到患者的生命。因此许多临床精神病学专家建议，精神分裂症的药物治疗应遵循下列治疗原则：

（1）应仔细确认治疗的靶症状；

（2）对过去效果好的药物应继续使用；

（3）判断一种抗精神病药物是否有效到治疗量至少应用4～6周；

（4）一般情况，尽量不要联合用药；

（5）患者应在达到治疗效果的最低治疗量上维持治疗。维持剂量往往低于急性发作期达到症状控制所需的剂量。

2. Classification of Antipsychotics Antipsychotics are classified as either typical or atypical, based on their pharmacologic effects.

(1) Typical antipsychotics are those that lead to extrapyramidal symptoms (EPS), such as chlorpromazine, perphenazine, and trifluoperaxine.

(2) Atypical antipsychotics, such as clozapine, olanzapine, risperidone, treat both positive and negative symptoms and cause little to no EPS. Usually, they are used for three reasons: lack of response to a typical antipsychotic agent; unmanageable side effects from the other antipsychotics, or presence of negative symptoms. Although clozapine has potential for greater therapeutic efficacy, it carries substantial risks that require careful client monitoring. Agranulocytosis, a life-threatening adverse effect associated with clozapine, requires weekly blood monitoring. Nurses also take an active role in monitoring side effects. Nurses should assess any signs of infection that signal a drop in white blood cell count, because clients may fail to observe or report these symptoms.

All of these medications have been shown to be better than a placebo (inactive treatment). However, some clients may respond better to atypical agents. Table 6-2 lists a comparison of haloperidol and commonly used atypical antipsychotic medications.

2. 抗精神病药物分类 通常抗精神病药物按照其药理作用的效果分为典型的抗精神病药物和非典型的抗精神病药物。

（1）典型的抗精神病药物：如氯丙嗪、奋乃静、三氟拉嗪等，其特点为有不同程度的镇静作用和抗M胆碱的作用，对控制兴奋、躁动、妄想有效，但对情感淡漠、抑郁、行为退缩等阴性症状效果不佳，容易引起锥体外系副作用。

（2）非典型抗精神病药物：如氯氮平、奥氮平、利培酮等，能有效控制患者的阴性症状，副作用较小。因此，患者对药物治疗的依从性较好。在临床上选用非典型抗精神病药物的指征包括：① 患者对典型抗精神病药物不敏感；② 不能承受其他药物的副作用；③ 有阴性症状存在。虽然非典型抗精神病药物的副作用较小，但是仍需要仔细监测药物的副作用，如氯氮平可导致患者出现强迫症状、粒细胞减少、抽搐发作、过度镇静等。所以，在非典型抗精神病药物的治疗中，护士同样扮演重要的角色，应仔细观察药物治疗的效果和副作用。

典型和非典型抗精神病药物都显示出较安慰剂明显的治疗效果，有的患者对典型的抗精神病药物治疗效果好，有的患者对非典型的抗精神病药物治疗效果好。应根据患者的反应选择药物，表6–2列出了各类抗精神病药物的主要治疗效果。

Table 6–2 Comparison of typical and atypical antipsychotics

Generic Name /Trade Name		Clozapine / Clozaril	Olanzapine/ Zyprexa	Risperidone / Risperdal	Serlect/ Sertindole	Haloperidol/ Haldol
Dose*	Initial dose	25-50	5-10	1-2	4	2-5
	Common dose	300-600	10-15	4-6	12-20	6-8
	Maximum dose	900	20	12	24	20
Common Side Effects	EPS	+	+	++	+	++++
	Anticholinergic	++++	++	+	+	++
	Sedation	++++	+++	++	+	++
	Hypotension	++++	+	+	+	+
	Weight gain	++++	++	++	++	++
	Seizure	++++	+	+	+	+

continued

Generic Name /Trade Name		Clozapine / Clozaril	Olanzapine/ Zyprexa	Risperidone / Risperdal	Serlect/ Sertindole	Haloperidol/ Haldol
Treatment Effect	Positive symptoms	Marked	Marked	Marked	Marked	Marked
	Negative symptoms	Marked	Moderate	Marked	Marked	Mild

* In mg, Key:+=very low, ++ =low, +++ = moderate, ++++ = high.

表 6-2　典型和非典型抗精神病药物比较

药名		氯氮平	奥氮平	利培酮	舍吲哚	氟哌啶醇
剂量 *	初始剂量 /mg	25 ~ 50	5 ~ 10	1 ~ 2	4	2 ~ 5
	一般剂量 /mg	300 ~ 600	10 ~ 15	4 ~ 6	12 ~ 20	6 ~ 8
	最大剂量 /mg	900	20	12	24	20
常见副作用	锥体外系作用	+	+	++	+	++++
	抗胆碱能作用	++++	++	+	+	++
	镇静作用	++++	+++	++	+	++
	体位性低血压	++++	+	+	+	+
	体重增加	++++	++	++	++	++
	癫痫发作	++++	+	+	+	+
治疗作用	阳性症状	显著	显著	显著	显著	显著
	阴性症状	显著	中等	显著	显著	不显著

注：+ = 非常低，++ = 低，+++ = 中等，++++ = 高。

There is no way to predict how a client might respond to an antipsychotic, unless the client has been on the medication before. If possible, ask the client about medications tried previously and his or her response to them. The nurse must remember the goal of pharmacotherapy: to achieve an adequate dosage with minimal side effects. Most clients require a moderate dose; for instance, a daily dose of 300 mg to 600 mg of clozapine, 8 mg to 10 mg of haloperidorhaloperidol, or 10 mg to 20 mg of olanzapine. Too low of a dose will be ineffective, whereas too high of a dose may lead to severe side effects and worsening of behavior. Because it takes several weeks for the antipsychotics to effectively treat positive symptoms, the client may not feel better initially and want to discontinue the medication. Nurse should teach clients and their families to wait, often for several weeks, to determine whether the drug will be effective. Monitor the potentially dangerous, uncomfortable, or embarrassing side effects that may occur in initial stages of treatment. Extrapyramidal symptoms are major side effects of typical antipsychotics.

ii. Extrapyramidal Symptoms: Side Effects of Typical Antipsychotics

1. Dystonia　Severe and involuntary contractions of muscles caused by antipsychotic drug therapy that may

没有一种方法可预测患者对哪种药物敏感，除非患者过去用过该药物。因此，应尽量询问患者过去用过什么药物以及对药物的反应。护士须明白药物治疗的目的是在副作用最小的情况下，获得最好的治疗效果。有许多患者要求尽量用小剂量或温和的药物来治疗，但太小剂量的药物达不到治疗效果，而剂量过大则药物副作用大。另外，抗精神病药物发挥治疗作用需要一段时间，通常需要几周的时间才能有效控制精神症状。在用药之初，患者并未感到药物治疗的益处，反而药物的副作用有可能比较明显，因而想终止治疗。所以，护士应做好患者及家属的指导工作，耐心等待药物治疗效果的出现。监测药物治疗初期可能出现的副作用。这些副作用可能发生在治疗的初期。锥体外系反应是典型抗精神病药物的主要副作用。

（二）抗精神病药物的常见副作用

1. 急性肌张力障碍　典型的抗精神病药物如氯丙嗪、氟哌啶醇、三氟拉嗪等容易出现急性肌张力障碍，临床主要表现为躯体某

include tics, problems with swallowing, and spasms in major muscle groups, for example, flexion of the trunk muscles or oculogyric crisis, prolonged fixation of the eyeballs in one place.

个肌群张力的突然增高，由此产生相应的功能障碍。如：面部、颈部、下颌部肌肉痉挛引起的面部怪相、扭曲和斜颈等；咽部肌肉痉挛引起吞咽困难；躯干肌肉痉挛引起角弓反张，躯体向一侧扭转；眼部肌肉痉挛引起动眼危象，眼球上翻或偏向一侧，不能转动。

2. Dyskinesia Difficulty and stiffness of voluntary movement, resulting in partial or incomplete movements.

2. 运动困难 肢体僵硬、随意运动困难，导致部分或不完全的运动障碍。

3. Akathisia Extreme restlessness and inability to still; often confused with anxiety. The clients may pace, constantly move the feet, and have difficulty in concentrating, reading or performing simple tasks. Clients often describe this feeling as if their bodies feel heavy, yet they feel like they could "jump out of their skin."

3. 静坐不能 不能静坐或静站，焦虑、踱步，不能集中注意力，不能静下来完成简单的工作。有患者描述“不是我想走，而是我的腿要走”。

4. Parkinsonism Syndrome Symptoms resembling Parkinson's disease that occur after the first week of treatment, but usually before entering the second month of treatment. The client's symptoms will resemble those of a Parkinson's patient, with fatigue, slowness, a feeling of heaviness, amotivation, muscular, rigidity, a flat, masklike facial expression, shuffling gait, drooling, pill-rolling movements of the fingers, tremors, and altered movement.

4. 帕金森综合征 患者在用药后一周或两个月时出现该综合征，症状非常类似帕金森病。患者表现为肌肉张力增高，活动减少、运动缺乏灵活性，走路时呈前冲步态，双手不摆动，面部肌肉强硬而出现“面具”脸。神经系统检查可发现双上肢有静止性震颤，有时肌肉的震颤可发生在唇、下颌以及下肢。

5. Akinesia Apathy, fatigue, slowness, lack of motivation. This can also be confused with the amotivation (negative symptom) of schizophrenia.

5. 运动不能 漠然、疲劳、缓慢、缺乏动力，该症状容易与精神分裂症的阴性症状相混淆，应注意区别。

6. Choreathetoid Movements Writhing, wormlike movements of limbs.

6. 舞蹈症状 肢体、四肢像虫一样扭曲、摆动。

7. Tardive Dyskinesia A syndrome that is seen after long-term use of antipsychotic medication. Symptoms include slow movements of lips, tongue, and mouth, with chewing, smacking. Sucking, tongue protrusion, or lip licking. Other symptoms may include puffing of the cheeks, blinking, and facial grimacing. Choreoform movements of the body and limbs may also be present. The symptoms may intensify with stress and are absent during sleep.

7. 迟发性运动障碍 一般发生于长期服用典型抗精神病药物的患者，表现为嘴、唇、舌等部位的不自主活动，像咀嚼、咋舌、吸奶等。四肢、躯干可出现舞蹈样动作，患者无法控制。其他常见症状，如鼓颊、眨眼、做怪脸等。

In the antipsychotic treatment, a key role of nurses is assessing the therapeutic and adverse response to medications. Nurses should distinguish the client's behavior due to worsening symptoms of psychosis or to a negative response to antipsychotic treatment. For example, an EPS symptom such as akinesia (lack of movement, stiffness) may be so disturbing to a client that it leads to noncompliance. Akinesia is also associated with the

在抗精神病药物治疗过程中，护士需要评估患者对药物治疗的反应，包括疗效和副作用，同时，应区别患者的行为是由于精神症状加重还是药物的不良反应。如肌张力障碍中的运动不能可能使患者表现不服从，而且运动不能的患者面部无表情，因此，应注意与情感淡漠区别。

appearance of a masklike face, which needs to be carefully distinguished from flat affect.

Clients must be adequately informed of their treatment, but not so frightened by the effects that they refused medication. Nurses should evaluate both the acute and long-term effects of antipsychotic agents, teach the knowledge of the medication, and assist the client in becoming responsible for personal medication management.

患者应对其治疗有所了解，但又不能被药物的副作用所吓倒而拒绝药物治疗。护士应评估药物治疗急性期和长期的反应，指导患者学习相关药物知识，帮助患者提高药物治疗的依从性和患者对药物的自我管理能力。

iii. Electroconvulsive Therapy

（三）电抽搐治疗

Electroconvulsive therapy (ECT) may sometimes be necessary for individuals with psychotic disorders. ECT is used along with antipsychotic medication for clients who show mood symptoms or catatonia. A rapid response may be obtained in severely ill psychotic clients who are at risk for dehydration or starvation. 6 to 12 ECT treatments are generally administered in the hospital. More than 12 treatments are not beneficial and will not prevent worsening or relapse of symptoms.

电抽搐治疗在精神分裂症的治疗中也起着重要作用。精神分裂症中严重兴奋躁动、冲动伤人、对药物治疗不敏感，伴有严重抑郁情绪的、紧张木僵的患者，电抽搐治疗效果比较满意，可有效控制患者症状，缩短病程。一般电抽搐治疗的疗程为 6～12 次一疗程。

III. Psychosocial Treatments and Rehabilitation

三、心理治疗

i. Cognitive-behavior Therapy

（一）认知行为疗法

The use of cognitive-behavior therapy (CBT) in schizophrenia is based on the rational that positive psychotic systems are amenable to structured reasoning and behavioural modification. With delusional beliefs,for example,individual ideas are traced back to their origin and alternative explanations are explored. However, direct confrontation is avoided. Similarly, it may be possible to modify a patient's beliefs about the omnipotence, identity, and purpose of auditory hallucinations, with a resulting decrease in the distress that accompanies the experience and, perhaps, in its frequency.

精神分裂症应用认知行为疗法（cognitive-behavior therapy，CBT）是基于理性的积极精神系统，结构化认知和行为的重塑。例如妄想信念，个人的想法要追溯到它们的起源和替代解释去进行探讨。然而，直接对抗是可以避免的。同样，它可能改变患者关于全能、身份和幻听企图的信念，因而降低伴随的痛苦体验，或者痛苦频率。

BOX 6-2 Learning More

Research Brief : CBT

In a British study, a group of researchers studied the effects of CBT using a randomized trial involving over 400 patients divided into two groups. One group received CBT from suitably trained community psychiatric nurses in addition to their standard treatment. The other (control) group received their standard treatment. The findings of the study showed that CBT had the potential to increase the individual's level of insight and that this could be achieved safely and effectively.

BOX 6-2 知识拓展

CBT 研究摘要

在英国，有学者将 400 例精神分裂症患者随机分为对照组和治疗组，治疗组在接受常规治疗同时加上 CBT 治疗，而对照组只接受常规治疗。其结果显示，CBT 治疗能够提高精神分裂症患者的自我认识能力，这将有助于患者获得更好的安全性和效能。

ii. Social Skill Training and Illness Self-managment

Social skill training uses a variety of approaches to teach complex interpersonal skill, including behavioural rehearsal, feedback, and training. Skills training may be combined with illness self-management in which patiens learn to adjust their own medication and organize their lives to minimize troublesome symptoms. The results of these interventions are generally positive but concerns remain about whether the gains are maintained when treatment ends and whether benefit is restricted to patients who have a good prognosis. Indeed, a meta-analysis concluded that social skills training does not produce reliable benefits and it was not recommended for routine use.

iii. Family-oriented Therapy

A variety of family-oriented therapies are useful in treatment of schizophrenia. The focus of the therapy should be on the immediate situation and should include identifying and avoiding potentially troublesome situations. When problems do emerge with the patient in the family, the focus of the therapy should be on the rapid resolution of the problem.

Subsequent to the immediate postdischarge period, an important topic to cover in family therapy is recovery process, particularly its length and its rate. The therapist must help the family and the patient understand schizophrenia without being overly discouraging. The therapist may discuss the psychotic episode itself and the events leading up to it. Openning discussion with the psychiatrist and the schizophrenic relative can often helpful for all parties. Subsequent family therapy can be directed toward the long-range implementation of reducing stress and coping strategies and toward gradual involvement of the patient in activities.

The excessive expression of emotion during a session of the family may damage the recovery process of a schizophrenic patient and can undermine the potential success of subsequent family therapy sessions. The therapist must control the emotional intensity of the session. Many studies have found family therapy to be especially effective in reducing relapse.

iv. Group Therapy

Group therapy for schizophrenia generally focuses on real-life plans, problems, and relationships. Groups may be behaviorally oriented, psychodynamically or insight-oriented, or supportive. Group therapy is effective in reducing social isolation, increasing the sense of cohesiveness, and improving reality testing for patients with schizophrenia. Groups led in a supportive manner,

（二）社会技能训练和疾病自我管理

社会技能训练运用多样化的方法去教授复杂的个人技能，包括行为排练、反馈和训练。技能训练可能结合疾病自我管理，患者学习去适应药物和组织他们的生活以减少令人困扰的症状。这些干预逐渐取得积极的结果，但是关注点依旧在于治疗结束时既得收获是否可以维持，或者拥有良好预后的患者的既得收获是否受到限制。实际操作中，一项 meta 分析表明社会技能训练没有取得可靠的收益，不推荐作为常规使用。

（三）家庭导向治疗

家庭导向治疗在精神分裂症的治疗中有一定的疗效。其要点是通过接近现实的场所帮助患者解决问题。

在家庭治疗的后期，治疗的重点应是帮助患者恢复家庭的功能，让患者及家庭清楚精神分裂症并不是不能解决的问题，与患者共同讨论有关精神分裂症的发病及其影响因素等。应重点注意帮助患者应对生活中的压力。

高情感表达的家庭可能影响精神分裂症患者的康复，并渐渐破坏家庭治疗的效果，因此作为治疗者一定要控制治疗过程中家庭的情绪表达。

（四）小组治疗

精神分裂症小组治疗的重心应集中在患者存在的现实问题、压力和人际关系上。它主要通过行为、精神动力和自知力方面，以及成员间的相互支持来发挥作用。小组治疗可减轻患者的社会隔离，增加患者与他人或社会接触的机会，增加凝聚力，提高患者对

rather than in an interpretative way, appear to be most helpful for schizophrenic patients.

v. Environmental Supports

Environmental supports focus on structuring the environment to compensate for or work around impairments in these cognitive functions. Therapies that mainly work through the systematic use of environmental compensatory strategies and supports are relatively uncommon for schizophrenia but have a growing evidence base. Compensatory strategies and environmental supports attempt to bypass cognitive deficits, negative symptoms, and disorganization by establishing supports in the environment that specifically cue and sequence adaptive behavior, and discourage maladaptive behavior. For example, checklists can be used to prompt specific behaviors that are necessary to live more independently. These techniques have been utilized for years in the rehabilitation of individuals with head injuries and with mental retardation. More recently, these supportive strategies have been extended to treatment of schizophrenia in an intervention known as cognitive adaptation training (CAT) with very encouraging results.

vi. Cognitive Rehabilitation

Cognitive rehabilitation is novel and has not yet been minutely examined. There is no consensus from its proponents on the language to describe the therapies or what their constituent parts should be. The underlying theory of how it works differs from one academic group to another, with suggestions about both compensating and repairing the cognitive system. But despite all these differences, many training packages do look similar, even if the emphasis within each package is different. Cognitive rehabilitation has been led by pragmatic studies that attempt to demonstrate individuals' cognitive improvement. The training programs adopted individuals have face validity, but there have been many different approaches: or group treatment, computer-driven presentation or paper-and-pencil tasks, therapist presentation or automated presentation (or both), frequency of therapy—either weekly or intensive daily sessions & type of training (rehearsal or strategic processing).

vii. Vocational Rehabilitation

The rate of unemployment for people with serious mental illness, and schizophrenia in particular, is approximately 85%. Employment provides a means for earning income, structuring daily schedules, building relationships, having opportunities to use personal talents and interests, and achieving recognition. Through employment, people increase their independence and

现实的感受和反应。

（五）环境支持

环境支持是指通过构建环境来弥补认知功能的缺陷。对于精神分裂症患者而言，那些主要是通过环境补偿策略的系统使用来产生作用的治疗相对稀有，却有增长的潜力。补偿策略和环境支持，顾名思义，是指建立环境中的支持，尤其是指试着通过整理和排序适应行为来绕过疾病的认知缺陷、阴性症状和混乱，从而减少适应不良行为。比如：为了更加独立地生活，一个清单可以被用来促进必要的独特的行为方式。这些技术近几年来已经被用于有头部损伤或者精神发育迟滞的个体康复。更近的，这些支持性策略已被扩展到精神分裂症的治疗中一个具有良好效果、被称为认知适应训练的干预措施。

（六）认知康复

认知康复是新提出的目前没有经过检验的方法。目前对描述认知康复疗法的术语及其组成没有一致的说法。关于此疗法如何运作，以及其补偿和修复认知系统的意见在不同的学派之间被强调的原理也大相径庭。但是尽管有这些不同，甚至强调的方式和工具重点不同，很多训练的方式和工具却看起来非常相似。实践主义学派领先尝试认知康复疗法去证实个体认知上的提高。被采用的训练程序直面有效性，但包括很多不同的方式：个体或小组治疗，电脑作业或纸笔作业，治疗师陈诉或自动化陈诉（或两者兼有），治疗频率——每周或每天不同会话与类型的培训（排练或战略性过程）。

（七）职业康复

严重精神疾患者，特别是精神分裂症人群的失业率85%左右。职业是提供赚钱，结构化日常生活，建立人际关系，发挥个人天赋和兴趣的机会，以及实现认可的一种方式。通过被雇佣，人们增加了独立感和群体生活的内容。职业支持的发展和确认通过提供给

inclusion in community life. Development and validation of supported employment have made work a realistic option for people with schizophrenia. Furthermore, in addition to increasing income, work helps to reduce disability, isolation, boredom, stigma, and discrimination.

精神分裂症人群一个现实的选择起作用。此外，除了增加收入外，工作有助于减少残疾、隔离、无聊、耻辱和歧视。

Section 6 Application of the Nursing Process

第六节　护理程序的应用

The behaviors of schizophrenic patients are difficult to understand and sometimes frightening. Patients who experience psychoses are also frightened by their experiences. They are usually unable to form close interpersonal relationships because of the demands of the illness for their attention and energy. Nursing care for schizophrenic patients is a challenge. Caring nurses must strive to make contact with psychotic patients and assist them to overcome or adapt to the effects of illness.

精神分裂症患者可能因疾病影响，行为很难被人理解，且攻击性强，很难与他人形成良好的人际关系。精神分裂症患者的护理对精神科护士来说极具挑战性。护士应运用有效的沟通交流技巧，与患者建立良好的治疗性关系，帮助患者克服疾病带来的障碍和不适应。

I. Nursing Assessment

一、护理评估

The first step of the nursing process is an assessment. The nurse gathers a database from which nursing diagnoses are derived and a plan of care is formulated. The first step of the nursing process is extremely important, for without an accurate assessment, problem identification, objectives of care, and outcome criteria cannot be accurately determined.

护理评估是护理程序的第一步，护士通过收集患者的资料，做出护理诊断和护理计划。护理评估直接关系到护理问题、护理目标和评价结果的准确性。

The assessment of the client with schizophrenia can be challenging and may be a complex process. Nurses should considered several factors and gather information of the client from a number of sources. Clients in an acute episode of their illness are seldom able to make a significant contribution to their history. Clients may refuse to communicate or communicate ineffectively as a result of impaired cognition or the presence of psychotic symptoms such as hallucinations or delusions. The data may be obtained from family members, from old records, or from other individuals who have been in a position to report on the progression of the client's behavior.

对精神分裂症患者的评估过程比较复杂，因为在急性期，患者由于认知功能受损或受精神症状（如幻觉、妄想等）的影响，不能与他人进行有效的交流，很难讲清楚其病史，有的患者甚至拒绝交谈。所以，护士应从多种渠道获得信息，并判断信息的真实性、可靠性。资料来源包括患者的家庭成员、以往的病历或其他重要相关人员等。

The nurse must be well-known behaviors common to the disorder in order to obtain an adequate assessment of the client with schizophrenia. Major disturbances of schizophrenic patients are in eight areas of functioning: thought, perception, affect, sense of self, volition, interpersonal functioning and relationship to the external world, psychomotor behavior and risk of self-injury and

从患者的行为中护士可发现很多重要信息。患者常见的问题主要表现在思维，感知，情感，自我认识，意志，人际关系，精神运动以及自杀、自伤和物质滥用八个方面。

substance abuse. These areas of functioning are employed to facilitate the presentation of background information on which to base the initial assessment of the client with schizophrenia. Additional impairments outside the limits of these eight areas also presented.

i. Thought

The nursing assessment of the person's thinking can provide significant information regarding nursing intervention. This method of assessment is based on the assumption that language is the vehicle of thought; that is, language mirrors the process of thinking-what we say is what we think. Obviously, language reflects only a part of thinking. There is a great deal of thinking that is not expressed verbally. However, a careful assessment of thinking requires that we first listen closely to the patient, and then that we question the patient to determine the subjective experience associated with his language to complete our impression of the "underlying processes".

1. Content of Thought Content of thought refers to beliefs, ideas and interpretations of actual internal and external stimuli. Delusions constitute the major disturbance in the content of thought. The delusions are most frequently bizarre, fragmented, and multiple in nature. Delusions are classified according to their content. Some more common delusions include delusion of persecution, delusion of grandeur, delusion of reference, delusion of control or influence, somatic delusion, nihilistic delusion, religiosity, paranoia, and magical thinking.

To assessment the patient's delusion is a technical skill. Does the client have ideas or beliefs that are untrue? Does the client have the belief that neutral cues in the environment refer to him? Does the client believe he has special talents and extraordinary power? Patients may report delusions spontaneously, but usually specific questioning is required. There are some questions that may help in eliciting delusional trends in the patient's thinking:

Do you feel that others might be responsible for your problems or the situation you are in?

Has anyone been paying particular attention to you, watching you, or talking about you?

Has anyone treated you badly or criticized you unfairly, annoyed you, or bothered you in any way that was unusual?

Have you felt that people on radio or TV were talking about you in their reports? What is the basis for these unpleasant experiences? Why are they happening to you?

Have you felt responsible for or blamed yourself for your illness or difficulties? Have you felt others blamed you?

（一）思维的评估

对患者思维方面的评估，可为护理干预提供重要信息和依据。语言是思维的表达工具，即语言反映了思维的过程。虽然有很多思想不能被口头语言所表达，但我们仍能够从患者的语言中获得他们部分的思想内容。因此，护士应小心、仔细地通过聆听和询问获得所需的信息和资料。

1. 思维内容 思维内容是指思想、信念以及对内外刺激的解释。妄想是精神分裂症患者主要的思维内容障碍，其内容常常奇异、片段、多样。一般根据妄想的内容可分为被害妄想、夸大妄想、关系妄想、影响（控制）妄想、疑病妄想、虚无妄想等，以及一些与宗教、偏执、着魔等有关的妄想。

护士要判断患者的一些想法或观念是否不切实际、是否与患者的文化或宗教有关。因许多患者不愿将自己的妄想告诉他人或者拒绝承认妄想，故护士应采用特定的提问方式，仔细评估，包括：

你是否认为其他人应对你的问题或你现在的情形负责？

是否有人特别注意你、看你或谈论你？

是否有人伤害你的身体？不公平的批评你？惹恼你？用一些异常的手段打扰你？

是否觉得他人、电视或广播都在谈论你？为什么发生在你身上？

是否感觉你应该对自己疾病或困难负责任，甚至认为自己该死？是否认为有人在谴责你？

是否感觉自己有一种不寻常的能力，可做任何活动或事情？

Have you felt unusually well or in very good spirits? Has this resulted in any activities on you part?

2. Processes of Thought The major features of alterations in thought processes include flow of thought, control of thought.

The disturbance in flow of thought can be see in other psychotic disorders, such as anxiety disorder, depression or organic brain disorder. In schizophrenic patients, they may show slowed or inhibited thinking, mutism, rapid thinking, circumstantiality, tangentiality, thought blocking, and perseveration in thinking.

Some schizophrenic patients say their thoughts, feelings, or actions have been controlled by other people or by something. The disturbance of thought control may appear as obsessional thinking, thought alienation, thought insertion, and thought broadcasting. There are some questions that may help nurses to elicit disturbance of thought control:

Have you felt forced to think, say, or do certain things?

Have you felt that your thoughts were not your own, that they were being broadcast?

Have your thoughts, feelings, or actions been controlled by other people? How?

3. Form of Thought Form of thinking traditionally refers to several features, which include the logical character, abstractness, coherence or connectedness, and association. Disturbances of thought form include asyndetin thinking, splitting of thought, incoherence of thought, symbolic thinking, illogical thinking, and neologisms.

ii. Perception Assessment

Perceptual disturbances may include hallucinations, illusions, and boundary and identity problems. Hallucination is a common perceptual dysfunction in schizophrenia. It involves any of the five senses (hearing, sight, taste, touch, smell), and can be identified as the following types: auditory, visual, tactile, gustatory, and olfactory hallucinations. Although hallucinations may occur in any of the senses, the most common are auditory hallucinations.

It is important for staff to thoroughly assess hallucinations, specially the command hallucinations, which may place the individual or others in a potentially dangerous situation. The "voices" may tell the client to

2. 思维过程 思维过程的改变主要表现在思维的速度、自主性方面。精神分裂症患者表现为思维迟缓、缄默症、思维奔逸、病理性赘述、思维中断及言语反复。思维速度障碍也可见于其他精神疾病，如焦虑障碍、抑郁障碍或器质性脑病等。

有些患者认为自己的思想、感受和行为被他人或事物所控制。思维控制障碍可表现为强迫性思维、异己思维、思维插入和思维播散等。应用下列提问可帮助护士发现患者思维控制障碍问题：

你是否感觉有一种力量或东西强迫你思考、说话或做事?

你是否感觉你的思想不是你自己的，你的思想是否被广播了?

你是否感觉你的思想、感受和行为被某人控制？是如何控制的?

3. 思维形式 思维形式的特征包括思维的逻辑性、抽象性、连贯性和联想性。思维形式的障碍主要包括思维散漫、思维破裂、思维不连贯、象征性思维、非逻辑思维和语词新作等。

（二）感知觉评估

感知觉障碍包括幻觉、错觉和界限及认定障碍。精神分裂症患者常见的感知觉障碍为幻觉。幻觉可涉及任何一个感觉器官（听觉、视觉、触觉、味觉、嗅觉），以听幻觉最常见。

护士应仔细评估患者的幻觉，特别是命令性幻听。因为这些"声音"可能是告诉患者伤害自己或他人，导致患者或其他人处于

harm self or others. The following questions may help staff to elicit hallucinations of the patient.

Do you see visions in the daytime?

Do you dream vividly?

Do you see flashes of light, patterns, figures, objects that others cannot see?

Do noises in your head, ears, or from the outside bother you?

Do you even hear your own thinking, your own thoughts, as if they were being spoken aloud?

Do you hear voices when there is no one else around who could be speaking? If so, whose voice? Is it clear? Abusive? Accusatory? Can you stop the voices from occurring?

In addition, Williams suggests that assessing hallucinations should consider the following factors regarding hallucination: identify all sensory aspects of the hallucination, including auditory, visual, tactile, and others. Assess how long the client has experienced hallucinations. If possible, ask the client to describe what happened and when the hallucinations were first experienced. Assess how real the hallucinations are to the client, as well as the ability to distinguish reality from the experience of the hallucination.Identify the major theme and underlying feelings of the hallucination. Assess whether command hallucinations are being experienced, whether the client follows the commands, and the potential for harm. Note the time of day or situations to the hallucinations, for most likely to experience hallucinations. Assess the client's response to the hallucinations. Determine the ways in which the individual has tried to cope with hallucination, both ineffectively and effectively. If the client denies hallucinations, but gives nonverbal indications suggesting them, ask gently if the voices are telling him not to discuss them, or to indicate by a nod if there is voice.

危险状态之中。护士应用下列问题提问可获得患者有关幻觉的信息：① 你在白天是否看见过一些别人看不见的东西？② 你是否做过一些非常生动的梦？③ 你是否看见一些东西，如光、图案、物体等，而其他人看不见？④ 在你的头脑中是否有声音，或有外界的声音烦扰你？⑤ 你是否听到你自已的思考和想法，好像它们被大声地讲出来？⑥ 当你周围没有人时，你是否听到有人说话的声音？如果有，是谁的声音？听得清楚吗？是辱骂的还是表扬你的？你能阻止声音发生吗？

另外，Walliams 认为，在评估患者的幻觉时，还应考虑下列因素：患者幻觉的类型（幻听、幻视、幻触和其他）；出现幻觉的时间、频率；首次产生幻觉的时间和体验；幻觉对患者的影响；患者区别幻觉和真实体验的能力；幻觉的主要内容及其潜在的危险；命令性幻听的内容、性质、对患者的影响；幻觉发生的时间、当时的情形；患者对幻觉的反应，应对幻觉的能力、方法等。

iii. Affect

Affect refers to feelings and emotions. In the normal state, feelings and emotions generally synchronize with the content of thoughts. When there is impairment of affect, this synchronization does not occur. The emotional response to what the person is saying is inappropriate and it does not match. In the schizophrenia, affect may be inappropriate, inconsistent, bland or flat, and apathy. In inappropriate affect, the individual's emotional tone is incongruent with the circumstances. In bland or flat affect, there is severe reduction in the intensity of affective expression. In flat affect, there is no sign of facial expression and the voice is usually monotonous. In apathy, the client with schizophrenia often demonstrates an indifference to or disinterest in environment.

（三）情感方面

情感反映了个人的情绪和感受。在正常状态，感受和情绪一般与当时的思想内容一致。当有情感障碍时，一致性就会丧失。患者当时的情绪状态可能与其当时的思想内容不符。在精神分裂症患者中，患者可能出现情感倒错、矛盾情感、情感平淡或淡漠等情况。情感倒错可表现为患者的情绪反应与当时的实际情况不符；情感平淡表现为情感反应明显降低，面无表情，语音单调；情感淡漠则表现为对周围环境或刺激缺乏情感反应或无任何反应。

iv. Sense of Self

Sense of self describes the uniqueness and individuality a person feels. Because of extremely weak ego boundaries, the schizophrenic person lacks this feeling of uniqueness and experiences a great deal of confusion regarding his or her identity.

v. Volition

Volition has to do with impairment in the ability to initiate goal-directed activity. In the individual with schizophrenia, this may take form of inadequate interest, drive, or ability to follow a course of action to its logical conclusion. The patient with schizophrenia may appear emotional ambivalence.

vi. Interpersonal Functioning and Relationship to the External World

The individuals with schizophrenia cling to others, intrude on strangers, and fail to recognize that excessive closeness makes other people uncomfortable and likely to pull away. Impairment in social functioning may also be reflected in social isolation, emotional detachment, and lack of regard for social convention. The patient with schizophrenia may appear autism and deteriorated appearance. They focus inward on a fantasy world, distort or exclude the external environment; personal grooming and self-care activities may become minimal.

vii. Psychomotor Behavior

There may be various disturbances in psychomotor behavior such as anergia, waxy flexibility, posturing, pacing and rocking.

viii. Risk of Self-injury and Substance Abuse

Because there is such a high rate of suicide and attempted suicides among patients with schizophrenia, it is important to assess for the risk of self-harm. The following questions will help the nurse assess risk of self-injury:

Does the client speak of suicide?

Does the client have delusional thinking that could lead to dangerous behavior?

Does the client have command hallucinations telling him to harm himself or others, or homicidal ideations?

Does the client have substance abuse?

II. Nursing Diagnosis and Nursing Objective

i. Nursing Diagnosis

From analysis of the assessment data, appropriate nursing diagnoses are formulated for the psychotic client. There are many nursing diagnoses that can be used with

（四）自我认识方面

自我认识是个人对自己个性特征的认识。由于患者的自我界限受损，因此患者在自我认识方面存在混乱。

（五）意志方面

意志是指个体自觉地确立目标，同时自觉地采取行动，并在行动中克服困难以最终达到目标的心理过程。意志活动的特点包括指向性、目的性、自觉性、果断性、自制性。意志障碍影响个体确立目标及对目标所采取的行动。精神分裂症患者可表现为病理性的意志增强、意志减退等。

（六）人际交往和人际关系

精神分裂症患者常常依赖（黏附）别人，不能与他人建立满意的亲密关系。社会功能的受损同样反映在患者的社会交往上，表现为社会退缩、情感分离、缺乏对社会或集体的关注。精神分裂症患者可能出现自闭，并且不注意外表的修饰和清洁，他们沉迷于一个幻想的世界，扭曲或忽视外部的环境，个人卫生和自我照顾能力下降。

（七）精神运动方面

精神分裂症患者可有各种精神运动方面的障碍，如肌肉无反应力、蜡样屈曲、僵直等。

（八）自杀、自伤危险和物质滥用

因为在精神分裂症患者中出现自杀、自伤和物质滥用的比率较高，因此评估患者自杀、自伤的危险度非常重要。护士可应用下列问题评估患者的自杀危险：① 患者是否提到过自杀？② 是否存在可导致患者危险行为的妄想？③ 是否有命令性幻听支配患者去伤害自己或他人？④ 患者是否存在物质滥用？

二、护理诊断和护理目标

（一）护理诊断

通过对所收集的有关患者信息的分析，可获得患者相关护理诊断。精神分裂症患者

schizophrenia as the other chapter described.

常见的护理诊断跟其他章节所列举的护理诊断一致。

ii. Nursing Objective

For each diagnosis, the nurse must establish appropriate and expected outcomes and goals. The expected outcomes will be different depending on whether the client is being treated in an acute or rehabilitative phase.

1. In the acute phase, the immediate goal of treatment is to bring symptoms under control. For example, for the diagnosis of alteration in thought processes, a stated outcome might be "with 4 days of initiating treatment, the patient will be able to answer simple direct questions." For the diagnosis of disturbance of sleep pattern, the stated outcome might be "within 3 days of hospital admission, the patient will sleep through the night".

2. In rehabilitative phase, the nurse will establish goals aimed at helping the patient and his family to make the best adjustment possible to a chronic illness and will take any measures possible to maintain the patient's independence to whatever degree possible. For example, for the diagnosis of impaired role performance, the nurse and patient together might determine work problems and might establish a goal that the patient will attend work regularly by going to work with his neighbor.

The following criteria may be used for measurement of outcomes in the care of the schizophrenic patient.

The patient:

Demonstrates an ability to relate satisfactorily with others.

Recognizes distortions of reality.

Has not harmed self or others.

Perceives self realistically.

Demonstrates the ability to perceive the environment correctly.

Maintains anxiety at a manageable level.

Relinquishes the need for delusions and hallucinations.

Demonstrates the ability to trust others.

Uses appropriate verbal communication in interactions with others.

Performs self-care activities independently.

（二）护理目标

针对患者的每个护理问题，护士应根据患者的情况和病程变化制订恰当的护理目标。

1. **急性期** 此期治疗和护理的重点是控制症状，如针对存在思维过程改变的患者，近期的护理目标可能是患者在治疗的第 4 天，能够回答简单直接的问题。又如对一个存在睡眠障碍的患者，近期的护理目标可能是患者在入院后第 3 天，睡眠得到改善，睡眠时间增加到每晚 8 个小时。

2. **恢复期** 此期的护理目标应注重帮助患者恢复自我照顾能力和独立能力，同时要帮助患者及家庭如何应对和调整适应慢性疾病。如针对一个存在角色功能障碍的患者，护士应和患者一起讨论患者工作上的问题，制订一个合适的目标，如在其同伴的协助下，逐渐恢复其工作等。

下列各项标准可用来评价和测量对精神分裂症患者的护理效果，患者将 : ① 能有与他人建立满意关系的能力；② 认识哪些是对现实的扭曲；③ 没有伤害自己或其他人的行为；④ 能真实地感受自己；⑤ 能够正确地感知周围环境；⑥ 焦虑控制在一个能够耐受的水平；⑦ 能从幻觉和妄想回到现实；⑧ 能够信赖其他人；⑨ 能使用恰当的语言与他人进行沟通；⑩ 有独立的自我照料的能力。

III. Nursing Plan and Implementation

In planning patient care, the nurse assesses each patient thoroughly, diagnoses nursing problems, establishes long and short-term goals, determines

三、护理计划和实施

护士根据患者的情况，制订合适的护理计划并实施。精神科护士在对患者护理的过

appropriate approaches of care for the particular patient, and then carries through with the specific nursing intervention. The role of the psychiatric nurse in the care of a person with schizophrenia must be flexible. Because the person communicates at various levels and is in control of himself at various times, the nurse has to be able to adjust the nursing care as the situation demands. It is important to observe each patient individually to determine the best nursing care.

程中一定要灵活。由于每个患者的沟通能力不同，而且对自己的控制能力也不同，护士必须根据具体情况及时调整护理措施，为每个患者提供最佳的护理。

Interventions for patients with schizophrenia include biologic, psychological, and social interventions.

对精神分裂症患者的护理干预包括生理、心理和社会文化等方面。下面从这几方面讨论为精神分裂症患者提供的护理措施：

i. Biologic Interventions

（一）生理方面的护理

Biologic interventions include monitor medications, minimize side effects, decrease impact of movement disorders, improve nutritional status, modify cognitive deficits, and improve sleep. In the acute phase of schizophrenia, the assessment, plan, and outcomes are all based on alleviating acute symptoms. Much of the nursing care will be collaborative and involve using of medications to bring symptoms under control. Independent nursing care will be done through interventions that establish a safe and trusting environment and provide an acutely ill client a space for sleep without interference from others.

The major biologic interventions during the initial acute phase of schizophrenia include:

a. Provide a safe, protective, quiet environment and establish a nurse-client relationship.

b. Assess and monitor the patient's health status. Inform administration of antipsychotic medications.

c. Attention to self-care needs and the patient's ability to maintain hygiene and adequate nutrition are important.

d. Developing a daily schedule of routine activities (showering, shaving, and so forth) can help the patient structure the day.

e. Assist the client to sleep and provide a space for sleep without interference from others.

f. Monitor the behavior of the patient and assess/monitor the risk to self and others.

对患者生理方面的护理干预包括药物监测、副作用的观察与处理、减少运动障碍的影响、改善营养状况、改善睡眠等。在精神分裂症急性期，护理工作的重点是改善患者的急性症状，许多护理措施能协助药物控制症状。另外，与患者建立信任关系和为患者建立一个安全的治疗和休息的环境也非常重要。具体的护理干预措施包括：① 提供安全舒适的治疗环境，与患者建立信任的护患关系；② 评估及监测患者的健康状态，为患者提供有关抗精神病药物治疗的信息；③ 关注患者自我照顾和维持个人卫生及营养的需要，提供及时的帮助；④ 帮助患者制订日常活动安排表，培养规律的生活；⑤ 提供安静的休息环境，帮助患者睡眠；⑥ 监护患者的行为，评估患者的自杀、伤人的危险性，必要时给予适当的保护。

ii. Psychological Interventions

（二）心理护理

The goal of psychological interventions include improve social skills, improve problem-solving skills, improve self-concept, increase stress management and relapse prevention skills, and improve family relationships.

心理护理在精神分裂症患者的护理中占有重要地位。护理目标包括提高患者社会技能和解决问题的能力；提高自我概念；增强应对压力和预防复发的能力；改善家庭关系等。

Psychological interventions such as cognitive therapy, self-monitoring and relapse prevention are useful to improve patient's social skills, problem-solving skills, self-concept, and relapse prevention skills. It also can

心理护理的内容包括认知治疗与护理，自我监护和预防复发。

increase their ability of stress management and symptoms management.

1. Cognitive Therapy Patients with schizophrenia experience several cognitive deficits including deficits in processing complex information, deficits in maintaining steady focus of attention, inability to distinguish between relevant and irrelevant stimuli, and difficulty in forming consistent abstractions, all of which can be a challenge to the nurse trying to teach these patients. Nursing education and skill training interventions must be used to help compensate for these cognitive deficits. When helping these patients to learn to process complex activities, such as preparing a meal, or shopping for food or clothes, nurse should break the activity into a series of small component or steps and list them for the patient' s reference. In addition, teaching and explaining should be done in an environment where distractions are minimized. Terminology should be clear and unambiguous. Visual aids can supplement verbal information but these draw attention away from important content. Most important of all, teaching should occur when the patient is ready.

2. Self-monitoring and Relapse Prevention Many studies prove that patients can greatly benefit by learning techniques of self-regulation, symptom monitoring, and relapse prevention. Self-monitoring and relapse prevention include:

a. Teaching patient regarding diagnosis, treatment options.

b. Assist patient with medication management, to identify effective, acceptable treatment plan.

c. Teach identification and management of symptoms.

d. Teach relapse planning and prevention, and identify symptom triggers.

e. Assist with avoidance of substance abuse.

f. Teach and assist with preventing sensory overload and sensory isolation.

iii. Social Interventions

Patients with schizophrenia have many social problems such as violence, risk of self-injury, ineffective cope, ineffective communication and relationships with others, deficit in life skills, have difficulty to use and establish kinship support, access appropriate community resources. There are some social interventions as following.

1. Interventions to Avoid Violence and Risk of Self-injury When hallucinations or delusions may put patients at risk of harming themselves or others, the patient who is hallucinating needs to be protected. The protection may include staff monitoring and providing safer environment. The nurse's best approach to avoiding violence or aggression is to administer medications

1. 认知治疗与护理 由于精神分裂症患者存在多方面的认知损害，如对复杂信息的处理、保持稳定注意力、区分相关的和不相关的刺激、形成一致的抽象思维等方面，因此对精神分裂症患者的心理治疗与护理对护士来说更具有挑战性。护士通过对患者进行教育指导、技能训练来帮助患者减轻或修正认知方面的损害。当训练患者学习处理复杂的活动时（如准备一餐，采购食品或衣物），护士应将这些活动分解，指导患者一步一步进行。另外，患者学习和训练的环境应尽量少被打扰，避免患者分心。护士的指导应清楚、不含糊。一些图像等辅助手段可对语言的教育起到促进作用，但应注意将患者的注意力引到重要的内容上。特别应注意要在患者做好充分的准备时，才开始对其进行教育指导。

2. 自我监护和预防复发 许多研究证明自我监护和预防复发技能的训练对精神分裂症患者的康复非常有利。自我监护和预防复发的训练包括：① 指导患者学习有关疾病的诊断、治疗等相关知识；② 帮助患者学习药物的管理，制订有效的可接受的治疗计划；③ 指导患者认识和处理精神症状；④ 指导患者学习预防复发的技术，识别疾病复发的先兆症状；⑤ 帮助患者避免精神活性物质滥用；⑥ 指导和帮助患者避免知觉超载或知觉隔绝。

（三）社会文化方面的护理干预

精神分裂症患者有较多的社会问题，如暴力危险、自伤的危险、无效应对、无效沟通和与他人建立关系困难、生活技能缺失、获取资源困难等。其社会干预措施如下：

1. 提供及时危机干预、避免暴力发生 当幻觉或妄想使患者处于危险状态（如命令性幻听、被害妄想、罪恶妄想等）时，应提供及时的危机干预，避免出现暴力危险和自杀自伤等危险。对严重幻听的患者可采用适当的保护，如专人监护、提供安全环境。同

as ordered, to assess and monitor for signs of fear and agitation, to demonstrate respect for the patient and the patient's personality, and to use preventive interventions before the patient loses control. In addition, reducing environmental stimulation is particularly important for individuals who are experiencing hallucinations.

时，保证患者按照医嘱进行治疗，观察患者恐惧、害怕、激动等情绪表现，尊重患者及其人格，并尽量减少环境的刺激。

2. Procedures for Violent Behavior If the patient loses control and is a danger to self or others, restraint and seclusion may be necessary. Staff should be trained in the proper use of seclusion and restraint.

2. 积极控制患者暴力行为 如果患者失去控制，使自己或他人处于危险状态，可采取保护和限制性措施，如身体保护、药物镇静、限制活动范围等。

3. Patient and Family Education Because a diagnosis of schizophrenia is a life-changing event not only for patients but also for the family and friends who must care and support them, educating patients and their families is crucial. Family's help and support are crucial to help patients maintain treatment. Education should include information about the disease course, importance of treatment regiments, support systems, and life management skills. Be attention to:

a. Facilitate effective communication and relationships with significant others including family.

b. Encourage and assist with developing life-skills, such as management of hygiene, health care, nutrition, sleep/rest patterns, exercise.

c. Assist to establish kinship support, to integrate into the community, and access appropriate community resources.

3. 患者及其家庭的健康教育 首次诊断为精神分裂症，对患者及家庭是一个重大的应激事件，所以，对患者及其家庭的健康教育尤为重要。家庭对患者的照顾和支持对患者能否坚持治疗起着至关重要的作用。针对患者和家庭的教育包括疾病病程、治疗管理的重要性、支持系统和生活管理技能等，同时应注意：① 鼓励患者与家人和朋友进行有效的沟通交流，建立友好关系；② 鼓励和帮助患者发展生活技能，如个人卫生的管理、卫生保健、营养－饮食的管理、睡眠/休息和运动的管理等；③ 协助建立亲属之间的支持关系和利用社会资源。

IV. Nursing Intervention for Three Types of Behaviors

四、针对特殊行为的护理

i. Nursing Care of the Patient with Altered Thought Process

The altered thought process is the most common problem in clients with schizophrenia. The main manifestation of patients is cognitive impairment. The factors that the altered thought process may be clients can not analyze, comprehensively deal with internal and external stimuli, the boundaries between themselves and others, self and environment, biological factors (neurological physiology, genetics, brain structure, etc.), perceived changes, and psychosocial stress. The altered thought process mainly manifests as unrealistic thinking, strange ideas, disengagement from reality, implicated ideas, thoughts being broadcast, thinking insertion, etc. Clients can't correctly accept and interpret information, and their abilities to judge, understand, and solve problems are impaired.

（一）思维过程改变患者的护理

思维过程改变是精神分裂症患者最常见的问题，患者主要表现为认知障碍。思维过程的改变与患者不能分析、综合处理内外刺激，患者自我与他人、自我与环境之间的界限混乱，生物因素（神经生理、遗传、脑结构等）、感知改变，以及心理社会压力等因素有关。其主要表现为非现实的思维、奇怪的想法、脱离现实、牵连观念、思维被广播、思维插入等，患者不能正确接受和解释信息，判断力、理解力、解决问题的能力受损。

1. Nursing Objective The problem of altered

1. 护理目标 应根据患者的具体情况

thought process is related to inability to trust, anxiety, possible hereditary or biochemical factors. Patients with thought disorders experience delusion, magical thinking, loose associations, ideas of reference, thought broadcasting, thought insertion, thought withdrawal, and impaired judgment, comprehension, perception, and problem-solving abilities.

制订相应的护理目标，下列护理目标可作参考：① 对妄想、幻觉和其他认知障碍的痛苦减轻；② 言语和行为上表现出接近现实的思维；③ 符合其年龄的抽象、推理和综合能力；④ 能够识别自我、他人和环境的界线；⑤ 符合其生长发育的自知、判断、应对技巧、解决问题的能力。

2. Nursing care of the patient with altered thought process includes following interventions.

2. 思维过程改变患者的护理措施

(1) Initiate a nurse-patient relationship by demonstrating an acceptance of patient as a worthwhile human being through the use of nonjudgmental statements and behavior.

（1）与患者建立信任性治疗关系。护士通过接受患者是一个有价值的人、尊重患者、对患者的行为不指责、不嘲笑等方法与患者建立信任关系。

(2) The nurse should accept the patients as a worthwhile individual without passing judgment. A person's self-image will improve when others see him as a worthwhile person. The nurse should be sensitive to the patient's feelings and should understand his needs for his fantasy world. When the patient realizes that he is accepted, he will find it easier to give up his autistic existence.

（2）接受患者是一个有价值的人，因为当个人被其他人所承认和尊重时，能够提高个人的自我认识。护士应该注重患者的各种感受，理解患者的需要。当患者明白自己被接受时，就容易走出自闭的圈子。

(3) The nurse should be consistent. The autistic patient is often frightened and bewildered. He needs to realize that the staff is not frightened by his behavior and that they can be counted on for help.

（3）安排相对固定的护士护理患者，保持护理的一致性。因为孤僻、自闭的患者容易被惊吓，感到不安全、迷惑等。患者需要一个了解自己，并且可信赖的护士来实施护理。

(4) The nurse should assist patient in differentiating between his own thoughts and reality. Validate the presence of hallucinations. Identify them as a part of the disorder and explain that they are present because of the metabolic changes that are occurring in his brain. Focus on reality-oriented aspects of the communication.

（4）护士应协助患者区别自己的想法和现实之间的差异，认识妄想是精神障碍的症状之一，是大脑功能障碍的表现。因此，护士在与患者的沟通中应重点强调现实，改善患者的现实感。

(5) The nurse should convey acceptance of patient's need for the false belief, but that you do not share the belief. Patient must understand that you do not view the idea as real.

（5）护士应该向患者传递患者错误的信念自己能理解，但不能赞同和分享这种错误的信念。

(6) The nurse should not argue or deny the belief. Use "reasonable doubt" as a therapeutic technique: "I find that hard to believe." Arguing or denying the belief serves no useful purpose, as delusional ideas are not eliminated by this approach, and the development of a trusting relationship may be impeded. If patient is highly suspicious, the following interventions may help:

（6）护士不要与患者争论或否认患者的信念，可使用某些治疗技巧，“合理地怀疑”患者的这些信念，如“我发现很难相信”。因为争论或否认患者的信念不仅不能消除患者的这些想法，反而会破坏护士与患者的信任关系。如果面对一个对别人有高度怀疑的患者，可采取下列干预措施：

1) To promote trust: use same staff as much as possible; be honest and keep all promises.

1）促进信任：① 尽可能安排固定的护士照顾患者，与患者真诚相待；② 遵守与患者的承诺。

2) To prevent the patient from feeling threatened: avoid physical contact; avoid laughing, whispering, or talking quietly where patient can see but cannot hear what is being said; provide canned food with opener or serve food family style; avoid competitive; use assertive, matter-of-fact, yet friendly approach.

2）防止患者感到威胁：① 避免与患者有身体的接触；② 避免在患者能够看见但听不见的地方嘻笑、耳语，使患者产生怀疑；③ 提供自助餐方式；④ 避免竞争；⑤ 使用肯定的、事实的、友好的方式与患者交流。

(7) The nurse should provide supervision so that the patient will not injure himself or others. The patient may experience "visions" or "voices" directing him to cause harm to himself or to other patients or staff. Patient needs the security of knowing that the nursing staff will not allow him to carry through with these dangerous impulses. A firm, directive, but gentle approach is best with the patient.

（7）护士应加强安全监护，避免患者发生自伤或伤人行为。患者可能诉说有声音命令他做一些伤害自己或他人的危险行为，因此，护士应了解患者是否存在命令性幻听，对患者的影响有多大，并指导患者当这些声音出现时，应寻求护士的帮助。

(8) The nurse should teach the patient techniques that will help stop the hallucinations. The interventions such as tell the voices to "go away"; have the patient sing, whistle, or play a musical instrument over the voices; have the patient seek another person in the environment for conversation; have the patient tell a staff member when the voices are bothersome; have the patient engage in an activity, exercise, or project when the voices begin.

（8）护士应指导患者学习终止幻觉的技巧，如当患者出现幻觉时，让患者唱歌、吹口哨或玩乐器等，使这些声音超过幻听；对声音说"走开"；在环境中寻找其他人进行交谈；让患者专注于一项活动，如锻炼、绘画等。

(9) The nurse should praise the patient's efforts to use learned techniques to distract from or manage hallucinations. Positive feedback will increase self-esteem and promotes repetition of successful behavior strategies.

（9）护士应该及时称赞患者对终止幻觉所做出的努力，因为正性的反馈能够提高患者的自信和自尊，并巩固和强化患者的正性行为。

(10) The nurse should teach the patient and family about the therapeutic effects of medications and the important role medications play in reducing psychotic symptoms. Discuss with patient and family the adverse effects of medication and how to manage them in accordance with the patient's treatment plan.

（10）护士应该向患者及家属进行有关药物治疗的知识教育，包括药物治疗的重要性，讨论家庭如何帮助患者管理和指导患者用药，保证治疗计划的实施。

(11) The nurse should increase social interaction for the patient gradually. As with the patient who is suspicious, this person also needs his activities to be increased in a gradual, non-threatening way. The nurse should provide group situations in which the patient can learn and practice activities of daily living, communication skills, social skills, and begin to improve interpersonal relatedness and independence.

（11）护士应该逐渐增加患者的社交活动，如面对一个对别人高度怀疑的患者，应在自愿、无威胁、安全的情况下逐渐增加人际交往。用团体活动可帮助患者学习人际交往技能，并学会相互谦让。患者也需要学习日常生活的自理、与人交流、建立关系、促进独立等方法及技能。

ii. Nursing Care of the Patient with Sensory/Perceptual Alterations

（二）感知觉改变患者的护理

The patient with sensory/perceptual alteration experiences a change in the amount or patterning of incoming stimuli accompanied by a diminished, exaggerated, distorted, or impaired response to such stimuli. The problem of sensory/perceptual alteration may be related to panic anxiety, extreme loneliness, and withdrawal into the self.

精神分裂症患者感知觉的改变主要表现为对客观刺激反应的程度及方式的改变，如刺激的反应减弱、反应增强、反应扭曲。感知觉的改变可能与严重的焦虑、极端寂寞和自我封闭有关。

1. The goal of nursing interventions is the patients will be able to define and test reality, eliminating the occurrence of hallucinations. When the patients feel anxious or when hallucinations begin, they may seek help of staff, refrains from harming self and others, and utilizes learned techniques for managing stress and anxiety.

2. There are some interventions of caring for sensory/perceptual alteration patients:

(1) The nurse should continue to observe patient's signs of hallucinations (listening pose, laughing or talking to self, stopping in midsentence). If the nurse can find the previous signs of hallucinations, the early intervention may prevent aggressive response to command hallucinations.

(2) The nurse should establish a therapeutic relationship with patients. The patient first trusts the nurse before being able to talk about hallucinations and other sensory/perceptual alterations.

(3) The nurse should avoid touching the patient without warning, because the patient may perceive touch as threatening and may respond in an aggressive manner.

(4) The nurse should use clear, concrete statement, and direct verbal communication with patients. Unclear directions or instructions may be confusing to patient and promote distorted perceptions or misinterpretation of reality.

(5) The nurse should refrain from judgmental or flippant comments about hallucinations, to avoid decreasing self-esteem of the patient. In addition, an attitude of acceptance will encourage the patient to share the content of the hallucination with nurse. It is important to prevent possible injury to the patient or others from command hallucinations.

(6) The nurse should not reinforce the hallucination. Use "the voices" instead of words like "they" that imply validation. Let patient know that nurse do not share the perception. Say, "even though I realize the voices are real to you, I do not hear any voices". Patient must accept the perception as unreal before hallucinations can be eliminated. The nurse should state her reality about the patient's hallucinatory experience using therapeutic response, such as "I don't hear the voices you describe, I know you hear voices, but with time they may go away". Nurses do not deny the existence of the patient's experience.

(7) The nurse should help patient understand the connection between anxiety and hallucinations. If patient

1. 患者将能够：① 认识和体验现实，消除幻觉的出现；② 当感到焦虑或当幻觉出现时，寻求医护人员的帮助，克制不要伤害自己或其他人；③ 运用所学的技巧应对压力和焦虑。

2. 感知觉改变患者的护理措施：

（1）仔细观察患者的幻觉症状，及时发现幻觉的一些先兆表现，如倾听的姿势、独自发笑或自言自语、突然终止谈话等，并及时进行早期干预，避免患者因命令性幻听而产生攻击性行为。

（2）与患者建立治疗性护患关系，使患者能够信赖护士，并愿意将自己的感受告知护士。

（3）护士应避免在患者不知晓的情况下接触患者，因为患者可能对这种突然的接触感到危险而产生攻击性行为。

（4）护士在与患者交谈时，应注意使用清楚、具体的陈述，避免患者产生误会和加重患者对现实的曲解。

（5）护士应注意克制，不要轻率批评患者的幻觉或向患者说明幻觉的不真实性，因为对患者幻觉的批评，可能伤害其自尊。另外，护士接受患者幻觉的态度，会鼓励患者与护士分享其幻觉的内容，从而可以预防患者因幻觉伤害自己或他人。

（6）护士应注意不要强化患者的幻觉，如患者说“他们在议论我”，护士可用“声音”代替“他们”，避免“他们”这样用词暗示和确认了患者的幻觉。应让患者意识到护士不认同其知觉，可这样说：“虽然我明白这声音对你来说是真实的，但是我确实未听见”。在患者幻觉未消除之前，护士应让患者明白其感受是不真实的，但不要否认患者的感受。如对患者说：“我确实未听见你所描述的声音，我知道你听见了这些声音，但是，这些声音过一会儿将会消失”。

（7）护士应帮助患者了解焦虑和幻觉之间的关系。如果患者能学习阻断焦虑的某些技

can learn to interrupt escalating anxiety, hallucinations may be prevented. In the same time, the nurse should modify the environment to decrease situations that provoke anxiety.

巧，就可能避免幻觉，并应注意减少环境中的刺激，避免患者焦虑增加。

(8) The nurse should try to distract the patient from the hallucination, because involvement in interpersonal activities and explanation of the actual situation may help bring the patient back to reality.

（8）护士应尽量转移患者对幻觉的注意力，因为在现实的情形下，人与人之间的活动可将患者从幻觉带回到现实。

(9) The nurse should explore the content of auditory hallucinations to determine the possibility of harm to self, others, or the environment (auditory command hallucinations) to prevent destructive behavior. When danger or violence is imminent, protect the patient and others by following facility procedures and policies for seclusion or chemical or mechanical restraint to prevent harm or injury to patient or others. When it is determined that the patient is not harmful to self or others, nurse may say "You look sad, Ms. Luo. You say the voices you hear keep telling you bad things about yourself. The staff is here to help you get relief from the voices."

（9）护士应清楚患者幻觉的内容、出现的频率、对患者或他人的影响程度等。当幻觉（命令性幻听）可能导致患者对自己或他人或环境有伤害时，应采取积极的干预措施，如适当隔离、药物或身体保护等控制患者的行为，避免危险行为的发生，以保证患者及他人的安全。如护士对某明显幻听的患者说："罗小姐，你看起来很忧愁，你说你听到有声音一直在说你的坏话，我们可帮助你减轻这些声音。"

(10) The nurse should teach the patient techniques that will help stop the hallucinations. Following techniques that nurse can use: have the patient sing, whistle, or play a musical instrument over the voices; tell the voices to "go away"; have the patient seek another person in the environment for conversation; have the patient engage in an activity, exercise, or project when the voices begin.

（10）护士应指导患者学习终止幻觉的技巧。如当患者出现幻觉时，让患者唱歌、吹口哨或玩乐器等，使这些声音超过幻听；对声音说"走开"；在环境中寻找其他人进行交谈；让患者专注于一个活动，如锻炼、绘画等。

(11) The nurse should praise the patient's efforts to use learned techniques to distract from or manage hallucinations.

（11）当患者努力学习和应用终止幻听的技巧时，应及时给予鼓励和表扬。

(12) The nurse should provide environmental opportunities to expand the patient's social network (start with one-to-one, add group activities when appropriate and the patient is able to tolerate them); provide a consistent, structured milieu that will promote trust, safety, and a sense of well-being for disorganized patient; provide group situations in which the patient can learn and practice activities of daily living, communication skills, social skills, and begin to improve interpersonal relatedness and independence.

（12）护士应该提供环境和机会，让患者学习人际交往技巧，扩大患者的社会网络，可从一对一的活动开始，当患者能够耐受后，逐步让患者参加一些团体活动。另外，提供一致的、安全的环境，可促进患者对护士的信任，并激励患者学习和应用应对幻听的技巧。提供集体活动让患者学习和练习日常生活技巧、沟通技巧、社会功能等，改良患者的人际关系和促进患者的独立。

iii. Nursing Care of the Withdrawn Patient

（三）退缩患者的护理

Some schizophrenic patients have negativistic behavior; they withdraw from their environment. Typical behaviors of withdraw patients are shy, aloof, lonely, apathetic, isolated, inadequate, inappropriate, autistic, and often very resistant to any form of suggestion from the environment. They are unable to invest emotional energy outside of themselves. Each person responds to stress

部分精神分裂症患者主要表现为抗拒性行为，他们表现孤僻、退缩、胆怯、与周围环境疏远、缺乏感情或情感平淡、冷漠等，对外界刺激选择退缩、回避、提防。

in different ways, many schizophrenic patients choose to withdraw from their environment because the world around them is too threatening.

1. In setting goals for this patient, the nurse must assess what is behind the withdraw behavior. Usually, the patient is so afraid of others and himself that he withdraws. Therefore, the nurse's long-term goal would be to increase the patient's self-esteem and help him to feel secure with other people. As a short-term goal, the aim would be establishing a therapeutic rapport with the patient in a one-to-one relationship.

1. **护理目标** 为患者设定恰当的护理目标，护士须认真评估患者阴性症状后面隐藏的因素。患者一般因害怕他人和自己，所以选择退缩。因此，长期护理目标是提高患者的自尊，帮助患者与他人建立关系。短期目标是帮助患者与护士建立一对一的治疗性关系。

2. Nursing interventions of the withdraw patient include:

2. **护理措施**

(1) Assess the extent of the patient's withdrawn behaviors and the related factors of withdraw behaviors, to plan strategies to break the pattern of withdrawal with interactions and activities.

（1）仔细评估患者的退缩行为和相关因素，制订护理计划阻断患者退缩的行为方式。

(2) Assess the patient to meet basic needs during times of withdrawal behavior (sleep, nutrition, personal hygiene) to promote the patient's physical health and well-being.

（2）仔细评估患者在退缩行为下的基本需要，如睡眠、营养、个人卫生等，满足患者的基本需要，促进患者的身体健康和自我照顾能力。

(3) Structure each day to include planned times for brief interactions and activities with the patient to help the patient organize times to engage with others and to let the patient know participation is expected and that he or she is worthwhile member of the community.

（3）制订患者每日生活安排表，包括日常生活、交往活动等时间安排。帮助患者组织和安排好日常活动，鼓励患者参与集体活动，让患者感受到自己是集体中的一员，大家都很欢迎和需要他。

(4) At the first time, the nurse should limit the environment for the patient. There is security in sameness, and so this patient does best on a small unit. Until the patient has had an opportunity to feel comfortable with the environment and himself, the nurse may take off the unit to occupational therapy or other activities.

（4）在患者第一次参加集体活动时，护士应考虑范围不要太大，避免使患者感到不安全，直到患者在小的团体活动中能够耐受和感到安全、舒适时，可让患者参加一些大的团体活动，如职业治疗或其他活动。

(5) The nurse should recognize that the patient tends to isolate himself from other patients and from the staff. In order for a patient to achieve psychological homeostasis, he must have interactions with other human beings. Thus, nurse's responsibility is to seek the patient out frequently. But the patient usually has had many painful experiences with people and so has found it easier to reject others than to risk being rejected, the nurse must adopt a nonjudgmental, accepting manner with this patient. It is important to understand that even if the patient gives no acknowledgment of the nurse's presence for a long period of time, consistent reaching out by the nurse will have an effect on the patient. The following is an example:

（5）护士应认识患者有独处和回避护士或其他人的趋向。为了帮助患者获得独处和交往的心理平衡，护士应鼓励和督促患者参加集体活动。但是，多数患者曾经有过失败的人际交往经验，对外界和他人有抵触和回避，护士应理解和接受患者，与患者一起共同制订目标，并向目标不断努力。即使短期很难看到目标的实现，护士也应坚持不懈地、反复地督促患者参加集体活动。下面是一个护生对一个回避患者的护理案例：

NURSE: Hello, Mr. Wang, I'm Xiaolin, a nursing student.

护生："你好，王先生，我叫小林，是护理系的学生"。

PATIENT: (No response).

患者：（没有回应）。

NURSE: I thought I'd sit with you awhile and we could talk.

护生:“我想坐在这和您谈一会儿话，好吗？”

PATIENT: I have nothing to say (Gets up and walks away).

患者:“我没有什么好谈的”，并起身走开。

In this case the student stalled the therapeutic process by requiring the patient to talk. If she only said, "I thought I'd sit with you for a while," the patient might not have felt threatened by her presence and might have been able to stay sitting with her.

从此案例中，我们可看出，护生过于着急与患者交谈，反而使患者感到紧张而离开。如果她只说，“我想在您旁边坐一会儿，好吗？”患者就可能不会感到有很严重的危险可能忍受护士在其身边坐下。对严重回避的患者，护士应有耐心，逐步引导患者。

(6) When with the autistic patient, the nurse should take note of how long the patient can tolerate her presence. She should be certain that the patient does not associate her with unpleasant feelings. Gradually, the time of visits can be lengthened and the patient may feel secure and can invest any energy beyond him in another individual or group.

（6）对于自闭的患者，护士应该注意患者能够忍耐护士出现在其身边多久。当护士确定患者对她的出现和拜访没有反感或不感到紧张害怕后，逐渐延长拜访患者的时间，并鼓励患者在护士的陪同下参加集体活动。

(7) The nurse should spend brief intervals with the patient each day, and engage in meaningful, nonchallenging interactions, to ease the patient out into the community by first developing trust, rapport, and respect. Also, the nurse should stimulate patient's interest in an activity or recreation and should try to find activities that patient will be able to succeed at, so as to increase patient's feeling of self-worth.

（7）护士应每天花一段时间去拜访患者，护士热情、诚恳和无威胁地与患者的互动有利于促使患者参加户外活动。在护士与患者的交往过程中，发展信任性关系，尊重患者非常重要。同时，护士应注意刺激和激励患者的兴趣，可选择一些患者喜欢的活动，以提高患者的自信和自尊。

(8) The nurse should initiate conversation that is reality-oriented and concrete, conversation in which the patient can participate, such as the weather, sports events, favorite activities, or hobbies, a magazine-any topic that is nonthreatening. The nurse should accept that initially the conversation may be very one-sided and limited.

（8）护士与患者交谈的主题应以对患者不构成威胁和挑战的话题做切入口，如运动、天气、爱好、习惯等。

(9) When the patient is provided positive experience, he will begin to feel better about himself and will have more energy to invest in his surrounding environment. When the patient begins to socialize more on the unit, the activities he is involved in should be gradually increased. The patient can be encouraged to attend occupational therapy and other activities. As the patient beings to feel good about his success, he will feel good about himself.

（9）当患者从与他人交往中获得正性的体验时，患者对自己有一种好的感受，更愿意融入到周围的环境中。此时，护士应逐渐增加患者的活动，可让患者参加职业训练或其他人较多的集体活动。

(10) The nurse should identify the patient's significant support persons and encourage them to seek out the patient for interactions, phone conversation, activities, and visits. A strong network of supportive individuals will increase the patient's social contacts, enhance social skills, promote self-esteem, and facilitate positive relationships.

（10）护士应帮助患者认识其社会支持系统，鼓励患者与他人沟通、交往。如让患者主动给朋友打电话、邀请朋友、拜访朋友等。因为社会支持系统可帮助患者与社会联系，提高社会技能、自尊，促进正性的人际关系。

(11) When the patient appears attempts to seek out others for interactions and activities and respond to

（11）当患者与他人交往取得进步时，护士应及时给予正性的反馈和鼓励。

others' attempts to engage the patient in interactions and activities, the nurse should praise the patient immediately.

iv. Interventions for Patient in the Community

Many of the acute interventions used for patients in the hospital are also helpful to those in the community. In the case of schizophrenia, nursing interventions are the keys in managing patients with long-term symptoms or those that are unresponsive to treatment. Despite adequate treatment and several medication trials, some patient will continue to suffer from positive and negative symptoms. Coping with ongoing symptoms is debilitating. The major role of the nurse in the community is to encourage patients to obtain and continue treatment while simultaneously assisting them to maintain structure and functional ability in their lives. Patients in the community usually require weekly home visit, supervised living arrangements such as halfway houses. Community nursing interventions can help patient rehabilitation. The key nursing interventions of community as following:

1. Assist with the Activities of Daily Living Assist patients with activities such as paying bills, buying groceries, and making meals. Ensure that patient gets physical, dental, and gynecological examinations and meets other health needs.

2. Watch for Signs of Relapse Continually monitor and assess the patient for signs of relapse. Prodromal symptoms may indicate a pending relapse. Stress the need for ongoing psychiatric care, including supportive psychotherapy and pharmacotherapy. Ensure opportunities for early intervention to prevent or lessen the severity of relapse. Daily structure and medication monitoring can help prevent acute exacerbation of the illness and prevent hospitalization.

3. Encourage Socialization Positive symptoms may be seen more often in early stages of the illness, whereas negative symptoms predominate in the long term. Motivating these patients is extremely challenging and requires a solid basis of trust and persistence. Help them develop social roles and social support network. Encourage patients' participation in client-based drop-in centers or self-help groups to promote social stimulation. Help patients to receive vocational training or return to a work environment adapted to their current level of functioning if possible.

4. Promote Communication Refer to group therapy. Groups may promote interpersonal connection, improve social skills, and diminish social withdrawal. It may also be an important educational tool in long-term management of symptoms. The mutual teaching

（四）社区精神分裂症患者的护理

许多针对住院患者的干预措施，同样适用于社区患者。社区精神分裂症患者的护理干预重点在于对患者长期存在的症状的管理和对患者治疗反应的观察与处理。护士的角色是鼓励患者坚持治疗，帮助患者维持和促进其社会功能。护士通常定期进行家庭访视，检查患者生活情况、药物治疗情况等，并为患者制订康复计划等。下列是一些具体的社区护理措施：

1. 评估患者日常生活情况 指导患者制订家庭经济计划，如家庭日常开销、购物、医疗支出等。

2. 持续观察患者的症状 留意有无复发迹象，重视精神障碍患者的持续照顾，包括支持性的心理护理、药物维持治疗，早期及时的干预可预防和避免疾病的复发，减少患者住院的次数。

3. 鼓励社会化 精神分裂症的阳性症状多在疾病的初期和急性期比较明显，然而，阴性症状一般长期存在。要求护士必须与患者形成牢固的信任基础，要有耐心和恒心。应帮助患者发展社会角色功能、社会支持系统，鼓励患者参加一些集体活动，如患者联谊活动、患者自助活动和社区康复活动等。帮助患者获得一些职业训练的机会和重新获得工作，提高患者的社会适应能力和社会功能，促进患者回归社会。

4. 促进沟通 提供集体治疗、团体活动等机会，促进患者与他人的联系，提高患者的社交能力，减轻患者的回避和退缩行为。

and learning among nurses and patients enhance their self-esteem and ability to communicate openly about auditory hallucinations. Participants achieve high levels of engagement and try new ways to manage symptoms and communicate with others.

5. Understand the Impact of Their Loss These patients and their family frequently face significant losses, including loss of future dreams of college, career, intimate relationships, and parenting. Financial loss is common, and the individual may need to receive long-term assistance.

6. Patient and Family Education Educate both patients and families about the diagnosis of major psychotic disorder, possible side effects of medication, positive and negative symptoms, resulting behaviors, possible causes, effective treatment, course, and prognosis.

When acute symptoms are controlled or moderated, the nurse should begin patient education. During this period, it is easier for the patient to learn about the disorder, medications, and symptoms management. Learning about and management of their illness can give patient a sense of control often absent during the acute stages of illness.

Family is the key to ensure that patient receives and maintains treatment. Some researchers offer helpful guidelines for assisting families to cope with the ill family member. The useful guidelines include clarify roles, work together, encourage input, expect intense feeling, use local support, recognize different beliefs, acknowledge family strengths, and recognize limitations.

5. 理解疾病给患者及其家庭带来的损失 如失去上大学的梦想、失去事业、失去亲密关系和父母养育等损失，有的患者可能导致长期的无能为力和需要别人的帮助。

6. 患者及其家庭的教育 是社区护理中重要的内容之一。它包括有关疾病的临床表现，诊断治疗，药物副作用的观察处理，疾病的进程、相关因素及预后。

当急性期主要症状被控制或缓解后，护士就应该开始对患者进行健康教育。通过学习有关疾病知识可帮助患者学会管理症状、遵从治疗，使患者获得控制症状的感受。家庭是保证患者能够获得并维持治疗的重要支持。有研究发现，对患者家庭成员提供帮助和指导对促进患者康复非常有益。对其家庭成员的指导包括帮助家庭成员澄清角色、协同努力、有效地利用社区资源，认识不同的信念，认识家庭的优势和不足。

BOX 6-3 Learning More

New Definition of Recovery

Recovery refers to the process in which people are able to live, work, learn, and participate fully in their communities. For some individuals, recovery is the ability to live a fulfilling and productive life despite a disability. For others, recovery implies the reduction or complete remission of symptoms. Science has shown that having hope plays an integral role in an individual's recovery. Definition of recovered as following:

1. Having a social life;
2. Holding a job;
3. Being symptom free;
4. Not taking medication.

(Li Xiaolin)

BOX 6-3 前沿知识

康复的新定义

康复是指患者有能力去生活、工作、学习和完全参与到社区活动的一种过程。对一些人来说，康复是指虽然带着疾病但仍然能去获得充实和丰富的人生。对另一些人来说，康复意味着减少或者消除症状。科学表明拥有希望在个人的康复中扮演了重要的角色。最新的康复定义如下：

1. 拥有社交生活；
2. 拥有工作；
3. 不受症状的完全约束；
4. 不吃药。

（李小麟）

Key Points

1. Of all mental illnesses, schizophrenia undoubtedly results in the greatest amount of personal, emotional, and social costs. It presents an enormous threat to life and happiness, yet it remains a puzzle to the medical community. In fact, for many years there was a little agreement as to a definition of the concept of schizophrenia.

2. The initial symptoms of schizophrenia most often occur in early adulthood, and development of the disorder can be viewed in four phases: the schizoid personality, the prodromal phase, the active phase, and residual phase.

3. The cause of schizophrenia remains unclear. Research continues, and many contemporary psychiatrists are giving more credence to the biologic theories and placing less emphasis on psychosocial influences. Integration of these theories support the idea that no single factor can be implicated in the etiology, but that the disease most likely results from a combination of influences including genetics, biochemical dysfunction, and physiological or environmental factors.

4. Various types of schizophrenic and related psychotic disorders have been identified. They are differentiated by their total picture of clinical symptomatology. They include simple schizophrenia, catatonic schizophrenia, paranoid schizophrenia, disorganized schizophrenia, undifferentiated schizophrenia.

5. Care of the patient with schizophrenia was presented in the context of the five steps of the nursing process which include nursing assessment, nursing diagnoses, nursing care plan and evaluation of patient.

6. There are various treatments for schizophrenia, including cognitive-behavior therapy, group therapy, family-oriented therapy, social skill training and illness self-management, environmental supports, cognitive rehabilitation and vocational rehabilitation

内容摘要

1. 精神分裂症可造成个人严重的认知、情绪、社会功能的损害，严重影响患者生活质量。事实上，有关精神分裂症的概念多年来一直有争议，是医学界的一个难题。

2. 精神分裂症常见于青壮年，有四个发展阶段：人格期、前驱期、活跃期和残留期。

3. 精神分裂症的病因未完全清楚，有关病因的研究仍在继续。有多种理论阐述了精神分裂症的有关因素，所有的理论都支持没有一种因素能够单独解释精神分裂症的起因。精神分裂症可能与多种因素有关，包括生物化学、遗传、心理社会因素等。

4. 精神分裂症根据其临床特点分为五类，包括单纯型精神分裂症、紧张型精神分裂症、偏执型精神分裂症、青春型精神分裂症、未定型精神分裂症。

5. 精神分裂症护理主要按照护理程序对不同类型精神分裂症患者提供整体的护理，包括护理评估、护理诊断、制订护理计划及预后评估。

6. 精神分裂症的治疗包括药物治疗、心理治疗和康复治疗、行为治疗、社会技能培训、家庭治疗等。

Exercises

(Questions 1 to 4 share the same question stem)

A patient, male, an unemployed 20 year-old, has suffered a gradual loss of attention over the past 5 years. He did not go to school after school weariness, and stayed at home all the time. He also did not want to go out. He lived a lazy and passive life style, and he did not brush his teeth or wash his face voluntarily, he only showers once every one or two months. He did not have a clear plan about his future.

1. What do you consider as the first diagnosis for this case?
2. What intervention should the nurses take first, if the

思考题

（1～4 题共用题干）

男性，20 岁，无业，近 5 年来逐渐出现注意力不集中，先厌学后不去上学，一直待在家里，不出门，不愿见人，生活懒散被动，不主动刷牙洗脸，1～2 个月不洗澡，对将来没有明确打算。

1. 针对该案例首先考虑的诊断是什么？
2. 患者入院后拒绝接受治疗，护士首先采取

patient refuses to accept treatments after he is admitted to hospital?

3. What should the nurses do to assess the patient's cognitive function?

4. Which aspect of rehabilitation exercises should be enhanced during the rehabilitation nursing?

(Questions 5 to 7 share the same question stem)

A patient, female, a 30-year-old company staff, has been ill for six months. After she was criticized by her boss, she had gradually become sensitive and suspicious. She thought that her boss was in the gang and wanted to harm her. She also thought that the people around her could know her thoughts. She was scared and afraid to go to work and she was suffering from insomnia.She had also reported her case to the police.

5. Ziprasidone was prescribed by the doctor. How could the patient take this medication accurately to achieve the best absorption for Ziprasidone?

6. Which is the most important nursing invention in the care for the patient's symptoms after she has been admitted to the hospital?

7. What does nurses provide to care for the safety of the patient?

(Questions 8 to 9 share the same question stem)

A patient, surname is Li, who is a 25-year-old female. Two months ago, after answering a congratulatory phone call about his birthday, she suddenly had an eerie feeling, and thought her classmate wanted to kill her. After which she suffer from insomnia and felt nervous and terrified. After this incident, she also felt that her colleagues had started to talk about her behind her back. She could hear the voice of a man which commanded and threatened her. She also felt that some people had monitored her phone. Recently her symptoms have progressed. She had stopped working and prefers staying in the room alone, and she also became angry every time the phone rang. She was in constant denial of her illness and refused therapy. Because of the difficulty of caring for her, so she was sent to hospital by her family.

8. Please put forward 4 main nursing diagnoses and related factors.

9. Please put forward the corresponding psychological nursing interventions.

的护理措施是什么？

3. 针对该患者的认知功能评估，应包括哪些方面？

4. 患者在治疗阶段的康复护理中，护士应该加强哪方面的训练？

（5～7题共用题干）

女性，30岁，公司职员，患病半年，主要原因是受老板批评后，渐出现敏感多疑，认为公司老板是黑社会的，要整自己害自己，认为自己的想法周围人能知道，恐惧害怕，不敢上班，找公安局报案，伴有失眠等。

5. 医嘱采用齐拉西酮治疗，请问该患者如何正确服用药物吸收效果更好？

6. 患者入院后护士在症状护理中，最重要的措施是什么？

7. 对该患者提供的安全护理是什么？

（8～9题共用题干）

患者，李某，女，25岁，2月前接一高中同学电话祝贺生日电话时，突然感觉不对头，认为对方要杀自己，夜里失眠，恐惧紧张。之后感觉周围同事议论自己，并在耳边能听到一个男人的声音，命令、威胁自己，并怀疑有人通过电话监控自己。近来病情加重，不上班，一个人关在房间里，听到电话铃声就生气，不承认有病，拒绝就诊。因治疗护理困难，由家人送入院治疗。

8. 请提出4个主要的护理诊断与相关因素。

9. 请提出相应的入院心理护理措施。

Chapter 7 Nursing Management for Clients with Mood Disorders

第七章 心境障碍患者的护理

Learning Objectives

Memorization

1. Describe concepts of mood disorder, mania and depression.
2. Sum up main points of the clinical characteristics of mania and depression.

Comprehension

1. Identify the risk factors of mood disorder
2. Describe the treatment of mania and depression

Application

1. Apply the nursing process to the care of a suicidal client.
2. Apply the nursing process to the care of clients with mania and depression.

学习目标

识记

1. 能准确描述心境障碍、躁狂症和抑郁症的概念。
2. 能正确概述躁狂症和抑郁症的临床表现。

理解

1. 能识别心境障碍危险因素。
2. 能具体说明心境障碍患者躁狂发作和抑郁发作的治疗。

运用

1. 能运用恰当的护理措施对自杀患者实施护理。
2. 能运用恰当的护理措施对躁狂发作和抑郁发作患者实施护理。

Lin Nan, male, 51-year-old, graduated from secondary vocational school, is admitted to hospital due to the alternative episodes between a depressed mood and a manic mood for about 5 years, an extremely depressive episode for about one month and one attempted suicide. Since January 2009, he was in a bad mood, loss of interest in daily work and life, feeling depressed, lonely and helpless, always said "I would just die", but never take any action, no he was not up to work. Lin Nan had poor appetite, always woke up early, he has been to a local hospital and asked for help with sleep problems. He was given medication (no details) and his sleep got a little improvement, but his mood and appetite were still in bad condition. He went to the local psychiatric hospital, got a diagnosis of depression disorder and the prescription "amitriptyline 150 mg/day, per os". After one month, the disease significantly alleviated.

Please think about the following questions based on the case:

1. What are the symptoms of the client in this case?
2. What might be the potential nursing diagnoses for Lin Nan? What might be the effective nursing interventions?

患者林楠，男，51岁，中专文化。因“反复情绪低落与情感高涨交替发作5年余，情绪低落加重一月并自杀未遂一次”入院治疗。患者始于2009年1月无明显诱因出现心情不好、对日常工作和生活丧失兴趣，感沮丧、孤独无助，觉得活着没有死了好，总说“死了算了”，但从未采取过行动，无法胜任工作。食欲缺乏，早醒，曾主动到当地医院求诊，要求解决睡眠问题，诊断不详，予以药物治疗（具体不详），睡眠虽略有改善，但情绪和食欲未恢复。至当地精神病院就诊，诊断为抑郁障碍，口服阿米替林150 mg/d，治疗一月后，病情明显缓解。

请思考：

1. 此病例中患者存在哪些精神症状？
2. 患者的主要护理诊断是什么？应采取哪些护理措施？

Mood is a persistent or predominant emotional state that colors the perception of the world and how one function in it. Variations or fluctuations in mood are a natural part of life. While mood swings is normal when people facing the pressure, it is abnormal when too intense or too weak emotional responses and inconsistency between the duration period and the intensity of outside environmental stimulus occur. If the abnormal emotion gets to such a degree that it influences the social and physiological function, then it develops into mood disorder. The World Health Organization (WHO) has ranked depression first in a list of the most urgent health problems worldwide in the 21st century. However, most clients with mood disorders remain hidden—not treated or talked about, especially in the early stage, which causes unnecessarily social burden, economic and individual costs. WHO works with health-care leaders to create options for managing and treating depression. Every country should have programs in place to help people with mood disorder. This chapter will introduce the concepts, epidemiology, etiology and treatment of mood disorder, and also the detailed nursing process of manic episode and depressive episode.

心境是一种持久或占主导地位的情绪状态，能显著地影响人们对自我和环境的感知与评价。作为对各种因素的反应，情绪的变化每天都会发生。人们面临压力时出现情绪波动是正常的情绪反应，情感反应过于强烈或过于平淡，持续的时间与外界环境刺激的强度不相符合，就是心理不健康的表现；情感异常如果达到一定程度，并影响了日常社会功能和生理功能，可成为心境障碍。WHO预计21世纪全球排在首位的公众健康问题是抑郁。目前大多数心境障碍的患者未能得到早期发现和早期治疗，从而造成不必要的社会负担、经济和个人损失。WHO已经与健康照护领导者创立了管理和治疗抑郁的方法。每个国家也应该有自己的项目来支持和帮助心境障碍的患者。本章将系统介绍心境障碍的概念、流行病学特点、病因与发病机制及治疗，同时根据护理程序重点介绍心境障碍中常见的躁狂发作和抑郁发作的护理。

Section 1 Introduction

I. Concepts

Mood disorders, which is known as affective disorders, is a group of conditions where pervasive alteration in the person's mood is the main underlying feature. Clinically, clients usually present elation or depression of mood, commonly associated with cognitive and behavioral changes. In severe cases, psychotic symptoms, such as hallucinations and delusions, may be observed. The disorders have a tendency to recur, but most recurrent episodes will eventually relieve without obvious personality changes.

II. Epidemiology

Depression is a significant contributor to the global burden of disease, and it affects people in all communities across the world. Nowadays, depression is estimated to affect 350 million people. The WHO World Mental Health Survey conducted in 17 countries including Africa (Nigeria; South Africa); the Americas (Colombia; Mexico; United States), Asia and the Pacific (Japan; New Zealand; Beijing and Shanghai in the Peoples Republic of China), Europe (Belgium; France; Germany; Italy; the Netherlands; Spain; Ukraine); and the Middle East (Israel; Lebanon) found that on average about 1 in 20 people reported having an episode of depression in the previous year. However, only 11.0% (China) to 62.1% (Belgium) of severe cases received any care in the prior year. The reported prevalence of mood disorders differs from country to country because of differences in the diagnostic criteria, investigation method, social-cultural background and conventional custom. Lifetime prevalence rates range from approximately 3 percent in Japan to 16.9 percent in the United States, with most countries falling somewhere between 8 to 12 percent. Suicide risk is high in mood disorder. Approximately one-third of clients with bipolar disorder report a lifetime history of suicide attempt. The lifetime risk of suicide in individuals with bipolar disorder is estimated to be at least 15 times that of the general population. In fact, bipolar disorder may account for one-quarter of all completed suicides.

第一节　概　述

一、概　念

心境障碍，又称情感性精神障碍，是以显著而持久地情感或心境改变为主要特征的一组疾病。临床上主要表现为情感高涨或低落，伴有相应的认知和行为改变，严重时可出现精神病症状，如幻觉、妄想。大多数患者有反复发作倾向，每次发作多可缓解，不遗留明显的人格改变。

二、流行病学

抑郁症是造成全球疾病负担重要因素，影响世界各地人们的健康。目前，世界范围的抑郁症患者大概有3.5亿人。WHO在非洲、美洲、亚洲及太平洋地区、欧洲和中东地区的17个国家进行的一项世界精神心理调查发现，平均每20人中就有1人在过去的一年中有抑郁发作。该调查还指出，在过去一年中，仅有11.0%（中国）到62.1%（比利时）的严重抑郁病例接受过医疗服务。由于诊断标准和调查方法的不同，社会文化背景、风俗习惯的差异，国内外心境障碍的流行病学报道结果差异悬殊。抑郁症的终生患病率大约在3%（日本）到16.9%（美国），多数国家在8%～12%。心境障碍患者的自杀率很高，约1/3双相障碍患者会有自杀企图。双相障碍患者的终生自杀风险至少是普通人群的15倍左右。实际上，双相障碍可以解释所有自杀行为的四分之一。

Section 2 Etiology

第二节　病因及发病机制

The etiology of mood disorders remains unclear. Current research shows that mood disorders may relate to genetic, neurochemical and psychosocial factors.

心境障碍的病因尚不清楚，现有研究发现可能的发病机制涉及遗传因素、神经生化因素和心理社会等因素等。

I. Biological Theories

一、生物因素

i. Genetic Theories

The mood disorders have a strong heritability. The rate of mood disorders may be as much as 5 to 10 times higher for people who have a relative with bipolar disorder than the rates found in the general population. Genetic factors may influence individual responses to events that trigger depression.

ii. Neurochemical Theories

Neurochemical influences of neurotransmitters (chemical messengers) focus on alterations of biogenic amines implicated in mood disorders, including serotonin, norepinephrine, and dopamine.

1. 5-hydroxytryptamine (5-HT) Hypotheses A decreased level of 5-hydroxytryptamine has been linked to depressed mood, appetite loss, insomnia, disturbance of circadian rhythm, endocrine dysfunction, sexual dysfunction, anxiety, reducted activities and ect in depression clients.

2. Norepinephrine Hypothesis Level of catecholamine norepinephrine at nerve center in the client with depression decreases obviously. Level of catecholamine norepinephrine at nerve center in the clients with mania are higher compared to the normal control.

3. Dopamine Hypotheses Level of dopamine in the brain of the clients with depression decreases, while client with mania increases.

iii. Neuroendocrine Influences

Hormonal fluctuations are being studied in relation to depression. Mood disturbances have been documented in people with endocrine disorders such as those of the thyroid, adrenal, parathyroid, and pituitary glands. Depression is associated with dysfunction of the adrenal cortex and is commonly observed in both Addison's disease and Cushing's syndrome. Other endocrine conditions that may result in symptoms of depression include hypoparathyroidism, hyperparathyroidism, hypothyroidism, and hyperthyroidism. Also, an imbalance of the hormones estrogen and progesterone has been

（一）遗传因素

心境障碍有较强的遗传性。心境障碍患者的一级亲属的患病率约是普通人群患病率的 5～10 倍。遗传因素可能影响了个体对诱发抑郁事件的反应。

（二）神经生化改变

神经递质（化学信使）的神经化学影响主要是与心境障碍有关的生物胺水平的变化，包括 5- 羟色胺，去甲肾上腺素和多巴胺。

1. 5- 羟色胺假说　5- 羟色胺功能降低与抑郁症患者的抑郁心境、食欲减退、失眠、昼夜节律紊乱、内分泌功能紊乱、性功能障碍、焦虑不安、不能对付应激、活动减少等密切相关。

2. 去甲肾上腺素假说　临床研究发现抑郁症患者中枢去甲肾上腺素明显降低；躁狂症患者中枢去甲肾上腺素水平比对照组增高，其增高与躁狂程度相关。

3. 多巴胺假说　研究发现抑郁症脑内多巴胺功能降低，躁狂症多巴胺功能增高。

（三）神经内分泌研究

激素的波动与抑郁症有关。在一些甲状腺、肾上腺、甲状旁腺、垂体等内分泌器官障碍的患者中可以观察到情绪波动。抑郁与肾上腺皮质功能低下有关，可见于艾迪生病和库欣综合征。其他内分泌疾病如甲状旁腺功能减退、甲状旁腺功能亢进、甲状腺功能减退和甲状腺功能亢进等也可能引发抑郁。雌激素和黄体酮分泌失衡可诱发经前期焦虑。

implicated in the predisposition to premenstrual dysphoric disorder.

II. Psychosocial Theories

Negative life events can induce mood disorder, especially depression. It is reported that, the occurrence of depression in person who undergoes great life events within 6 months, is 6 times more than that in general people, and occurrence of suicide is 7 times more than that in general persons. 37% of adolescents from divorced family can suffer from depression.

二、心理社会因素

负性生活事件对心境障碍的发病起着“扳机”的作用，特别是首次发作的抑郁症较为明显。据报道在最近六个月内有重大生活事件发生者，其抑郁发作的危险率增高6倍，自杀率增高7倍。离婚家庭中的儿童和青少年中37%可能患抑郁症。

Section 3 Clinical Manifestation of Mood Disorders

第三节 心境障碍患者的临床特点

The *CCMD-3* classified mood disorders into several subtypes, including manic episode, depressive episode, bipolar disorder, and persistent mood disorder, etc. However, in *DSM-5* (APA, 2013) bipolar and related disorders are separated from the depressive disorders and both are placed as the one-level classification. Box 7-1 shows the DSM-5 diagnostic criteria of major depression disorder. *ICD-10* still has the classification of manic episode. In this chapter, we will follow the classification criteria of *ICD-10* and *CCMD-3* and introduce the clinical manifestation of manic episode, depressive episode and bipolar disorder.

*CCMD-3*中将心境障碍分为几种亚型，包括躁狂发作、抑郁发作、双相障碍和持续性心境障碍等。然而，*DSM-5* (APA, 2013) 中把双相障碍及其相关障碍从抑郁症中分离出来，使得双相障碍和抑郁障碍各自独立为一级分类，提高了它们在分类中的地位，Box 7−1 列出了抑郁障碍的诊断标准。*ICD-10*中也保留单相躁狂发作的分型。本书遵循*ICD-10*和*CCMD-3*的分类原则，介绍躁狂发作、抑郁发作和双相障碍的临床特征。

BOX 7-1 Learning More

Criteria for Major Depressive Disorder

Five or more of the following symptoms during the same two week period representing a change from normal; at least one of the symptoms is either (1) depressed mood or (2) loss of pleasure.

1. Depressed mood;
2. Markedly diminished interest or pleasure in all, or almost all, activities;
3. Significant weight loss (a change of 5% or more in a month);
4. Insomnia or hypersomnia;
5. Psychomotor agitation or retardation;
6. Fatigue or loss of energy;

BOX 7−1 知识拓展

抑郁障碍的诊断标准

在同一个2周内出现5个或以上下列症状并且表现为既往功能改变；其中至少一项症状为（1）情绪低落或（2）愉快感下降。

1. 情绪低落；
2. 明显的对全部或几乎全部活动失去兴趣；
3. 显著的体重下降（一月内体重改变超过5%或更多）；
4. 失眠或嗜睡；
5. 精神运动性兴奋或迟滞；
6. 疲劳或无精打采；

7. Feelings of worthlessness or excessive or inappropriate guilt;
8. Diminished ability to think or concentrate, or indecisiveness;
9. Recurrent thoughts of death, recurrent suicidal ideation without a specific plan, or a suicide attempt or a special plan for committing suicide.

7. 无价值感，过度或不恰当的自责；

8. 思维、注意力或决策力下降；
9. 反复出现的自杀念头，反复出现的没有具体计划的自杀观念，自杀企图或明确的自杀计划。

I. Manic Episode

The typical clinical manifestation of manic episode includes elevated mood, thought racing, and increased activities. Typically, this period lasts about 1 week.

i. Elevated Mood

Manic episodes are characterized by a predominantly elevated, expansive or irritable mood that presents as a prominent or persistent part of the illness. People experiencing a manic state may laugh, joke, and talk in a continuous stream, with uninhibited familiarity. They often demonstrate boundless enthusiasm, treat others with confidential friendliness, and incorporate everyone into their plans and activities. Some clients experience unstable mood, only have the predominant presentation of irritability. The irritability and belligerence may be short-lived and change quickly to joy.

ii. Thought Racing

Thought racing is a characteristic clinical signs of manic clients. Someone experiencing idea flight shows a nearly continuous flow of accelerated speech with abrupt changes from topic to topic that are usually based on understandable associations or plays on words. Speech is rapid, verbose, and circumstantial. When the condition is severe, speech may be disorganized and incoherent. Clients can be overly self-confident and become preoccupied with political, personal, religious, and sexual themes. They may exhibit an inappropriate increase in self-esteem and open grandiosity. Their judgment is impaired significantly, resulting in buying sprees, sexual indiscretions, and unwise business investments. The clients are easily distracted.

iii. Increased Activities

Manic clients classically have abundant resources of energy and engage in multiple activities and ventures. At baseline and between episodes, the manic client may indeed function at a high level of productivity, particularly

一、躁狂发作

躁狂发作的基本临床表现是心境高涨，思维奔逸和精神运动性兴奋，即典型的“三高”症状。如果上述症状一次发作的持续时间在一周以上，称为躁狂发作（或称躁狂症）。

（一）心境高涨

心境高涨是躁狂发作的必备症状，是一种强烈而持久的喜悦与兴奋。患者整天显得喜气洋洋，兴高采烈，讲话时眉飞色舞，表情生动。精力充沛，热情洋溢，具有一定的感染力，往往能引起周围人的共鸣。也有一部分患者表现情绪不稳定，以易激惹为主，稍有不如意便大发雷霆，常以敌意或暴怒来对待别人的干涉和反对，但转瞬即逝，患者很快转怒为喜。

（二）思维奔逸

思维奔逸是躁狂发作的特征性症状。患者思维联想非常迅速，涉及范围广，引经据典，高谈阔论，口若悬河，滔滔不绝，声音提高。新的概念不断涌现，常常可以从一个概念迅速联系到其他概念，形成“意念飘忽”。言语跟不上思维活动的速度。甚至可出现音联（音韵相联）和意联（词意相联）。有些患者由于联想过程过快，谈话的内容往往显得肤浅和表面化，给人以信口开河之感。患者常表现出不恰当的自尊增强且更加自大。患者常常被环境的变化所吸引而转移话题（随境转移）。

（三）精神运动性兴奋

患者精力显得异常旺盛，兴趣范围扩大，投入到很多活动中，整天忙忙碌碌。在基线水平或发作间歇期，躁狂患者可能有较高水

in areas requiring creative talent. However, as the investment in these activities becomes excessive, the client losses the capacity to behave with reasonable caution and judgment, and conforms to social expectations and norms. Clients are social, outgoing, and talkative and can be difficult to interrupt. They know no strangers, and energy and self-confidence seem boundless. They may present to an emergency room setting dressed in colorful, flamboyant, and inappropriate clothing. In severe episode, they may be aggressive. Some may have a characteristics of excitement, grandiosity, emotional lability, psychosis and insomnia characteristic of mania, altered consciousness.

平的工作效率，特别是在需要创造性人才的领域。但是，当投入活动过多，患者会丧失合理谨慎的判断力以及遵守社会期望和规范的能力。有的患者表现爱交际，健谈，很难被打断。能与陌生人一见如故，精力充沛，自信满满。他们可能会穿着色彩鲜艳、艳丽和不合适的衣服出现在急诊室里。病情较重者，可出现攻击性和破坏性行为。当躁狂发作严重时，患者呈重度兴奋状态，行为活动明显紊乱，无目的性和指向性，易产生暴力行为，甚至还可出现时间、地点定向障碍，意识障碍，错觉，幻觉及思维不连贯等症状。

iv. Psychotic Symptoms

Some clients may have hallucination, especially auditory hallucination. The content of hallucination mainly describes the clients' special abilities and rights, which is corresponding with the clients' emotion.

（四）精神病性症状

部分患者可能出现幻觉，多见于幻听，内容大多是称赞自己的才能和权利的，与其情绪相符合。

v. Somatic Symptoms

Clients have few uncomfortable somatic symptoms. They usually present flushing, fiery eyes, increasing heart rate, increasing appetite and increased libido. But they can become thin because of overactivity.

（五）躯体症状

患者较少表现不舒适的躯体症状。可有交感神经功能兴奋症状，表现面色红润，双目有神，瞳孔轻度扩大，心率增快，食欲、性欲增强，睡眠减少。另外，患者因体力过度消耗，多有体重减轻。

II. Special Clinical Manic Situation

二、特殊的躁狂状态

i. Hypomania

Hypomania is defined as that the mood elevation is of a milder nature, either in severity or in duration, and is unassociated with a marked impairment in function and psychotic symptoms such as delusion and hallucination. The clients do not need in-patient care. The main manifestations include more talkative than usual or pressure to keep talking, flight of ideas or subjective experience that thoughts are racing, inflated self-esteem or grandiosity, increase in goal-directed activity (either socially, at work or school, or sexually) or psychomotor agitation, increased libido, decreased need for sleep. Clients may notice the changes.

（一）轻躁狂

轻躁狂是躁狂发作较轻，社会功能无损害或轻度受损，不伴妄想、幻觉的状态。患者无需住院治疗。主要表现为言语活动增多，思维奔逸，情感高涨，高度自信且自我感觉良好，社交能力增加，对人过分热情。性欲增强，睡眠需要减少。有些患者知道心情有改变，但认为这种改变是正常现象。

ii. Delirious Mania

Delirious mania is the most serious kind of mania. The clients may have conscious disturbance and severe psychomotor excitement. The clients may have disorientation of time and place. The obvious disturbance of behavior without any aim and the inclination of violent behavior may be present in some clients. Some psychotic

（二）谵妄型躁狂

谵妄型躁狂为病情严重的躁狂发作，伴有明显的意识障碍和严重的精神运动性兴奋。患者出现时间、地点定向障碍，行为明显紊乱而毫无目的，易产生暴力冲动行为，出现错觉、幻觉、思维不连贯。有的患者甚至出现躯体消耗性衰竭。此时的症状往往失去了

symptoms, such as illusion, hallucination and incoherence of thought, can be observed. The severe clients appear somatic exhaustion and can be easily misdiagnosed as schizophrenia.

情感的色彩，给人以分裂的印象，容易误诊为精神分裂症。

III. Depressive Episode

Depressive episode typically involves 2 or more weeks of a sad mood, slow thought or lack of interest in life activities with at least four other symptoms of depression such as anhedonia and changes in weight, sleep, energy, concentration, decision making, self-esteem, and goals.

三、抑郁发作

抑郁发作的典型临床症状是情绪低落、思维迟缓和意志活动减退，可为单次发作，也可为反复发作。如果抑郁症状一次发作持续存在2周以上即为抑郁发作。它可伴有下述症状四种或以上：快感缺失及体重、睡眠、精力、注意力、决策、自尊和目标性的改变。

i. Depressed Mood

Depressed mood is the basic characteristic symptom. The client usually describes himself or herself as feeling sad, low, empty, hopeless, gloomy, or down in dumps. The quality of mood is likely to be portrayed as different from a normal sense of sadness or grief. Clients make self-deprecating remarks, criticizing themselves harshly and tend to ruminate, which is repeatedly going over the same thoughts focusing only on failures or negative attributes. Many depressed clients state that they are unable to cry, whereas others report frequent weeping spells that occur without significant precipitants. A small percentage of clients do not report a depressed mood, usually refer to as masked depression. An inability to enjoy usual activities is almost universal among depressed clients. The client or his or her family may report markedly diminished interests in all, or almost all, activities previously enjoyed such as sex, hobbies, and daily routines.

（一）情绪低落

情绪低落是必备的症状。患者的情感基调是低沉灰暗的，可以表现为忧心忡忡、闷闷不乐、无精打采、愁眉苦脸、唉声叹气，且此种低落的情绪不为喜乐的环境而改变。患者自我评价很低，总是过分自责，并且有反刍思维，即反复思考失败的和不愉快的事情。对孩子、挚友失去热情，漠然置之。患者自诉“高兴不起来，活着没意思”。有时患者也会察觉到自己与别人不同，因而尽力掩饰伪装，称之为“微笑性抑郁”。有些患者在情感低落的基础上伴有焦虑，表情紧张、恐惧，坐立不安，搓手顿足、来回踱步等症状。

ii. Thoughts Retardation

About one half of depressed clients complain of or exhibit a slowing of thought. They may feel that they are not able to think as well as before, that they cannot concentrate, or that they are easily distracted. Frequently they will doubt their ability to make good judgments and find themselves unable to make even small decisions.

（二）思维迟缓

患者联想速度缓慢，约有一半的患者觉得自己思想困难、反应迟钝、思路闭塞，常称“脑子好像是生锈了”“脑子不灵了，什么都想不起来了”，患者感到脑子不够用、不能用。临床表现为主动言语减少、语速减慢、回答问题拖延很久、难以出口，患者常常会怀疑自己做出正确判断的能力，甚至发现自己无法做出哪怕是很小的决定。

iii. Decreased Activities

Clients may have obvious and persistent decrease of activities. Depressed clients may develop a slowing, or retardation, of the normal level of activity. They may exhibit slowness in thinking, speaking, or body movement or a decrease in volume or content of speech, with long pauses before answering. In about 75% of depressed

（三）意志活动减退

患者少有甚至是缺乏意志活动，呈显著、持久、普遍的抑制。临床表现为行为缓慢，反应迟钝，生活被动、疏懒，不想动，不愿做事，也不愿和周围人接触交往，在集体活动中常独处一隅。约有75%的女性患者，50%

women or 50% of depressed men, anxiety is expressed in the form of psychomotor agitation, with pacing, an inability to sit still and hand-wringing. Some serious clients may present no care of personal health and have no speaking, no activities and no eating, which can be called inhibited stupor. But after careful examination, the clients' expression and posture are consistent with the internal emotional experience and depressive mood can also be observed.

的男性患者会出现焦虑症状，可有坐立不安、手指抓握、搓手顿足或踱来踱去等症状。严重时连个人卫生都不料理，蓬头垢面、不修边幅；甚至发展为不语、不动、不食，可达木僵状态。此种“抑郁性木僵”状态，经仔细地精神检查，可发现患者仍会流露痛苦、悲观的情绪。

iv. Somatic Symptoms

The clients with depressive episode usually have some somatic symptoms, including poor appetite, weight loss, constipation, decreased libido, impotence; menoschesis, etc. Somatic symptoms can involve every organ. The disturbance in automatic nerve system is also common. About 80% of depressed clients complain of some type of sleep disturbance, the most common being insomnia. Insomnia is a group of syndromes including problems in falling asleep, problems of staying asleep with frequent awakenings throughout the night, early morning awakening. The most common and unpleasant form of sleep disturbance in depressive clients is awakenings in the early morning associated with significant worsening of depressive symptoms in the first part of the day. In contrast, insomnia of problems in falling asleep is especially common in those with significant comorbid anxiety. Some clients complain of hypersomnia rather than insomnia; hypersomnia is common in atypical depression and seasonal mood disorder and is often associated with hyperphagia.

（四）躯体症状

情绪反应不仅表现在心境上，并且总是伴有机体的某些变化。躯体不适可涉及各个脏器，表现食欲下降、体重减轻、便秘，可有性欲减退，男性出现阳痿，女性有性感缺失和闭经。躯体症状可能涉及各个器官，自主神经系统紊乱也很常见。约 80% 的抑郁症患者抱怨自己有睡眠障碍。睡眠障碍则主要表现为早醒，一般比平时早醒 2～3 小时，醒后不能再入睡，这对抑郁发作具有特征性意义。有的患者表现为入睡困难，睡眠不深，夜间多次醒转；失眠在共病焦虑的患者中更加明显。少数患者表现为睡眠过多。嗜睡在非典型抑郁症和季节性情绪障碍中很常见，常与嗜睡症有关。

v. Suicide

Severe depressive clients experience recurrent thoughts of death, ranging from transient feeling that others would be better off without them, to the actual planning and implementing of suicide. Up to 15% of clients with severe depressive disorder are likely to die by suicide. The risk of suicide is present throughout a depressive episode but is probably highest immediately after initiation of treatment and during the 6-9 months period following symptomatic recovery.

（五）自杀观念和行为

严重的抑郁发作患者常反复出现自杀的观念或行为，自杀观念和行为是抑郁患者最危险的症状。重型抑郁障碍中可有 15% 的患者死于自杀。自杀的风险存在于整个重型抑郁发作的过程中，但在开始治疗的初期及症状消失后的 6～9 个月内危险性最高。

IV. Bipolar Disorder

Bipolar disorder is characterized by repeated episodes in which the client's mood and activity levels are in significant disturbance. The disturbance (at least 2 times) consists of at least one episode of any type of mania, and another episode of any type of depression. Client has mood shifts from serious depression to extreme euphoria (mania), with normal mood in the remission period. If the

四、双相障碍

双相障碍指反复（至少 2 次）出现心境和活动水平紊乱的发作，有时表现为情感高涨、活动增加等躁狂或轻躁狂症状；有时表现为心境低落、活动减少等抑郁症状，发作间期基本缓解。如果在目前疾病发作中，躁狂和抑郁症状同时存在，临床表现都很突出，

current episode is characterized by co-existence or rapid alternation of manic and depressive symptoms for at least 2 weeks, a diagnosis of Bipolar disorder, current episode mixed should be considered.

如情感高涨而运动减少，情感低落而思维奔逸，持续病期不短于 2 周，诊断为双相障碍混合发作。

V. Persistent Mood Disorder

五、持续性心境障碍

Persistent mood disorder describes recurrent elated and/or depressed mood, but the criteria of manic or depressive episode are not fulfilled, without or only mild impairment of social function. Usually an episode can persist for many years even the rest of whole life.

持续性心境障碍表现为反复发作的兴奋和 / 或抑郁情绪。每次发作极少严重到躁狂或抑郁的程度，且社会功能受损较轻。一般一次发作要持续数年，有时甚至占据一生中的大部分时间。

Section 4 Treatment

第四节 治 疗

I. Treatment Principles

一、治疗原则

Mood disorder cannot be cured currently. Various therapies can only relieve or modify the symptoms, reduce the complication and mortality, and promote the return of social function.

心境障碍目前还无法根治，但通过各种治疗可以减轻或缓解症状，减少并发症及病死率，逐渐恢复其社会功能。

i. Treatment Principles of Mania

Treatment for maina involves a lifetime regimen of medications. Other treatments include psychotherapy, and ECT (electroconvulsive therapy).

（一）躁狂发作的治疗原则

各类躁狂发作均以药物治疗为主，特殊情况下可选用无抽搐电痉挛治疗、心理治疗。

ii. Treatment Principles of Depression

Treatment for depression involves a lifetime regimen of medications. ECT is also a choice for severe depression. Psychotherapy is throughout all the other treatments.

（二）抑郁发作的治疗原则

各类抑郁发作均以药物治疗为主，特殊情况下可选用无抽搐电痉痉治疗，心理治疗贯穿其中。

II. Treatment of Mania

二、躁狂发作的治疗措施

i. Psychopharmacology

1. Lithium Lithium is the most common drug to treat manic clients especially lithium carbonate. There is a narrow margin between the therapeutic and toxic levels, and onset of lithium action is 7 to 14 days until the therapeutic level is reached around 0.6-1.2 mmol/L, and then monthly during maintenance therapy. Because lithium toxicity is a life-threatening condition, monitoring of lithium levels is critical. Lithium use during pregnancy is not recommended because it can lead to first-trimester

（一）药物治疗

1. 碳酸锂 是目前治疗躁狂发作的首选药，口服是唯一的给药途径。急性躁狂发作时治疗剂量，一般从小剂量开始给药，锂盐治疗一般在 7 ~ 14 天内显效，经治疗血锂浓度达到治疗浓度 0.6 ~ 1.2 mmol/L，并保持 2 ~ 4 周后，病情无改善，则应更换其他治疗。碳酸锂用于维持治疗，可以减低复发的风险。

developmental abnormalities.

维持治疗量为治疗剂量的一半，疗程至少1年。锂中毒会危及生命，使用时监测锂的水平是至关重要的。急慢性肾炎、肾功能不全、严重心血管疾病中枢神经系统器质性疾并急性感染、电解质紊乱、低盐饮食患者禁用。年老体弱、怀孕及哺乳期妇女、12岁以下儿童慎用。

2. Anticonvulsants Anticonvulsants such as carbamazepine and valproate can used in the treatment of mania and the prevention of manic episode, especially the clients who cannot tolerate the side effect of lithium carbonate or when lithium carbonate is ineffective.

2. 抗惊厥药 丙戊酸盐和卡马西平等适用于碳酸锂治疗无效或不能耐受碳酸锂治疗的患者。Freeman等的研究显示，在抑郁性症状存在、冲动性、高活动性和多次提早复发这些情况下，丙戊酸盐的治疗反应较锂盐好。Weisler的研究提示卡马西平在治疗躁狂急性发作时是有效的。

3. Antipsychotics Antipsychotics such as chlorpromazine, haloperidol and clozapine, can be effective for excitement, impulsive behavior, some psychotic symptoms including hallucination, delusion and weird behavior in manic episode. Antipsychotics take effect faster than lithium.

3. 抗精神病药 一般不单独使用，常与碳酸锂等合用。对严重兴奋、激惹、攻击或伴有精神病性症状的急性躁狂发作患者治疗早期可短期联用抗精神障碍药物。代表药物有氯丙嗪、氟哌啶醇、氯氮平、奥氮平等。

4. Manic episode has a tendency to recur. So it is important to prevent the recurrence. The dosage and duration of drugs to prevent the recurrence depend on the different situations, for example, whether the client is the first episode or relapse, or whether the client has psychotic symptoms.

4. 其他药物 如氯硝西泮、可乐定和维拉帕米等，用于药物治疗无效或效果不好的患者。与药物合用时，药物剂量不宜太大，尤其与锂盐合用时需防止意识障碍。急性症状控制后仍需抗躁狂药巩固维持疗效。

ii. Electroconvulsive Therapy (ECT)

Electroconvulsive therapy (ECT) is the induction of a random (generalized) seizure through the application of electrical current to the brain. ECT can be applicable for severe manic clients or manic clients who are irresponsive to lithium, which can be used singly or combined with medication. Clients usually take ECT every other day and a period of treatment includes 8 to 12 ECT.

（二）无抽搐电痉挛治疗

无抽搐电痉挛治疗对严重躁狂有一定治疗效果，其作用机制可能与药物作用相同，即纠正中枢神经递质的代谢异常。在有严密监护措施的情况下可单独应用或合并药物治疗。若合并药物治疗，应减少给药剂量。一般隔日一次，8～12次为一疗程。

iii. Psychotherapy

Psychotherapy is usually used combined with medication for manic clients, including psychodynamic therapy, cognitive behavioral therapy, ect.

（三）心理治疗

主要配合药物治疗使用，如心理动力学治疗、认知行为治疗等。

III. Treatment of Depression

三、抑郁发作的治疗措施

i. Psychopharmacology

There are many kinds of antidepressants. The doctor should be cautious to select the drug in clinic according to the most effective drugs in clients' history or the clinical

（一）药物治疗

抗抑郁药物品种繁多，临床选择用药应谨慎。可根据以往病史中最有效的治疗药物，

manifestation and the drugs' side effect, to see figure 7-1.

1. Tricyclic Antidepressants (TCAs) and Tetracyclic Antidepressants The tricyclic antidepressants (TCAs) have been the most widely prescribed drugs used to treat depression, which are also cheap. TCAs such as imipramine, clomipramine, amitriptyline and doxepin are used in the acute depressive episode or the maintenance therapy. For about 70%-80% of the clients, TACs are effective. The curative effect may not occur until 2-4 weeks after taking TCAs, associated with a few side effects. Maprotiline, which belongs to tetracyclic antidepressants, is similar to TCAs. It takes effect faster than TCAs, only 4-7 days after taking medicine, and has fewer side effects. But overdosage of TCAs and tetracyclic antidepressants can cause death, which is the most serious side effect.

2. Monoamine Oxidase Inhibitors (MAOI) Moclobemide is a new type of reversible and selective monoamine oxidase (MAO) A inhibitor, which can overcome the hypertensive crisis, toxicity to liver and orthostatic hypotension caused by other irreversible and non-selective MOAI. It is applicable for depressive clients who cannot be treated by TCAs, especially the depression with psychomotor inhibition. It is also effective to elderly

如无资料，可根据患者的典型症状及药物的副作用来选择（图7-1）。

1. 三环类及四环类抗抑郁药物 是抗抑郁的传统药，价格便宜。三环类如米帕明（丙咪嗪）、氯米帕明（氯丙咪嗪）、阿米替林及多塞平（多虑平）是临床上常用于治疗抑郁急性期和维持期患者，总有效率70%～80%，一般用药后2～4周起效，不良反应较多。马普替林为四环类抗抑郁药，作用与TCA相似，起效快，约4～7天，不良反应少。但三环类和四环类过量会致死是其最严重的副作用。

2. 单胺氧化酶抑制剂 吗氯贝胺是一种新型的可逆性、选择性单胺氧化酶A抑制剂，克服了非选择性、非可逆性MAOI的高血压危象、肝脏毒性及体位性低血压等不良反应的缺点，适用于三环类抗抑郁药物治疗无效的患者，对精神运动性迟滞的抑郁症尤其适用，

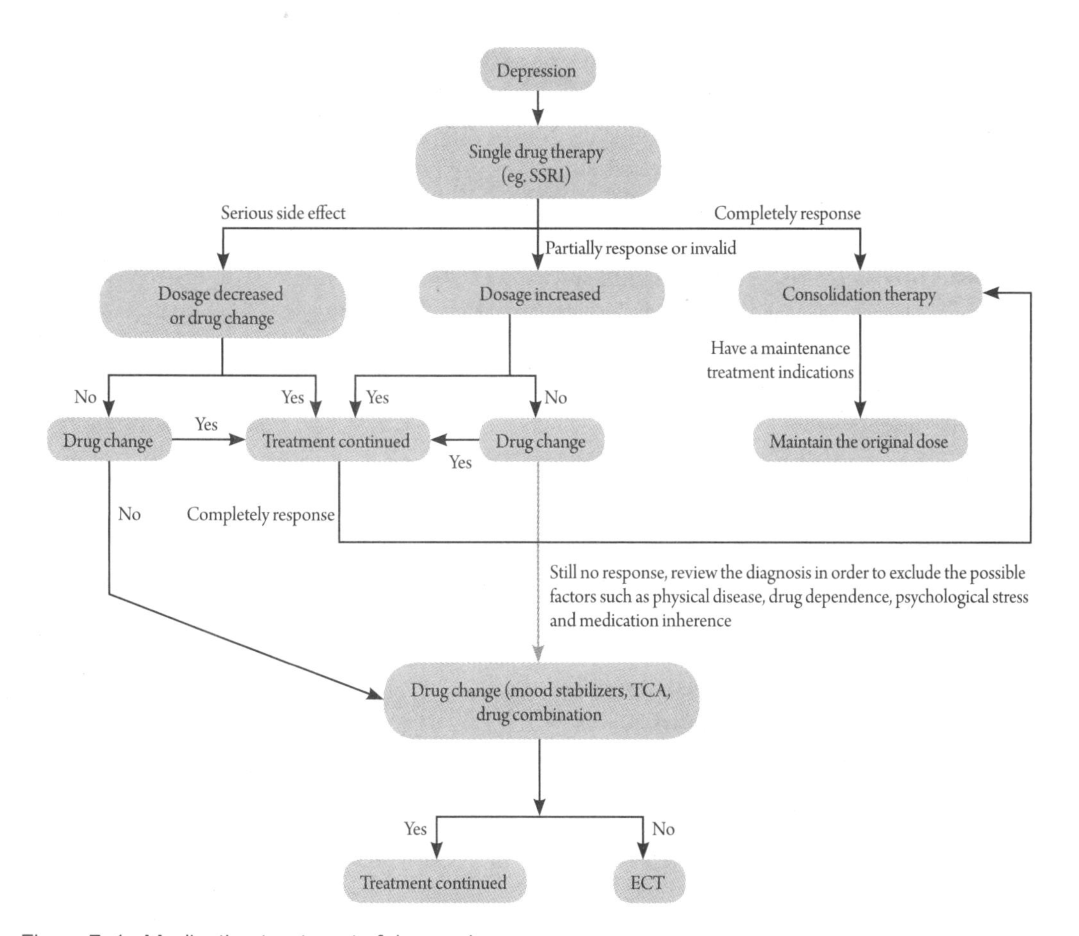

Figure 7-1 Medication treatment of depression

clients. Moclobemide can be absorbed completely after being taken orally and have mild side effects. Most clients can tolerate it.

也适用于老年人。口服后迅速完全地吸收，副作用较轻，患者的耐受性好。

3. Other Medicines　Selective serotonin reuptake inhibitors (SSRIs) including fluoxetine, paroxetine and sertraline are applicable for various depressive episodes, which have few side effects. Clients usually can tolerate them. The half-life of SSRIs is relatively long. Clients only need to take medicine once a day. So SSRIs can be easily accepted by the clients. In addition, anti-anxiety drugs and antipsychotics are effect to some depressive clients.

3. 其他药物　选择性5-羟色胺再摄取抑制剂，这类药物的品种主要有氟西汀、帕罗西汀、舍曲林等。它适用于治疗各种类型的抑郁症，副作用较小，一般均能耐受，清除半衰期较长，1天只需给药1次，易被患者接受。此外，抗焦虑药、抗精神病药等也可用于若干亚型患者。

4. Drug Treatment of Depressive Episode of Bipolar Disorder　Don't use antidepressant treatment alone. Mood stabilizers and atypical antipsychotics with mood stabilizing effect should be taken as the inevitable choice. Based on clinical practice, it is also need to be taken into consideration the mechanism of drugs, therapeutic basis, clinical symptoms to be resolved, the common adverse reactions and drug interactions when providing a combined medication.

4. 双相障碍抑郁发作的药物治疗　不主张单独使用抗抑郁药物治疗。心境稳定剂及具有心境稳定作用的非典型抗精神病药物应作为必然选择。联合用药时应在实践基础上考虑药物的作用机制、治疗学基础、需解决的临床目标症状、常见不良反应及药物间相互作用。

ii. Psychotherapy

Psychotherapy should be throughout the treatment. The goals of combined therapy are symptom remission, psychosocial restoration, prevention of relapse or recurrence, reduced secondary consequences. Commom psychotherapy includes interpersonal therapy, behavior therapy and cognitive therapy.

（二）心理治疗

贯穿于整个治疗过程，目的在于减少应激性生活事件，使患者消除不必要的顾虑和悲观情绪，主动配合治疗。常用的心理治疗方法有人际关系疗法、行为疗法和认知疗法等。

Interpersonal therapy focuses on difficulties in relationships, such as grief reactions, role disputes, and role transitions. For example, a person who, as a child, never learned how to make and trust a friend outside the family structure has difficulty establishing friendships as an adult. Interpersonal therapy helps the person to find ways to accomplish this developmental task.

人际关系疗法目的在于解决患者的人际关系问题，包括痛苦反应、角色冲突和角色转变等问题。如一个人儿童时期没有学会如何与家庭成员之外的人建立朋友关系，成人后与他人建立朋友关系就比较难。人际关系疗法可以帮助这类患者完成该发展任务。

Behavior therapy seeks to increase the frequency of the client's positively reinforcing interactions with the environment and to decrease negative interactions. It also may focus on improving social skills.

行为疗法指通过对个体反复训练，学习适应新的环境，达到矫正不良行为的目的。注重改善社交技能，认为是治疗重性抑郁者的有效方法。

Cognitive therapy focuses on how the person thinks about the self, others, and the future and interprets his or her experiences. This model focuses on the person's distorted thinking, which, in turn, influences feelings, behavior, and functional abilities.

认知疗法关注患者如何看待自我、看待自己的所作所为以及未来。治疗的目标就是转变患者的消极的认知，用更接近现实的解释替代消极的认知，使患者更好地面对现实，应对现实问题。

iii. Electroconvulsive Therapy

Psychiatrists may use Electroconvulsive therapy (ECT) to treat depression in select groups, such as clients

（三）无抽搐电痉挛治疗

患者对抗抑郁药不耐受或者副作用较强时选用无抽搐电痉挛治疗。此外，孕妇进行

who do not respond to antidepressants or those who experience intolerable side effects at therapeutic doses (particularly true for older adults). In addition, pregnant women can safely have ECT with no harm to the fetus. Clients who are actively suicidal may be given ECT if there is concern for their safety while waiting weeks for the full effects of antidepressant medication.

无抽搐电痉挛治疗不会对胎儿造成不良影响。对强烈自杀观念及使用药物治疗无效的抑郁症患者，电抽搐疗法亦有效。电抽搐治疗后仍需要药物维持治疗。

Section 5 Application of the Nursing Process

第五节 护理程序的应用

When caring the mood disorder clients, the nurse should assess the clients from physiology, psychology and social cultural aspects then make a detailed plan to assure the safety and meet clients' physiological need. Emergency measures should be taken in time when the clients have impulsive behavior and suicide ideas. Family members and available social support system should be taken into consideration when the clients are in the difficulty of receiving treatment.

心境障碍患者的护理，应按照护理程序的工作原理和思维方式，从护理评估入手，观察和系统分析患者的心理、生理、社会文化等多层面信息，制订详细的护理计划。当患者出现冲动、自杀企图等危险行为时，应及时采取应急措施，以保证患者的安全；当患者出现不能接受治疗的困境时，还应针对患者的家庭、生活环境、可利用的社会支持系统等情况进行周密策划，以保证患者治疗和康复的预期效果。

I. Mania

一、躁狂发作的护理程序

i. Nursing Assessment

1. Biological Assessment Biologic assessment involves with health history including history of personal growth, past history, lifestyle, special hobby, family history, history of allergies, ect. also the client's nutrition status, the presence of high appetite, increased libido, sleep disturbance including insomnia and hypersomnia.

2. Psychiatric Assessment Psychiatric assessment includes self-consciousness and treatment cooperation. Whether the clients have delusion of reference or delusion of persecution and impaired concentration. Whether the clients have agitation, excitement, elevated mood, grandiosity, and conceit. Whether the clients have overactivity, reckless or irresponsible behavior, and condemnation over others.

3. Psychosocial Assessment Psychosocial assessment includes personalities, life events, coping style, social function, and supporting system.

（一）护理评估

1. 生理状况的评估 健康史，包括个人成长发展史、既往史、生活方式、特殊嗜好、家族史、过敏史等；患者的营养状况，有无食欲旺盛、性欲亢进；睡眠情况，有无入睡困难、早醒、醒后难以入睡等。

2. 精神症状的评估 包括对疾病的自知力，治疗护理配合情况。有无意念飘忽、语速加快、意联等思维联想过程加快，以及有无自我评价过高、夸大观念、夸大关系、被害妄想等思维内容障碍。患者的情绪变化和行为举止，是否易激惹，有无冲动、攻击、破坏行为。

3. 心理社会状况的评估 包括患者的既往的性格特征、生活事件、患者应对挫折与压力调节的方式及效果、社会功能和可利用社会支持系统等情况。

Box 7-2 shows hypomania check list.

Box 7-2 列出了轻躁狂的临床评估方法。

BOX 7-2 Learning More

Hypomania Check List

Everyone experiences changes in mood at different times in their life. Please answer whether the following conditions exist?

1. I need less sleep.
2. I feel more energetic and more active.
3. I am more self-confident.
4. I enjoy my work more.
5. I am more sociable (make more phone calls, go out more).
6. I want to travel and/or do travel more.
7. I tend to drive faster or take more risks when driving.
8. I spend more money/too much money.
9. I take more risks in my daily life (in my work and/or other activities).
10. I am physically more active (sport etc.).
11. I plan more activities or projects.
12. I have more ideas, I am more creative.
13. I am less shy or inhibited.
14. I wear more colorful and more extravagant clothes/make-up.
15. I want to meet or actually do meet more people.
16. I am more interested in sex, and/or have increased sexual desire.
17. I am more flirtatious and/or am more sexually active.
18. I talk more.
19. I think faster.
20. I make more jokes or puns when I am talking.
21. I am more easily distracted.
22. I engage in lots of new things.
23. My thoughts jump from topic to topic.
24. I do things more quickly and/or more easily.
25. I am more impatient and/or get irritable more easily.
26. I can be exhausting or irritating or others.
27. I get into more quarrels.
28. My mood is higher, more optimistic.
29. I drink more coffee.
30. I smoke more cigarettes.

BOX 7-2 知识拓展

轻躁狂的临床评估

每个人在人生的不同时期会经历情绪的改变，请回答是否存在下列问题？

1. 我需要的睡眠时间比平时少。
2. 我感觉精力充沛或活动增多。
3. 我更加自信。
4. 我更加享受工作。
5. 我更加喜欢交往（打更多电话、外出更加频繁）。
6. 我喜欢旅行并且确实旅行得很多。
7. 我喜欢开快车或在驾驶中寻求刺激。
8. 我花钱比平时更多。
9. 我的日常生活更加地冒险。
10. 我的活动量会增多（如花较多时间体育活动）。
11. 我计划去做更多的活动或项目。
12. 我有很多想法，思如泉涌。
13. 我不腼腆也不前怕狼后怕虎。
14. 我穿着鲜艳，打扮时尚。
15. 我希望接触更多人或的确结识了很多人。
16. 我对性更加感兴趣或者性欲明显增加。
17. 我更喜欢找异性聊天。
18. 我更加健谈。
19. 我思维更加敏捷。
20. 我讲话时，经常讲笑话或开玩笑。
21. 我比较容易分心。
22. 我喜欢做新奇的事情。
23. 我的思维经常跳跃。
24. 我感到思维更加迅速或者思考问题更加容易。
25. 我更加没有耐心和/或更容易对别人发怒。
26. 我常常令他人疲惫不堪或恼怒。
27. 我经常与人争吵。
28. 我情绪激昂，更加乐观。
29. 我喝更多的茶或咖啡。
30. 我抽更多的烟。

31. I drink more alcohol.
32. I take more drugs (sedatives, anti-anxiety pills, stimulants).

31. 我喝更多的酒。
32. 我吃过诸如镇静剂，兴奋剂等之类的药物。

ii. Nursing Diagnosis

1. Risk for violence related to lack of normal social control, and delirium, illusion, agitation and provocation due to mental disorders.

2. Risk for injury related to overactivity, evidenced by increased agitation and grandiosity, and lack of self-control.

3. Sleep pattern disturbance related to persistent excitement and no sleep needs.

4. Altered nutrition: Less than body requirements related to overexcitement, overactivity, large wastage and reduced ingestion.

5. Self-care deficit: hygiene/clothing/feeding related to the symptom itself.

6. Personal identity disturbance related to the content of grandiose delusion.

7. Constipation related to irregular daily life, lack of water.

（二）护理诊断

1. **有对他人施行暴力的危险**　与易激惹、好挑剔、过分要求受阻有关。

2. **有受伤的危险**　与易激惹、活动过多有关。

3. **睡眠型态紊乱**　与精神运动性兴奋、精力旺盛有关。

4. **营养失调：低于机体需要量**　与兴奋消耗过多、进食无规律有关。

5. **自理缺陷：卫生/穿着/进食**　与躁狂兴奋、无暇料理自我有关。

6. **自我认同紊乱**　与夸大妄想的具体内容有关。

7. **便秘**　与生活起居无规律、饮水量不足有关。

iii. Nursing Care Plan

1. Outcome Identification

(1) The client will learn to control his or her elevated mood or anxiety so as not to injure self or others.

(2) The client can identify and analyze the pathological behavior and be responsible for consequences of his or her behavior, and will show disappear of elevated mood and racing thought.

(3) The client can fall asleep within 30 minutes and sleep for 6 to 8 hours without taking medicine that is the client's sleep is improved.

(4) The client will keep a balanced diet and good nutrition.

(5) The client can live a regular life and get self-care ability improved.

(6) The client will develop ego identity by time of discharge from treatment.

(7) The client can maintain passage of soft, formed stool at a frequency perceived as "normal".

2. Nursing Intervention

(1) Physiological nursing: (a) Providing quite and safe environment. The client should be in a quiet, simple-decorated ward with little stimulus. The sweet light and feint color in the ward can tranquilize the clients.

（三）护理计划及措施

1. 预期目标

（1）患者在住院期间能控制自己的情感，不因冲动攻击行为造成人与物的损害。

（2）患者对疾病有正确认识，情绪高涨、思维奔逸等症状得到基本控制。

（3）患者能在30分钟内入睡，每晚睡眠逐步达到8小时左右。

（4）患者过多的活动量减少，营养和水分摄入能满足机体需要。

（5）患者生活起居有规律，生活自理能力显著改善。

（6）患者能在治疗后形成自我认同。

（7）患者能以正常频率排成形软便。

2. 护理措施

（1）基础护理：①提供安静、安全的环境，室内物品力求简单。室内灯光柔和，物品颜色淡雅，具有镇静作用，可以安定患者

Hazardous objects and substances (including smoking materials) should be kept in safe places. Nurses educate the client to obey the security regulations and some knowledge about safety. Windows and doors should be repaired immediately after being destroyed. Stay with the client who is hyperactive and agitated. Encourage clients to participate in some physical activities. (b) Provide adequate food,water and encourage maintain personal hygiene. Provide clients with their favorite food, which is also high-nutritional, high-calorie, and easily digested high-protein and moderate quantity of fruit to supplement vitamins and minerals, keep the balance between hydro-electrolyte. Record accurately input and output, total calorie, and weight, and monitor regularly laboratory values. Stay with clients and help them to eat. If the client is highly exciting, the nurse should feed him or her patiently and explain the harm of irregular diet. (c) Sleep guidance: when possible, try to direct energy into productive and calming activities (e.g., pacing to slow, soft music; slow exercise; drawing alone; or writing in quiet area). Provide nursing measures at bedtime that promote sleep—warm milk, soft music.

的情绪。教育患者自觉遵守和执行安全管理和检查制度，门窗、门锁有损坏及时修理。对患者及其家属进行安全知识的宣传和教育。活动亢进和激动不安的患者，护士应多陪伴，凡是有患者活动的场所都应有护士看护。引导患者参与他喜爱的体育活动，并给予支持和鼓励。② 帮助患者维持足够的营养、水分、保持良好的个人卫生状况：躁狂患者可能过度忙碌于他所认为的伟大事业，易忽略最基本的生理需求。患者活动增多、体力消耗大、说话滔滔不绝，易造成口干舌燥，营养差，衣着不整，护理人员应提供高热量、高蛋白、营养丰富的食物，以保证患者足够的营养与水分摄入，并督促或协助患者做好个人卫生、仪表修饰。③ 指导患者重建规律有质量的睡眠模式：知道并督促患者每日养成定时休息习惯，如有入睡困难，应做好睡眠管理，以保证患者足够的休息时间。

(2) Psychosocial intervention: Psychosocial interventions are particularly important to improve medication effect, which include client and family education on suicide prevention, and limitation of clients with mania and Hypomania. Some experts emphasize communication and psychoeducation: listening to clients' concerns about taking medication and any side effects they may experience, visiting clients frequently, and educating clients and their families verbally and with written materials. An extremely important component in client and family education for mood disorders is the importance of medication maintenance and side effects. Clients taking lithium should be fully informed about expected side effects and some interventions that can help to prevent and control them. It is clear that pharmacotherapy alone does not meet needs of many clients with mania. A comprehensive therapy should be developed to treat mania.

（2）心理护理：社会心理干预对提高药物治疗效果尤其重要，包括对患者和家庭进行自杀预防教育，限制躁狂和轻躁狂患者。一些专家强调沟通和心理教育：倾听病人对服药及其可能产生的副作用的担忧，经常关心患者，用语言和书面材料对患者及其家人进行教育，尤其是告知维持用药和药物副作用。服用锂盐的患者应该充分了解其副作用以及有助于预防和控制副作用的措施。很明显，单靠药物治疗并不能满足许多躁狂患者的需求。应该发展一种综合疗法来治疗躁狂。

(3) Safety care and prevent from violence: Provide clients quiet environment, reduce the stimulus outside and put the client in isolation ward when necessary. Observe client's behavior once per 15 minutes. Intensify the management of dangerous materials and ensure that all sharp objects, glass, belts, ties, smoking materials have been removed from client's environment. Encourage clients to participate in some physical activities. The application of communication skills in the interaction between nurses

（3）安全护理，防范患者的暴力行为：① 给患者提供安静的生活环境，必要时安置在安静的隔离房间，减少外界环境中的不良刺激。② 密切观察患者的病情和行为，每15分钟巡视一次。③ 加强危险品的管理，确保患者活动的范围内无玻璃、带子、吸烟物品及其他锐利的物品等。④ 引导患者参与他喜

and clients: maintaining a kind attitude to clients without judgment of clients' abnormal behavior and being cautious to contact with clients' body. Educate clients to search for help from doctors and nurses rather than use violence. Educate clients skills to control and vent moods. Offer tranquilizer according to prescription. If clients refuse, use of mechanical restraints may be necessary.

爱的活动，并给予支持和鼓励。⑤ 接触患者过程中，注意沟通交流技巧的应用：护士态度和蔼，不用刺激性的语言，对患者的过激行为不做评判，但不轻易迁就，对其打抱不平行为必须婉言谢绝。在沟通、治疗和护理中，与患者发生躯体接触时应谨慎，必要时要有他人陪同。⑥ 教育患者应主动求医而非使用暴力。⑦ 教给患者控制和发泄情绪的技巧。⑧ 可遵医嘱给予镇静药，必要时应用约束措施。

(4) Medication care: Medication management and prevention of side effects are a major nursing responsibility during nursing care of inpatients. For clients treated with lithium, blood concentration should be measured frequently to determine an effective dosage within the therapeutic range. Therapeutic blood concentration of lithium is 0.5 to 1.2 mEq/L. There are several drugs and substance interactions and interventions to help control side effects with which the nurse must be familiar. The relationship between lithium and sodium in the body remains a crucial issue in the safe and effective use of lithium. It is not necessary to control sodium in the diet, but clients need to understand how changes in sodium levels affect lithium blood levels and how this might affect therapeutic results. For instance, if sodium level drop significantly due to hot environment, vomiting, or drastic reduction of sodium in the diet, then lithium level in the blood can rise sharply, which can induce a severe side effect and develop to lethal lithium toxicity.

（4）用药护理：应帮助患者正确认识自身疾病，保证药物治疗准确实施。保证药物治疗并控制其副作用是护士护理住院患者的主要职责。对接受锂盐治疗的患者，需经常监测患者的血药浓度，能在药物使用剂量的范围中选出一个最为有效的剂量。锂盐的治疗性血药浓度是 0.5 ~ 1.2 mEq/L。护士应熟悉药物之间的相互作用，并采取相应的措施最大限度地降低副作用对患者的影响。通过指导患者合理饮食，使体内锂和钠维持在一定水平，让锂盐发挥最佳疗效。让患者理解钠的水平的改变可以影响锂盐的血药浓度，进而影响药物疗效。例如患者在很热的环境出汗过多、呕吐或饮食中钠的摄入量减少，体内钠的水平明显下降，血液中锂盐就会急剧上升，从而导致重症副作用，最终发展至锂盐中毒。

iv. Nursing Evaluation

1. Whether the client does harm to body or articles due to unsuitable behavior, whether the client has learned to control his or her elevated mood or anxiety and has not injured self or others.

2. Whether the client can identify and analyze the pathological behavior and be responsible for consequences of his or her behavior.

3. Whether the client can fall asleep within 30 minutes and sleep for 6 to 8 hours without taking medicine, which is the client's sleep has been improved.

4. Whether the client has a balanced diet and good nutrition.

5. Whether the client has established a good interpersonal relationship.

（四）护理评价

1. 患者是否有伤害他人、冲动的行为，是否学会控制和宣泄自己高涨或焦虑的心境。

2. 患者是否能认识和分析自己的病态行为，对自己的行为负责。

3. 患者睡眠是否改善，能否在 30 分钟内入睡。在不服药物的情况下睡 6 ~ 8 小时。

4. 患者是否维持营养、水分、排泄等方面的适当生理功能。

5. 患者是否能恰当地与人交往，在需要时能主动寻求支持和帮助。

II. Depression

i. Nursing Assessment

1. Biological Assessment Biological assessment include history of personal growth, past history, lifestyle, special hobby, family history, history of allergies, ect. Assessment of appetite and weight aims to know whether the client has altered nutrition or obvious loss of weight. Sleep assessment examines whether the clients have sleep disturbance, such as problems in falling asleep, problems of staying asleep with frequent awakenings throughout the night, early morning awakening, hypersomnia, etc.

2. Psychiatric Assessment Psychiatric Assessment include: (a) Emotion: whether the clients have loss of interest and enjoyment, depression, anxiety, lower self-evaluation, guilty, despair, decreased libido. (b) Cognition: whether the clients have distorted cognition, over concentration on self and neglecting of outer environment, hallucination or illusion, thinking disturbance, difficulty in memory, hypomnesia. (c) Behavior: whether the clients have self-mutilation or suicide behavior. The frequency of occurrence, intensity, lethality of suicide ideas should also be assessed.

3. Psychosocial Assessment Psychosocial assessment includes family history, educational background, previous personality characteristics, social participating, and supporting system.

ii. Nursing Diagnosis

1. Risk for self-mutilation related to pessimistic mood, self-blame or a sense of guilt, suicide idea or behavior, a sense of worthless.

2. Self-care deficit: hygiene/clothing/feeding related to the symptom itself.

3. Sleep pattern disturbance related to difficulty in falling asleep, early morning awakening due to pessimistic mood.

4. Altered nutrition: less than body requirements related to decreased ingestion due to self-blame and a sense of guilt, poor appetite, immovableness, and stupor.

5. Ineffective individual coping related to helplessness, lack of energy.

6. Personal identity disturbance related to the depressed mood, low self-evaluation.

7. Anxiety related to depression mood, self-blame.

8. Constipation related to decreased activity, slow gastrointestinal peristalsis.

二、抑郁发作的护理程序

（一）护理评估

1. 生理状况的评估 健康史，包括个人成长发展史、既往史、生活方式、特殊嗜好、家族史、过敏史等；患者的营养状况，有无食欲低下、性欲减退；睡眠情况，有无入睡困难、早醒、醒后难以入睡等。

2. 精神症状的评估 评估抑郁表现、程度和持续时间，具体包括以下几方面：① 情绪方面是否对日常活动丧失兴趣、无愉快感、精力减退、自我评价过低、自责等。② 认知方面是否有联想困难，注意力下降，自责、罪恶、虚无、疑病、贫穷妄想，有无轻生意念。③ 行为方面是否有行动缓慢、少语少动；是否焦虑不安，躁动易激惹，有无自杀企图与行为，出现频率，强度等。

3. 心理社会状况的评估 包括患者家庭史、教育背景、病前个性特点、患者社交活动和支持系统。

（二）护理诊断

1. 有自伤（自杀）的危险 与自我评价低、悲观绝望等情绪有关。

2. 自理缺陷：卫生 / 穿着 / 进食 与精神运动性迟滞、兴趣减低、无力照顾自己有关。

3. 睡眠型态紊乱 与情绪低落、沮丧、绝望等因素有关。

4. 营养失调：低于机体需要量 与抑郁致食欲下降及自罪妄想内容有关。

5. 应对无效 与无助感、精力不足等因素有关。

6. 自我认同紊乱 与抑郁情绪、自我评价过低、无价值感有关。

7. 焦虑 与无价值感、罪恶感、内疚、疑病等因素有关。

8. 便秘 与日常活动减少、胃肠蠕动减慢有关。

iii. Nursing Care Plan and Intervention

1. Outcome Identification

(1) The client has experience no physical harm to self.

(2) The client can care for self, for example bathing, washing, combing, and dressing without assistance.

(3) The client can sleep for 6 to 8 hours per night without taking medicine.

(4) The client can eat a well-balance diet with snacks, to prevent weight loss and maintain nutritional status.

(5) The client can control his mood, and concentrate, reason and solve problems.

(6) The client is no longer afraid to attempt new activities and can express personal satisfaction and search for spiritual support.

(7) The client can verbalize positive aspects about self, past accomplishment or future prospects.

(8) The client can maintain passage of soft, formed stool at a frequency perceived as "normal".

2. Nursing Interventions

(1) Physiological nursing: (a) Help client to keep a well-balanced diet and appropriate rest. Lack of appetite and constipation are common in depressed patients. Clients should eat foods rich in cellulose. Sitting quietly with clients during meals can promote eating. If clients feel no value, not worth and refused to eat, clients can engage in some activities for others, so as to assist clients to accept food. Nasal feeding or infusion may be needed if necessary. Monitoring food and fluid intake may be necessary until clients are consuming adequate amounts. (b) Encourage maintain personal hygiene. The ability to perform daily activities is related to the level of psychomotor retardation. To assess ability to perform activities of daily living independently, the nurse first asks the client to perform the global task. The nurse helps clients to dress only when they cannot perform any of the above steps. This allows clients to do as much as possible for themselves and to avoid becoming dependent on the staff. (c) Improving sleep style. Promoting sleep may include the short-term use of a sedative or giving medication in the evening if drowsiness or sedation is a side effect. It is also important to encourage clients to remain out of bed and active during the day to facilitate sleeping at night. Early waking up is common, while suicide, self-injury tend to occur during early waking up. It is important to monitor the number of hours clients sleep as well as whether they feel refreshed on early awakening. For clients with severe stupor state, or

（三）护理计划及措施

1. 护理目标

（1）患者住院期间不伤害自己，在出现自杀意念时能向工作人员诉说。

（2）患者生活恢复自理，不需他人帮助能自行洗澡、洗涤、梳头、更衣等。

（3）患者在不用药物时，每晚有6~8小时的睡眠时间，对睡眠有自我满足。

（4）患者摄入营养均衡的食物，体重未下降。

（5）患者能够控制自己的情绪，集中注意力分析和解决问题。

（6）患者能在治疗后形成自我认同。

（7）患者不再害怕参加新的活动，能够表达自我满足和寻求精神支持。

（8）患者能以正常频率排成形软便。

2. 护理措施

（1）基础护理：① 帮助患者维持适当的营养、水分、排泄、休息，保持良好的个人卫生状况。食欲缺乏、便秘是抑郁患者常出现的胃肠道反应。可选择患者平时较喜欢的含纤维素丰富的食物，陪伴患者进餐，少量多餐。若患者因觉得自己没有价值，不值得吃饭而拒食时，可让患者从事一些为别人做事的活动，如此可以协助患者接受食物。若患者坚持不吃或体重持续减轻，则必须采取进一步的措施，如喂食、鼻饲、输液等。进食粗纤维食物、供给足够水分，进行足够的活动后，仍无法解决便秘时，需给予缓泻剂或灌肠处理。应监测患者食物和液体的摄入量。② 抑郁患者常不注重自己的衣着，外观及个人卫生。对轻度抑郁患者可鼓励其在能力范围内自我料理；重度抑郁患者则应帮助其洗脸、洗脚、口腔护理、会阴护理、更衣、如厕、仪表修饰，使患者感到整洁、舒适。允许患者适度的依赖，有助于减轻心理压力。③ 改善睡眠模式。不易入睡、易醒、早醒的患者，应鼓励或陪伴患者白天多活动，不要长时间卧床。入睡前喝些热饮料，洗热水澡

completely in bed without any movement, the prevention of pressure ulcers is also important.

等。抑郁患者的睡眠障碍主要表现为早醒，而患者发生的许多意外事件，如自杀、自伤等，多发生在这种时候，清晨应加强护理巡视，对早醒者应予以安抚，使其延长睡眠时间，对重度抑郁木僵、完全卧床不动的患者，需要协助患者翻身及被动运动，预防压疮。

(2) Psychological interventions: (a) Be accepting of client and spend time with him or her even though pessimism and negativism may seem objectionable. Focus on strengths and accomplishments and minimize failures. (b) Promote attendance in therapy groups that offer clients simple methods of accomplishment. Encourage clients to be as independent as possible. Encourage clients to recognize areas of change and provide assistance toward this effort. Techniques include activity scheduling, self-control therapy, social skills training, and problem-solving, which are within the scope of basic nursing practice. In the process of behavior therapy, nurses can help clients to build a good interpersonal communication skill. (c) Nurses are exceptionally well positioned to engage clients and their families in the active process of recovery and rehabilitation by focusing on knowledge and skill acquisitions to achieve recovery and maintain remission. Motivation is developed when a person sees a discrepancy between his or her present state and anticipated future state. This discrepancy or difference between the present and future is called a motivating gap. The focus of self-care management is to help the client develop a motivating gap so that the client has a goal, sees alternatives and can choose the action best for himself or herself to achieve recovery or rehabilitation.

（2）心理护理：① 指导患者肯定自己的优点、长处，让其对自身价值有信心 抑郁患者对自己或外界事物常不自觉地持否定的看法（负性思考），护理人员必须协助患者确认这些负性思考，然后设法打断这种负性循环，可以协助患者回顾自身的优点、长处、成就来增加患者对自身或外界的正向认识，培养正确的认知方式。② 鼓励患者多参与治疗性小组活动，培养患者的独立人格。在护理过程中，要积极营造、利用一切个人会团体的人际交往机会，改善患者以往消极被动的交往方式，逐步建立积极健康的人际交往方式，增加社交技巧。③ 应教会患者自我照顾的知识和技巧，以促进患者尽快康复。患者健康状况的改善，是患者接受治疗的推动力。这种治疗前后的差距被称为是动机差距。自我照顾的目标是让患者发展这种动机差距，这样患者有了明确的目标，会促使患者选择最适合自己的行为以尽快地康复。④ 向患者家属了解患者的兴趣爱好，鼓励患者参加其喜爱的活动，以疏泄抑郁情绪。

(3) Safety care: The first priority is to determine whether a client with depression is suicidal. If a client has suicidal ideation or hears voices commanding him or her to commit suicide, measures to provide a safe environment are necessary. If the client has a suicide plan, the nurse asks additional questions to determine the lethality of the intent and plan. The nurse reports this information to the treatment team. Create a safe environment for the client. Supervise closely during meals and medication administration. Perform room searches as deemed necessary. Store items that client uses frequently within easy reach. Remove potentially harmful articles from client's room: cigarettes, matches, lighters, sharp objects. Pad side rails and headboard of client with history of seizures. Prevent physical aggression and acting out behaviors by learning to recognize signs that client is

（3）安全护理：护理人员应做好安全护理，预防患者可能伤害自己的行为。① 将患者置于工作人员视线下，置于患者群体及安全环境中，避免单独居住、单独活动。② 严密观察患者的病情变化，特别是异常的言行，如流露厌世的想法、收藏危险品等，以便及早发现自杀先兆。③ 在交接班时间，吃饭时间，清晨、夜间或工作人员较少时，要特别注意密切观察，需 15 分钟巡视患者一次。④ 安排患者床位靠近护士站，必要时 24 小时严加管理。⑤ 使用腋下或肛表测量体温，并加强看护，严防口腔测温吞服体温表。⑥ 做好并取得安全管理工作，提供安全的治疗环

becoming agitated.

境，撤除所有的危险品。⑦ 外出检查、洗澡或户外活动时，要有工作人员重点看护。

(4) Medication care: Careful observation of curative effect and side effect of drugs: antidepressant medications are a primary intervention for most clients experiencing a major depressive disorder. So it is important for nurses to observe curative effect and side effect of drugs. Nurses should ensure that clients take all medicines and observe the clients after taking medicine. Outpatients with severe depression should visit doctor weekly within the first 6 to 8 weeks of acute treatment. The drug should not be changed frequently because it usually doesn't take effect until 4 to 6 weeks after medication. Once depression symptoms relieve, clients can visit doctor every 4 to 12 weeks. Clients with mild depression can visit doctor every 10 to 14 days within the first 6 to 8 weeks or more frequently if required.

（4）用药护理：抗抑郁药物对抑郁症的治疗非常重要，因此，护士需要密切观察药物的疗效和副作用。护士应确保患者将药物全部服用，并密切观察服后行为。在院外治疗的患者，抑郁症状严重者，在前 6～8 周应每周就诊一次，应密切观察药物疗效，不宜频繁更换药物，药物的效果应观察 4～6 周；抑郁症状得到控制，每 4～12 周复查一次是合理的。症状轻者，在前 6～8 周 10～14 天就诊一次，必要时可增加次数。

The side effect of drugs is the primary reason why clients cannot persist in medication. The nurse must be familiar with the medications, dosage range, therapeutic blood levels, and side effects of all current antidepressants. Clients should be fully informed of main side effects of antidepressants before medication. Nurses should also try to reduce the impact of side effect on the clients. The common side effects of antidepressants include fatigue, orthostatic hypotension, gastrointestinal distress, and weight gain. The evaluation of curative effect of medicine should be made from physiological and psychological aspects.

治疗药物的副作用是患者不能坚持服药的原因。护士应该熟悉目前常用抗抑郁药的用药剂量、疗效及副作用等，并将常见的不良反应告诉患者，让其有心理准备。护士应采取适当措施最大限度地降低药物的不良反应对患者造成的不良影响。常见的不良反应，如疲乏、直立性低血压、胃肠道抑制、体重增加等。护士通过观察、监测生命体征、评估患者的主观描述，来监测药物疗效。同时了解患者使用药物前后的心理反应。

It is important to establish personalized therapeutic dosage levels because therapeutic blood levels vary among individuals. Some of traditional antidepressants have prescribed therapeutic range. However, some of the new antidepressants, the therapeutic ranges vary so widely and there are no standardized therapeutic ranges. So it is important to identify specific ranges for each individual. Individualizing the medication regimen is crucial for clients taking antidepressants. Nurses can inform the doctor of tuning medication dosage according to careful observation and communication with clients.

由于个体差异性，每个患者的有效血药浓度可能有所不同。有些传统的抗抑郁药有规定的有效血药浓度范围，有些新型的抗抑郁药有效浓度范围很宽，这时需要识别每个患者的有效药物范围。药物治疗的个体化非常重要。护士通过对患者的密切观察和与患者的沟通交流，及时告知医生调整药物剂量。

iv. Nursing Evaluation

1. Whether the client has experience no physical harm to self.

2. Whether the client can verbalize positive aspects about self, past accomplishment or future prospects.

3. Whether the client is no longer afraid to attempt new activities.

4. Whether the client can express personal satisfaction and search for spiritual support.

（四）护理评价

1. 患者住院期间是否没有发生伤害自己的行为。

2. 患者是否能用言语表达与自我、过去和未来有关的正性事件。

3. 患者是否不再害怕参加新的活动。

4. 患者是否能够表达自我满足和寻求精神支持。

5. Whether the client can control his or her mood.

6. Whether the client can interact willingly and appropriately with others.

7. Whether the client can eat a well-balance diet with snacks, to prevent weight loss and maintain nutritional status.

8. Whether the client can concentrate, reason and solve problems.

9. Whether the client can care for self, for example bathing, washing, combing, and dressing without assistance.

10. Whether the client can sleep for 6 to 8 hours per night without taking medicine.

(Dong Fanghong)

5. 患者是否能够控制自己的情绪。

6. 患者是否能无拘无束地与他人交往。

7. 患者是否营养均衡，无体重下降。

8. 患者是否能集中注意力分析和解决问题。

9. 患者是否能生活自理，无他人帮助下进行洗澡、洗涤、梳头、更衣等。

10. 患者是否在不服用药物时，每晚有6~8小时的睡眠时间。

（董方虹）

Key Points

1. Mood disorders or affective disorders are a group of mental disorders characterized by obvious and persistent elation or depression of mood (elated or depressed mood). The mood disturbance is commonly associated with cognitive and behavioral changes. In severe cases, psychotic symptoms, such as hallucinations and delusions, may be observed.

2. Manic episode is characterized by elated and expansive mood that is out of keeping with the individual's circumstances (*CCMD-3*). The major symptoms are elevated mood, thoughts racing, and increased activities.

3. Depressive episode is characterized by depressed mood that is out of keeping with the circumstances (*CCMD-3*). The major symptoms are depressed mood, thoughts retardation, and decreased activities.

4. Lithium is used to treat clients with mania. It is helpful for bipolar mania and can partially or completely eradicate cycling toward bipolar depression. Lithium has a narrow range of safety; thus, ongoing monitoring of serum lithium levels is necessary to establish efficacy while preventing toxicity. Clients taking lithium must ingest adequate salt and water to avoid overdosing or underdosing because lithium salt uses the same postsynaptic receptor sites as sodium chloride does. Other drugs include sodium valproate, carbamazepine, and other anticonvulsants.

5. Major categories of antidepressants include cyclic antidepressants, monoamine oxidase inhibitors (MAOIs), selective serotonin reuptake inhibitors (SSRIs), and atypical antidepressants.

6. Nursing care of mood disorder clients should focus on how to protect the clients from suicide or other accidents,

内容摘要

1. 心境障碍是以显著而持久的心境或情感改变为主要特征的一组疾病。临床上主要表现为情感高涨或低落，伴有相应的认知和行为改变，可有精神病性症状。

2. 躁狂发作的基本临床表现是典型的“三高”症状，即情感高涨、思维奔逸和活动增多。

3. 抑郁发作的典型症状是“三低症状”，即情感低落、思维迟缓、意志活动减退为主要特征。

4. 躁狂发作的首选药物是锂盐（碳酸锂），既可用于躁狂的急性发作，也可用于缓解期的维持治疗，对躁狂的复发也有预防作用。碳酸锂的治疗量与中毒量接近，在急性治疗期间除严密观察病情变化和治疗反应外，应每周检测血锂浓度。此外，还可使用心境稳定剂（锂盐、丙戊酸盐、卡马西平）。

5. 抗抑郁药物有三环类及四环类抗抑郁药、单胺氧化酶抑制剂、选择性5-羟色胺再摄取抑制剂和非典型抗抑郁药。

6. 心境障碍患者的护理重点在保证患者安全，防止自杀等意外事件的发生，还应加强饮食

still the nurse must monitor food and fluid intake, rest and sleep, and pharmaceutical and psychological need.

护理、睡眠护理、用药护理和心理护理等。

Exercises

(Questions 1 to 2 share the same question stem)

June, 46 years old, is divorced with three children. She works in the county clerk's office and has called in sick four times in the past 2 weeks. June has lost 8 kg in the past 2 months, is spending a lot of time in bed, but still feels exhausted "all the time." During the clinical examination, June looks overwhelmingly sad, is tearful, has her head down, and makes little eye contact. She answers the nurse's questions with one or two words.

1. Identify three nursing diagnoses on the basis of the available data.

2. Discuss nursing interventions that would be helpful for June.

(Questions 3 to 4 share the same question stem)

A client with mania begins dancing around the day room. When she twirled her skirt in front of the male clients, it was obvious she had no underpants on. The nurse distracts her and takes her to her room to put on underpants.

3. Discuss the nurse acted as she did to do.

4. Identify possible nursing diagnoses for the patient.

思考题

（1～2题共用题干）

朱恩，46岁，离异后带着三个孩子生活。她在政府办公室工作，近两周病了4次，而且在过去的两个月内瘦了8公斤。每天大部分时间都躺在床上，还是感觉很累。体检发现，患者表情很悲伤，总是哭，低着头，很少有眼神接触；只用一两个词来回答护士的问题。

1. 根据该病例的情况给出三个护理诊断。

2. 讨论对患者有利的护理措施。

（3～4题共用题干）

某躁狂患者围着休息室跳舞，当她在男患者面前转裙子时，很明显她没穿内裤，护理人员分散她的注意力并将她带回病房穿好内裤。

3. 讨论护理人员当前的做法的目的。

4. 给出该患者目前可能的护理诊断。

Chapter 8 Nursing Management for Clients with Personality Disorders

第八章 人格障碍患者的护理

Learning Objectives

Memorization

1. Describe the characteristics of personality disorders.
2. Summarize the clinical manifestations of the common personality disorders.

Comprehension

1. Understand the importance of genetic, biological, psychological, social-environmental factors in relation to personality disorders.
2. Differentiate the borderline personality disorder and impulsive personality disorder.

Application

Provide corresponding nursing interventions to the client with personality disorders.

学习目标

识记

1. 能准确描述人格障碍患者的共同性格特征。
2. 能正确简述常见人格障碍的临床表现。

理解

1. 能正确理解遗传、生物学、心理、社会环境因素与人格障碍的关系。
2. 能区别边缘型人格障碍和冲动型人格障碍。

运用

能针对性应用相应的措施护理人格障碍患者。

08章

The patient is 38 years old, lives alone, and is a writer. She goes out every night, only at night, to a nearby grocery store (because "their magic does not work at night"). She dresses in several layers of multicolored and mismatched clothes even in warmer weather. She wears a turban on her head to "keep them from seeing my thoughts" . Each night she tells grocer in a flat and formal manner that she is going to be a famous director and star. She knows this because "It hasn't snowed yet, and that means the coast is clear."

患者，38岁，是一位独居的作家。她喜欢独处，仅每晚出现在附近的一家杂货店（因为她认为"晚上其他人的魔法失灵"）。她经常穿着五颜六色的衣服，即使是在暖和的天气，也会穿好几层衣服，并且戴着头巾以免他人看到自己的想法。每次她都会郑重地告诉店员，她将会成为一名著名的导演和演员，而她之所以可以提前预知是"因为没有下雪，所以海岸是干净的。"

Please think about the following questions based on the case:

1. What is the most likely clinical and nursing diagnosis?

2. How do psychiatric mental health nurses provide effective care for the patient?

请思考：

1. 患者最有可能的医疗诊断和护理诊断是什么？

2. 护理人员应如何为患者提供有效的护理措施？

Personality traits are enduring patterns of perceiving, relating to, and thinking about the environment and oneself that are exhibited in a wide range of social and personal contexts. They determine how an individual reflects upon and responds to life events, as well as many dynamics of personal behavior. A "healthy personality" might be described as one that allows an individual to live harmoniously in society, develop positive self-concepts and body images, and experience a sense of worth and an ability to relate openly and honestly with others. Only when personality traits are inflexible and maladaptive and cause significant functional impairment or subjective distress do they constitute personality disorders.

人格指个体在遗传与环境的交互作用下所形成的稳定而独特的心理结构，在社会与生活环境中具有固有的行为模式和待人处事的习惯方法。若个体与社会生活相适应，形成正性的自我概念和体像，并具有自我价值感及与他人坦诚交往的能力，称为正常人格；反之，若个体的适应不良与社会生活产生严重冲突，明显影响社交和职业功能者（时）则称为人格障碍。

Individual with personality disorder has behavioral pattern that deviates from the "norms" of his social/cultural background. It is related to genetic, biological, psychological, and social-environmental factors. Personality disorders frequently emerge early in childhood or adolescence and persist throughout the individuals life. Because the treatment of personality disorders is often extremely difficult and time consuming, preventive interventions are critical. This chapter describes 8 personality disorders listed in *ICD-10* in details: paranoid personality disorder, schizoid personality disorder, dissocial personality disorder, emotionally unstable personality disorder, histrionic personality disorder, Anankastic personality disorder, avoidant personality disorder, and dependent personality disorder.

人格障碍患者的行为表现多背离本身所处社会文化背景，其形成与遗传、生物、心理和社会环境因素有关。人格障碍通常在儿童或青少年期表现出来，多伴随终身，治疗相对困难，所以重在预防。本章重点介绍*ICD-10*列出的八种人格障碍，即偏执型人格障碍、分裂样人格障碍、社交紊乱型人格障碍、情绪不稳型人格障碍、表演型人格障碍、强迫型人格障碍、回避型人格障碍、依赖型人格障碍。

Section 1 Introduction

I. Definition

Personality disorders are a class of mental disorders characterized by enduring maladaptive patterns of behavior, cognition, and inner experience, exhibited across many contexts and deviating markedly from those accepted by the individual's culture. Once these maladaptive behavior patterns are formed, it is difficult to correct by medical treatment, education or punishment, only a few patients may be improved to some extent in adult. The onset of the disorder is usually in childhood or adolescence and is stable over times.

BOX 8-1 Learning More

Personality Disorder and Personality Change

Personality disorders should not be confused with personality changes. Personality change is acquired, which refers to a person has normal personality originally and appears after severe or prolonged stress, severe mental disorder and brain diseases or injuries occurred, but they may recover from illness with condition improvement. There is no clear onset time in personality disorder, which often began in childhood or adolescence and lasts for a lifetime. The reference of personality change is the original personality, and the main judgment criteria for personality disorder come from the general criteria of the society and the psychology.

II. Characteristics of Personality Disorders

The essential feature of personality disorder is an enduring pattern of inner experiencing and behavior that deviates markedly from the expectations of the individual's culture and is manifested in at least two of the following areas: cognition (how the patient perceives and interprets self, others, and events), affect (appropriateness, intensity, liability, and range of emotions), interpersonal functioning, or impulse control. This enduring pattern is inflexible and pervasive across a broad range of personal and social situations and leads to clinically significant distress or impairment in social, occupational, or other important areas of functioning. The common characteristics of personality disorders are as follows:

1. The maladaptive behaviors usually begin during childhood or adolescence, but are almost universally

第一节 概 述

一、概 念

人格障碍是指一类行为表现显著偏离所处文化背景，行为、认知和内心体验持久适应不良的精神障碍。一旦适应不良的行为模式形成，通过医疗、教育或惩罚措施很难矫正，仅少数患者成年后可能在一定程度上有所改善。人格障碍通常在童年期或青少年期开始形成，并长期持续发展至成年或终生。

BOX 8-1 知识拓展

人格障碍与人格改变的区别

人格障碍和人格改变不能混为一谈。人格改变是指一个人原本人格正常，而在严重或持久的应激、严重的精神障碍、脑部疾病或损伤之后发生的人格偏离，为获得性人格障碍，随着疾病痊愈或境遇改善可恢复或部分恢复。人格障碍没有明确的起病时间，始于童年或青少年且持续终生。人格改变的参照物是病前人格，而人格障碍主要的评判标准来自于社会、心理的一般准则。

二、人格障碍的共同特征

人格障碍的基本特点是患者至少在以下两方面具有显著偏离其文化背景的固有行为模式，即认知（患者如何感知和理解自我、他人以及事件），情感（恰当程度、强烈程度、易变性、情感范围等），人际交往功能或冲动控制力。患者的这种异常行为模式往往固定，而且渗透到其生活的各个方面，常明显影响其社会、职业和其他重要功能。通常具有以下共同特征：

1. 人格障碍起始于儿童或青少年时期，但大多于18岁前发病，并一直持续到成年或

manifested before 18 years old as a way of coping and remain throughout most of his or her adulthood or whole life, the time of onset is not clear.

2. The person always denies that the behaviors are maladaptive; the behaviors have become a way of life for the individual, although, at times, he/she may experience distress or impaired work, social, or personal functioning and promise to change his/her future behavior. Because personality disorders are so pervasive in the make-up of the individual, such promises are useless.

3. There is no obvious pathological change of the nervous system.

4. The maladaptive behaviors are inflexible and hard to be changed. There are no obvious intelligent or consciousness changes.

5. Psychiatric help is rarely sought because the person is unaware of his/her behaviors or denies that they are maladaptive. Though he or she has difficulty in dealing with the reality of his/her culture and society, he/she remains in contact with reality.

6. The person generally can cope with daily life and work.

终生，起病时间不明确。

2. 缺乏自知之明，有时会对自己的行为感到痛苦，保证自己今后不再犯，但保证往往无效。

3. 一般没有明显神经系统形态学病理变化。

4. 异常行为固定且难以改变，但其智能和意识状态无明显缺陷。

5. 主动求医者少，患者常忽略其行为或否认其行为异常，虽然他 / 她很难融入于其所处社会和文化中，但仍坚持接触现实生活。

6. 人格障碍者多数能应付日常工作和生活。

III. Epidemiology

Studies of prevalence rates vary from region to region and country to country. A screening survey across 13 countries by the World Health Organization, reported in 2009 a prevalence estimate of any personality disorder was 6.1%, 4.1% in China, 2.4% in Western Europe and 7.6% in American.

三、流行病学

人格障碍患病率的报告差异很大。世界卫生组织 2009 年对全球 13 个国家进行筛选调查，发现人格障碍的患病率约为 6%，其中中国的患病率为 4.1%，西欧国家为 2.4%，美国为 7.6%。

IV. Etiology and Mechanism

The cause of personality disorders is not so clear, which involving genetic, biological, psychological, and social aspects. At present, it is considered that formed on the basis of congenital defect of the brain and influenced by the environmental harmful factors (especially the psychosocial factors). It is generally recognized that the following factors may contribute to the development of personality disorders.

1. The Genetic Factors Researches indicated that the incidence of a personality disorder is related to genetic factors. Statistically significantly higher correlation rates have consistently been found among identical twins than among fraternal twins. Moreover, relatively greater correlation rates have been found among members of families with members who experience personality

四、病因及发病机制

人格障碍的病因迄今仍不甚明确，可能涉及遗传、生物、心理、社会等各个方面。目前认为它是在大脑先天性缺陷的基础上，遭受环境有害因素（尤其是心理社会因素）的影响而形成。一般认为以下因素与人格障碍的发生密切相关。

1. 遗传因素 研究发现人格障碍的发生与遗传有关。同卵双生子同时发生人格障碍的几率高于异卵双生子。患者的亲属中常常也有人格障碍患者。

disorders.

2. Biological Factors It was indicated by some researchers that cerebral development in person with personality disorder is later than that of the normal person. Infection, poison, malnutrition in early childhood, trauma during or after birth, and other factors can cause injury to cerebral function, which may affect cerebral development.

3. Psychological Factors Some theorists contend that unpleasant childhood experience, e.g. parental divorce, conflicted intra-family relationships, and inappropriate or ineffective child-rearing practices may provoke abnormal psycho/social reactions and provoke personality disorders.

4. Social-environmental Factors Personality disorder is associated with cultural maladjustment from the view of social culture. Because the ability of children to influence their environments is quite limited, children's personality is subject to the influences of their cultures and social settings in ways that may contribute to the development of personality disorders.

2. 生物学因素 研究表明人格障碍患者的大脑发育成熟程度较正常人有所延迟。大脑发育不成熟可能与婴幼儿时期感染、中毒、营养不良、出生时或出生后脑损伤有关。

3. 心理发展因素 童年时期生活经历对个体人格的形成具有重要作用。重大精神创伤或刺激，如父母离异、家庭关系紧张、家庭教育方式不当等对儿童人格的发育有着不利的影响，并可最终导致人格障碍。

4. 社会环境因素 从社会文化角度来看，人格障碍与文化适应不良有关，不同的社会和文化塑造不同的性格。由于儿童自制力相对较差，易受周围环境影响，如受到不利于儿童青少年身心成长的文化媒介和社会环境的影响，可导致其产生不良心理并发展至人格障碍。

Section 2 Types and Clinical Manifestation

第二节 常见类型及临床表现

Although the behavior of individuals with personality disorder may deviate significantly from social/cultural norms, it is inappropriate and unprofessional to label such individuals as "immoral" or "bad". It may, however, be appropriate to label the behaviors of such individuals with dissocial personality disorder. The major effects of other personality disorders are manifested as problems of interpersonal relationship and social adaptation. The types of personality disorder are shown in figure 8-1.

虽然人格障碍患者的行为明显偏离社会文化标准，但不能将这些患者视为“不道德的”或者“坏”人。在人格障碍中，只有社交紊乱型人格障碍与道德伦理观念沦丧或犯罪倾向有一定关系，会危害他人及社会秩序，其余各型主要影响人际关系与社会适应（见图 8-1）。

I. Paranoid Personality Disorder

Paranoid personality disorder is a personality disorder characterized by extreme suspiciousness and paranoia. This pattern begins at early adulthood and is present in a variety of contexts. It is occurs more commonly in males. It is characterized by at least three of the following:

1. Excessive sensitivity to setbacks, and rejections;

一、偏执型人格障碍

偏执型人格障碍以过分的猜疑和偏执为特点。始于成年早期，男性多于女性。此种人格障碍的表现至少具备以下中的三点：

1. 对挫折与拒绝过分敏感；

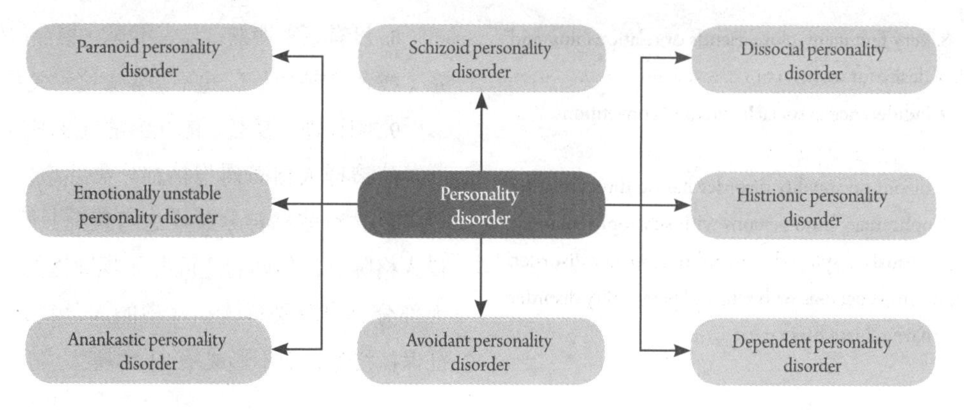

Figure 8-1　Types of personality disorder

2. Tendency to bear grudges persistently, i.e., refusal to forgive insults and injuries or slights;

2. 容易长久地记仇，即不肯原谅侮辱、伤害或轻视；

3. Suspiciousness and a pervasive tendency to distort experience by misconstruing the neutral or friendly actions of others as hostile or contemptuous;

3. 猜疑和将体验歪曲的一种普遍倾向，以及把他人无意的或友好的行为误解为敌意或轻蔑；

4. A combative and tenacious sense of personal rights out of keeping with the actual situation;

4. 与现实环境不相称的好斗及顽固地维护个人的权利；

5. Recurrent suspicions, without justification, regarding the sexual fidelity of the spouse or sexual partner;

5. 极易猜疑，毫无根据地怀疑配偶或性伴侣的忠诚；

6. Tendency to experience excessive self-importance, manifest in a persistent self-referential attitude;

6. 将自己看得过分重要的倾向，表现为持续的自我援引态度；

7. Preoccupation with unsubstantiated "conspiratorial" explanations of events both immediate to the patient and in the world at large.

7. 将其周围事件以及世间的形形色色都解释为"阴谋"的无根据的先占概念。

II. Schizoid Personality Disorder

二、分裂样人格障碍

Schizoid personality disorder is a personality disorder characterized by preoccupations of bizarre appearance, behaviors and ideas, apathy, and impairment in interpersonal relationship. It is more common in men than in women. It is characterized by at least four of the following:

分裂样人格障碍以外表、行为、观念的古怪，情感冷漠以及人际关系明显缺陷为特点。男性略多于女性。此种人格障碍的表现至少具备以下中的四点：

1. Taking pleasure in few, if any, activities;
2. Emotional coldness, detachment or reduced affect;
3. Limited capacity to express feelings either positive or negative emotions towards others;
4. Indifference to either praise or criticism;
5. Little interest in having sexual experience with another person (taking age into account);
6. Consistent preference for solitary activities;
7. Preoccupation with fantasy and introspection;

1. 几乎没有可体验到的愉快的活动；
2. 情绪冷淡，隔膜或平淡的情感；
3. 对他人表达温情，体贴或愤怒情绪的能力有限；
4. 无论对批评或表扬都无动于衷；
5. 对与他人发生性接触毫无兴趣（要考虑年龄）；
6. 几乎总是偏爱单独行动；
7. 过分沉湎于幻想和内省；

8. Very few, if any, close friends or relationships, and a lack of desire for such;

9. Indifference to social norms and conventions.

Schizoid personality disorder has no direct relation to schizophrenia. Some persons with schizophrenia may have previously displayed schizoid personality disorder. However, most persons with schizoid personality disorder will not have schizophrenia.

8. 没有亲密朋友，与人不建立相互信任关系（或者只有一位），也不想建立这种关系；

9. 明显地无视公认的社会常规及习俗。

分裂样人格障碍与精神分裂症之间无直接关系。有些精神分裂症患者病前具有分裂样人格障碍，但两者之间并无规律性的联系。大部分具有分裂样人格障碍的人，其人格特征保持终生，而不形成精神分裂症。

III. Dissocial Personality Disorder

Dissocial personality disorder, also known as antisocial personality disorder, is a pervasive pattern of disregard for others and violation of social norms, which begins in childhood or early adolescence (usually before the age of 18 years) and continues into adulthood. It is diagnosed significantly more often in male. It is characterized by at least three of the following:

1. Callous unconcern for the feelings of others;

2. Gross and persistent attitude of irresponsibility and disregard for social norms, rules, and obligations;

3. Incapacity to maintain enduring relationships, though having no difficulty in establishing them;

4. Very low tolerance to frustration and a low threshold for discharge of aggression, including violence;

5. Incapacity to experience guilt or to profit from experience, particularly punishment;

6. Marked readiness to blame others or to offer plausible rationalizations for the behavior that has brought the person into conflict with society.

三、社交紊乱型人格障碍

社交紊乱型人格障碍又称为反社会型人格障碍，其以无视社会责任、冷酷无情为特点，往往在儿童或青少年期（18 岁以前）发生品行障碍，成年后习性不改。男性多于女性。此种人格障碍的表现至少具备以下中的三点：

1. 对他人感受漠不关心；

2. 全面、持久的缺乏责任感，无视社会规范与家庭义务；

3. 尽管建立人际关系并无困难，却不能长久地保持；

4. 易激惹，对挫折的耐受性低，微小刺激便可引起攻击，甚至暴力行为；

5. 无内疚感，不能从经历中特别是从惩罚中吸取教训；

6. 很容易责怪他人，或者当他们与社会冲突时，对行为作似是而非的合理化解释。

BOX 8-2 Learning More

Ethical Issues in the Diagnosis of Antisocial Personality Disorders

There are very serious ethical issues in relation to the concept of personality disorder as a diagnosis. Some psychiatrists are vehemently opposed to the principles underlying the process categorizing certain individuals in this way. What is considered acceptable behavior by society is partly dependent upon the individual's behavior but also depends upon the degree of tolerance the society has towards variance. There are many examples of behavior that has been considered "deviant" at certain time in the past and is now considered part of normal variation. The more intolerant the society, the greater the number

BOX 8-2 知识拓展

人格障碍诊断中的伦理问题

一些精神病学家强烈反对现有的人格障碍的诊断分类。他们认为社会可接受的行为，不但取决于个人行为，而且取决于社会的宽容程度。有很多这样的例子，许多过去被认为是离经叛道的行为，现在则被认为是正常行为变化中的一部分。社会越不能容忍，越多的人则被划为异类，进而被诊断为人格障碍。目前，政府赋予了精神科医生更大的权力以用于扣留反社会人格障碍的患者。人格

of people who will be classified as aberrant and likely to have a personality disorder. These issues are particularly important at present, as the government is seeking to provide psychiatrists with greater powers to detain patients with antisocial personality disorders. It illustrates the difficult balance between protecting the human rights of individuals versus society. The diagnosis of personality disorder is not an exact science and is dependent upon the judgment of individual psychiatrists. It is, therefore, impossible to exclude bias in this process, although all psychiatrists should strive to be as objective as possible.

障碍的诊断不是一门精准科学，依赖于精神科医生的判断，因此，即使所有的精神科医生尽力保持客观，也不能完全排除偏见。

IV. Emotionally Unstable Personality Disorder

Emotionally unstable personality disorder characterized by a definite tendency to act impulsively and without consideration of the consequences; the mood is unpredictable and capricious. There is a liability to outbursts of emotion and incapacity to control the behavioral explosions. There is a tendency to quarrelsome behavior and to conflicts with others, especially when impulsive acts are thwarted or censored. This kind of personality disorder has two specific subtypes.

i. Impulsive Type

This type characterized by at least three of the following:

1. Marked tendency to act unexpectedly and without consideration of the consequences;
2. Marked tendency to engage in quarrelsome behavior and to have conflicts with others, especially when impulsive acts are thwarted or criticized;
3. Liability to outbursts of anger or violence, with inability to control the resulting behavioral explosions;
4. Difficulty in maintaining any course of action that offers no immediate reward;
5. Unstable and capricious (impulsive, whimsical) mood.

ii. Borderline Type

This type characterized by at least two of the following:

1. Disturbances in and uncertainty about self-image, aims, and internal preferences;
2. Liability to become involved in intense and unstable relationships, often leading to emotional crisis;
3. Excessive efforts to avoid abandonment;
4. Recurrent threats or acts of self-harm;
5. Chronic feelings of emptiness.

四、情绪不稳型人格障碍

情绪不稳型人格障碍有一个突出的倾向，即行为冲动，不计后果，伴有情感不稳定，强烈的愤怒暴发常导致暴力或“行为爆炸”，当冲动行为被人批评或阻止时，极易诱发上述表现。此类人格障碍有两个特定的亚型：

（一）冲动型

此种人格障碍的表现至少具备以下中的三点：

1. 明显的行为冲动，不计后果的倾向；
2. 明显好斗的倾向，尤其是冲动的行为遭到反对或批评时；
3. 愤怒或暴力暴发的倾向，没有控制行为暴发的能力；
4. 难以维持没有提任何奖励的活动；
5. 情绪不稳、反复无常（冲动，古怪）。

（二）边缘型

此种人格障碍的表现至少具备以下中的两点：

1. 对自己自我形象、目的及内心的偏好常常模糊不清；
2. 易于卷入强烈及不稳定的人际关系，可能会导致连续的情感危机；
3. 竭力避免被人遗弃；
4. 经常发生威胁或自伤行为；
5. 持续的空虚感。

V. Histrionic Personality Disorder

Histrionic personality disorder is characterized by pervasive and excessive emotionality and attention-seeking behaviors. The clients usually display shallow and labile affectivity, self-dramatization, theatricality, exaggerated expression of emotions, suggestibility, egocentricity, self-indulgence, lack of consideration for others, easily hurt feelings, and continuous seeking for appreciation, excitement and attention, and so forth. There are no differences in prevalence based on sex, race, or education. In the results of different studies, the ratios of gender are not consistent. It is occurs more commonly in females.

五、表演型人格障碍

表演型人格障碍以过分的感情用事或夸张言行吸引他人的注意为特征。患者常常表现出肤浅或易变的情感，戏剧化，夸张的情绪表达，暗示性高，以自我为中心，自我放纵，缺乏对他人的尊重，感情易受伤害，不停地追求他人的赞赏，追求刺激以及注意等。此种人格障碍与性别、种族和教育背景关系不大。男女比例在不同的研究中结果不一致，临床上以女性多见。

VI. Anankastic Personality Disorder

Anankastic personality disorder is a personality disorder characterized by a general pattern of concern with orderliness, perfectionism, excessive attention to details, mental and interpersonal control, and a need for control over one's environment, at the expense of flexibility, openness, and efficiency. It is approximately twice as common in men as in women. It is characterized by at least three of the following:

1. Feelings of excessive doubt and caution;
2. Preoccupation with details, rules, lists, order, organization, or schedule;
3. Perfectionism that interferes with task completion;
4. Excessive conscientiousness, scrupulousness, and undue preoccupation with productivity to the exclusion of pleasure and interpersonal relationships;
5. Excessive pedantry and adherence to social conventions;
6. Rigidity and stubbornness;
7. Unreasonable insistence by the individual that others submit exactly to his or her way of doing things or unreasonable reluctance to allow others to do things;
8. Intrusion of insistent and unwelcome thoughts or impulses.

六、强迫型人格障碍

强迫型人格障碍以整洁，完美主义，过分的注重细节，控制内心及人际关系，有控制其外部环境的需求，损害其灵活性、坦率和效率为特征。男性是女性2倍。此种人格障碍的表现至少具备以下中的三点：

1. 过分疑虑及谨慎；
2. 对细节、规则、条目、秩序、组织或计划过分关注；
3. 完美主义，以至影响了工作的完成；
4. 道德感过强，谨小慎微，过分看重工作成效而不顾乐趣和人际关系；
5. 过分迂腐，拘泥于社会习俗；
6. 刻板和固执；
7. 患者不合情理地坚持他人必须严格按自己的方式行事，或即使允许他人行事也极不情愿；
8. 有强加的，令人讨厌的思想或冲动闯入。

VII. Avoidant Personality Disorder

Avoidant personality disorder or anxious personality disorder is a behavior characterized by persistent feelings of tension, insecurity, and inferiority. The prevalence appears to be equally common in men and women. It is characterized by at least four of the following:

七、回避（焦虑）型人格障碍

回避型人格障碍，又称焦虑性人格障碍，是以持久和广泛的内心紧张、不安全、忧虑体验及自卑为特征。此种人格障碍的表现至少具备以下中的四点：

1. Persistent and pervasive feelings of tension and apprehension;

2. Belief that one is socially inept, personally unappealing, or inferior to others;

3. Excessive preoccupation with being criticized or rejected in social situations;

4. Unwillingness to become involved with people unless certain of being liked;

5. Restrictions in lifestyle because of need to have physical security;

6. Avoidance of social or occupational activities that involve significant interpersonal contact because of fear of criticism, disapproval, or rejection.

7. Overly sensitive to rejection and criticism.

1. 持续和泛化的紧张感与忧虑；

2. 相信自己在社交上笨拙，没有吸引力或不如别人；

3. 在社交场合总过分担心被人指责或拒绝；

4. 除非肯定受人欢迎，否则不肯与他人打交道；

5. 出于维护躯体安全感的需要，在生活风格上有许多限制；

6. 由于担心批评，指责或拒绝，回避那些与人密切交往的社交或职业活动；

7. 对拒绝与批评过分敏感。

VIII. Dependent Personality Disorder

Dependent personality disorder is defined as a pattern of relying excessively on others, lack of confidence and obedience. It is characterized by at least three of the following:

1. Encouraging or allowing others to make most of one's important life decisions;

2. Subordination of one's own needs to those of others on whom one is dependent, and undue compliance with their wishes;

3. Unwillingness to make even reasonable demands on the people one depends on;

4. Feeling uncomfortable or helpless when alone, because of exaggerated fears of inability to care for oneself;

5. Preoccupation with fears of being abandoned by a person with whom one has a close relationship, and of being left to care for oneself;

6. Limited capacity to make everyday decisions without an excessive amount of advice and reassurance from others.

八、依赖型人格障碍

依赖型人格障碍是以极端缺乏自信，顺从和依赖的行为模式为特征。此种人格障碍的表现至少具备以下中的三点：

1. 请求或同意他人为自己生活中大多数重要事情做决定；

2. 将自己的需求附属于所依赖的人，过分顺从他人的意志；

3. 不愿意对所依赖的人提出即使是合理的要求；

4. 由于过分害怕不能照顾自己，在独处时总感到不舒服或无助；

5. 沉陷于被关系亲密的人所抛弃的恐惧之中，害怕只剩下他一人来照顾自己；

6. 没有别人过多的建议和保证时做出日常决定的能力很有限。

Section 3 Treatment and Prevention

The treatment of persons with personality disorders is difficult and may seem impossible in some instances. Therapeutic interventions in the treatment of personality disorders include pharmacological therapy, and psychological interventions focused on the rebuilding

第三节 治疗和预防

人格障碍的治疗比较困难，其原则是在药物治疗和心理治疗的基础上着重强调人格重建，而且治疗年龄越早越好。

of the personality. The younger the client is at the time of intervention, the more positive the potential outcome.

I. Treatment

1. Psychological Therapy Psychotherapy is essential in the treatment of personality disorders and its application should be based on specific psychological data. The main purpose about psychotherapy is not to help the clients recover completely. It is expected to help the clients realize their defects of behavior, maintain stable emotions, and help them change gradually to establish healthy behavior patterns and develop better relationships with others.

2. Pharmacology Therapy At present, no special medication is available for the treatment of personality disorder. Although medications have no immediate effect on the treatment of personality disorders, they can provide some symptomatic relief of specific symptoms. Medications may be helpful in specific cases, including in the reduction of anger, impulsiveness, and mood instabilities. Carbamazepine and epamin can be used in the treatment of impulsive personality disorders. Antipsychotic medications can be used in the treatment of clients with dissocial personality disorder and obvious agitation. Anxiolytics are sometimes helpful for the clients with anxiety. Pharmacology therapy is generally not recommended for long-term and routine use.

II. Prevention of Personality Disorders

It is very difficult to change the behavior pattern of a client with personality disorder. The prevention of personality disorder is more important than the treatment after its development. Children should be provided health family and academic environments and allowed to grow-up in warm and friendly settings, with minimal stress and violence. Children should be provided with opportunities to develop open and trusting friendships and relationships.

一、治　疗

1. 心理治疗 心理治疗是本病的基本治疗方法，在应用时需注意根据患者的具体心理学资料进行个体化治疗。其主要目的不是帮助患者完全恢复，而是在稳定患者心理状况的前提下，促进患者性格的改变，帮助患者认识其人格的缺陷，帮助患者建立良好的行为模式以发展良好的人际关系。

2. 药物治疗 目前尚未发现对人格障碍有特效的药物，药物治疗只能对症治疗，改善症状，但不能解决根本问题。治疗主要针对冲动、攻击行为、情绪不稳定等极端行为。对冲动性人格障碍伴有脑电图改变者可试用苯妥英钠或卡马西平；社交紊乱型人格障碍出现兴奋躁动时，可给予抗精神病药；对具有焦虑表现者可用抗焦虑药物等。药物治疗一般不主张长期和常规使用。

二、预　防

事实表明，人格障碍形成后，很难矫正，因此预防尤其重要。应重视儿童早期教育，家庭、幼儿园、学校能对孩子的不良行为进行及时纠正，这对孩子的人格发展十分有益；社会应大力开展心理健康知识的宣传，实现家庭和睦，减少或消除家庭暴力和家庭纠纷，给孩子一个温暖的家，使孩子在民主、和谐的家庭中健康成长；学校教育要提倡团结友爱、互相帮助，在社会上创造一个良好的人际关系和生活氛围，有利于人格的健康成长和不良行为的纠正。

Section 4 Application of the Nursing Process

第四节 护理程序的应用

Nursing care of the clients with personality disorders is accomplished using the steps of the nursing process. All nurses, not just those working in psychiatric settings, should be familiar with the characteristics associated with personality-disordered individuals. More often than not, the personality disorder is not the reason for clients to seek medical or nursing attention; rather, clients present for the care of concurrent conditions. Clients with a personality disorder may present in a clinic with vague complaints or may present at a counseling center with depression. Nurses should initially recognize the personality disorder and, then, provide care to minimize the negative impact of the client's behaviors.

应用护理程序对人格障碍患者进行护理，除了医院的医务工作者外，社区及其他卫生部门也应该对人格障碍的特点有所了解。人格障碍患者常以其并存症状前来就诊，多表现出愤怒不满或抑郁。护士应首先认识到人格障碍患者的主要问题，然后再提供帮助，减少患者异常行为所导致的负面影响。

I. Nursing Assessment

一、护理评估

i. Biologic Assessment

The assessment of clients with personality disorders includes history of any prenatal and prenatal problems, diseases at childhood, nutrition status, sleep pattern, and abuse of psychoactive substance (time, types, amount, route).

（一）患者生理状况

患者出生时的情况，包括产前及围产期是否有问题，儿童青少年时期的疾病史，营养状况、睡眠情况、精神活性物质滥用情况（时间、种类、量、方法）。

ii. Psychological Assessment

1. Motivation Motivation should be assessed in order to determine possible causes of impulsive, self-destructive, anti-social and violent behaviors. To the fullest extent possible, the motivations, if any, for client behaviors should be assessed and evaluated.

（二）患者心理状况

1. 动机 评估引起患者冲动、自我破坏、反社会以及暴力行为的可能原因和动机。

2. Cognition The levels of client cognitive functioning (IQ), as well as attitudes of suspiciousness, paranoia, obsessive ideations, ability to make correct judgments, and senses of morality, shyness and remorse/guilt, should all be evaluated.

2. 认知 评估患者的认知功能（智力水平），患者是否有多疑、偏执、强迫观念，有无判断缺损、道德心、羞耻感、内疚感等。

3. Affectivity An evaluation of the client's generalized levels of affective functioning should include irritability, unstable emotions, indifference, vindictiveness, and hostility.

3. 情感方面 患者是否易激惹、情感不稳、冷漠、愤怒、敌视、后悔等。

4. Behavior Behavioral assessments should include consideration of the client's impulsive, aggressive, violent, self-injuring, and suicidal behavior patterns. Impulsivity should also be assessed. It can be identified by asking the clients if they have done things impulsively or spur of moment, have been hurt by their actions or have later regretted things they did impulsively. It is critical that clients with some types of personality disorders be assessed for the risk of suicide and self-injury, including

4. 行为 患者的行为有无目的性、有无恶作剧行为、好冲动、攻击行为、暴力行为，有无自杀、自伤行为等。评估患者是否在冲动时有伤害自己的行为，是否事后感到过后悔；对某些人格障碍的患者，评估其自杀和自伤的行为，包括药物、酒精成瘾或依赖等至关重要。护士应该直接询问患者是否有自

drug and alcohol abuse/dependence. The nurses should ask patients directly whether or not they have thought about or engaged in suicidal or self-injurious behaviors. If so, the nurses should continue to explore the behaviors: what is done, how it is done, its frequency, and the circumstances surrounding the self-injurious behavior.

5. Self-assessment It can be assessed if the client can realize self-defects, or improper behavior.

iii. Social Assessment

Individuals with personality disorders frequently have difficulty in maintaining intimate relationships, keeping long-term employment, and avoiding criminal behavior. They may have family/personal histories marked by parental discipline that was either absent or excessively authoritarian; family discipline may also have been erratic or inconsistent; and, some individuals may never have been held responsibility for the consequences of their behaviors. These individuals may also have chaotic personal and family histories. Assessment should consider all of these factors, as well as the possibility of mental disorders and levels of cognitive functioning among members of the client's family should also include evaluations of past and present functioning. The assessment should also reflect the familial, social, and community support available to the client, including friendships and frequency of contact with friends and family members.

II. Nursing Diagnosis

The common and possible nursing diagnoses for clients with various personality disorders are listed as following:

1. Anxiety related to empty inside, low self-esteem and unconscious conflict based on fear of abandonment.

2. Risk for other-directed violence related to irritability, negative role-modeling, and inability to tolerate frustration.

3. Risk for self-directed violence related to unstable emotion, irritability and distorting self-consciousness.

4. Risk for compromised human dignity related to sensitivity and suspiciousness.

5. Disturbed personal identity related to lack of self-confidence.

6. Impaired social interaction related to incorrect self-evaluation and lack of interpersonal skills.

7. Ineffective coping related to less self-control, unstable emotions, and an ineffective supportive system.

杀、自伤的想法或曾实施过自杀、自伤行为，如果患者有过这样的行为，护士需要进一步询问患者做了什么，怎样做的，发生的次数以及当时的周围环境等。

5. **自知力** 患者是否意识到自身个性缺陷与不适当的行为方式。

（三）社会因素

人格障碍的患者常无法维持亲密关系，无法长期维持工作，无法避免犯罪行为，应评估患者在青少年期有无品行问题，患者是否被公安、司法部门强制管教及判刑情况；患者与家人、亲友、邻居、共事者的人际关系；患者生活学习的周边环境、学校教育方式等；其行为对工作及角色功能的影响；患者的工作形式、工作表现如何；患者的家庭氛围，父母的教育方式，父母及家庭对患者的影响，以及家庭成员中有无犯罪、吸毒人员。

二、护理诊断

人格障碍患者常见的护理诊断如下：

1. **焦虑** 与内心空虚、低自尊和害怕被抛弃有关。

2. **有对他人施行暴力的危险** 与易激惹、负面榜样影响以及不能承受挫折有关。

3. **有对自己实行暴力的危险** 与情绪不稳定、易冲动及自我认识扭曲有关。

4. **有个人尊严受损的危险** 与敏感多疑有关。

5. **自我认同紊乱** 与缺乏自信心有关。

6. **社会交往障碍** 与不正确的自我评价和缺乏人际沟通技巧有关。

7. **应对无效** 与个人不能控制冲动、不能调节情绪、支持系统不足有关。

8. Hygiene/dressing self-care deficit related to excessive dependence on others and lack of confidence in life.

8. **卫生/穿着自理缺陷** 与过分依赖他人、对生活缺乏自信有关。

III. Nursing Care Plan

三、护理计划

i. Outcome Identification

（一）护理目标

The following criteria may be used for expectation of outcomes in the care of clients with personality disorders:

人格障碍的患者护理目标一般包含下列内容：

1. The client can identify the feeling of ease and anxiety and ease the anxiety in a suitable way;

1. 患者能识别轻松、焦虑的感觉，能够用适宜的方式来减轻焦虑；

2. The client can express anger and frustration in language, abreact impulsive mood in the way that the society could accept and has not hurt others;

2. 患者能用语言表达愤怒和受挫感，采用社会能接受的方式发泄冲动情绪，不发生伤人和毁物行为；

3. The client can express emotion in an appropriate way and remove the thought of self-mutilation from one's mind;

3. 患者能用合适的方式表达心中的感受，消除任何自我伤害的想法；

4. The client can confirm the behavior of low self-esteem, evaluate himself/herself correctly, to confirm their value, enhance self-confidence and self-esteem;

4. 患者能确认引起低自尊的行为，能够正确评价自己，确认自己的价值，增强自信及自尊；

5. The client can gradually accept the closeness from the medical personnel and others, evaluate the life situation according to the facts, and enhance mutual trust with others;

5. 患者能逐步接受医务人员及他人对自己的接近，能够据实评价生活情形，增加与他人的相互信任；

6. The client can evaluate himself/herself according to the facts, engage in daily activities with others, and enhance communication with others;

6. 患者能够据实进行自我评价，能与其他人从事一些日常活动，增加与他人的沟通；

7. The client can recognize his/her own manipulative behaviors, meet the needs in other appropriate ways, and no longer manipulate others to increase the sense of self-value;

7. 患者能承认自己的操纵行为，并能通过其他合适的方式满足其需求，不再以操纵别人来增加自我价值感；

8. The client can strengthen the self-confidence gradually and conduct basic daily activity with the help of the others.

8. 患者的自信心逐渐增强，并能在外界的帮助下进行简单的生活自理。

ii. Nursing Interventions

（二）护理措施

In formulating a care plan, the nurse analyzes and synthesizes the assessment data into a working hypothesis about central concerns for the client and his family, and if possibly, the community in which the client lives.

护士在全面分析和综合评估资料的基础上，制订针对患者及其家庭，包括其所居住社区在内的护理计划和措施。

1. Biologic Interventions These interventions will focus on the wide-ranging of client's biological/medical needs, including his ability to assume responsibility for personal hygiene and self-care. The evaluation should serve to highlight possible areas of concerns, including nutrition, sleep, medication management, and the management of psychotic episodes in patients with multiple needs.

1. 生理方面的护理 生理方面的护理措施应注重满足患者全面的生理或医疗需要，包括患者的个人卫生和自我照顾等。应注意评估患者的营养状况、睡眠状况、服用药物，对精神症状发作的处理等。

(1) Nutrition: Because many patients with

（1）营养：由于人格障碍的患者常常无法

personality disorders fail to maintain healthy diets, this aspect of the biological evaluation/intervention should consider all of the dynamics of the patient's diet and facilitate appropriate dietary interventions.

坚持健康饮食，护士应提供并协助患者摄入足够的营养。

(2) Sleep: Because many patients with personality disorders live unscheduled and disengaged lives, they frequently have scattered or irregular sleep patterns. This dynamic of assessment/intervention is designed to evaluate the patient's sleep patterns, educate the patient on issues of sleep, and design appropriate measures for establishing healthy sleeping patterns/routines.

（2）休息：由于许多患者生活无计划，睡眠不规律，护士应评估患者的睡眠形态，教育患者保证规律而充足的睡眠，并提供安静、舒适的睡眠环境。

(3) Medication security: It is critical that patients with personality disorders be educated about the medications prescribed for them and their possible interactions with legal and illegal substances. Clients who rely on medication to deal with stress or who are periodically suicidal are at high risk for the abuse of medications. Clients who experience significant side effects from medications are at high risk for noncompliance. The nurse must determine whether or not the client is following the prescribed regimen of medication, the effects of medication on the targeted symptoms, and whether or not the client is using other drugs-including over-the-counter medications-that are not prescribed and may interact with prescribed medications. The nurse must also assist the client in establishing an appropriate routine for taking prescribed medications, reporting side effects, and developing effective coping strategies for dealing with daily stress as an alternative to medication.

（3）保证用药安全：对人格障碍患者进行有关药物方面的教育至关重要，教育患者认识所服用药物，识别违禁药物。那些依靠药物来减轻压力的患者，或有自杀行为的患者常常会出现药物滥用，而那些出现过药物副作用的患者则常常不能坚持服用药物。护士必须明确患者是否遵医嘱服用药物，药物治疗效果如何，以及患者是否同时服用其他药物，包括是否过量服用药物等。护士应协助患者规律服药，教育患者及时报告药物副作用，并帮助患者应用有效的应对技巧以应对日常压力，而不是依赖药物。

2. Psychological Interventions

2. 心理干预

(1) Establishment of good interpersonal relationship: Individuals with personality disorders have difficulty in establishing healthy relationships. Therefore, nursing interventions designed to establish a therapeutic relationship require patience and planning. The purpose of the therapeutic relationship is to allow the client to experience model of health interactions. Clients with personality disorders, especially those who experience low self-esteem, will benefit from the experience of unconditional positive regard and the genuine respect of the nurse and other members of the therapeutic team. It should, however, be noted that such interventions often demand a great deal of time.

（1）与患者建立良好人际关系：人格障碍的患者常常无法建立健康的人际关系，因此，要与患者在治疗护理过程中建立治疗性护患关系，就需要护士的耐心和周密计划。治疗性护患关系的目的是能够让患者体验到健康的人际交往，特别是让那些自尊心差的患者恢复自信，并学会真正尊重护士及其他医务人员，一般需要护士花费很多的时间和精力。

(2) Positive encourage: Individuals with personality disorders frequently have problems recognizing and controlling their feelings and often respond quickly without thinking. Therefore, one of the primary therapeutic goals of intervention is to help patients learn to tolerate their feelings without acting on them. Therapy

（2）正性激励：人格障碍的患者常常很难认识和控制其情感，反应迅速但不假思索。因此，护理干预的目的之一是帮助患者学会控制情感，学会体验强烈的情感，但并不采取针对自己或他人的行动，为此，护士应对

is designed to help patients experience intense emotions without feeling compelled to act out-either against themselves or another person. In part, this is accomplished by providing patients with positive feedback or rewards for acceptable behavior.

患者可以接受的行为予以表扬和奖励。

(3) Nursing for client with trend of suicide: Clients who tend to entertain and/or act upon suicidal ideations can be taught to identify and cope appropriate with situations that lead to self-destructive behaviors. Because some clients are impulsive and may respond without thinking in stressful situations, it is important that clients learn and develop techniques for self-observation and how to use those in order to limit or eliminate dangerous behaviors.

（3）对有自杀倾向的患者：护士教育患者认识和恰当应对导致其自我破坏性行为的环境，因为一些患者往往在压力环境下很冲动，不假思索地做出反应。护士应教导患者学会并发展自我观察的技巧，在无法应对压力时采取这些行为以减少或消除危险行为。

3. Social Interventions

3. 社会干预

(1) Group therapy: Group therapy and milieu therapy are especially appropriate for clients with dissocial personality disorder, who respond more adaptively to support and feedback from peers; in group and milieu therapy, feedback from peers is more effective than in one-to-one interaction with a therapist. These modalities are helpful in overcoming social anxiety and developing interpersonal trust and rapport in clients with avoidant personality disorder. Feminist consciousness-raising groups can be useful in helping dependent clients struggling with social-role stereotypes.

（1）团体治疗：团体治疗或环境治疗尤其适合于社交紊乱型人格障碍的患者，治疗过程中同伴支持和反馈性团体治疗，效果明显好于治疗师一人对患者的干预。此治疗形式，可帮助回避型人格障碍的患者克服社会焦虑，建立信任和谐的人际关系。在团体治疗中强调男女平等的意识，有助于帮助依赖性人格障碍的患者承担其应有的社会角色。

(2) Social and family support: Social and family support offers reinforcement for positive change and may be useful for clients with dissocial, obsessive-compulsive, avoidant, and passive-aggressive personality disorders. Social skills training and assertiveness training teach alternative ways to deal with frustration. Some clients may be dependent on their family members. They need help in maintaining a separate identity, while staying connected to family members for social support. Family members sometimes help. The nurses can help them explore new relationships that can provide additional social contacts and support.

（2）社会家庭支持治疗：社会和家庭的支持能促进患者的行为产生积极的改变，尤其适合社交紊乱型人格障碍、回避型人格障碍以及依赖型人格障碍的患者。社会技能和患者的自信训练有助于患者应对生活中的挫折。一些患者也许过分依赖其家庭成员，应该帮助其能够保持自我独立，护士可帮助他们建立新的社会关系和支持。

4. Health education Client education within the context of a therapeutic relationship is one of the most important and empowering interventions. Teaching client's skills to better interact with others, resist suicidal urges, improve emotional self-regulation, enhance interpersonal relationships, tolerate stress, enhance overall quality of life, and provide the foundation for long-term behavioral changes. The nurses must keep in mind to remind the clients that change occurs slowly.

4. 健康教育 患者教育是最重要和有效的干预措施之一，护士应指导患者与他人友好交往的技巧，抵制自杀的欲望，提高患者情感自我调节能力，促进其人际关系，正确面对挫折和压力，提高患者的生活质量。所有这些患者教育可成为患者长期行为改变的基础，护士应时刻牢记并提醒患者，其行为改变是缓慢发生的。

IV. Nursing Evaluation

Effective behavior changes in clients with personality disorders are only accomplished over time. Therefore, both short-and long-term goals must be established and must reasonably reflect the realities of the client's life and circumstances. For a client with severe symptoms or a history of repeated self-inflicted injuries, client safety should be a realistic and primary goal. It is also important to recognize the necessity of maintaining the client's family and support systems as active members of the therapeutic process even after the client's discharge from the hospital.

Evaluation of the nursing interventions for the clients with personality disorders may be facilitated by gathering information using the following types of questions:

1. Can the client ease the anxiety in a suitable way?
2. Has injury to others been avoided?
3. Has injury to self been avoided?
4. Can the client evaluate himself/herself correctly and enhance self-confidence?
5. Can the client evaluate the life situation according to the facts and enhance mutual trust with others?
6. Can the client evaluate himself/herself according to the facts and enhance communication with others?
7. Does the client manipulate others in an attempt to have his or her own desires fulfilled?
8. Can the client conduct basic daily activity?

Treatment for individuals with personality disorders involves long-term therapy. Hospitalization is sometimes necessary during acute episodes. It is important for clients to continue with treatment in either in-patient or out-patient settings. They may need continued follow-up and long-term therapy including psychological education, individual therapy, pharmacological therapy and especially the establishment of effective family support systems.

(Wang Xiaoqin)

四、护理评价

由于人格障碍的特点，患者偏离正常的行为方式改变非常缓慢。治疗及护理的目标应注重长期目标。长期及短期目标必须与现实情况相符合。如有反复自残行为的患者，保证患者安全和生命为首要目标。若治疗期间目标未达到，应将情况介绍给家属和社会相关机构，使治疗能继续下去。评价内容主要包括：

1. 患者是否能用适宜的方式减轻焦虑？
2. 患者是否发生伤人和毁物？
3. 患者是否发生自伤行为？
4. 患者是否能正确评价自己，增强自信？
5. 患者是否据实评价生活情形，增加与他人的相互信任？
6. 患者是否能据实进行自我评价，增加与他人的沟通？
7. 患者是否不再以操纵别人来达到自己的目标？
8. 患者是否能进行简单的生活自理？

总之，人格障碍的治疗是一个长期的过程，入院治疗在急性发作期是必要的，更重要的是患者在出院后仍保持继续治疗，包括心理指导、个人应对措施的指导、药物治疗，最好能建立有效的家庭支持系统。

（王小琴）

Key Points

1. Personality traits are enduring patterns of perceiving, relating to, and thinking about the environment and oneself that are exhibited in a wide range of social and personal contexts.
2. Personality disorders are collections of traits that have become rigid and work to the individual's disadvantage, to the point that they impair functioning or cause distress. Once

内容摘要

1. 人格指个体在遗传与环境的交互作用下形成的稳定而独特的心理结构，在社会与生活环境中固有的行为模式和待人处事的习惯方法。
2. 人格障碍指人格特征明显偏离正常，使患者形成了一贯的反映个人生活风格和人际关系的异常行为模式。患者虽然无智能障碍，

these maladaptive behavior patterns are formed, it is difficult to correct by medical treatment, education or punishment.

3. The cause of personality disorders is not so clear, which involving genetic, biological, psychological, and social factors.

4. The subtypes of personality disorders include paranoid personality disorder, schizoid personality disorder, dissocial personality disorder, emotionally unstable personality disorder, histrionic personality disorder, Anankastic personality disorder, avoidant personality disorder, and dependent personality disorder.

但适应不良的行为模式一旦形成，通过医疗、教育或惩罚措施很难矫正。

3. 人格障碍的病因迄今尚不明确，可能涉及遗传、生物、心理、社会各个方面。

4. ICD-10列出的八种主要的人格障碍有偏执型人格障碍、分裂样人格障碍、社交紊乱型人格障碍、情绪不稳型人格障碍、表演型人格障碍、强迫型人格障碍、回避型人格障碍、依赖型人格障碍。

Exercises

(Questions 1 to 2 share the same question stem)

A 23-year-old librarian has been exceedingly shy and fearful of people since childhood. She longs to make friends but even casual social interactions cause her a great deal of shame and anxiety. She has never been at a party and she has requested to work in the least-active section of her library, even though this means lower pay. She cannot look at her rare customers without blushing and she is convinced that they see her as incompetent and clumsy.

1. What is the correct clinical diagnosis?

2. What is the anxiety disorder that is most likely to be confused with this personality disorder?

(Questions 3 to 4 share the same question stem)

A 24-year-old man is brought to the A&E Department after he has been arrested by the police for threatening behavior toward his ex-girlfriend. The man said that he has been killing his family pets for the last 5 years. The man has a long history of violence towards women. He has attacked girlfriends in the past, but they have never brought charges against him. He has never worked and continues to abuse cannabis, amphetamines and alcohol.

3. What is the correct clinical diagnosis?

4. What is the main nursing diagnosis for him?

(Questions 5 to 6 share the same question stem)

A 16 years old boy was appointed monitor when entering the high school, but his position was displaced after half semester due to he did not get on well with other classmates. He suspected the other boy framing him and thought he was suppressed and treated unfairly. Therefore, he often conflicts with teachers and classmates, and even sued to the headmaster and his parents. Although everybody tried to persuade him, he was always eager to

思考题

（1～2题共用题干）

患者，女，23岁，图书管理员，自诉从童年时期开始就非常害羞和怕人。即使她非常渴望交朋友，但即使平常的社会交往也会使她非常害羞和焦虑。她从来没有参加过聚会，并且要求在图书馆最不活跃的部门工作，这也意味着她的工资很低。她看到不太熟的读者总是会脸红，并且深信别人认为她很无能和笨拙。

1. 该患者正确的临床诊断是什么？

2. 最易与此种人格障碍混淆的焦虑障碍是什么？

（3～4题共用题干）

患者，男，24岁，因为威胁其前女友被警察带到急诊科。他陈述说他已经持续5年杀死他家中的宠物。他对妇女有着很长时间的暴力史。他过去对他的女朋友施暴，但是没有人控诉他。此外，他从不工作，长期滥用大麻、冰毒和酒精。

3. 该患者正确的临床诊断是什么？

4. 该患者目前最主要的护理诊断是什么？

（5～6题共用题干）

患者，男，16岁，刚升入高中被老师指定为班长，半学期后由于与同学关系不和，被撤掉班长一职。该生怀疑是另外一位同学因为嫉妒他而搞的鬼，认为自己受到压制及不公平待遇，为此该生经常与老师、同学发生冲突，甚至状告到校长和家长那里。虽然大家都耐心劝解他，但他总是急于辩解、对大家

explain who did not wait for you finish and his hostility to everyone. He threatened to appeal and revenge, which has no fundamental change until the end of semester.

5. What is the correct clinical diagnosis?

6. What is the major nursing diagnosis?

充满敌意，并且扬言要上告、伺机报复等，此种情形持续至学期末也无根本性变化。

5. 该患者正确的诊断是什么？

6. 患者目前存在最主要的护理问题是什么？

Chapter 9 Nursing Care of Clients with Trauma and Stressor-Related Disorders

第九章 创伤与应激相关障碍患者的护理

Learning Objectives

Memorization

1. Describe the concepts of stress, cognitive appraisal, stress responses, coping resources, and coping mechanisms.
2. Describe the types of crisis, phases in the development of a crisis, and steps in crisis intervention.
3. Describe appropriate nursing interventions for trauma and stressor-related disorders.

Comprehension

1. Discuss the importance of cognitive appraisal in experiencing stress.
2. Discuss various modalities relevant to treatment of trauma and stressor-related disorders.
3. Examine crisis intervention techniques to provide crisis intervention for a client experiencing crises.

Application

1. Apply the nursing process to clients experiencing trauma and stressor-related disorders.
2. Apply the nursing process to clients experiencing crises.
3. Evaluate nursing care of clients with post-traumatic stress disorder.

学习目标

识记

1. 能准确描述应激、认知评价、应激反应、应对资源和应对机制的概念。
2. 能准确描述危机的种类、危机发展的阶段以及危机干预的步骤。
3. 能准确说出创伤与应激相关障碍的护理干预措施。

理解

1. 能讨论认知评价在应激发展过程中的重要性。
2. 能讨论创伤与应激相关障碍的治疗方式。
3. 能准确分析恰当的危机干预技巧。

运用

1. 能运用护理程序为创伤与应激相关障碍的患者提供恰当的护理措施。
2. 能运用护理程序为经历危机的患者提供恰当的护理措施。
3. 评价创伤与应激相关障碍护理措施的效果。

Lily, age 23, witnessed the death of her younger brother in a car accident. During the past week, she has been having frequent flashbacks of the scene of the accident. She is having nightmares which result in her waking up frequently, is afraid of going out of her home, and becomes fearful when she hears loud noises.

Please think about the following questions based on the case:

1. What is the priority nursing diagnosis for Lily?
2. What are the most appropriate nursing interventions for Lily?

患者，莉莉，23岁，在一周前目睹弟弟车祸身亡。一周来脑海里不断闪现车祸现场的情形，晚上睡觉时噩梦连连，极易被惊醒，不敢出门，一听到声响就极度恐惧。

请思考：

1. 莉莉首要的护理诊断是什么？
2. 目前首先应当采取的护理措施是什么？

Stress is a natural part of life, and crises are inevitable in everyone's life. Mild forms of stress can motivate people to change, deal with everyday issues, or seek help for major life problems. However, in its severe forms, stress may create a substantial burden on the individual. Such trauma may come from child abuse or neglect, domestic violence, natural disasters, or warfare. Extreme stress can lead to severe and enduring reactions. Sometimes successfully coping with stress and surviving crises makes the difference between being mentally healthy and mentally ill. This chapter will explore a basic understanding of stress and crises, nursing management of trauma and stressor-related disorders and crisis intervention.

应激是日常生活中不可避免的现象，每个人在一生中有可能经历不同形式的应激。轻度应激能够促进个体成长，更好地应对日常生活事件，或者通过寻求帮助，有效地解决问题。然而，过度应激将对个体产生严重而持久的反应，甚至造成创伤。此类创伤可来自儿童期遭受虐待的经历、家庭暴力、自然灾害或战争等。成功地应对应激和危机是预防心理疾病、保持心理健康的关键。本章将主要介绍应激和危机的基本理论知识、创伤与应激相关障碍的护理及危机干预。

Section 1 Introduction

第一节 概 述

Understanding the basis of stress is the foundation for nursing management of trauma and stressor-related disorders. This section will introduce the concepts of stress, cognitive appraisal, stress responses, coping resources, and coping mechanisms.

了解应激是护理创伤和应激相关障碍的基础。本节将介绍应激、认知评估、应激反应，应对资源和应对机制的概念。

I. Stress

一、应 激

Various researchers of this century have contributed to different concepts of stress. Three of these concepts include stress as a biological response, stress as an environmental event, and stress as a transaction between the individual and the environment. The latter offered a new approach to understanding stress, which is consistent with the biopsychosocial perspectives of psychiatric mental health nursing practice, and is usually as a framework for understanding stress. The experience

应激是一个复杂的概念，不同学科对应激有不同的解释。但目前普遍认为应激可以从三个不同的层面来解释：应激是一种生理反应；应激是一种环境事件；应激是个体和环境之间的互动。其中强调互动的“应激、应对与适应”模型提供了理解应激的新视角，与精神心理实践中的生物－心理－社会模型

of stress, the individual's responses, coping, and the adaptation model are depicted in figure 9-1. Lazarus and Folkman (1984) define stress as a relationship between the person and the environment that is appraised by the person as taxing or exceeding his or her resources and endangering his or her well-being. This definition of stress emphasizes the relationship between the individual and the environment. Personal characteristics as well as the nature of the environmental event are considered. This illustration parallels the modern concept of the etiology of disease. No longer is causation viewed solely as an external organism; whether or not illness occurs depends on the receiving organism's susceptibility. Similarly, to predict psychological stress as a reaction, the properties of the person in relation to the environment must be considered.

一致，是现代应激理论最为常用的一种框架（图 9-1）。在本章中，应激被认为是个体与环境之间的互动，个体认识到需求与实际的或满足需求的能力不平衡，觉察到威胁时所作出的适应过程。Lazarus 和 Folkman（1984）认为，应激既不是环境刺激，也不是人的性格或反应，而是人与环境相互作用的产物。当人对内外环境刺激做出判断，认为它超过自身应对能力及应对资源时，就会产生压力。因此，压力是由于内外需求与有机体应对资源的不匹配，从而破坏了人体的平衡所致。Lazarus 和 Folkman 强调，应激源作用于有机体后，能否产生压力，主要取决于两个重要的心理学过程：认知评价和应对。

II. Cognitive Appraisal

Determination that a particular personal/environmental relationship is stressful depends on the individual's cognitive appraisal of the situation. Cognitive appraisal is an individual's evaluation of the personal significance of the event or

二、认知评价

认知评价是指个体觉察到情境对自身是否有影响的认知过程。主要的心理活动包括感知、思考、推理及决策等。认知评价影响

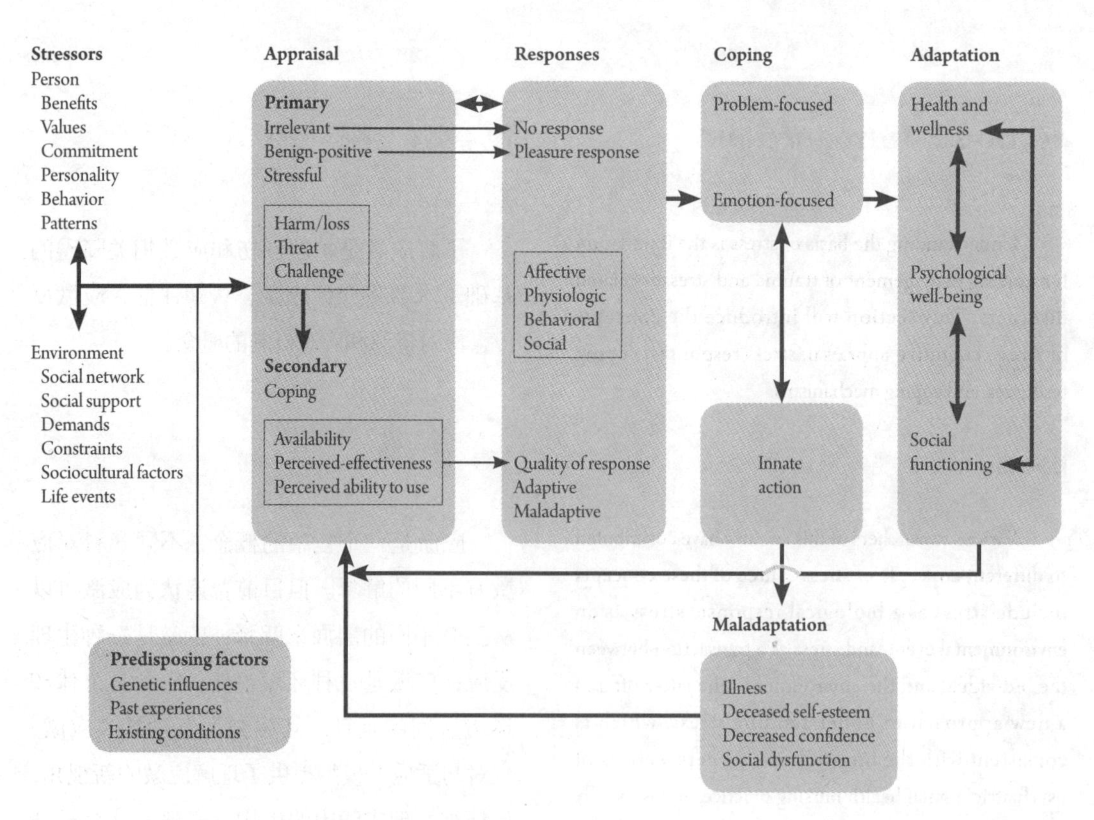

Figure 9-1 Stress, coping, and adaptation model

occurrence. Cognitive factors play a central role in adaptation. They affect the impact of stressful events; the choice of coping patterns used; and the emotional, physiological, and behavioral reactions. The cognitive response consists of a primary appraisal and a secondary appraisal.

i. Primary Appraisal

Lazarus and Folkman (1984) identified three types of primary appraisal including irrelevant, benign-positive, and stressful. Stressful appraisals include harm/loss, threat, and challenge. Harm/loss appraisals refer to damage or loss already experienced by the individual. Appraisals of a threatening nature are perceived as anticipated harms or losses. When an event is appraised as challenging, the individual focuses on potential for gain or growth, rather than on risks associated with the event. Those who view stress as a challenge are more likely to transform events to their advantage and thus reduce their level of stress.

ii. Secondary Appraisal

When stress is produced in response to harm/loss, threat, or challenge, a secondary appraisal is made by the individual. This secondary appraisal is an assessment of skills, resources, and knowledge that the person possesses to deal with the situation. The individual evaluates what coping strategies are available to me, will the option I choose be effective in this situation, and do I have the ability to use that strategy in an effective manner.

The interaction between the primary appraisal of the event that has occurred and the secondary appraisal of available coping strategies determines the individual's quality of adaptation response to stress.

III. Stress Responses

i. Affective Responses

An affective response is the arousal of a feeling. In the appraisal of a stressor, the predominant affective response is a nonspecific or generalized anxiety reaction. This generalized anxiety response becomes expressed as emotions. These may include joy, sadness, fear, anger, acceptance, distrust, anticipation, or surprise.

个体生理、心理和行为反应，最终会影响应激的结局。认知评价包含两种方式：原发性评价与继发性评价。

（一）原发性评价

发生于个体觉察到自身濒临某种事件或情境时，是对事件或情境本身的评价，它所关注的是所遇到事件的结果对个人是有益的还是有害的。初级评价的结果有三种：与个人无关、有益的或应激的。应激的评价包括伤害、威胁及挑战。伤害性评价的性质一般与真实或预期的丧失有关，这种损伤一般对个体的身心健康或资源有较大的损害；当个体评价应激事件是威胁性的，说明预期的丧失将要发生；当事件被评价为具有挑战性时，其感情基调是兴奋及期待，也包含焦虑与不安的成分。

（二）继发性评价

当应激被个体感知为丧失、威胁或挑战时，个体就会进行继发性评价。它是对个体应对能力及资源的评价，判定个体的应对技巧与情境事件之间的匹配程度。它所要回答的问题是“在这种情况下我应该作什么”“所选择的方法是否有效”“我是否有能力运用该策略取得有效结果”等。继发性评价可以改变初评的结果。对应激事件的初级评价和对应对策略及资源的继发性评价相互影响，共同决定个体适应性反应的质量及水平。

三、应激反应

（一）情绪反应

在应激过程中，如果机体的应对能力不能适应环境的变化，不能有效地控制应激，就会产生心理挫折，而引起一系列情绪反应。情绪反应主要有焦虑、愤怒、恐惧、情绪消沉、失望、抑郁等负性行为，甚至发生攻击性行为（包括攻击事物、他人或自身），严重时可发生自杀行为，也会产生如快乐、接受等正性情绪。

ii. Physiological Responses

Physiological responses reflect the interaction of several neuroendocrine axes involving growth, hormone, prolactin, adrenocorticotropic hormone (ACTH), luteinizing and follicle-stimulating hormones, thyroid-stimulating hormones, vasopressin, oxytocin, insulin, epinephrine, norepinephrine, and a variety of other neurotransmitters in the brain. The fight or flight physiological response stimulates the sympathetic division of the autonomic nervous system and increases activity of the pituitary-adrenal axis. Additionally, stress can affect the body's immune system, and the ability to defend the individual's body against disease.

iii. Behavioral Responses

Behavioral responses reflect emotions and physiological changes as well as cognitive analysis of the stressful situation. Caplan (1981) described the following four phases of an individual's response to a stressful event:

Phase 1 Shock　It is characterized by behaviors that change the stressful environment or allow the individual to escape from it.

Phase 2 Transaction　Behaviors that allow the individual to change the external circumstances and their aftermath are present.

Phase 3 Emotional changes　This is characterized by intrapsychic behaviors to defend against unpleasant emotional arousal.

Phase 4 Rebalance　It is characterized by intrapsychic behaviors to come to terms with the event and its consequences by internal readjustment.

iv. Social Responses

Social responses to stress include three aspects. The first aspect is the search for meaning in which people

（二）生理反应

在应激状态时，下丘脑－垂体－甲状腺轴、肾上腺轴以及性腺轴均受到影响，导致腺体功能亢进，激素分泌增多。表现为心率加快、血压升高、胃肠蠕动减慢，伴出汗、呼吸加快、手足发凉等现象。此外，垂体前、后叶兴奋，垂体前叶兴奋能使肾上腺皮质系统大量释放糖皮质激素和盐皮质激素，影响机体的免疫功能和抗病能力。

（三）行为反应

行为反应是个体对应激环境的评价以及情绪及生理变化产生的结果。Kaplan将个体应激的行为反应分为四期：

第一期－冲击期　当个体遭受应激后，处于一种“茫然”休克状态，表现出某种程度的定向力障碍和注意力分散，一般持续数分钟到几小时。这时，个体主要采取改变环境或远离应激源的行为。在应激状态下，人们可采取逃避或回避的方式来应对应激源。

第二期－混乱期　以明显的混乱及变化不定为特点，并伴有情绪障碍，如焦虑、抑郁或暴怒等表现。此时，个体行为表现以改变外部环境（应激源而不是自身）及其影响为特点。它包括消除或减弱应激源的条件活动。例如，工作环境、家庭环境、人际环境的改善等或采取否认、投射、隔离等机制对抗不愉快情绪反应。

第三期－情绪影响期　个体主要通过内心自我调试以适应应激所带来的情绪反应。

第四期－再平衡期　包括重建和再度平衡。个体可通过调整自己的想法、行为、应对策略等，对环境挑战，对应对效果做出新的解释，以减轻应激所引起的紧张和内心痛苦。其结果是可出现功能的增强，也可出现心理的、躯体的或人际关系之间的障碍，甚至可能慢性迁延。

（四）社会反应

应激的社会反应主要分为三方面。第一方面为寻找有关问题的信息，以采取应对性

seek information about their problem. This is necessary for devising a coping strategy because only through understanding what is occurring can a person come up with a reasonable response. The second aspect is social attribution, in which the person tries to identify the factors that contributed to the situation. Clients who see their problem as resulting from their own negligence may be blocked from an active coping response. They may see their problems as a sign of their personal failure and engage in self-blame and passive, withdrawn behavior. The third aspect of social response is social comparison, in which people compare skills and capacities with those of others with similar problems. A person's self-assessment depends heavily on those with whom comparisons are made. The outcome is an evaluation of the need for support from the person's social network or support system. Predisposing factors such as age, developmental level, and cultural background, as well as the characteristics of the precipitation stressor, determine the perceived need for social support.

策略。只有了解问题的实质，才能找到合理的应对方法。第二方面为寻找导致目前状况的影响因素。如果认为是由于自身疏忽造成，个体将处于极大的自责之中，并产生消极和退缩行为。第三方面从技巧、能力等方面与有过同样问题的人进行对比。比较的结果将有助于判断需要帮助和支持的程度。年龄、发展水平、文化背景、应激源的特点等都决定了社会支持的情况。

IV. Coping Resources and Coping Mechanisms

i. Coping Resources

Coping resources include economic assets, abilities and skills, defensive techniques, social supports, and motivation. Other coping resources include health and energy, positive beliefs, problem-solving and social skills, social and material resources, and physical well-being.

Viewing oneself positively can serve as a basis of hope and can sustain a person's coping efforts under the most adverse circumstances. Problem-solving skills include the ability to search for information, identify the problem, weigh alternatives, and implement a plan of action. Social skills facilitate the solving of problems involving other people, increase the likelihood of getting cooperation and support from others, and give the individual greater social control. Finally, material assets refer to money and the goods and services that money can buy. Obviously, monetary resources greatly increase a person's coping options in almost any stressful situation. Knowledge and intelligence are other resources that allow people to see different ways of dealing with stress. Finally, coping resources also include a strong ego identity, commitment to a social network, cultural stability, a stable system of values and beliefs, a preventive health orientation, and genetic or constitutional strength.

ii. Coping Mechanisms

Coping mechanisms can be defined as any efforts

四、应对资源及应对机制

（一）应对资源

应对资源主要包括个人的经济状况、能力和技巧、社会支持情况。另外，个体的健康状况、问题解决技巧、积极的自我认识、社会交往能力等也是影响应激的资源。

对自身持有积极评价是个体怀抱希望的基础，使其在困难情况下也不放弃努力。解决问题的技巧包括寻求信息，确认问题、权衡不同方法的利弊、实施计划等方面。社会技能主要指通过与他人合作，寻求支持，促进问题的解决，提高个体社会控制力。当然，经济状况，如金钱、物质等资源也会增加应激情境下个体应对选择的机会。知识和智力水平也能作为应激资源，使个体在处理应激时能灵活采用不同的应对方法。另外，应对资源还包括自我认知、良好的社交网络体系结构、稳定的文化环境、稳定的价值和信仰系统、预防为主的健康取向以及遗传的优势等。

（二）应对机制

应对机制主要指为了适应应激而采取的

directed at stress management. There are two main types of coping mechanisms:

1. Problem Focused Coping Mechanisms These involve tasks and direct efforts to cope with the threat itself. Examples include negotiation, confrontation, and seeking advice.

2. Emotion Focused Coping Mechanisms These include the perspective by which the client is oriented to moderating emotional distress. Examples include the use of ego defense mechanisms such as denial, suppression, or projection.

各种措施及方法。根据应对的指向性可以将应对机制分为问题取向和情绪取向两种：

1. **问题取向机制** 主要指个体针对已察觉的问题采取积极的努力，寻求解决问题，或者回避问题。如协商、勇敢地面对、寻求建议等。

2. **情绪取向机制** 侧重于调节和控制应激时的情绪反应，从而降低心理不适状态。如启动否认、压抑或投射等自我防御机制。

Section 2 Trauma and Stressor-Related Disorders

第二节 创伤与应激相关障碍

I. Introduction

一、概 述

Trauma and stressor-related disorder is a condition of mental disorder caused by psychosocial elements. The factors determining the occurrence, development, duration and clinical manifestations of this disorder are life events or conditions, such as severe super-strong mental trauma of life events or continuous difficult situations; social cultural background; personality traits, level of intelligence, attitudes toward life and creed; excluding hysteria, neurosis, and physiologic disorders associated with psychological factors and psychotic disorders.

创伤与应激相关障碍指一组主要由心理、社会（环境）因素引起的异常心理反应，导致的精神障碍，也称心因性精神障碍。其共同特点为心理社会因素是发病的直接原因；症状表现与心理社会因素的内容有关；病程、预后与精神因素的消除有关；病因大多为剧烈或持久的精神创伤因素，如战争、亲人突然死亡、经历重大灾害事故、罹患重大疾病、被强奸、失恋、家庭矛盾等；一般预后良好，无人格方面的缺陷。它不包括癔症、神经症、心理因素所致生理障碍，及各种非心因性精神病性障碍。

According to *ICD-10*, trauma and stressor-related disorder is divided into three types including acute stress disorder, post-traumatic stress disorder, and adjustment disorder.

在我国，根据*ICD-10*标准，将创伤与应激相关障碍主要分为急性应激障碍（acute stress disorder，ASD）、创伤后应激障碍（post-traumatic stress disorder，PTSD）和适应性障碍三种类型。

i. Definition

（一）定义

1. Acute Stress Disorder (ASD) It is a transient psychotic disorder which is directly caused by exceptionally severe or continued psychological traumatic events, and the onset occurs within an hour.

1. **急性应激障碍** 又称急性心因性反应，是由于突如其来且异乎寻常的强烈应激性生活事件所引起的一过性精神障碍。在受刺激后立刻（1小时之内）发病。常在几天至一周内恢复。如应激源及时消除，症状缓解完全，预后良好。

2. Post-Traumatic Stress Disorder (PTSD) also known as delayed psychogenic reaction, arises as a delayed and/or protracted reaction to a stressful event or situation of an exceptionally threatening or catastrophic nature. PTSD is characterized by the development of a long-lasting anxiety response following a traumatic or catastrophic event.

3. Adjustment Disorder is defined as having affective symptoms, behavioral symptoms with poor adjustment and physiological disorders, which is caused by prolonged presence of a stressor or difficult situation, and the client's personality deficit.

2. **创伤后应激障碍** 又称延迟性心因性反应，是由异乎寻常的威胁性或灾难性心理创伤，导致延迟出现和/或持久的精神障碍，以持续出现的创伤体验及焦虑为特点。

3. **适应性障碍** 是一种短期的和轻度的烦恼状态及情绪失调，常影响到社会功能，但不出现精神病性症状。

ii. Epidemiology

Rates of trauma and stressor-related disorders vary depending upon the definitions and diagnostic criteria being used. ASD occurs in individuals of all ages, with young people being affected most frequently. The prevalence rate of PTSD must take into consideration the characteristics of the event. Men have a higher rate of exposure to more traumatic events but the incidence rate of PTSD in females versus males is about 2 to 1. According to the *DSM-Ⅳ*, the prevalence rates of PTSD are 5% and 10.4% across the lifespan for male and female clients, respectively, between 15 and 24 years of age, and 60.7% and 51.2% after exposure to traumatic events. Adjustment disorder is most frequently diagnosed in adolescents but may occur at any age. In the adult population, single women are generally overly represented as being the most at-risk group. Adjustment disorder is one of the most common psychiatric diagnoses among clients hospitalized for medical/surgical problems.

（二）流行病学

由于概念和诊断标准不一致，创伤与应激相关障碍发病率的统计结果也有差异。ASD可发生于任何年龄，青年人多见。同一创伤性事件中，年龄较大更可能患PTSD，但也有研究不支持这一观点。男性比女性更多暴露于创伤性事件，但女性的PTSD发病率是男性的两倍。依据*DSM-IV*诊断标准，美国一项针对15～24岁的社区人群的调查显示，终生患病率男性为5%，女性为10.4%；暴露于创伤性事件后PTSD的发生率男性为60.7%，女性为51.2%。国内在张北（中国，河北省）地震受灾群体中的调查发现，3个月和9个月内PTSD的发生率分别为18.8%和24.2%。适应障碍可发生于任何年龄，但以青春期少年为主，在成年人群中，单身妇女被认为发病危险因素最高。同时，适应障碍是住院治疗的内、外科患者最常见的心理问题。

iii. Prognosis

Social support, family history, childhood experiences, personality style, and other disorders may influence recovery. The overall prognosis of trauma and stressor-related disorder is generally favorable with appropriate treatment. If treated in time, a client with an acute stress disorder can recover, and the individual's mental condition can be normal. PTSD tends to have a chronic, fluctuating course, often associated with other problems, including substance abuse and mood disorders. Individuals often use illicit substances or alcohol to escape or to enhance numbing from the emotional pain. For those clients having PTSD, 30% will recover completely, 40% will have persistent minor symptoms, 20% will have persistent major symptoms, and the remaining 10%

（三）预后

社会支持、家庭历史、儿童时期的经历、个性心理特征等都会影响疾病的康复。一般预后良好，无人格缺陷。ASD经及时治疗，预后良好，精神状态可完全恢复正常。PTSD病程多为慢性、波动性，同时伴有物质滥用和情绪障碍等，约30%会完全恢复，约40%余有轻微症状，约20%余有重度症状，约10%症状不变或恶化。适应障碍患者经过适当治疗后的预后通常较理想，大多数人可以在几周或几个月内恢复到以往的功能状态。然而，慢性应激源，如患病等可使病程延长；青春

will have no relief of symptoms or their condition will deteriorate. Once identified, the course of adjustment disorder is usually limited to weeks or months. However, chronic stressors, such as ongoing medical illness or chronic marital stress, may result in a longer course. Adolescents usually require a longer time to recover than do adults. Some people may be at risk for suicide because of the nature and severity of their responses. Left untreated, clients with these disorders may progress to mood and anxiety disorders.

期少年恢复需更多时间；部分人可能有自杀倾向。如果不经治疗，适应障碍可发展为情绪障碍或焦虑障碍。

II. Etiology and Mechanism

二、病因及发病机制

The mechanism of trauma and stressor-related disorder is complicated and not clear. Three factors which influence its occurrence, development, course and manifestations are as follows: a. stressful life events (their degree, quantity, duration, and reversibility) and an unhappy environment; b. individual susceptibility, including family history and past history of mental disorders, psychological trauma during childhood (sexual abuse, parents divorced when child is younger than 10 years of age), personality changes or history of neurosis, other negative life events before or after traumatic events, low family economic status and poor physical health; c. cultural tradition, education background and beliefs.

创伤与应激相关障碍的发病机制比较复杂，至今仍未完全阐明。影响创伤与应激相关障碍的发生、发展、病程及临床表现的因素大致可归纳为三个方面。① 应激性生活事件（如程度、数量、持续时间、可逆性等）或不愉快的处境。② 个体易感性包括精神障碍的家族史与既往史；童年时代的心理创伤（如遭受性虐待、10 岁前父母离异）；性格内向及有神经质倾向；创伤性事件前后有其他负性生活事件；家境差；躯体健康状态欠佳等。③ 文化传统、教育水平及生活信仰等。

Severe psychological traumatic events, stressing life events, and continued difficult situations are the direct causes of ASD. In PTSD, the events are extremely stressful, life threatening, and beyond most individuals' usual experience. The traumatic event involves a personal experience of threatened death, injury, or threat to physical integrity. It may also include witnessing such an event happening to another person or learning that a family member or close friend has experienced such an event. Adjustment disorder is a maladaptive reaction to a significant life change or stressful event. The occurrence and degree of severity of adjustment disorder are affected by stressors, the environment and the client's personal context.

剧烈的精神创伤或应激性生活事件，或持续的艰难处境是 ASD 发病的直接因素。PTSD 发生多与经历创伤性事件有关，应激源一般较为激烈，危及个人生命安全。同时，当目睹他人，或听说自己家人和朋友经历创伤性事件时，也可导致 PTSD 的发生。适应障碍的发生是对某一明显的生活变化或应激性生活事件所表现的不适反应，适应障碍的发生及其程度，除了受应激源特点影响外，还受环境及个性心理特征的制约。

III. Types and Clinical Manifestations

三、常见类型和临床表现

i. ASD

（一）急性应激障碍

By definition, acute stress reaction disappears within days and often within hours of the stressor. Individual vulnerability and coping style may affect the severity and occurrence of acute stress reaction since most individuals

急性应激反应发病急，一般在遭受超强应激性生活事件的影响后几分钟出现症状。临床表现有较大变异性，受个体易感性和应

who are exposed to major stressors do not develop this disorder. The symptoms usually are transient, with favorable prognosis, and complete remission, if the stressor is delimited. The traumatic events that can lead to an acute stress reaction are of similar severity to those involved in post-traumatic stress disorder.

对能力等综合因素的影响。

In the acute stage, ASD is characterized by:

1. Conscious disorder which includes symptoms such as a mixture of an initial state of "daze", narrowing of attention, reduced levels of consciousness, disorientation and amnesia.

在急性发病期，主要表现为：

1. 以意识障碍为主的表现。患者多表现为定向力障碍、注意狭窄、言语缺乏条理、动作杂乱、对周围事物感知迟钝、可有人格解体、偶见冲动行为、有的可出现片段的心因性幻觉。患者事后常对发病情况出现部分遗忘。

2. Psychomotor inhibition with affective vlunting which includes symptoms of dull appearance of the eyes, loss of expression, emotional slowness, behavior withdrawal, limited movement and vocalization, or even stupor.

2. 以伴有情感迟钝的精神运动性抑制为主的表现。患者表现为目光呆滞、表情茫然、情感迟钝、行为退缩、少语少动，甚至出现缄默、对外界刺激毫无反应的木僵状态。此型历时短暂，一般不超过一周。有的可转入兴奋状态。

3. Psychomotor hyperactivity with excessive fear which includes symptoms of agitation, excitement, impulsivity and destructive behavior.

3. 以伴有强烈恐惧体验的精神运动性兴奋为主的表现。患者表现为激越、兴奋、活动过多、有冲动、毁物行为。

4. Severe emotional problems, such as depression and anxiety (eg, sweating, increased heart rate, and flushing).

4. 部分患者可伴有严重的情绪障碍，如焦虑、抑郁；也可同时伴有自主神经症状，如大汗、心悸、面色苍白等。以上症状可单独出现，也可混合出现，在不同患者的表现上有较大差异。

ii. PTSD

PTSD is a set of reactions to an extreme stressor. These reactions include intense fear, helplessness, or horror that leads individuals to relieve the trauma. Individuals with PTSD develop three groups of symptoms containing intrusive re-experiencing of the trauma, hyperarousal, and avoidance behaviors. Symptoms can develop acutely, within 3-6 months of exposure to the traumatic event, or chronically, several years later. Three variables have been identified as affecting the development of PTSD involved in preexisting personality, extent, duration and intensity of trauma involved, and environment. Higher levels of anxiety, lower self-esteem, and existing personality difficulties may increase the likelihood, as may the severity of the event. If trauma survivors have a strong support network, and if they were able to aid others during the trauma or disaster, they may handle stressful events better and be less prone to develop PTSD. The onset of mental disorders follows the

（二）创伤后应激障碍

PTSD 是对重大应激源的一组反应，包括严重害怕、无助或者恐惧，使个体远离创伤。它主要包括三大表现，即闯入性症状、回避症状和警觉性增高症状。精神障碍可急性发生，在遭受创伤后 3~6 个月出现，也可延迟到数年之后才发生。影响 PTSD 发生的因素包括个性特点，创伤的范围、持续时间及强度以及环境因素。一般来讲，焦虑程度高、自尊低、有现存人格障碍者，创伤事件对其影响的严重程度较高；具有良好的支持系统，或自己曾帮助他人度过创伤或灾难者，能够更好地处理应激事件，相对不易发展为 PTSD。

trauma with a latency period ranging from a few days to months. Sometimes, the duration may be over many years.

Symptoms of PTSD include:

1. Intrusive symptoms which has primary manifestations of repeated reliving of the trauma in intrusive memories (flashbacks), dreams or feelings of affiliation and involuntary repeated recall when faced with situations similar or related to the original stimulus, and nightmares.

(1) Flashbacks: that is, without the influence of any factors or related objects, traumatic scenarios repeatedly appear in the patient's associations and memories involuntarily, or cause the patient to experience illusions, hallucinations, as if completely in the trauma situation. Reappear the various strong emotional reactions and obvious physiological reactions that accompanied the trauma, such as rapid heartbeat, sweating, and pale complexion. The duration can vary from a few seconds to a few days.

(2) Involuntary repeated recall when faced with situations similar or related to the original stimulus: strong emotional pain or physical reaction when exposed to a traumatic event or similar events, situations or other clues. Such as the anniversary of the event, similar weather and various scene factors may trigger the patient's psychological and physical reactions.

(3) Nightmare: The symptoms of intrusion will appear in the form of nightmare during sleep, manifested as recurring traumatic events or nightmares in the patient's dream.

2. Sustained avoidance which includes avoidance of cues which act as reminders of the traumatic event, the response to general events appears numb, reflecting the patient's attempts to stay away from trauma physically and emotionally. Mainly manifested as:

(1) Avoidance: avoiding things and environments that may evoke scary memories, avoiding talking about topics related to trauma. Media interviews after traumatic events and the process of obtaining evidence involving legal procedures often bring great pain to patients. selective amnesia of some important aspects of traumatic events is also one of the manifestations of avoidance. Other factors, such as personality changes, or some patients with a history of neurosis, have severe symptoms due to limited coping strategies.

(2) Numbness: the patients dominated with numbness in general. It is manifested as slow response to general stimuli in the surrounding environment. The patient himself feels that it is difficult to be interested in anything. The activities that he was passionate about in the past are not interested now. The patients have social

创伤后应激障碍的症状包括：

1. 闯入性症状具体表现为无法控制地以各种形式重新回忆创伤经历和体验，包括闯入性记忆（闪回），严重的触景生情反应和梦魇。

（1）闪回：即在无任何因素或相关物体的影响下，创伤情景经常不由自主地出现在患者的联想和记忆中，或使患者出现错觉、幻觉，仿佛又完全置身创伤性事件发生时的情景，重新表现出事件发生时所伴发的各种强烈情感反应和明显的生理反应，如心跳加快、出汗、面色苍白，持续的时间可从数秒钟到几天不等。此种短暂“重演”性发作的现象称为“闪回”。

（2）严重的触景生情反应：暴露于与创伤性事件相关联或类似的事件、情景或其他线索时，出现强烈的情感痛苦或生理反应。如事件发生的周年纪念日、相近的天气及各种场景因素都可能促发患者的心理与生理反应。

（3）梦魇：闯入性症状还会在睡眠状态中以梦魇的形式出现，表现为患者梦中反复重现创伤性事件或做噩梦。

2. 回避症状　回避与创伤性事件有关的刺激，对一般事件的反应显得麻木，反映了患者试图在生理和情感上远离创伤。主要表现为：

（1）回避表现：回避可能勾起恐怖回忆的事情和环境，回避谈及与创伤有关的话题。在创伤性事件后的媒体访谈及涉及法律程序的取证过程往往给患者带来极大的痛苦。对创伤性事件的某些重要方面选择性遗忘也是回避的表现之一。另外一些其他因素，如个性改变，或者有神经症病史的个别患者，由于应对能力的限制，症状较重。

（2）麻木表现：在总体上给人以木然、麻痹的感觉。表现为对周围环境的一般刺激反应迟钝，患者自己感到似乎难以对任何事情发生兴趣，过去热衷的活动现在都不感兴趣，感到与外界疏远、隔离，甚至格格不入，难以表达及感受各种细腻的情感，对未来失去

withdrawal, isolated, or even incompatible with the outside world. It is difficult to express and feel various delicate emotions, loss of longing for the future, and even committed suicide.

3. Sustained hypervigilance which includes intense arousal and anxiety on exposure to trauma cues, reflecting the patient's long-term "fighting" or "flight" state against the traumatic event. Symptoms of hypervigilance are most common in the first month after trauma exposure. The specific manifestations are: (a) it is being easily startled and disturbance of sleep, difficult for people to sleep or wake up easily; (b) startle reactions, such as encountering some similar scenes or slight sensory stimuli, showing that they are easily frightened, and there are panic reactions, such as nervousness, fear, palpitation, and heartbeat, Pale, cold sweats; (c)It's difficult to be focused. There are several scales are used to assess the clinical manifestations of PTSD. Figure 9-2 shows one of them.

信心，甚至自杀。

3. 警觉性增高症状表现为自发性的高度警觉状态，反映患者长时间处于对创伤事件的“战斗”或“逃跑”状态。警觉性过高的症状在创伤暴露后的第一个月最为普遍。具体表现为：① 难以入睡或易醒。② 易产生惊跳反应，如遇到一些类似的场面或轻微的感觉刺激表现出容易受惊吓，出现惊恐反应，如紧张、恐惧、心慌、心跳、面色苍白、出冷汗等；或表现为易激惹。③ 难以集中注意。目前已有较多量表用于评估PTSD的临床表现，图9–2展示了其中一种。

PTSD 筛查量表-城市居民版（PTSD Checklist Clvilian Version, PCL）

PCL-M for DSM-IV (11/1/94)

Name:____

INSTRUCTIONS TO PATIENT: Below is a list of problems and complaints that people sometimes have in response to stressful experiences. Please read each one carefully, put an X in the box to indicate how much you have been bothered by that problem in the past mouth.

1. Repeated, disturbing *memories, thoughts or images* of a stressful experience?
   1. Not at all 2. A little bit 3. Moderately 4. Quite a bit 5. Extremely
2. Repeated, disturbing *dreams* of a stressful experience?
   1. Not at all 2. A little bit 3. Moderately 4. Quite a bit 5. Extremely
3. Suddenly *acting or feeling* as if a stressful experience were *happening again* (as if you were reliving it)?
   1. Not at all 2. A little bit 3. Moderately 4. Quite a bit 5. Extremely
4. Feeling *very upset* when *something reminded you* of a stressful experience?
   1. Not at all 2. A little bit 3. Moderately 4. Quite a bit 5. Extremely

Figure 9–2 PTSD checklist civilian version (PCL)

BOX 9-1 Learning More

DSM-V Diagnostic Criteria for Posttraumatic Stress Disorder

A. Exposure to actual or threatened death, serious injury, or sexual violence.

B. Presence of one (or more) ng intrusion symptoms associated with the traumatic event(s), beginning after the traumatic event(s) occurred.

C. Persistent avoidance of stimuli associated with the traumatic event(s), beginning after the traumatic event(s) occurred.

BOX 9–1 知识拓展

DSM–V 诊断标准：创伤后应激障碍

A. 患者以一种（或多种）方式接触真正的或者被威胁的死亡，严重创伤，或性暴力等创伤事件。

B. 在创伤事件发生后，存在一种（或多种）与创伤事件有关的重新体验症状。

C. 创伤事件后开始持续地回避与创伤事件有关的刺激，出现一种或两种回避情况。

D. Negative alterations in cognitions and mood associated with the traumatic event(s), beginning or worsening after the traumatic event(s) occurred.

D. 与创伤性事件有关的认知和心境方面的消极改变，在创伤事件发生后开始出现或加重，具有两种（或更多）情况。

E. Marked alterations in arousal and reactivity associated with the traumatic event(s), beginning or worsening after the traumatic event(s) occurred.

E. 与创伤事件有关的警觉性或反应性有显著的改变，在创伤事件发生后开始或加重，表现为两项（或更多）情况。

F. Duration of the disturbance (Criteria B, C, D, and E) is more than 1 month.

F. 病期（诊断标准 B、C、D、E）超过 1 个月。

G. The disturbance causes clinically significant distress or impairment in social, occupational, or other important areas of functioning.

G. 此障碍产生了临床上明显的痛苦，或导致社交、职业、或其他重要功能方面的缺损。

H. The disturbance is not attributable to the physiological effects of a substance (e.g., medication, alcohol) or another medical condition.

H. 此障碍的产生排除了物质滥用导致的躯体影响（例如药物、酒精）或其他疾病的影响。

iii. Adjustment Disorder

（三）适应障碍

The onset of adjustment disorder is usually within 1-3 months of the occurrence of the stressful event or life change, and the duration of symptoms does not usually exceed 6 months, except in the case of prolonged depressive reaction. Adjustment disorder is expected to remit soon after the stressor ceases or, if the stressor persists, a new level of adaptation is achieved. The response is maladaptive because of impairment in social or occupational functioning or because of symptoms or behaviors that are beyond the normal, usual, or expected response to such a stressor.

发病多在应激性事件发生后 1～3 个月之内。当应激源消失，或者新的适应水平达到时，症状可缓解或消失。患者的反应表现为适应不良，因为患者常有社会或职业功能受损表现，或者其症状或行为常超出正常的应激反应限度。

Changes in mood and behavior are common. The manifestations vary, and include fearful, depressed, angry, anxiety, worried, guilty, or a mixture of these states. The stressor may interfere with their ability to think and concentrate. Lower confidence and decreased self-esteem frequently occur. Some individuals experience sleep disruption and have difficulty in falling or staying asleep. Others withdraw from the world and have little energy to accomplish things. Difficulties in interpersonal relationships may emerge, including tension, irritability, and frequent arguments. The individual may feel liable to dramatic behavior or outbursts of violence, but these rarely occur. However, conduct disorders (e.g. aggressive or dissocial behavior) may be an associated feature, particularly in adolescents. In children, regressive phenomena such as return to bed-wetting, babyish speech, or thumb-sucking are frequently part of the symptom pattern.

主要表现为情绪障碍，亦可出现适应不良的行为或生理功能的障碍，常见焦虑、烦恼、抑郁、胆小害怕、注意力不集中、易激惹等；还可伴有心慌、震颤等躯体症状；可出现适应不良的行为而影响到日常活动。有时患者发生酒精或药物滥用。其他较为严重的症状包括兴趣索然、无动力、快感缺失和食欲缺乏等，但较少见。有报道指出，临床表现与年龄之间有一定的联系，如老年人可伴有躯体症状；成年人多出现抑郁或焦虑症状；青少年以品行障碍常见；儿童多出现退化现象，如尿床、幼稚语言或吮拇指等形式。

IV. Treatment

i. ASD

Treatment for acute stress disorder usually includes a combination of antidepressant medications and short-term psychotherapy. Alternative treatment is also used in a clinical setting. Acupuncture has been recommended as a treatment for acute stress disorder. Some other alternative approaches, including meditation, breathing exercises, and yoga, may be helpful when combined with short-term psychotherapy. Homeopathic treatment and the use of herbal medicine and flower essences also can help the person with acute stress disorder rebalance on physical, mental, and emotional levels. Environment therapy is also essential to ASD. Decreasing or eliminating the stimuli in the environment can help the client feel safe and decrease traumatic feelings.

ii. PTSD

The suggested treatment methods include psychopharmacology, psychotherapy, and/or a combination of both.

1. Psychopharmacology A wide variety of medications have been tried for symptoms of PTSD. Clinical reports indicate the best response is from the tricyclic antidepressants. Other optional medications include anxiolytics, anticonvulsants and lithium. Unless the client is experiencing excessive excitement or violent episodes, antipsychotics are not generally suggested.

2. Psychotherapy Crisis intervention is the primary psychotherapy approach for clients with PTSD. Individual or group support is provided to help clients to identify their feelings and learn adaptive coping strategies. Health education of the client's family to improve their knowledge and understanding is also important, and strong family social support can improve the recovery process. Exposure therapy and psychological desensitization therapy are also common methods of psychological therapy.

3. Combination Therapy A combined approach with medications and psychotherapy is the treatment method most advocated by mental health professionals. PTSD clients often feel the environment is unsafe and unpredictable and they can easily lose control. Therefore, establishment of a solid therapeutic relationship

四、治　疗

（一）急性应激障碍

急性应激障碍的治疗通常包括抗抑郁药物治疗及短程心理治疗。在临床上也会采取针灸一类的替代性疗法。其他替代疗法包括冥想、呼吸训练和瑜伽等同短程心理治疗结合疗效更佳。结合草药及香薰的顺势疗法也可以帮助处于急性应激障碍的患者恢复躯体、心理和情感的平衡。环境治疗也非常重要，为了减弱或消除引起发病的应激处境的不良影响，应尽可能离开或调整当时的环境，消除创伤性体验，有助于整个治疗取得良好的效果。

（二）创伤后应激障碍

建议的治疗方法包括药物治疗，心理治疗和/或两者结合。

1. 药物治疗　除改善睡眠、抑郁焦虑症状外，抗抑郁药物还能减轻闯入和回避症状。但目前还没有对PTSD的各种症状都能产生满意疗效的药物。根据患者症状特点，可以考虑选用的药物包括抗焦虑药、抗痉挛药、锂盐等。除非患者有过度兴奋或暴力性的发作，一般不主张使用抗精神病药物。

2. 心理治疗　各种形式的心理治疗在PTSD都有应用的报告。对于PTSD主要采用危机干预的原则与技术，主要通过提供支持，帮助患者接受所面临的不幸与自身的反应，鼓励患者面对事件，表达宣泄与创伤性事件相伴随的情感。治疗者要帮助患者认识其所具有的应对资源，同时学习新的应对技巧。另外，还应为患者及其亲属提供有关PTSD知识，动员家庭及社会的力量，强化社会支持。暴露疗法和心理脱敏疗法也是常见的心理治疗法方法。

3. 心理治疗合并药物治疗　PTSD的首选治疗尚无一致意见，较为肯定的是心理治疗合并药物治疗效果更佳。PTSD患者往往感觉外部世界不安全、不可预测、无从把握，因此，建立稳固的治疗关系是治疗的基础。首

is the basis for treatment. First, mental health professionals must stabilize the client's panic response. When planning to use medications with psychotherapy, it is best to discuss the problem with the client at the planning stage of treatment, allowing the patient to participate in the treatment process and regain control.

先要做稳定化工作，让患者从惊恐中安定下来。如果计划在心理治疗中合并用药，最好在治疗的计划阶段就与患者讨论有关问题，使患者参与到治疗过程，重获控制感。

iii. Adjustment Disorder

（三）适应障碍

The general recommendation for treatment of adjustment disorder is for brief treatment with periodic reassessments. The primary goals of treatment are to relieve symptoms and assist clients in achieving a level of adaptation that at least equals their functioning before the stressful event. A secondary goal is to foster positive change whenever possible, particularly in areas still vulnerable to recurrent stress-related disorders.

适应障碍的治疗目标是增进患者的适应水平以期恢复到患病前功能状态，以及帮助患者产生积极变化，弥补自身个性不足，防止再发。

1. Biomedical Treatment Methods The judicious use of medications can help clients with adjustment disorder, but they should be prescribed for brief periods. A client may respond to an antianxiety agent or to an antidepressant, depending on the type of adjustment disorder. When they are used, clinicians should prescribe the lowest effective dosage for the shortest possible duration, together with frequent monitoring of efficacy and side effects;

1. 药物治疗 对情绪异常明显的患者，为加快症状的缓解，可根据病情选用抗焦虑药和抗抑郁药。以低剂量、短疗程为宜。在药物治疗同时，心理治疗应继续进行，特别是对恢复较慢的患者更为有益。

2. Psychosocial Treatment Methods Mental health professionals most commonly recommend some form of psychosocial treatment for clients with adjustment disorder. Since adjustment disorder is generally thought to arise from vulnerabilities in psychosocial functioning, treatment measures are designed to have an impact on whatever habits, conflicts, developmental inadequacies, or disturbing social symptoms are thought to be the source of the client's problem. Psychotherapy can help the person adapt to the stressor if it is not reversible or time-limited and can serve as a preventive intervention if the stressor does remit. Individual psychotherapy is the most common psychosocial treatment for adjustment disorder. After successful therapy, clients sometimes emerge from adjustment disorder stronger than in the premorbid period. Family therapy is the second most common treatment for adjustment disorder. Self-help groups are also being used in the treatment of adjustment disorder.

2. 心理治疗 因为适应障碍通常被认为是由于个体的易感性所致，因此通过心理治疗帮助患者认识问题，同时通过采取措施对其习惯、冲突、发展缺陷等施加影响，帮助患者提高适应水平，防止复发。个别心理治疗是最常用的针对适应障碍患者的治疗手段，除此之外，还可通过家庭治疗和自我帮助团体来进行。

V. Application of the Nursing Process

五、护理程序的运用

Nurses provide service to individuals who are currently experiencing stress and those who are high risk for stress. The overall goals for those with active stress responses are to eliminate the unfavorable person-environment situations (when possible), reduce the stress

护士在为正在经历应激或有发生应激可能的人群提供护理服务的过程中，对于前者，护理目标为消除不良的环境因素，减轻应激反应，提高积极的应对技巧；对于后者，护

response, and develop positive coping skills. The goal for those who are high risks for stresses (experiencing recent life changes, vulnerable to stress, or have limited coping mechanisms) are to recognize the potential for stressful situations and strengthen positive coping skills. These persons benefit from education and practice of new coping skills. They often access the nurse through health promotion services. Those actually experiencing stress require a more intense level of intervention than those who are high risk for stress. This section explains nursing management for those experiencing a stress response.

理目标为帮助其认识潜在的应激情境，加强积极的应对机制，防止应激的发生。通过健康促进项目，如提供健康教育和发展新的应对技能等方式，可以帮助创伤与应激相关障碍患者。本部分内容主要介绍对正在经历应激反应人群的护理。

i. Nursing Assessment

Stress responses vary from person to person. Some people have primary somatic responses, such as headaches, dermatitis, flushing, or stomach pains. Others experience fear and apprehension or withdraw from social situations. Usually, the person becomes emotionally upset and is unable to think clearly for a short time period. Nursing assessment in these situations is fairly complex because many aspects must be considered: the situation, the biologic responses, the emotions, and the coping responses. From the assessment data it is possible to determine the presence of illnesses, the intensity of the stress response, and the effectiveness of coping strategies. Nurses typically identify stress responses in persons or family members. Information from significant others or school or business colleagues may help determine problems with social or occupational functioning.

（一）护理评估

应激反应因人而异。一些人可有基本的躯体反应，如头痛、皮炎、面部潮红、胃疼等。另一些人可有害怕、忧虑或者退缩的表现。通常，应激中的个体在短期内会有情绪紊乱和思维混乱的表现。在这种情况下，护理评估应该包括对个人和家庭成员的评估，调查对象还应包括重要关系人、学校老师或同学以及单位同事等，以全面确定患者是否存在社会或职业等问题。总体而言，护理评估的内容应包括生理、心理和社会三方面。

1. Biologic Assessment Biologic assessment include three areas. a. Review of systems: highlights the susceptibility of different biologic areas. Because physiologic responses to stress result from the activation of the sympathetic nervous system and the immune system, the person may experience symptoms from any of the body systems. A systems review can elicit the person's own unique response to stress. A systems review can also provide important data on the effect of chronic illnesses. Thus, biological data are useful for analyzing the person-environment situation and the person's stress reactions, coping responses, and adaptation. b. Physical functioning: usually changed during a stress response. Typically, sleep is disturbed, appetite is changed, body weight fluctuates, and sexual activity changes. Physical appearance may be uncharacteristically disheveled--a projection of the person's feelings. Body language expresses muscle tension, which conveys a state of anxiety not usually present. Because exercise is an important strategy in stress reduction, the amount of physical activity, tolerance for exercise, and usual exercise patterns should be assessed. c. Pharmacologic assessment: in assessing a person's coping

1. 生理评估 生理评估过程中包括系统回顾，身体功能的评估以及用药评估。① 系统回顾：因为对应激的生理反应主要因交感神经系统和内分泌系统的激活引起，所以，个体可有各个器官系统的表现，如心血管系统、呼吸系统、胃肠道系统、肌肉骨骼系统、泌尿生殖系统以及皮肤系统等。② 身体功能评估：在应激过程中身体功能通常发生改变。典型的表现为睡眠障碍、食欲改变、体重波动和性行为改变。从个体的外表也可反映其内在的感觉，如不注意衣着、头发凌乱等。身体语言上常有肌紧张，是个体紧张的表现。另外，体育锻炼的情况，如形式、数量、耐受力等也应加以评估，因为锻炼是一种重要的减压策略。③ 用药评估：护士应询问个体有否使用酒精、烟草、大麻或其他成瘾物质的历史。因为物质滥用常发生在应激人群中，这种行为反过来又加重了应激行为。另外，

strategies, the nurse should ask about the use of alcohol, tobacco, marijuana, and any other addictive substances. Many people begin using these substances or increase their frequency of use as a way of coping with stress. In turn, substance abuse contributes to the stress behavior. Knowing details about the person's use of these substances (number of times a day or week, amount, circumstances, side effects, etc.) helps in determining the role these substances play in overall stress reduction or management. Stress often prompts people to use anxiolytics without provider supervision. Use of over-the-counter sleep medications for sleep disturbances is common. The use of any drugs to manage stress symptoms should be carefully assessed.

个体还经常未经医生允许自行使用抗焦虑药或购买非处方镇静安眠药物来自行解决睡眠障碍问题，这些情况均应仔细评估。

2. Psychological Assessment Unlike assessment for other health problems, psychological assessment of the person under stress does not ordinarily include a mental status examination. Instead, psychological assessment focuses on the person's emotions and their severity and coping strategies. (a) Emotions: the assessment elicits the person's appraisal of risks and benefits, the meaning of the situation to the client personally, and the person's commitment to a particular outcome. (b) Cognitive: after identifying the client's emotions, the nurse determines how the person reacts initially to them. For example, does the person who is angry respond by carrying out an urge to attack someone whom the person blames for the situation? Or does the person respond by thinking through the situation and overriding the initial urge to act? (c) Cognitive appraisal and coping: according to the stress, coping, and adaptation model, there are two types of coping: problem-solving coping and emotion-focused coping. In an assessment interview, the nurse can determine if the person uses coping strategies effectively.

2. 心理评估 与其他健康问题不同，对应激人群的心理评估通常不包括对其精神状态的评估。心理评估主要针对其情绪及应对策略的评估。① 情绪反应：主要关注情绪状态及严重程度，常见的情绪反应有焦虑、愤怒、恐惧、抑郁和敌意等；可以观察患者平时情绪表现，也可以与患者讨论此时此刻的感受，了解患者的内心想法。② 认知反应：评估患者的注意力、记忆力、智力、逻辑思维和判断能力是否受影响，是否存在认知歪曲或负性思维。③ 认知评价及应对方式：了解患者对应激事件的看法和打算，患者所面临的威胁及机遇；患者通常的应对方式。

3. Social Assessment The assessment should include discovering the person's social network, social support, and underlying sociocultural attitudes and beliefs that relate to the current stress. Assessment should include use of the social readjustment rating scale to determine the number and importance of life changes that the client has experienced within the past year. Both the supportive and non-supportive relationships within the client's environment should be assessed. The client specifies who is helpful in his or her environment and who is not, and also assesses the helpfulness of those who most and least affect his or her life and determines those who are members of the client's formal and informal groups (eg, work, clubs, religious organizations). Nurses should assess the following aspects: who is in the client's

3. 社会评估 主要对与目前应激有关的个体的社会关系网、社会支持、社会文化态度和信仰等方面进行评估。可以应用生活事件变化量表对个体过去一年中经历的生活事件数量及重要性进行评估。同时，个体周围所有支持性的或非支持性的关系均应加以评估。了解哪些是对个体有帮助的人；哪些是最有可能影响其生活的人。护士应评估以下方面，即个体的社会网络中都有谁？与个体的关系如何？都能为个体提供哪些帮助？帮助的程度如何？所期待的帮助程度如何等。

network; their relationship to the client (spouse, child, minister, etc.); what each relationship provides: the degree of helpfulness; and the expected degree of helpfulness.

4. Safety Assessment Assess whether there is a potential for self-injury and risk for suicide. Some patients' coping styles include substance abuse, aggressive and suicidal behaviors. Depression is also a common symptom in many patients with PTSD.

4. 安全评估 评估是否有潜在的自伤、自杀风险。有些患者还会表现出滥用成瘾物质、攻击性行为、自伤或自杀行为等，这些行为往往是患者心理行为应对方式的表现。同时抑郁症状也是很多PTSD患者常见的伴随症状。

ii. Nursing Diagnosis

A variety of nursing diagnoses can be generated from assessment data. Any nursing diagnosis that involves the person-environment interaction related to a stress response (anxiety, powerlessness, fear, fatigue, low self-esteem) or a coping process (ineffective coping, family coping, altered role performance) should be supported by the data. The challenge of generating nursing diagnoses is to make sure that they are based on the person's appraisal of the situation.

Common nursing diagnoses for a client's underlying stress are listed below.

1. Risk for injury or suicide, related to individual's maladaptive coping style and in crisis situation.

2. Post trauma syndrome, related to stressful events out of control.

3. Risk for post trauma Syndrome, related to stressful events threaten to self and significant others.

4. Complicated grieving, related to self-concept injury in stressful event.

5. Ineffective coping, related to stressful events and lack of support system.

（二）护理诊断

在评估的基础上，综合个体对应激的反应、应对的过程以及个体对应激的评价，可提出存在的或潜在的护理问题。

常见的护理诊断有：

1. **有自伤或自杀的危险** 与个体应对失调，陷入危机状态有关。

2. **创伤后综合征** 与应激事件超出可以应对的范围有关。

3. **有创伤后综合征的危险** 与应激事件威胁到自身或重要他人有关。

4. **复杂性悲伤** 与创伤性事件中自我概念受损有关。

5. **个人应对无效** 与应激性事件的发生、支持系统缺乏有关。

iii. Nursing Planning and Implementation

1. Nursing Outcomes For the individual with stress-related disorders, improvement will be demonstrated by the ability to:

(1) Remain safe, and not engage in self-destructive or mutilating behaviors.

(2) Demonstrate adequate sleep, activity patterns and regular daily life.

(3) Understand and recognize the presence of stress-related behaviors.

(4) Demonstrate diminished fear, anxiety, and depression which due to complicated grieving, or show appropriate expression of affect.

(5) Substitute more effective ways to promote

（三）护理计划

1. 护理目标 针对创伤与应激相关障碍的患者，护理目标是患者能够：

（1）保证安全，没有发生自残行为；戒酒或停止药物滥用；

（2）展现充足的睡眠、活动形态，保持规律日常生活；

（3）理解并认识应激相关行为的存在，确认应激发生时的症状；

（4）与复杂性悲伤相关的恐惧、焦虑和抑郁减少，能够适当表达情感；

（5）采取更有效的方法以促进有效适应。

healthy adaptation.

2. Nursing Interventions Successful stress management leads to positive health status, psychological well-being, and improved social functioning. Stress management interventions target biologic, psychological, and social dimensions.

(1) Biologic interventions: persons under stress usually can benefit from several biologic interventions. Their activities of daily living are usually interrupted, and they often feel that they have no time for themselves. The stressed client who is normally fastidiously groomed and dressed may appear disheveled and unkempt. Simply reinstating the daily routine of shaving (for a man) or applying makeup (for a woman) can improve the person's outlook on life and ability to cope with the stress.(a) Stress is commonly manifested in the areas of nutrition and activity. During stressful periods, a person's eating patterns change. To cope with stress, a person may either overeat or become anorexic. Both are ineffective coping behaviors and actually contribute to stress. Educate the client about the importance of maintaining an adequate diet during the period of stress.(b) Exercise can reduce the emotional and behavioral responses to stress. In addition to the physical benefits of exercise, a regular exercise routine can provide structure to a person's life, enhance self-confidence, increase feelings of well-being, and explore the client's personal beliefs about the value of activity. (c)The person under stress tends to be tense, nervous, and on edge. Simple relaxation techniques will help the person relax and may improve coping skills. If these techniques do not help the client relax, distraction or guided imagery may be taught to the client. Referral to a mental health specialist for hypnosis or biofeedback should be considered for clients who have severe stress response.

(2) Psychological interventions: numerous interventions help reduce stress and support coping efforts. These interventions are best carried out within the framework of a supportive nurse-client relationship. Six classes of useful generalist and specialist nursing interventions are included: behavior therapy, cognitive therapy, communication enhancement, coping assistance, client education, and psychological comfort promotion. Depending on the nursing diagnosis, any one of these interventions may be used. (a) Behavioral therapy: aims to reinforce or promote desirable behaviors or alter undesirable behaviors. Generalist interventions include assertiveness training, behavior management, behavior modification, limit setting, mutual goal setting, client contracting, self-modification assistance, self-responsibility assistance, smoking cessation assistance,

2. 护理措施 成功的应激管理可以带来积极的健康状况，促进心理健康，改善社会功能。应激管理干预措施包括生理、心理和社会方面。

（1）生理干预：应激中的个体通常可以从几种生理干预措施中受益。应激中的个体通常表现为没有时间照顾自己，日常生活行为受到严重干扰。有的表现为不拘小节，衣着凌乱；此时，通过恢复简单的日常常规，如男性剃须，女性化妆等，可以改善外观，增强应对压力的能力。① 应激通常体现在营养和活动领域。应激中的个体饮食习惯会发生变化。为了应对压力，会出现暴饮暴食或厌食。两者都是无效的应对行为，也会加剧应激状况。因此，需要向处于应激中的个体介绍应激期间保持适当饮食的重要性。② 运动可以减少应激的情绪和行为反应。锻炼会促进身体健康，定期锻炼还可以促进生活常规的恢复，增强自信心，增加幸福感，并有益于探索个体对活动价值的个人看法。③ 应激中的个体处于紧张和不稳定的状态。简单的放松技巧可以帮助人们放松并提高应对能力。如果简单的放松技巧不能帮助应激中的个体放松，可以进一步分散注意力和实施引导性意念想象。对于应激反应严重的个体，应考虑转介精神卫生专家，进行催眠或生物反馈等。

（2）心理干预：有很多心理干预措施可以达到减轻应激和加强应对的目的。所有的护理干预必须建立在支持性的护患关系基础上。常用的心理干预措施包括六个方面：① 行为干预主要为了加强、促进、完善适应性行为，改变非适应性行为。一般的干预措施包括自信训练，行为管理，行为矫正，制订限制，确定共同目标、建立合约，帮助戒烟，避免物质滥用以及帮助进行体育锻炼等。特殊的进一步干预措施包括心理治疗，咨询，动物辅助性治疗，物质滥用治疗，以及艺术治疗等。② 认知干预主要用以加强或促进适应性的认知功能，或者改变非适应性的功能状态。

substance use prevention, and activity therapy. Specialist (advanced practice) interventions include psychotherapy, consultation, animal-assisted therapy, substance use treatment, and art therapy. (b) Cognitive therapy: aims to reinforce or promote desirable cognitive functioning or alter undesirable functioning. Generalist interventions include anger control, bibliotherapy, and reality orientation. Specialist (advanced practice) interventions include psychotherapy, consultation, cognitive restructuring, cognitive stimulation, memory training, and reminiscence therapy. (c) Communication enhancement: aims to facilitate interaction or receive or deliver verbal or nonverbal messages. Generalist interventions include active listening, communication enhancement, and socialization enhancement. Specialist (advanced practice) interventions include psychotherapy, consultation, complex relationship building, music therapy, art therapy, play therapy and animal-assisted therapy. (d) Coping assistance Interventions: aim to help a client to build on own strengths, adapt to a change in function, or achieve a higher level of function. Generalist interventions include anticipatory guidance, body image enhancement, counseling, grief work facilitation, guilt work facilitation, decision-making support, care of the dying, emotional support, hope instillation, humor, role enhancement, recreation therapy, self-awareness enhancement, spiritual support, support system enhancement, and values clarification. Specialist (advance practice) interventions include psychotherapy (individual and group), consultation, genetic counseling, grief therapy, guilt work, sexual counseling, and touch therapy. (e) Health education: aims to facilitate learning. General interventions include learning facilitation, learning readiness enhancement, parent education, teaching disease process, teaching (group, individual), teaching (activity, exercise, diet, medication, procedure/treatment), and psychomotor skills. (f) Psychological comfort promotion: aims to promote comfort using psychological techniques. Generalist interventions include anxiety reduction, calming technique, distraction, simple guided imagery, and simple relaxation therapy. Specialist (advanced practice) interventions include psychopharmacologic agents prescribed, autogenic training, biofeedback, hypnosis, and meditation.

(3) Social and family interventions: People who are coping with stressful situations can often benefit from interventions that facilitate family unit functioning and promote the health and welfare of family members. For the nurse to intervene with the total family, the stressed person must agree for the family members to be involved.

一般的干预措施包括愤怒控制，阅读疗法和现实导向等。特殊的干预措施包括心理治疗，咨询、认知重建、认知刺激、记忆训练、回忆治疗等。③ 交流能力训练主要用以促进语言和非语言的交往。常用的措施包括积极的倾听，加强交流，加强社会化功能等。特殊的措施包括心理治疗、咨询、复杂关系的建立、音乐治疗、艺术治疗、游戏治疗、动物辅助性治疗。④ 辅助应对性干预主要用以帮助个体建立自己的优势，适应各种功能变化，或者达到更高的功能水平。一般的干预措施包括引导想象，完善个人形象，咨询以及对悲哀、哀伤及内疚感的应对。同时它包括决策支持、临终护理、情绪支持、希望建立、幽默、角色强化、娱乐治疗、自我意识加强、精神支持、支持系统的加强、价值的澄清等。特殊的措施包括心理治疗、咨询、悲痛治疗、内疚心理护理、性咨询以及触摸治疗等。⑤ 患者教育主要用以促进学习。一般的措施包括学习的促进，学习信心的加强，父母教育，疾病过程的教育，对疾病相关治疗，如饮食、锻炼、用药、治疗等的教育，以及心理动力学技巧等。⑥ 促进心理舒适主要应用心理学技巧促进舒适。一般的措施包括减轻焦虑、平静技巧、转移、简单的指导想象、放松技巧等。特殊的措施包括药物治疗、生物反馈、自我训练、催眠及沉思等。

（3）社会及家庭干预：在对应激的干预过程中，家庭成员的参与十分必要。护理措施应促进家庭功能的完善与提高。可采用的护理措施包括支持照护者，促进家庭完整性，促进及动员家庭参与，保持良好的家庭过程

If the data gathered from the assessment of supportive and non-supportive relationships indicate that the family members are not supportive, expansion of the social network should be considered. If the family is the major source of support, interventions should be designed that support the functioning of the family unit. The following generalist interventions are included in family care intervention: caregiver support, family integrity promotion, family involvement, family mobilization, family process maintenance, family support, respite care, and home maintenance assistance.

以及家庭支持等。

(4) Communications and general support: (a) Assign the same staff as often as possible. Use a nonthreatening, matte of fact, but friendly approach. Respect client's wishes regarding interaction with individuals of opposite sex at this time (especially important if the trauma was rape). Be consistent; keep all promises; convey acceptance; spend time with client. (b) Stay with client during periods of flashbacks and nightmares. Offer reassurance of safety and security and that these symptoms are not uncommon following a trauma of the magnitude he or she has experienced. (c) Obtain accurate history from significant others about the trauma and the client's specific response. (d) Encourage the client to talk about the trauma at his or her own pace. Provide a nonthreatening, private environment, and include a significant other if the client wishes. Acknowledge and validate client's feelings as they are expressed. (e) Discuss coping strategies used in response to the trauma, as well as those used during stressful situations in the past. Determine those that have been most helpful, and discuss alternative strategies for the future. Include available support systems, including religious and cultural influences. Identify maladaptive coping strategies (eg, substance use, psychosomatic responses) and practice more adaptive coping strategies for possible future post-trauma responses. (f) Assist the individual to try to comprehend the trauma if possible. Discuss feelings of vulnerability and the individual's "place" in the world following the trauma.

（4）沟通及一般性支持：针对有创伤后综合征得患者，沟通及一般性支持包括：① 尽量由同一个护士提供连续性护理；态度耐心和蔼，实事求是沟通，避免威胁性语言或姿态；遵守承诺，前后一致。② 在患者出现闪回或梦魇的时候陪伴患者；做稳定化工作，让患者从惊恐中安定下来；让患者感到他已经脱离了危险境地或可以克服现在的危机状况；通过让患者自由选择座位、是否关闭窗户、拉上窗帘、是否与医生接触等行为重获控制感。③ 与患者保持适当的距离，减少可能引发的焦虑。④ 从患者的家人和朋友处获取尽可能多的与病史以及患者反应相关的信息，避免追问患者，以免进一步刺激患者。⑤ 鼓励患者谈论自身的感受，不评判，帮助患者确认自身的感受并引导表达。⑥ 讨论既往使用过的应对方式以及当前可以采取的适应性的应对策略；帮助患者识别自身的非适应性应对方式（如物质滥用等）以及可能的替代性选择，如寻求支持系统。

BOX 9-2 Learning More

Key Elements of Psychological First Aid (PFA) for PTSD

1. Contact and Engagement Respond to contacts initiated by affected persons, or initiate contacts in a non-intrusive, compassionate, and helpful manner.

2. Safety and Comfort Enhance immediate and ongoing safety, and provide physical and emotional comfort.

BOX 9-2 知识拓展

PTSD 的紧急护理要点

1. 联系和参与 回应受影响者发起的联系，或以非侵入性、同情和有帮助的方式主动发起联系。

2. 安全和舒适 改善当下的安全及持续的安全状况，并提供身体和情绪的舒适。

3. Stabilization (if needed)　Calm and orient emotionally overwhelmed or distraught survivors.

4. Information Gathering　Current Needs and Concerns - Identify immediate needs and concerns, gather additional information, and tailor PFA interventions.

5. Practical Assistance　Offer practical help to the survivor in addressing immediate needs and concerns.

6. Connection with Social Supports　Help establish opportunities for brief or ongoing contacts with primary support persons or other sources of support, including family members, friends, and community helping resources.

7. Information on Coping　Provide information (about stress reactions and coping) to reduce distress and promote adaptive functioning.

8. Linkage to Collaborative Services　Link survivors with needed services and inform them about available services that may be needed in the future.

3. 稳定化（如果需要）　为处于惊慌失措或心神不宁状态下的幸存者提供安抚。

4. 信息收集（当前需求和关注）　确定即时需求和关注，收集更多信息，并调整紧急干预措施。

5. 实际援助　为幸存者提供实际帮助，解决眼前的需求和关切。

6. 建立与社会支持系统的联系　帮助建立与主要支持人员或其他支持来源，包括家庭成员，朋友和社区帮助资源的短暂或持续联系的机会。

7. 应对信息　提供信息（关于压力反应和应对），以减少痛苦和促进适应性功能。

8. 与协作服务的联系　将幸存者与所需的服务联系起来，并告知他们未来可能需要的可用服务。

iv. Nursing Evaluation

The following questions may be asked during the nursing evaluation process.

(1) Have nursing actions provided for the client's safety been sufficient to prevent injury?

(2) Has the client had an improved sleep, activity pattern and daily life arrangement?

(3) Has the client understood and recognized the presence of stress-related behavior?

(4) Has the client demonstrated diminished emotional disorder and shown appropriate expression of affect?

(5) Has the client identified support sources to facilitate coping? Has the client been able to perform role functions appropriately?

（四）护理评价

在评价阶段，护士可提出如下问题：

（1）护理措施是否有效地保护了服务对象的安全？

（2）服务对象的睡眠、活动型态及日常生活安排是否得到了改善？

（3）服务对象是否理解并认识应激相关障碍行为的存在？

（4）服务对象情绪问题是否减少？情绪表达是否恰当？

（5）服务对象是否确认了促进应对的支持资源？是否掌握了有效的应对策略？

Section 3　Crisis Intervention

第三节　危机干预

Stressful situations are a part of everyday life. Any stressful situations can precipitate a crisis. Crises result in a disequilibrium from which many individuals require assistance to recover. Crisis intervention requires problem-solving skills that are often diminished by the level of anxiety accompanying disequilibrium. Assistance with problem-solving during the crisis period preserves

个体在一生中不可避免地面对应激情况的发生，而应激将导致危机的出现。应激是在生活的各个方面都能感受到的一种身心反应，是普遍存在的。而危机不同，属于生活中的偶发事件。危机造成个体失衡，

self-esteem and promotes growth with resolution. This section examines the phases in the development of a crisis and the types of crises that occur in people's lives. The methodology of crisis intervention, including the role of the nurse, is explored.

必须借助于帮助才能恢复。创伤与应激障碍患者通常需要接受危机干预。本节将介绍危机发展阶段，危机种类等。危机干预方法，护士在危机干预中的角色等也将在此探讨。

I. Introduction

一、概 述

The term crisis was defined by Caplan (1964) as the psychological disequilibrium in a person who confronts a hazardous circumstance that for him constitutes an important problem which he can for the time being neither escape nor solve with customary problem-solving resources.

Individuals who are in crisis feel helpless to change. They do not believe they have the resources to deal with the precipitating stressor. Levels of anxiety rise to the point that the individual becomes nonfunctional, thoughts become obsessional, and behavior is aimed at relief of the anxiety being experienced. The feeling is overwhelming and may affect the individual physically, as well as psychosocially.

It is assumed that crises are acute, not chronic, situations that will be resolved in one way or another within a brief period. Barrell (1974) stated, "Crises are defined as self-limiting and generally last from 4 to 6 weeks." During this brief period the person is psychologically vulnerable and is, consequently, ready for the learning and growth opportunity. Crises can become growth opportunities when individuals learn new methods of coping that can be preserved and used when similar stressors recur.

危机研究专家 Gerald Caplan 认为，危机是一个人重要的生活目标遇到障碍，利用常规的解决问题的方法而无法解决问题时，引起的日常生活的混乱及瓦解。简单地说，危机是人体的平衡状态突然遭到破坏后的反应。

处于危机中的个体常有无助感，他们通常感到自己无能为力。焦虑水平的上升使其各种功能受损，思维混乱，甚至发生生理、心理的损害。危机具有急性发展的特征。应在短时间内通过一种或几种方法解决危机情景。情绪危机一般具有自限性，危机期通常发生在 4 到 6 周。

遇到危机，人们多会将它与“危险”联系起来，Caplan 认为危机除了破坏原有的平衡外，也预示着机会或转机。如果个体采用不恰当的方法去应付和解决危机，往往可导致心理及社会功能下降；在危机的关键时刻，如果处理得当，不仅可以扭转危机的局面，转危为安，而且人们会在经历特殊的危机事件后更加成熟，学习到更多的处理危机的技巧，进一步成长，恢复到比危机之前更高的平衡状态，以迎接未来可能出现的同样的或更严重的挑战。

II. Types of Crisis

二、危机的种类

There are three types of crisis: maturational, situational, and adventitious. More than one type of crisis can occur at the same time.

危机有三种：发展性危机、事故性危机和偶然性危机。危机可以其中一种形式出现，或几种形式同时并存。

1. Maturational Crises Maturational crises are developmental events requiring role changes. For example, successfully moving from early childhood to middle childhood requires the child to become socially involved

1. **发展性危机** 发展性危机主要是指个人在不同生命发展阶段面临角色变换时出现的危机。如随着年龄的增长，人们要面临、

with people outside the family. Both social and biological pressures to change can precipitate a crisis.

解决不同阶段带来的生理、心理和社会任务所带来的危机，如青春期危机及更年期危机。这些阶段的社会或生理变化的应激加剧危机的发生。

2. Situational Crises Situational crises occur when a life event upsets an individual's or group's psychological equilibrium. Examples of situational crises include loss of a job, loss of a loved one, unwanted pregnancy, onset or worsening of a medical illness, divorce, school problems, and witnessing a crime.

2. 事故性危机 事故性危机主要指导致个体或群体心理失衡的生活事件。如失业、意外怀孕、失恋、患病或疾病加重、离婚、学业问题及目击犯罪等。

3. Adventitious Crises Adventitious crises are accidental, uncommon, and unexpected. Multiple losses with gross environmental changes result. Unlike maturational and situational crises, adventitious crises do not occur in the lives of everyone. When they do occur, however, they challenge every coping mechanism because of the severity of the stress. Cultural crisis is a situation where a person experiences culture shock in the process of adapting/adjusting to a new culture or returning to one's own culture after being assimilated into another.

3. 偶然性危机 偶然性危机主要指偶然的、少见的、不可预知的危机。通常带来多种损失及重大的环境改变。这类危机，虽然并不是在每一个人身上发生，但由于其严重性的原因，对个体的应对机制带来较大的挑战。除此之外，还有文化性危机，是由文化的变迁所产生的。

III. Phases in the Development of a Crisis

三、危机的发展阶段

The development of a crisis situation follows a relatively predictable course. Caplan (1964) has outlined four specific phases through which an individual progress in response to a precipitating stressor and which culminate in the state of acute crisis.

Caplan 认为，危机的发生与发展主要经历以下四个阶段：

Phase 1 The individual is exposed to a precipitating stressor. Anxiety increases; previous problem-solving techniques are employed.

第一阶段 当事人暴露于逆境及创伤性应激事件，焦虑水平明显上升，并影响日常生活、工作及学习。个体表现为生理变化及心理紧张，并不断加重与恶化，社会适应功能明显受损及减退。个体主要采取以往的问题解决技巧来应对。

Phase 2 When a previous problem-solving technique does not relieve the stressor, anxiety increases further. The individual begins to feel a great deal of discomfort at this point. Coping techniques that have worked in the past are attempted, only to create feelings of helplessness when they are not successful. Feeling of confusion and disorganization prevail.

第二阶段 常用的防御方式不能解决目前所存在的问题，创伤性应激反应持续存在，生理及心理等紧张表现加重并恶化，个体的社会适应功能受损或减退。以往有效的应对技巧不再有效时，使人产生无助感。个体常处于混乱、无序状态。

Phase 3 All possible resources, both internal and external are called upon to resolve the problem and relieve the discomfort. The individual may try to view the problem from a different perspective, or even to overlook certain aspects of it. New problem-solving techniques may be used, and, if effectual, resolution may occur, with the

第三阶段 各种可能的内部和外部资源都被运用以解决问题和缓解不舒适。个体尝试从不同角度重新审视问题，甚至忽略问题的某一方面。新的问题解决技巧被应用，如

individual returning to a higher, a lower, or the previous level of premorbid functioning.

Phase 4　If resolution does not occur in previous phases, Caplan states that the tension mounts beyond a further threshold or its burden increases over time to a breaking point. Major disorganization of the individual with drastic results often occurs. Anxiety may reach panic levels. Cognitive functions are disordered, emotions are labile, and behavior may reflect the presence of psychotic thinking.

Aguilera suggests that whether or not an individual experiences a crisis in response to a stressful situation depends upon the following three factors: (a) Individual's perception of the event: if the event is perceived realistically, the individual is more likely to draw upon adequate resources to restore equilibrium. If the perception of the event is distorted, attempts at problem solving are likely to be ineffective, and restoration of equilibrium goes unresolved. (b) Availability of situational support: Aguilera states, "situational supports are those persons who are available in the environment and who can be depended on to help solve the problem". Without adequate situational supports during a stressful situation, an individual is most likely to feel overwhelmed and alone. (c) Availability of adequate coping mechanisms: when a stressful situation occurs; individuals draw upon behavioral strategies that have been successful for them in the past. If these coping strategies work, a crisis may be diverted. If not, disequilibrium may continue and tension and anxiety increase.

果有效，危机可望在这一阶段得到解决。个体重新恢复较高的或较低的，或者以往的功能水平状态。

第四阶段　如果在前一阶段没有找到解决问题的方法，个体的认知、情绪、行为状态进一步恶化，超出个体的防御限度。如果问题长期存在，个体可出现明显的人格障碍、行为退缩、精神异常、甚至自杀。

Aguilera 认为，面对应激事件，个体是否经历危机反应，还要考虑以下三方面因素：① 个体对事件的感知是现实的还是扭曲的。如果个体对事件的感知是现实的，个体将更有可能寻求足够的资源以恢复平衡状态；如果感知是扭曲的，问题解决将趋向于无效，平衡不能恢复。② 是否能够得到足够的情境性支持。情境性支持是指在特定的环境下能够随时帮助解决问题的人。危机情况下缺乏足够的支持，个体将倍感压抑、无助及孤独感。③ 有效应对机制的可获得性。当危机发生时，个体通常运用以往成功的经验来应对，当这些应对策略有效时，危机将被逆转；如果无效，失衡状态将持续，应激和焦虑水平将增高。

IV. Crisis Intervention and the Role of the Nurse

i. Content of Crisis Intervention

Crisis intervention is a brief, focused, and time-limited treatment strategy that has been shown to be effective in helping people adaptively cope with stressful events. It can offer a person in critical need, immediate help. It is an inexpensive, short-term therapy focused on solving the immediate problem, and it is usually limited to 6 weeks. The goal of crisis intervention is for the individual to return to a pre-crisis level of functioning. Often the person advances to a level of growth that is higher than the pre-crisis level because new ways of problem solving have been learned. Knowledge of crisis intervention techniques is an important clinical skill of all nurses, regardless of their clinical setting or practice specialty.

四、危机干预及护士的角色

（一）护士危机干预的角色及内容

危机干预能够立即对处于危机中的人提供帮助。它花费少、时间短，主要针对当前问题的快速解决，通常在 6 周之内完成。其目的在于使个体重返危机前功能状态。通常，由于个体学到了新的解决问题的方法而使其发展水平得到更大的提高。

Nurses respond to crisis situations on a daily basis. Crises can occur on every unit in the general hospital, in the home, in a community health care setting, in schools, offices, and private practice. Medical hospitalizations are stressful for clients and their families and are often precipitating causes of crises. The diagnosis of an illness, the limitations imposed on one's activities, and changes in body image because of surgery can all be viewed as losses or threats that may precipitate situational crisis. Simply the stress of being dependent on nurses for care can precipitate a crisis for the hospitalized client. Strain and Grossman identified the following categories of psychological stress in hospitalized clients: threat to narcissistic integrity; fear of strangers; separation anxiety; fear of loss of love and approval; fear of loss of control of developmentally achieved functions; fear of loss or injury to body parts; reactivation of feelings of guilt and shame and fear of retaliation.

Nurses who work in obstetric, pediatric, geriatric, or adolescent settings can readily observe clients or family members undergoing maturational crises. The anxious new mother, the acting-out adolescent, and the newly retired depressed client are all possible candidates for crisis therapy. If physical illness is an added stress during maturational turning points, the client is at an even greater risk. Emergency room settings are also flooded with crisis cases. People who attempt suicide, psychosomatic clients, and crime and accident victims are all possible candidates for crisis therapy. If the nurse is not in a position to work with the client on an ongoing basis, a referral for crisis therapy can be made.

Community health nurses can observe clients in their own environments and can often spot and intervene in family crises. The child who refuses to go to school, the man who refuses to learn how to give himself an insulin injection, and the family with a member dying at home is possible candidates for crisis therapy. Community health nurses are in a position to evaluate the needs of high-risk families for crisis therapy. Families with new babies, ill members, recent deaths, and a history of difficulty coping are all possible high-risk families.

危机干预在帮助个体更好地适应危机事件时非常有效，对于工作在不同场所的所有护士来说，掌握危机干预的知识和技巧是非常重要的。

护士每时每刻都面临着对危机情境的处理。危机可发生在各个场所，如综合医院的各个病房、家庭、社区、学校、办公室等。工作在各个领域的护士都会面对处于危机中的个体，因病住院对患者及其家庭来讲通常是危机的原因。疾病的诊断、对个体行为的限制或者外科手术带来的体像的改变等均可成为事故性危机的诱因，甚至依赖护士完成日常活动都会导致住院患者危机的发生。Strain 和 Grossman 列出了以下住院患者的心理应激情况：对个体完整性的威胁、对陌生人的恐惧、分离性焦虑、对缺乏爱与赞许的恐惧、对发展性功能失去控制的恐惧、身体损伤或部分器官失去的恐惧，以及犯罪感和羞耻感等。

在妇产科、儿科以及老年病房等的患者或其家庭成员常面临发展性危机，如过分担忧初为人母/父的夫妻、刚刚退休的抑郁患者都可能成为危机干预的对象，加之生理上疾病的困扰，更加大了其发生危机的可能性。另外，急诊室里的急诊患者，一些企图自杀者，心身疾病者，犯罪或事故中的受害者，都可成为危机干预的对象。如果护士不能为其提供持续性护理，应该指导并推荐其进行危机干预。

Community-oriented crisis intervention modalities have been developed. These are based on the philosophy that the health care team must be aggressive and go to the clients rather than wait for the clients to come to them. Two such modalities are mobile outreach services and psychiatric home care services. Nurses working in these modalities intervene in a variety of settings, ranging from homes to street corners.

社区保健护士应对高危家庭的干预需要进行评估，并对家庭危机进行干预。拒绝上学的孩子，拒绝学习自行注射胰岛素的患者，临终患者的家庭都可能成为危机干预的对象。

ii. Phases of Crisis Intervention

（二）危机干预的过程

Roberts and Ottens (2005) provide a seven-stage model of crisis intervention，which is one of the most often used to provide crisis intervention. This model is summarized in table 9-1.

Roberts 和 Ottens（2005）总结出了七阶段危机干预模型，这一模型是当前危机干预当中被广泛运用的干预模型之一（表 9–1）。

Aguilera (1998) describes four specific phases in the technique of crisis intervention. These phases are clearly comparable to the steps of the nursing process.

Aguilera（1998）将危机干预过程分为 4 个阶段。这些阶段将按照护理程序的步骤介绍如下：

1. Assessment In this phase, the crisis helper gathers information regarding the precipitating stressor and the resulting crisis that prompted the individual to seek professional help. A nurse in crisis intervention might perform the following assessments: (a) Ask the individual to describe the event that precipitated this crisis. (b) Determine when it occurred. (c) Assess the individual's physical and mental status. (d) Determine if the individual has experienced this stressor before. If so, what method of coping was used? Have these methods been tried this time? (e) If previous coping methods were tried, what was the result? (f) If new coping methods were tried, what was the result? (g) Assess suicide or homicide potential, plan, and means. (h) Assess the adequacy of support systems. (i) Determine level of pre-crisis functioning. Assess the usual coping methods, available support systems, and ability to problem solve. (j) Assess the individual's perception of personal strengths and limitations. Assess the individual's use of substances.

1. 评估阶段 在评估阶段，危机干预者将对危机的原因和结果进行评价，具体内容如下：① 询问个体导致这次危机的事件是什么？② 确定危机发生的时间。③ 评估个体的生理和精神状态。④ 确认个体以前是否经历过同样的危机。如果经历过，以往应用的应对方法如何，本次危机发生是否尝试了上述方法。⑤ 如果运用了以往的应对方法解决这次危机，结果如何？⑥ 如果运用了新的应对方法解决这次危机，结果如何？⑦ 评估个体有无自杀或杀人的可能，计划或方式如何？⑧ 评估个体是否有足够的支持系统。⑨ 个体危机前的功能水平如何，常用的应对方法，可得到的支持系统，以及问题解决能力。⑩ 个体对自身优势和缺陷的感知，物质滥用情况。

2. Planning of Therapeutic Interventions In the planning phase of the nursing process, the nurse selects the appropriate nursing actions for the identified nursing diagnoses. In planning the interventions, the type of crisis, as well as the individual's strengths and available resources for support, are taken into consideration. Goals are established for crisis resolution and a return to, or increase in, the pre-crisis level of functioning.

2. 计划阶段 在这一阶段，护士针对确定的护理诊断，选择恰当的护理措施。措施的选择同时应考虑到危机的种类，个体的优势以及可得到的支持资源。

3. Intervention The third phase of crisis intervention is implementing the intervention itself. The intervention can take place on many levels using a variety of techniques. Shield has described four specific levels of crisis intervention, which represent a hierarchy

3. 实施阶段 实施阶段，针对危机干预的方法很多。Shield 将危机干预分为 4 个水平，即环境干预、全面支持、一般性方法以及个别化方法。

Table 9-1 Robert's seven-stage crisis intervention model

Stage	Interventions
Stage I. Psychosocial and lethality assessment	● Conduct a rapid but thorough biopsychosocial assessment.
Stage II. Rapidly establish rapport	● The counselor uses genuineness, respect, and unconditional acceptance to establish rapport with the client. ● Skills such as good eye contact, a nonjudgmental attitude, flexibility, and maintaining a positive mental attitude are important.
Stage III. Identify the major problems or crisis precipitants	● Identify the precipitating event that has led the client to seek help at the present time. ● Identify other situations that led up to the precipitating event. ● Prioritize major problems with which the client needs help. ● Discuss client's current style of coping, and offer assistance in areas where modification would be helpful in resolving the present crisis and preventing future crises.
Stage IV. Deal with feelings and emotions	● Encourage the client to vent feelings. Provide validation. ● Use therapeutic communication techniques to help the clients explain his or her story about the current crisis situation. ● Eventually, and cautiously, begin to challenge maladaptive beliefs and behaviors, and help the client adopt more rational and adaptive options.
Stage V. Generate and explore alternatives	● Collaboratively explore options with the client. ● Identify coping strategies that have been successful for the client in the past. ● Help the client problem-solve strategies for confronting current crisis adaptively.
Stage VI. Implement an action plan	● There is a shift at this stage from crisis to resolution. ● Develop a concrete plan of action to deal with the current crisis. ● Having a concrete plan restores the client's equilibrium and psychological balance. ● Work through the meaning of the event that precipitated the crisis. How could it have been prevented? What responses may have aggravated the situation?
Stage VII. Follow-up	● Plan a follow-up visit with the client to evaluate their post-crisis status. ● Beneficial scheduling of follow-up visits include 1-month and 1-year anniversaries of the crisis event.

表 9-1 Roberts 七阶段危机干预模型

阶段	干预
I. 心理社会及自杀危险性评估	● 进行一个快速彻底的生理 - 心理 - 社会全面评估
II. 快速建立和谐氛围	● 真诚、尊重、无条件接受以建立和谐的治疗信任关系 ● 保持眼神接触，不评判，使用灵活的技巧，保持积极的精神状态
III. 识别主要问题或危机的促发因素	● 识别促使个体当前寻求帮助的主要促发性事件 ● 识别导致促发性事件的其他情形 ● 确定个体需要帮助的主要问题 ● 讨论个体当前的应对方式，帮助个体修正最相关的领域，以解决当前存在的危机或预防危机的进一步发生
IV. 处理感受及情绪问题	● 鼓励个体表达自身的感受并帮助其确认 ● 使用治疗性沟通技巧，帮助个体更好地理解导致当前危机状况的一些“故事” ● 最终，谨慎地挑战个体的非适应性信念和行为，并帮助个体采取更合理的适应性选项
V. 探讨替代选择	● 和个体合作，共同探讨合理选项（替代性方法） ● 识别个体曾经成功采取过的应对策略 ● 帮助个体合理采取“问题取向型”策略以战胜当前的危机

续表

阶段	干预
VI. 实施一项行动计划	● 这个阶段是一个从危机向解决问题转变的阶段 ● 制订一个详细的行动计划以处理当前的危机 ● 在详细的行动计划中，帮助个体恢复保持平衡的能力，实现心理平衡 ● 帮助个体理解危机促发性事件。探讨如何预防，讨论哪些反应使事情恶化
VII. 随访	● 设计一个随访计划，评估个体危机后的状态 ● 随访计划的设定应遵循有益原则，应当包含危机时间后 1 月或一周年随访等具体计划

from the most superficial to the most in-depth. They are environmental manipulation; general support; generic approach; and, individual approach. Each step includes the lower levels of intervention. The progressive order of the steps also indicates the degree of knowledge and skill needed by the nurse for application.

(1) Environmental manipulation: It includes interventions that directly change the client's physical or interpersonal situation. These interventions provide situational support to remove stress. For example, a client who lives alone may move in with his closest sibling for several days.

（1）环境干预：主要通过消除应激源，改变当事人所处的物理或人际环境。如一名独自生活的人，可帮助其与同胞在一起居住一段时间以解决此时的危机情境。

(2) General support: It includes interventions that provide the client with the feeling that the nurse is on his side and will be a helping person. The nurse uses warmth, acceptance, empathy, caring, and reassurance to provide this type of support.

（2）全面支持：通过对个体各方面的支持使其感到护士时刻在其左右，随时准备为其提供各种帮助。因此，需要护士以温暖、接受、移情、关心的方法提供服务。

(3) A generic approach: It is a type of crisis intervention that is similar to the public health model. It is designed to reach high-risk individuals and large groups as quickly as possible. It applies a specific method to all individuals faced with a similar type of crisis. The course of the particular type of crisis is previously studied and mapped out. The intervention is then set up to ensure that the course of the crisis results in an adaptive resolution.

（3）一般性方法：是一种与公共卫生保健模式相似的干预方法。它能在高危个体或人群面临危机时迅速提供帮助，对面临同样类型的危机人群提供特殊的干预方法。一般性方法是假设在多数危机发生时，都会有某些被确认的行为反应。这些危机，如悲伤反应、早产儿母亲的反应等在发生时都有其特定的反应出现。危机的过程已被事先预知，干预方法也被事先指定，最终达到适应性解决危机的方法。

(4) Individual approach: It is a type of crisis intervention similar to the model of diagnosis and treatment of a specific problem in a specific client. The nurse must understand the client's psychodynamics that led to the present crisis and must use the intervention that is most likely to help the client to a healthy resolution to his crisis. This type of crisis intervention can be effective with all types of crisis. It is particularly useful in combined situational and maturational crises. The individual approach is also beneficial when symptoms include homicidal and suicidal risk. The individual approach

（4）个别化方法：此方法相当于对于特定患者给予特殊的诊断和治疗的过程。这种方法的应用要求护士首先必须理解导致现存危机的患者的心理动力学因素，然后选择最有可能帮助患者顺利度过危机的措施。个别化方法对所有类型的危机均有效，尤其适合于发展性危机和事故性危机并存的情况。当个体有自杀或杀人倾向，或者危机的过程不可预料，或者一般性方法无效时，个别化方法

should be applied if the course of the crisis cannot be determined. It also should be applied to crises that have not responded to the generic approach. It is often helpful to consult with others when deciding which approach to use for a specific client.

将具有较好的作用。

4. Evaluation The fourth step of crisis intervention is evaluation. During this phase the nurse and client evaluate whether the intervention resulted in the desired effect--a positive resolution of the crisis. To evaluate the outcome of crisis intervention, a reassessment is made to determine if the stated objective was achieved: (a) Has the client returned to his pre-crisis level of functioning? (b) Have the client's original needs, which were threatened by the precipitating or stressful event, been met? (c) Have the client's symptoms, which demonstrated ineffective use of coping mechanisms, subsided? (d) Have the client's useful coping mechanisms begun to function again? (e) Does the client have a strong support system to rely on now? (f) Have positive behavioral changes occurred? (g) Has the individual developed more adaptive coping strategies? Have they been effective? (h) Has the individual grown from the experience by gaining insight into his or her responses to crisis situations? (i) Does the individual believe that he or she could respond with healthy adaptation in future stressful situations to prevent crisis development? (j)Can the individual describe a plan of action for dealing with stressors similar to the one that precipitated this crisis?

4. 评价阶段 在这一阶段，护士和患者共同评价措施是否达到了预期的结果，即危机是否被积极解决。

在评价阶段，通常需要提出以下问题：①个体是否恢复到了危机前的功能水平？②受危机事件威胁的个体的最初需要是否得到了满足？③个体由于应对无效而表现出的症状是否消退？④个体有效的应对机制是否又开始发挥作用？⑤个体现在是否有强大的支持系统可依赖？⑥积极的行为改变是否已发生？⑦个体是否发展了更为适应性的应对策略？这些策略是否有效？⑧个体是否通过对危机情境反应的洞察得到了个人的成长？⑨个体是否确信他/她在今后遇到应激情境时能够用健康性适应性方式应对，从而预防危机的发生？⑩面对类似的危机情境，个体是否能够计划出具体的应对措施？

During the evaluation period, the nurse and client summarize what has occurred during the intervention. They review what the individual has learned and "anticipate" how he or she will respond in the future. A determination is made regarding follow-up therapy; if needed, the nurse provides referral information.

总之，在评价阶段，护士和个体共同总结在干预阶段所发生的事情，对个体已经学到的内容进行回顾，对未来的反应进行展望。评价的结果将用来指导随后的干预措施，必要时，提供可供利用的信息。

iii. Crisis Intervention Techniques

（三）危机干预的技巧

The nurse uses techniques that are active, focal, and exploratory to carry out the interventions. The intervention must be aimed at achieving quick resolution. The nurse also must be active in guiding the crisis intervention through its various steps. A more passive approach is inappropriate for this type of psychotherapy because of the time limitations of the crisis situation.

护士运用积极的、围绕主要问题的探索性技巧实施危机干预。干预的目的是迅速解决问题。同时，护士必须通过各种步骤指引危机干预的进程。由于时间的有限性，不适合采用消极的方法。

The nurse is creative and flexible, trying many different techniques. Some of these include abreaction, clarification, suggestion, manipulation, reinforcement of behavior, support of defenses, raising self-esteem, and exploration of solutions. A brief description of these techniques follows.

护士可以富有创造力和灵活度，尝试多种技巧。其中一些包括发泄、澄清、建议、操纵、行为强化、防御性支持、提高自尊和探索解决问题的方法。这些技巧的简要说明如下。

1. Abreaction It is the release of feelings that takes place as the client talks about emotionally charged

1. 发泄 是一种情感的释放。当一个人意识到自己对某一事件的感觉时，应激将减

areas. As he becomes aware of his feelings about the events, he experiences tension reduction. The nurse encourages abreaction by asking the client how he feels about his situation, recent events, and significant people involved in his crisis. The nurse asks open-ended questions and reflects the client's words back to him so that he will further ventilate his feelings. The nurse does not discourage crying or angry outbursts but rather sees them as a positive release of feelings. Only when feelings seem out of control, such as in extreme rage or despondency, should the nurse discourage abreaction and help the client concentrate on thinking rather than feeling. For example, if a client angrily talks of wanting to kill a specific person, it is better to help him focus on thinking through the consequences of carrying out the act rather than encouraging free expression of the angry feelings.

轻。护士通过询问个体对所处情境、最近事件以及危机牵涉的重要关系人的感觉，从而鼓励个体的发泄。护士通过提出开放式问题，或者重述个体的话语来证实对患者的理解。护士不鼓励痛哭或者愤怒，但是也应将其看作积极的情感释放。但是，一旦感情爆发失去控制，护士应帮助个体集中精力思考，代替以往的情感发泄。例如，当一名个体气愤地谈及想要杀人时，护士应该帮助其思考这种行为的后果，而不能盲目地鼓励其自由发泄气愤的情感。

2. Clarification It is used when the nurse helps the client to identify the relationship between certain events in his life. For example, helping a client see that it was after he was passed over for a promotion that he began feeling too sick to go to work is clarification. Clarification helps the client gain a better understanding of his feelings and how they led to the development of a crisis. In crisis intervention the clarification of unconscious processes is minimal.

2. 澄清 护士应用澄清的方法帮助个体明确生活中一定事件之间的关系。例如，帮助个体明确，是由于升职失败，他才有厌倦工作的情绪。澄清可帮助个体更好地理解自己的感觉，以及这些是如何影响危机发展的。

3. Suggestion It is the process of influencing a person so that he accepts an idea or belief. In crisis intervention the nurse influences the client to see him or her as a confident, calm, hopeful, empathic leader who can help. By believing the nurse can help, the client feels optimistic and in turn will feel less anxious. He also may want to please the nurse by fulfilling his or her expectations of getting better.

3. 建议 即影响一个人使其接受一种观点或信念的过程。在危机干预中，护士通过对个体施加的影响，使个体感到护士是可以信赖的、沉着的且令人充满希望的、同理的引导者，是能够提供所需帮助的人。如果个体对护士产生了信任感，就会寻求帮助，因此情绪乐观，焦虑水平下降。同时，个体也愿意做得更好，努力实现护士的期望。

4. Manipulation It is a technique in which the nurse uses the client's emotions, wishes, or values to his benefit in the therapeutic process. Like suggestion, manipulation is a way of influencing the client. For example, the nurse may want to point out to the client who prides himself on his independence that he is responsible for much of the work of solving his problems.

4. 操纵 是一种利用个体的情绪、希望或价值观等达到良好治疗效果的技巧。与建议相似，操纵也是一种影响患者的途径。例如，护士通过告诉个体，有人对他的独立性大加赞赏，从而影响个体更好地独立解决问题。

5. Reinforcement Behavior It occurs when healthy and adaptive behavior of the client is reinforced. The nurse strengthens positive responses made by the client by agreeing with or complimenting him on those responses. For example, when a client who has passively allowed himself to be criticized by his boss states that he asserted himself in an interaction with his boss, the nurse

5. 行为强化 指当个体表现出健康的、适应性行为时，护士通过同意或称赞达到积极强化。例如，当一个通常以消极态度允许上司无端批评的个体告诉护士他今天与上司据理力争时，护士应表示对他的行为的赞许。

can tell him she is pleased with his assertiveness.

6. Support of Defenses It occurs when the nurse encourages the use of healthy defenses and discourages those that are unhealthy. Defense mechanisms are indirect behaviors used to cope with stressful situations. The purpose of defense mechanisms is to maintain self-esteem and ego integrity. When defenses deny, falsify, or distort reality to the point that the person cannot deal effectively with reality, they are maladaptive. The nurse should encourage the client to use adaptive defenses and discourage those that are maladaptive. For example, when a client denies the fact that her husband wants a separation despite the fact that he has told her what he wishes, the nurse can point out to her that she is not facing facts and dealing realistically with the problem. This is an example of discouraging the use of the defense mechanism of denial. If a client who is furious with his boss writes a letter to his boss's supervisor rather than assaulting his boss, the nurse should encourage his adaptive use of the defense mechanism of sublimation.

In crisis intervention, defenses are not attacked but rather are more gently encouraged or discouraged. When defenses are attacked, the client cannot maintain his self-esteem and ego integrity. There is not enough time in crisis intervention to help replace the attacked defenses with new healthier defenses. Returning the client to his previous level of functioning is the goal of crisis intervention, not the restructuring of defenses.

7. Raising Self-esteem It is a particularly important technique. The client in a crisis feels helpless and may be overwhelmed with feelings of inadequacy. The fact that he has found it necessary to seek outside help for his problem may further increase his feelings of inadequacy. The nurse should help the client regain his feelings of self-worth. She does this by communicating her confidence that the client can participate actively in finding solutions to his problems. The nurse also communicates to the client that he is a worthwhile person by listening to him, accepting his feelings, and relating to him with respect.

8. Exploration of Solutions It is essential because crisis intervention is geared toward solving the immediate crisis. The nurse and client actively explore solutions to the crisis. Answers that the client had not thought of before may become apparent as he talks to the nurse and his anxiety decreases. For example, a client who has lost his job and has not been able to find a new one may become aware of the fact that he knows many people in his field of work that he could contact to get information regarding the job market and possible openings.

6. 防御性支持 指护士对健康的防御机制进行鼓励，消除不健康的防御机制。当个体应用否认、歪曲等防御机制时，将不能有效地应对现实，这种机制即为适应不良。护士应鼓励适应性防御的应用，避免不适应性防御机制的应用。例如，当丈夫告诉妻子他想与她分开的事实，而妻子却否认时，护士应向妻子指出她并没有面对现实和解决问题。这是一个对不恰当防御机制的否认。又如一个对上司不满的人用给上级管理者写信的方法，而不是用攻击方法，应该得到护士的鼓励，因为他的防御机制为适应性防御机制。

在危机干预中，个体的防御机制不应受到攻击，而应温和地鼓励或劝阻。当防御机制受到攻击时，个体将无法维持其自尊心和自我完整性。危机干预过程中没有足够的时间来重构新的、更健康的防御机制以替代原有的自我防御机制。危机干预的目标是使个体恢复到以往的功能水平，而非重组防御机制。

7. 提升自尊 危机中的人们通常感觉无助和自卑，只有通过他人帮助才能解决问题的事实更加重了其自卑感。护士应该帮助个体找回自我价值感。护士应通过交流使个体确信他能够通过积极参与找到问题的解决办法。同时，护士通过倾听、接受其情感以及尊重等也能表达对个体自我价值的认可。

8. 探索解决问题的方法 危机干预的最终目的是为了达到危机的尽快解决，所以解决问题的方法最重要。护士应该和个体共同探讨问题的解决办法。通过交谈，可以使得个体以往从未设想过答案的问题变得清晰，从而减轻焦虑感。例如，一位失去工作而又找不到新工作的人可能会意识到，他认识许多工作领域的人，可以联系他们以获得有关

In addition to using these techniques, attitudes are essential for the crisis worker. The crisis worker should see this work as the treatment of choice with persons in crisis rather than as a second best treatment. Assessment of the present problem should be viewed as necessary for treatment, but complete diagnostic assessment should be viewed as unnecessary. The goal and time limitations of crisis intervention should be kept in mind, and unrelated material should not be explored. An active directive role must be taken, and flexibility in the approach is essential.

It is important for the nurse to remember that cultural attitudes strongly influence the communication and response style of the crisis worker. These attitudes are deeply ingrained in the processes of asking for, giving, and receiving help. They also affect the victimization experience, so it is essential to understand and respect the cultural values of the victim. Specific cultural factors to be considered in crisis intervention include the following: migration and citizenship status, gender, and family roles.

Stress and crisis are inevitable throughout everyone's life. Nurses are more frequently being placed in the role of providing primary health care and therefore are becoming more involved in the direct practice of stress management and crisis intervention. This trend seems to be continuing and will grow as certification procedures for nurses further develop. Nurses are also involved in indirect services in the field of stress management and crisis therapy. The theory and practice of stress and crisis intervention are taught by nurses to other nurses in various settings and also to paraprofessionals, and to members of the community whose work frequently brings them in contact with persons in stress and crisis.

It is elementary for nurses to grasp theoretical knowledge, such as basic concepts, etiology, clinical manifestations, etc. Cognitive appraisal is very important to consider when faced with stress and crisis. Nurses can apply the nursing process in problem identification, nursing intervention implementation and evaluation. Nurses should try effective strategies such as physiological, psychological and social supports to help clients restore or reach higher levels of function in addition to avoiding maladaptive coping or to cope successfully.

(Yang Bingxiang)

就业市场和可能的职位空缺的信息。

除了使用上述技巧外，对探索解决问题的方法持有积极态度对于危机工作者也至关重要。危机工作者应该将探索个体当前面临的首要问题的解决方法视为优先任务，而非次要任务。在危机状况下，对个体进行全面的诊断评估反而是非必需的。危机干预工作者应牢记危机干预的目标和时间限制，不应探索无关的信息，在危机干预的过程中发挥积极的指导作用，并且保持方法灵活性。

护士应明确，文化态度影响个体和危机工作者的交流和反应形式，进而影响危机个体的经历。所以，危机干预中的护理工作者必须理解并尊重个体的文化价值。同时，还应考虑影响危机干预的特殊文化因素，如移民和居民的状态、性别和家庭角色等。近来，新的社区危机干预形式已被建立。典型的有活动性服务，以及精神护理之家。在这里工作的护士，其活动场所可从患者的家庭扩展到街区的每一个角落。

应激和危机在每个人一生的各个阶段都是难以避免的。对于承担初级卫生保健任务的护士来说，应更多地主动承担应激和危机的直接干预者角色。这是一种发展趋势。另外，通过对同行、辅助人员、社区工作人员等进行有关应激和危机知识的介绍，护士也间接地承担应激护理和危机干预的职责。

护士应掌握应激及其相关障碍；危机的理论知识，如概念、原因、临床表现等基本知识。通过护理程序的应用，护士应能够确认或预测问题，并采取生理、心理和社会等方面的护理措施解决问题，以使个体避免或尽快度过应激和危机期，获得功能的恢复和提高。

（杨冰香）

Key Points

1. Concepts of stress include stress as a biological response, an environmental event, and a transaction between the individual and the environment.

2. Stress, coping, and the adaptation model are consistent with the biopsychosocial perspectives of psychiatric mental health nursing practice, and are used as a framework for understanding stress.

3. Cognitive appraisal is an individual's evaluation of the personal significance of the event or occurrence.

4. Trauma and stressor-related disorders are caused by psychosocial elements.

5. Post-traumatic stress disorders arise as a delayed and/or protracted stressful event or situation of an exceptionally threatening or catastrophic nature.

6. Nurses provide service to individuals who are currently experiencing stress and those who are high risk for stress. The overall goals for those with active stress responses are to eliminate the unfavorable person-environment situations, reduce the stress responses, and develop positive coping skills. The goals for those who are high risk for stress are to recognize the potential for stressful situations and strengthen positive coping skills.

7. A combination of biological, psychological, and social interventions is used to help the client with trauma and stressor-related disorders.

8. There are three types of crisis: maturational, situational, and adventitious.

9. Roberts and Ottens (2005) provide a seven-stage model of crisis intervention，which is one of the most often used to provide crisis intervention

10. There are four specific levels of crisis intervention, which represent a hierarchy from the most superficial to the most in-depth; they are environmental manipulation, general support, generic approach, and individual approach.

内容摘要

1. 应激的三个概念包括应激作为一种生理反应；应激作为一种环境事件；以及应激作为个体和环境之间的互动。

2. 应激、应对与适应模型提供了理解应激的一种新视角，与精神心理实践中的心理－社会－社会模型一致，是现代应激理论最为常用的一种框架。

3. 应激评价指个体对应激事件对于自身重要性的评价。

4. 创伤与应激相关障碍指一组主要由心理、社会（环境）因素引起的异常心理反应。

5. 创伤后应激障碍是由异乎寻常的威胁性或灾难性心理创伤，导致延迟出现和长期持续的精神障碍。

6. 护士担负着为正在经历应激或有发生应激可能的人群提供护理服务的职责。对于前者，护理目标为消除不良的环境因素，减轻应激反应，提高积极的应对技巧；对于后者，护理目标为帮助其认识潜在的应激情境，加强积极的应对机制，防止应激的发生。

7. 生物、心理以及社会干预方法被联合应用于创伤与应激相关障碍个体的护理。

8. 危机的种类主要有三种，即发展性危机、事故性危机和偶然性危机。

9. Roberts 和 Ottens 的危机干预七步骤模型是当前危机干预当中被广泛运用的干预模型之一。

10. 从基本到深入，危机干预分为 4 个水平，即环境干预、全面支持、一般性方法以及个别化方法。

Exercises

(Questions 1 to 2 share the same question stem)

Amy, who lives in Maine, hears on the evening news that 25 people were killed in a tornado in south Texas. Amy experiences no anxiety on hearing of this stressful situation.

Amy regularly develops nausea and vomiting when faced

思考题

（1～2 题共用题干）

艾米，居住于美国缅因州，在晚间新闻中听到一则消息说 25 位南得克萨斯居民在一场飓风中遇难。听到这一应激性事件后，艾米并未感到焦虑。

艾米在遇到一些应激性事件后，总是会有规

with a stressful situation.

1. Describe the most likely reason Amy experiences no anxiety.

2. Describe the most likely predisposing factor to this maladaptive response.

(Questions 3 to 4 share the same question stem)

Li Wen, a 28-year-old single woman, has been admitted to an inpatient psychiatric unit. She was transferred to the unit from the emergency room, where she was treated for a drug overdose. She is sullen when she is introduced to her roommate and refuses to answer questions by the nurse as part of the admission procedure. The nurse tells Li Wen that she will return later to see how she is feeling. A few minutes later, Li Wen approaches the nurses' station and asks in a demanding tone to talk with someone and complains that she has been completely ignored since she came to the unit.

3. What interventions might the nurse choose to help Li Wen behave in a manner that is consistent with the norms of this inpatient unit?

4. When a nurse minimizes verbally abusive behavior by a client, family member, or health care colleague, what implicit message does she or he send?

律地恶心呕吐。

1. 艾米做出了何种初级评价以致她并未感到焦虑?

2. 艾米在遇到应激性事件后产生非适应反应的最可能的诱发因素是什么?

（3～4题共用题干）

李文，28岁的单身女性，因服用过量药物到急诊科接受治疗，目前从急诊科转入精神科住院病房。当她被介绍给室友时，她闷闷不乐，并且在入院评估时拒绝回答问题。护士告诉李文，她稍后会回来，继续对她进行评估。几分钟后，李文走近护士站，用命令式的口吻与他人教谈，并抱怨自从她入院以来就被完全忽略了。

3. 李文当前的首要的护理诊断是什么?

4. 护士当前应首要采取哪一个水平的危机干预措施?

Chapter 10 Nursing Management for Clients with Neurosis

第十章 神经症患者的护理

Learning Objectives

Memorization

1. Define the concepts of normal anxiety and pathological anxiety.
2. Describe various types of anxiety disorders and obsessive compulsive disorder.
3. Define the concepts of somatization disorder and hypochondriasis.

Comprehension

1. Discuss etiological implications in the development of neurosis.
2. Identify symptomatology associated with anxiety disorders, obsessive compulsive disorder, dissociative disorders and conversion disorders.
3. Explain various modalities relevant to treatment of individuals with neurosis.

Application

1. Formulate nursing diagnoses and outcome identification for clients with neurosis.
2. Implement appropriate nursing interventions for behaviors associated with neurosis.
3. Evaluate nursing care of clients with neurosis.

学习目标

识记

1. 能分别说出正常焦虑和病理性焦虑的概念。
2. 能描述不同类型焦虑障碍和强迫障碍的基本概念。
3. 能正确概述躯体化障碍和疑病障碍的概念。

理解

1. 能归纳神经症病因学方面的影响因素。
2. 能识别焦虑障碍、强迫障碍、分离性障碍和转换性障碍的症状表现。
3. 能具体说明神经症患者的主要治疗方式。

运用

1. 能提出神经症患者常用的护理诊断并归纳护理目标。
2. 能为神经症患者实施恰当的护理干预。
3. 能评价神经症患者的护理干预效果。

A 30-year-old woman has experienced panic episodes since age 23. Attacks usually began spontaneously, characterized by tachycardia, nausea, dizziness, discomfort, sweating, trembling, and a fear of doing something uncontrolled. Early severe episodes included symptoms associated with hyperventilation, including "smothering", choking, chest discomfort, faintness, and paresthesias. She has experienced a feeling of panic on several occasions, and found no reliable pattern of the attacks. She neither smoked or used alcohol and had discontinued use of caffeine for 3 years because it made her feel jittery. The client reported increased frequency but not severity of panic attacks in the premenstruum. Family history was positive for similar episodes in her mother and for depression on both sides of her family.

患者，女性，30岁，23岁时诊断为惊恐障碍。惊恐发作时主要表现为心动过速、呕吐、头晕、不舒服、出汗、发抖及恐惧。早期惊恐发作时的症状还包括过度通气、窒息感、胸部不适、乏力以及感觉异常等。惊恐发作在很多场合发生，没有规律可循。患者没有饮酒史及抽烟史，因使用咖啡因后感到紧张已停止使用3年。患自诉月经前期惊恐发作频率有所增加但症状未明显加重。患者有抑郁症家族史，母亲曾诊断为惊恐障碍。

Please think about the following questions based on the case:

1. Which psychotherapies could be suggested in this client?
2. How can the client be taught to recognize symptoms of onset of anxiety and to intervene?

请思考：

1. 建议对该患者应用何种心理治疗？
2. 有哪些措施可以帮助患者及时识别焦虑的前期症状并采取干预方法？

Neurosis is a group of mental disorders with certain personality basis, without any demonstrable organic basis, usually onset after psychosocial factors and last for a long time. The main manifestations are anxiety, depression, phobia, obsession-compulsion, hypochondriasis, somatic systems, or neurasthenic symptoms, which are disproportional to the client's actual situation. The clients have insight of the illness, but feels affliction and no significance. "Neurosis" was first mentioned by an English doctor named William Cullen in 1769, and the concept was gradually generated until 20 century. As a set of mental disorders combined artificially, opinions on neurosis of academics from different countries in the world are not accordance. Various diagnosis system including *ICD* (*International Classification of Diseases*), *DSM* (*Diagnostic and Statistical Manual of Mental Disorders*), and *CCMD* (*Chinese Classification and Diagnostic Criteria of Mental Disease*), also has integrated or separated them occasionally. Although they have some common clinical features, they still have different complicated etiology and pathogenesis, and inconsistent clinical manifestation and treatment. This chapter will discuss the major types of neurosis according to *ICD*, which include anxiety disorders, obsessive-compulsive disorder, somatoform disorders and dissociative [conversion] Disorders.

神经症是一组精神障碍的总称，该障碍多有一定的人格基础，起病常与社会心理因素有关。症状主要表现为焦虑、抑郁、恐惧、强迫、疑病症、各种躯体不适感等。症状没有任何可证实的器质性病变，与患者的现实处境不相称，但患者的疾病痛苦感明显并对此感到无能为力，病程大多持续迁延。1769年，英国医生William Cullen首次提出“神经症”这一术语，直至20世纪，神经症的概念和内涵才逐渐形成，作为一组人为合并起来的精神障碍。世界不同国家的学者们对神经症的看法不尽一致，各诊断系统包括《国际疾病分类系统》、《美国精神障碍诊断和统计手册》、《中国精神疾病分类方案与诊断标准》等也把它时分时合。神经症所涉及的疾病虽然具有共同的临床特征，但仍有着各自复杂的病因与发病机制，也有着一些不一致的临床表现、治疗方法等。本章参考国际精神疾病分类系统的特点，主要介绍焦虑障碍、强迫障碍、躯体形式障碍及分离（转换）性障碍患者的护理。

Section 1 Nursing Management for Clients with Anxiety Disorders

第一节 焦虑障碍患者的护理

Anxiety disorders is a type of neurosis predominated by anxiety. The main categories are panic disorder and generalized anxiety disorder. It is necessary to distinguish pathological anxiety and normal anxiety in the diagnosis of anxiety disorders.

焦虑障碍是以焦虑为主要特征的一种神经症，包括惊恐障碍与广泛性焦虑障碍两种主要形式。在判断患者是否患有焦虑障碍时，首先应区分正常情况下的焦虑和病理性焦虑。

I. Normal Anxiety and Pathological Anxiety

一、正常焦虑与病理性焦虑

Anyone may suffer from anxiety in their life. Anxiety is a common experience of man. It is a basic mood that has developed from the conflict between man and environment and in the course of adaptation. Not all types of anxiety are clinical disorder. Pathological anxiety must have some features.

每个人在生活中或多或少都会受到焦虑的影响，焦虑是人们的共同经历，是人类在与环境互相作用及生长适应过程中发展起来的基本情绪。焦虑并不都具有临床意义，只有在具备某些特征时，才成为病理性焦虑。

i. Normal Anxiety

Individuals face anxiety on a daily basis. Anxiety, which provides the motivation for achievement, is a necessary force for survival. Anxiety can be a healthy adaptive response when it serves to alert a person of impending threat. Normal anxiety is described as being of realistic intensity and duration for the situation and is followed by relief behaviors intended to reduce or prevent more anxiety. A normal emotional state of anxiety consists of three parts: physiologic arousal, cognitive processes, and coping strategies (Peplau, 1989).

The term anxiety is used to describe feelings of uncertainty, uneasiness, apprehension, or tension that a person experiences in response to an unknown object or situation. A "fight-or flight" decision is made by the person in an attempt to overcome conflict, stress, trauma, or frustration. Anxiety is often used interchangeably with the word stress. However, they are not the same. Stress is an external pressure, which is brought to bear on the individual. Anxiety is the subjective emotional response to a stressor.

Anxiety may be distinguished from fear in that the former is an emotional process, whereas fear is a cognitive one. Fear is defined as an emotional and physiological response to a recognized external threat. Anxiety is an unpleasant emotional state, the sources of which are less readily identified. Fear involves the intellectual appraisal of a threatening stimulus, and anxiety involves the emotional response to that appraisal.

（一）正常焦虑

每个人都会面临焦虑，焦虑可以提供成就的动机，是一种必要的生存力。当危险临近时，焦虑可为人们提供危险预警，是一种健康的适应性反应。正常焦虑是对现实情境持续的反应并伴有减轻和防止更加焦虑的一些行为。Peplau 在 1989 年提出，正常状态的焦虑反应包括三个部分：生理的觉醒、认知过程和应对。

焦虑是一种不确定的、不舒适的、恐惧或忧虑的感受，或是对未知事物或场景的一种紧张体验。当个体试图克服冲突、压力、创伤或挫折时，须决定是“面对”还是“逃避”。焦虑常常被人们描述为紧张，但是两者的意义却不相同。紧张是一种外在压力，而焦虑是对压力源的主观情绪反应。

焦虑与害怕的内涵也不相同，焦虑是一种情绪过程，是个人内在意识的感觉，而害怕是一种认知过程，有具体的外在刺激源，所表现的是对现实客观威胁的一种情绪及心理反应，且这种情绪反应与现实威胁相适应。焦虑是一种令人不愉快的情绪状态，所担心的事情可能不确定。害怕涉及对威胁刺激的

ii. Pathological Anxiety

It is difficult to draw a precise line between normal and abnormal anxiety. Normality is determined by societal standards. What is considered normal in China may not be considered so in other countries. They may have differences within a different country, culture, or region. So what criteria can be used to determine if an individual's anxious response is normal? Beck and Emery (1985) have offered the following guidelines. Anxiety is considered abnormal or pathological if:

1. The response is greatly disproportionate to the risk and severity of the danger or threat.
2. The response continues beyond the existence of a potential danger or threat.
3. Intellectual, social, or occupational functioning is impaired.
4. The individual suffers from a psychosomatic effect (e.g., colitis or dermatitis).

BOX 10-1 Learning More

Degrees of Anxiety

Peplau identified several degrees of anxiety in persons. Mild anxiety creates a state of heightened senses and an acute awareness that is helpful in resolving issues and learning more positive behavior. Perceptual field widens slightly. Able to observe more than before and to see relations. Moderate anxiety decreases the patient's perceptual field so that problem-solving and behavior modification become possible only with outside assistance. At this level, perceptual field narrows slightly. Sees, hears, and grasps less than previously. Usually able to state "I am anxious now." Severe anxiety involves feelings of extreme fear or dread that eliminates the patient's ability to focus on any task. This type of anxiety may also manifest itself physically through excessive perspiration, chest pains and a faster heartbeat. Perceptual field is greatly reduced. Sees, hears, and grasps far less than previously. Attention is focused on a small area of a given event. Inferences drawn may be distorted because of inadequacy of observed data. Panic anxiety is completely debilitating and may involve hallucinations, delusions, physical immobility and irrational thought. Perceptual field is reduced to a detail, which is usually "blown up," i.e., elaborated by distortion (exaggeration), or the focus is on scattered details.

认知评价，而焦虑则是对此评价的情绪反应。

（二）病理性焦虑

明确区分正常焦虑和病理性焦虑有一定的困难，其程度通常由一些社会标准来决定，如在中国属于正常焦虑，而在其他国家可能就不这样认为，这与不同的社会文化背景、宗教信仰等有关。因此 Beck 和 Emery（1985）提出确定个人的焦虑反应是否属于正常反应，需考虑以下因素：① 情绪反应的强度与实际危险是不相称的，大大地超过实际的危险或威胁；② 持续的焦虑反应，远远超过其可能的或潜在的危险或威胁；③ 认知、社会或职业功能常常有受损或削弱；④ 个体身心受到影响（如肠炎、皮肤炎等）。

BOX 10-1 知识拓展

焦虑的程度划分

Peplau 将焦虑划分为不同的程度。轻度焦虑能使敏感性和警觉性增高，其有助于解决问题和学习更积极的行为。知觉领域略有扩大，能够观察到比以前更多的事物并分析其关系。中度焦虑将减少个体的知觉领域，导致解决问题和行为矫正可能需要外部援助。此时，知觉领域略有缩小，看到、听到和掌握的比以前偏少，通常能够表述"我现在处于焦虑状态"。严重焦虑涉及极端恐惧或害怕的感觉，其将影响个体关注任何事物的能力。这种类型的焦虑通常有一些躯体表现如过度出汗、胸痛、心动过速。知觉领域大大降低，看到、听到和掌握的比以前少得多，通常注意力仅集中在特定事件的某个很小的区域。因所获得的观察数据不足可能得出歪曲的推论。恐慌性焦虑是指个体完全衰弱，可能出现幻觉、妄想、身体不能移动和非理性想法。知觉领域极度降低，通常称之为"爆发"，即知觉领域被扭曲或夸大的事实充斥，或者是将着重点集中于分散的细节。

II. Panic Disorder

Panic is an extreme overwhelming form of anxiety often experienced when an individual is placed in a life-threatening situation. Panic is a normal response in such real situations. However, in panic disorder, people experience panic in situations that do not pose any real danger or alter the person's general behavior. The frequency with which clients with panic disorder experience panic attacks varies from multiple attacks during a single day to only a few attacks during the course of a year. About 35% of the population experiences a panic attack in the course of a year, but a much smaller proportion will develop panic disorder. The 2001-2002 National Epidemiologic Survey on Alcohol and Related Conditions (NESARC) revealed a 1-year and lifetime prevalence of panic disorder of 2.1% and 5.1% respectively. Females are more frequently affected than males, at a rate of approximately 2∶1. Being female, middle-aged, widowed/separated/divorced, and of low income, increases the risk for panic disorder, whereas being Asian, African American, or Hispanic decreases risk. In addition, a meta-analysis of studies on anxiety disorder prevalence of Chinese people in 1982-2012 showed that the point prevalence rate of panic disorders was 0.2%. Another study on mental illness survey in China's four provinces (2001-2005) revealed that the prevalence of panic disorder was 0.12%.

二、惊恐障碍

惊恐是指当个体处于危险的场所或情境时，产生的一种极度焦虑反应。在真实的危险场景中，惊恐是一种正常的反应，然而，惊恐障碍患者发生惊恐时所处的场景却并非能构成真正的威胁或改变个体的行为。惊恐发作的频率可一日发作多次或一年仅发作几次。大约有35%的人在一年中经历过惊恐发作，但是只有很少一部分人会发展成为惊恐障碍。2001—2002年美国国家流行病学调查显示惊恐障碍的一年和终身患病率分别为2.1%和5.1%，女性比男性更多地受到影响，其比例约为2∶1。女性、中年、鳏寡/分居/离婚和低收入增加了患惊恐障碍的风险，然而亚洲人、非洲裔美国人或西班牙人风险较低。中国普通人群1982—2012年焦虑障碍患病率的荟萃分析结果显示惊恐障碍的时点患病率为0.2%，而2001—2005年中国四省精神疾病调查结果显示惊恐障碍的月患病率为0.12%。

i. Etiology and Mechanism

1. Biological Theories There are a number of biological theories of panic disorder, which argue strongly against the notion that panic is a reaction to nonspecific distressing stimuli and suggest more specific biological bases. These theories are as follows: overreaction of the locus coeruleus; the panicogen sodium lactate; decreased γ-aminobutyric acid (GABA)-benzodiazepine receptor complex binding; abnormality of serotonergic system adjustment; hypersensitive brain stem CO_2 chemoreceptors; abnormally sensitive fear network centered in the amygdala; and moderate genetic influence. But the underlying pathophysiology of panic disorder has not been elucidated.

2. Psychodynamic Theories Psychoanalytic theories conceptualize panic attacks as resulting from an unsuccessful defense against anxiety-provoking impulses. The research indicates that the cause of panic attacks is likely to involve the unconscious meaning of stressful events and that the pathogenesis of the panic attacks may

（一）病因及发病机制

1. 生物学理论 有关惊恐障碍的生物学理论有很多，这些理论有力地反驳了惊恐是对非特定痛苦刺激的反应，并提供了惊恐障碍的许多生物学基础。这些生物学理论包括蓝斑的过度反应；引起惊恐的乳酸钠；γ-氨基丁酸-苯二氮䓬受体复合体捆绑力下降；血清素能调控紊乱；脑干二氧化碳化学受体敏感性增高；敏感性增高状态下的恐惧网络集中于扁桃体；以及中等程度的遗传因素影响等。但是有关惊恐障碍的病理生理学尚不清楚。

2. 心理动力学理论 精神分析理论认为焦虑与早期发展有关，惊恐发作是由于对潜意识冲突不成功防御的结果。有研究发现，对压力事件的无意识反应是惊恐发作的原因，惊恐发作的发病机理或许与心理反应所引起

be related to neurophysiological factors triggered by the psychological reactions.

3. Learning Theories and Traumatic Antecedents Behavioral theories posit that anxiety is a learned response either from modeling parental behavior or through the process of classical conditioning, and anxiety is conditioned by the fear of certain environmental stimuli. Moreover, childhood interpersonal trauma also appears to make a contribution to the likelihood that individuals will manifest panic disorder.

ii. Clinical Manifestation

Panic disorder is also called acute anxiety. It refers to recurrent unexpected panic attacks. Although the first attack generally strikes during some routine activity, several events are often associated with the early presentation of panic disorder, which could be a life-threatening illness or accident, the loss of a close interpersonal relationship, or a separation from family. The major mental symptoms are extreme fear and a sense of impending death and doom; feelings of going crazy or losing control and desperation are common. Cognitive symptoms also include disorganized thinking, irrational fears, and decreased ability to communicate verbally. Clients are usually not able to name the source of their fear. The clients may feel confused and have trouble in concentrating. Several of a group of associated symptoms, mostly physical, are also experienced: tachycardia or palpitations, nausea, dizziness, chest pain or discomfort, dyspnea, paresthesias, trembling or shaking, sweating and sensation of suffocation or shortness of breath. Clients often try to leave whatever situation they are in to seek help. The attack often begins with a 10-minute period of rapidly increasing symptoms, lasts 20 to 30 minutes and rarely more than an hour. Somatic concerns of death from a cardiac or respiratory problem may be the major focus of clients' attention during panic attacks. Clients may believe that the palpitations and the pain in their chest indicate that they are about to die. About 20 percent of such clients actually have syncopal episodes during the onset of panic attack. Approximately 60% of the clients develop avoidance behavior due to fearing no help during the panic attack, such as not go out alone, not go to crowded place. Some clients have expectancy anxiety during the intervals of the attacks.

iii. Treatment

The two most effective treatments are pharmacotherapy and cognitive-behavioral therapy. Family and group therapy may help affected clients and their families adjust to the face that clients have the disorder and to the psychosocial difficulties the disorder

的神经生理学因素的改变有关。

3. 学习理论与创伤经历 行为或学习理论认为焦虑是学习而得到的反应，许多人可能是从其双亲或共同生活者的角色示范中学会焦虑，焦虑是以对某些环境刺激的恐惧为条件的。此外，儿童时期的人际创伤似乎也对个体表现惊恐障碍的可能性有促进作用。

（二）临床表现

惊恐障碍又称为急性焦虑症，其基本特征是严重焦虑的反复发作，具有不可预测性。首次惊恐发作常出现于日常活动中，但惊恐发作也通常与一些重大生活事件相关，如重大疾病或事件、亲密关系的丧失或与家庭分离等。惊恐发作时，患者常突然感到一种突如其来的恐惧体验，觉得死亡将至，并伴有濒死感或失控感，以及绝望感。在认知方面患者可能出现思维紊乱、不合理的恐惧和言语沟通能力下降等。患者通常不能明确说明恐惧的来源，可能感到困惑、不能集中注意力。惊恐发作常伴随一些躯体症状，包括心动过速或心悸、恶心、头晕、胸痛不适、呼吸困难、皮肤感觉异常、震颤或发抖、出汗、窒息感或气短等。惊恐发作通常起病急骤，10分钟内达到高峰，一般历时20～30分钟，发作很少超过1小时。当惊恐发作时，患者最关注心脏和呼吸系统方面的症状，胸部不适和心悸常使患者相信即将面临死亡。约20%的患者在惊恐发作时有眩晕的症状。约60%的患者由于担心发病时得不到帮助而产生回避行为，如不敢单独出门，不敢到人多热闹的场所，发展为场所恐惧症，有些患者发作间期有害怕再次发作的期待性焦虑。

（三）治疗

惊恐障碍的主要治疗方法包括药物治疗和认知行为治疗，而家庭和小组治疗也可以帮助患者和家属正确面对疾病、适应和克服疾病所导致的心理社会方面的问题。

may have precipitated.

1. Pharmacotherapy Most antidepressants (tricyclics, selective serotonin reuptake inhibitors, monoamine oxidase inhibitors, and others) substantially reduce the frequency and severity of panic attacks and often completely prevent them. Benzodiazepine anxiolytics are also effective antipanic drugs (including alprazolam and clonazepam, but do not appear to be unique) and work quicker than the antidepressants, although they have a risk of dependence. For clients with severe anxiety, it can be helpful to initially prescribe a concomitant benzodiazepine that can be gradually tapered and discontinued after several weeks of antidepressant treatment. All antipanic drugs should be started at low dosages such as what would be given to depressed clients and increased gradually until an effective dosage level is achieved.

1. 药物治疗 很多抗抑郁剂，如三环类抗抑郁药、选择性5-HT再摄取抑制剂、单胺氧化酶抑制剂等，都能够很好地控制惊恐发作的频率及强度，减轻焦虑，并预防再次发作。此外，使用苯二氮䓬类药物治疗惊恐障碍也有肯定疗效，该类药物比抗抑郁剂起效更快，通常不单独使用，常用的药物有阿普唑仑、氯硝安定等，但此类药物容易产生药物依赖。针对严重焦虑患者，在抗抑郁治疗的同时，可以同时使用苯二氮䓬类药物并逐渐减少剂量直至停用。惊恐障碍治疗药物均应从低剂量开始并逐渐增加至有效剂量。

2. Cognitive and Behavioral Therapies Cognitive therapy is an effective treatment for panic disorder, and behavioral therapy such as exposure therapy, can substantially reduce the frequency and severity of panic attacks. A combination of medication and cognitive-behavioral therapy is most beneficial for many clients. Relapse rates following withdrawal from medication may be substantially lower when the two therapies are combined.

2. 认知行为治疗 认知治疗是惊恐障碍的有效治疗方法，行为治疗如暴露治疗能帮助降低惊恐发作的频率和强度。而药物治疗联合心理治疗能够更好预防停药后的复发，获得更为持续的效果。

(1) Cognitive therapy: The two major foci of cognitive therapy for panic disorder are instruction regarding the client's false beliefs and information regarding panic attacks. The instruction regarding false beliefs centers on the client's tendency to misinterpret mild bodily sensations as indicative of impending panic attacks, doom or death. The information about panic attacks includes explanations that panic attacks. Cognitive therapy is mainly to help the client to recognize the relationship between their own specific ideas and the realized anxiety, and to find cognitive process of special internal or external cues with anxiety.

（1）认知治疗：认知治疗惊恐障碍的两个主要焦点为纠正患者关于惊恐障碍的错误信念与理解，错误信念常使患者倾向于误认为不舒适的躯体感觉代表即将到来的惊恐发作、厄运或死亡，而有关惊恐发作的理解主要指对于惊恐发作的解释。认知治疗主要帮助患者认识到自己的某些特殊想法与所体验到的焦虑之间的关系，发现特殊的内在或外界的线索与其焦虑情绪之间的认知过程。

(2) Applied relaxation: The goal of applied relaxation is to instill a sense of controlling in clients regarding their levels of anxiety and relaxation. Through the use of standardized techniques for muscle relaxation and the imagining of relaxing situation, clients learn techniques that may help them through a panic attack.

（2）放松训练：应用放松的目的是营造一种氛围，帮助患者控制焦虑水平并进行放松，通过肌肉放松及想象放松训练，特别是患者掌握这些技术后，能帮助他们减少惊恐发作。

(3) Breathing retraining: Since the hyperventilation associated with panic attacks is probably related to some symptoms, such as dizziness and faintness, one direct approach to control panic attacks is to train clients how to control both acute and chronic hyperventilation.

（3）呼吸训练：患者在惊恐发作时常伴有过度通气或呼吸困难，其可能与头晕、虚弱无力等症状有关，可以教会患者在惊恐发作时如何进行呼吸控制，包括急性与慢性的过度通气。

3. Supportive Psychotherapy Despite adequate treatment of panic attacks with medication, phobic avoidance may remain. Supportive psychotherapy and education about the illness are necessary to urge the client to confront the phobic situation. Clients who fail to respond may then need additional psychotherapy, either dynamic or behavioral. Encouragement from other clients with similar conditions is often quite helpful. Yet supportive psychotherapy alone is not adequate treatment for panic disorder.

3. 支持性心理治疗 尽管给予患者足够的药物治疗，患者的恐惧性回避仍可能存在。支持性心理治疗和疾病知识教育对促使患者面对恐惧性场景非常必要，但有些治疗效果较差的患者可能需要额外的心理治疗，如动力学或行为治疗。此外，来自病友的鼓励对恢复非常有帮助。然而单纯的支持性心理治疗对于惊恐障碍不是有效的治疗方法。

III. Generalized Anxiety Disorder

三、广泛性焦虑障碍

Generalized anxiety disorder (GAD) is defined as a kind of anxiety disorder predominated by breathlessness with anxiety and nervousness which are not restricted to clear objects and concrete content, and accompanied by autonomic symptoms (dizziness, chest tightness, palpitation, dyspnea, etc.), muscular tension, and motor intranquility. The clients often feel affliction but are unable to get rid of it. The essential feature of generalized anxiety disorder is excessive anxiety and worry (apprehensive expectation) about a number of events or activities. The intensity, duration, or frequency of the anxiety and worry are out of proportion to the actual likelihood or impact of the anticipated event.

The National Comorbidity Survey found the 12-month prevalence of generalized anxiety disorder to be 2.0% in males and 4.3% in females. Women are approximately twice as likely to experience GAD as men. Higher rates of the disorder were also found in the elderly. In China, a meta-analysis of studies on anxiety disorder prevalence of Chinese people in 1982-2012, showed that the point prevalence of generalized anxiety disorders is 0.6%. An investigation of mental illness in China's four provinces (2001-2005) revealed that the prevalence rate of generalized anxiety disorder was 1.3%. The age of onset is difficult to specify, since most clients with disorder report that they have been anxious for as long as they can remember. There are some reports that half of adults with GAD report onset in childhood.

广泛性焦虑障碍又称慢性焦虑症，其特征是对没有明确的客观对象和固定内容的过分担心、紧张不安等，常伴随自主神经功能紊乱症状（头晕、胸闷、心悸、呼吸困难等）、肌肉紧张、运动性不安等，患者常感到痛苦，但又无法摆脱。广泛性焦虑障碍的患者常对于诸多事件或活动产生过度的焦虑和担心（焦虑性期待），其紧张度、持续时间或焦虑和担心出现的频率都与现实可能性或预期事件的冲击不成比例。

美国疾病调查发现广泛性焦虑障碍12个月患病率男性为2.0%、女性为4.3%。女性患广泛性焦虑障碍的概率是男性的2倍，此外，老年人中也发现较高的患病率。中国普通人群1982—2012年焦虑障碍患病率的荟萃分析结果显示广泛性焦虑障碍的时点患病率为0.6%，2001—2005年中国四省精神疾病调查结果显示广泛性焦虑障碍的月患病率为1.3%。广泛性焦虑障碍的发病年龄很难界定，大多数患者称自能记事起就出现焦虑，也有报道显示一半的成年广泛性焦虑障碍患者在儿童时期开始出现焦虑。

i. Etiology and Mechanism

（一）病因及发病机制

1. Biological Theories The GABA-benzodiazepine system may be more active in generalized anxiety disorder. Benzodiazepines are known to reduce anxiety, whereas flumazenil (Romazicon) (a benzodiazepine receptor antagonist) and the β-carbolines (benzodiazepine receptor antagonist) are known to induce anxiety. Moreover, Studies suggest that a tendency for anxiety may

1. 生物学理论 广泛性焦虑障碍患者中γ-氨基丁酸-苯二氮䓬受体可能更活跃，因此苯二氮䓬类药物具有抗焦虑作用，而氟马西尼（一种苯二氮䓬受体拮抗剂）也能降低焦虑。此外，遗传研究发现，焦虑的发生有遗传倾向，广泛性焦虑障

be inherited, about 25 percent of first-degree relatives of clients with generalized anxiety disorder are also affected. Some twin studies report a concordance rate of 50 percent in monozygotic twins and 15 percent in dizygotic twins.

2. Psychological Theories There are two major schools of thought regarding the psychosocial factors leading to the development of generalized anxiety disorder. One is cognitive-behavioral school, which hypothesizes that clients with generalized anxiety disorder are responding to perceived danger incorrectly and inaccurately. The inaccuracy is generated by selective attention to negative details in the environment, by distortions in information processing, and by an overly negative view of one's own ability to cope. The other one is the psychoanalytic school, which hypothesizes that anxiety is a symptom of unresolved unconscious conflicts about dangerous emotions, behaviors, or states.

ii. Clinical Manifestation

The essential feature of generalized anxiety disorder is persistent anxiety and excessive worry lasting at least 6 months. The symptoms of this type of anxiety fall within two broad categories: apprehensive expectation and worry, and physical symptoms. Clients with GAD are constantly worried over minor matters, fearful, and anticipating the worst. Muscle tension, motor tension, a "keyed up" feeling, difficulty concentrating, insomnia, irritability, and fatigue are typical signs of GAD. The motor tension is most commonly manifested as shakiness and restlessness. GAD is often accompanied by autonomic hyperactivity symptoms, such as dry mouth, excessive sweating, palpitations, shortness of breath, and various gastrointestinal symptoms. Motor tension and hypervigilance better differentiate GAD from other anxiety states than autonomic hyperactivity.

iii. Treatment

The most effective treatment of clients with generalized anxiety disorder is probably one that combines psychotherapeutic, pharmacotherapeutic, and supportive approaches.

1. Pharmacotherapy The two major drugs to be considered for the treatment of generalized anxiety disorder are benzodiazepines and buspirone. Other drugs that may be useful are the tricyclic drugs.

(1) Benzodiazepine antianxiety drugs are effective in reducing or alleviating symptoms of generalized anxiety in many clients. Sedation is the major side effect, and physiological dependence will occur in most clients taking benzodiazepines steadily over several months.

(2) Buspirone, an azapirone, is most likely effective

碍患者的一级亲属中约25%患病，而有关孪生子患病的研究发现，单卵双生子的同病率为50%，双卵双生子的同病率为15%。

2. 心理学理论 关于广泛性焦虑障碍的心理社会因素有两种学说。一种是认知－行为学说，认为患者患病与对危险的不正确和不切实际的认知有关。患者的这种不正确的感受是源于选择性地关注环境中的负性信息，信息过程扭曲，或只看到自己应对能力弱的方面。另一种学说是以弗洛伊德为代表的精神分析理论，认为焦虑是潜意识中未解决的、无意识的冲突表现。

（二）临床表现

广泛性焦虑障碍的基本特征是持续存在的焦虑与过度担心，持续时间至少6个月以上。其临床症状主要包括两大类：焦虑性期待与担心、躯体症状。广泛性焦虑障碍患者总是持续担心一些小问题、感觉恐惧，并进行最坏情况的预测。其特征性症状包括肌肉紧张、运动不安、“紧张”的感觉、注意力不集中、失眠、易怒和疲劳等，运动不安的症状主要为轻微震颤、坐立不安等。广泛性焦虑障碍常伴有自主神经功能紊乱等躯体症状，如口干、出汗、心悸、气短及各种消化道症状等。运动不安及过度焦虑相较于自主神经功能亢进能更好地将广泛性焦虑障碍从其他焦虑障碍中区分出来。

（三）治疗

广泛性焦虑障碍患者的治疗通常采用心理、药物和支持性治疗等联合治疗方式。

1. 药物治疗 苯二氮䓬类药物和丁螺环酮是治疗广泛性焦虑障碍最主要的两类药物，其他有效治疗的药物主要为三环类药物。

（1）苯二氮䓬类药物：对广泛性焦虑障碍有肯定的抗焦虑作用，副作用主要为镇静，在使用数月后可造成患者对药物的依赖。

（2）丁螺环酮：对60%～80%的广泛性

in 60 to 80 percent of clients with generalized anxiety disorder. Data indicate that buspirone is more effective in reducing the cognitive symptoms of generalized anxiety disorder than in reducing the somatic symptoms. It does not have sedative effects, does not interact with alcohol, and does not lead to dependence. The major disadvantage of buspirone is that its effects take two to three weeks to become evident, in contrast to the almost immediate anxiolytic effects of the benzodiazepine. Buspirone is not effective treatment for benzodiazepine withdrawal.

(3) Tricyclic antidepressants and venlafaxine have been shown to be effective treatment for GAD, the latter having recently been approved for this condition by the Food and Drug Administration (FDA). They avoid risks of physical dependency associated with benzodiazepine treatment, but usually cause more side symptoms.

2. Psychotherapy The major psychotherapeutic approaches to generalized anxiety disorder are cognitive-behavioral, supportive, relaxation and insight-oriented. Cognitive approaches directly address the client's hypothesized cognitive disorder, and behavioral approaches address the somatic symptoms directly. The major techniques used in the behavioral approaches are relaxation and biofeedback. Supportive therapy offers clients reassurance and comfort, although its long-term efficacy is doubtful. Insight-oriented psychotherapy focuses on uncovering unconscious conflicts and identifying ego strengths.

焦虑障碍患者有效。数据显示，丁螺环酮在减轻认知症状方面的作用优于减轻躯体症状。它没有镇静的副作用，也不与酒精相互作用，并且不产生依赖性，最主要的缺点是药物疗效须经过 2～3 周才能显现出来，抗焦虑作用不同于苯二氮䓬类药物的迅速起效。对于苯二氮䓬类药物的戒断反应，丁螺环酮是无效的。

（3）其他：三环类抗抑郁药物和文拉法辛对治疗广泛性焦虑有肯定疗效，后者已经被美国食品药品监督管理局认证。这两类药物都可以避免苯二氮䓬类药物的成瘾作用，但是却可能引起其他一些副作用。

2. 心理治疗 广泛性焦虑障碍患者常用的心理治疗包括认知 – 行为治疗、支持性心理治疗、松弛治疗和心理教育认知。认知治疗主要针对患者对疾病的不恰当认识和曲解，进行心理治疗和教育，行为治疗直接针对躯体症状，主要的训练方法为放松训练和生物反馈。支持性治疗主要为患者提供舒适，尽管其长期疗效存在争议。心理教育认知治疗主要帮助患者认识和解决潜意识的冲突和矛盾。

Ⅳ. Application of the Nursing Process

Often, physiologic symptoms are the primary reason for the client to seek medical assistance. In addition, anxiety disorder can mimic the symptoms of other medical and psychiatric illness. From a thorough biologic, psychological, and social assessment, nurses provide significant contributions to accurate diagnosis.

i. Nursing Assessment

1. Biologic Assessment

(1) Symptom assessment

1) Symptom assessment of panic disorder: Clients with panic disorder often present with a confusing array of symptoms. There are high correlations between panic disorder and some medical conditions such as cardiac disease, asthma, and some gastrointestinal disorders. Physical symptoms associated with panic attacks may cause the nurse to draw incorrect conclusions.There are some questions will help nurse to ask the clients as

四、护理程序的应用

躯体症状常常是焦虑障碍患者寻求治疗的主要原因，而焦虑障碍的症状常常又与其他躯体疾病和精神疾病的一些临床表现类似。通过系统评估，护士可获得准确完整的信息资料，帮助确立护理问题，进而提出恰当的护理措施。

（一）护理评估

1. 生理方面

（1）症状评估

1）惊恐障碍：惊恐障碍的患者通常主诉一些容易使人混淆的症状，其症状与某些躯体疾病如心脏病、哮喘、胃肠疾病等有相似之处，容易导致护士做出错误的判断。以下一些提问可帮助护士了解患者的情况：① 当您处在惊恐发作期和间隔期时有什么样的体

following:(a)What do you experience proceeding and during a panic episode, including physical symptoms, feelings, thoughts, and behaviors?(b)When did the symptoms begin? Were there precipitants (e.g., events, environmental conditions, or substance exposure)?(c)Have you experienced these symptoms in the past? If so, under what circumstances?(d)Has anyone in your family had similar symptoms?(e)What actions have relieved these symptoms? Did they resolve without intervention?

验，包括身体的、感知的、思想的和行为方面的？② 这些症状是什么时候开始的，是突发的吗，有无突发事件、环境因素或物质暴露？③ 您曾经经历过这些症状吗，如果有，是在什么样的情况下发生的？④ 您的家族中还有谁有同样的问题？⑤ 使该症状减轻或消失的措施有哪些，症状能够自己缓解吗？

2) Symptom assessment of GAD: Assessment of the client's individual anxiety symptoms should include the following questions:(a) How does the client experience symptoms?(b)Are the client's symptoms primary physical, psychological, or both?(c) Is the client aware when he or she is becoming anxious?(d)Is the client even aware that the symptoms are anxiety induced?(e) What coping mechanisms does the client routinely use to deal with anxiety?(f)What life stressors add to these symptoms? What changes can be made to reduce these stressors?

2）广泛性焦虑障碍：评估患者的焦虑症状时，应注意以下问题：① 患者是如何感受这些症状的？② 患者最初出现的是躯体方面的不适，还是精神心理方面的症状，或者两者同时都有？③ 患者是否清楚何时出现焦虑？④ 患者是否清楚这些症状是焦虑所致？⑤ 患者通常采用的焦虑应对策略有哪些？⑥ 有哪些生活压力可能加重症状，而有哪些措施可减轻这些压力？

(2) Substance use: It is important to assess for substance use, such as sources of caffeine, pseudoephedrine, amphetamines, cocaine, or other stimulants. Cigarette consumption and alcohol must also be considered as a stimulant as well as a condition that may increase carbon dioxide and thus contribute to the onset of anxiety.

（2）物质滥用评估：评估患者是否存在物质滥用，如咖啡因、伪麻黄碱、安非他明、可卡因或酒精、烟草等物质，这些刺激性物质均可能诱发焦虑发作。

(3) Sleep patterns: Sleep is often disturbed in anxiety disorder. Individuals who experience spontaneous panic attacks during sleep may have particular fears regarding going to sleep. Sleep difficulties also occur more frequently for individuals with other coexisting psychiatric disorder, such as depression. Nurse should closely assess the impact of sleep disturbance because fatigue may increase anxiety and susceptibility to panic attack.

（3）睡眠型态：焦虑障碍的患者常常存在睡眠障碍，特别是对那些在睡眠中出现惊恐发作的患者，常因为担心惊恐发作而害怕睡觉。另外，伴发其他精神障碍如抑郁的患者也常存在睡眠问题，睡眠障碍可加重患者的焦虑和导致惊恐发作。

(4) Nutrition: Eating poorly or infrequently can contribute to the occurrence of a panic attack and aggravated anxiety. In addition, some of the physical symptoms of hypoglycemia such as sweating, nausea, palpitations, and tremors are similar to those of panic attack and can also trigger fears that an attack is about to begin.

（4）营养情况：如果患者进食过少或进食次数太少都可能导致惊恐发作或焦虑加重。此外，低血糖的一些临床表现如出汗、恶心、呕吐、心悸、震颤等与惊恐发作的症状类似，其常会引起患者害怕再次惊恐发作。

(5) Physical activity: Physical exercise can diminish the occurrence of panic attacks and anxiety. Regular exercise reduces muscle tension, increases metabolism, and discharges emotional frustrations. Nurse should ask the client if regular exercise is part of their schedule. If not, what are the barriers?

（5）活动：体育活动能够缓解惊恐发作及焦虑，有规律的体育活动可放松肌肉，增加新陈代谢、释放焦虑。护士应了解患者是否能够进行有规律的活动，如不能，有什么原因。

(6) Menstrual cycle: With women, nurse should assess whether the client experiences increased episodes

（6）月经周期：对于女性患者，护士要询问患者的月经周期，并了解惊恐发作、焦

of panic or severe anxiety during the days before the onset of menses. Premenstrual hormonal changes produce a number of physical sensations that may appear to be the beginning of panic symptoms, and influence the degree of anxiety possibly.

虑水平与月经周期之间的关系，是否存在月经前期惊恐发作频率增加、焦虑加重的现象。因月经前期体内激素水平的变化可导致身体及精神的变化，而这些变化与惊恐发作的前期症状相似，进而影响患者的焦虑水平。

2. Psychological Assessment Except assessment of characteristic symptoms of anxiety, a more comprehensive assessment should include the client's responses to the anxiety, suicidal tendencies and thoughts, cognitive thought patterns, and avoidance behavior patterns.

(1) Mental status examination: Even without the presence of a panic attack, individuals with panic disorder often exhibit symptoms of anxiety, restlessness and irritability, watchful or worried facial expression, decreased attention span, and apprehensive behavior or helplessness. During a panic attack the individual may exhibit disorganized thinking, irrational fears, and decreased ability to communicate verbally. Some clients have proven to be at greater risk for suicide. The nurse should assess the risk of suicide, including information from family and significant others.

(2) Cognitive thought patterns: Although catastrophic thinking alone does not cause panic attacks, such catastrophic misinterpretations can aggravate panic and anxiety symptoms. This type of thinking includes: "Something terrible is happening to me," or "I'm dying."

(3) Avoidance behavior patterns: Individuals with panic attack may have learned to avoid certain physical conditions or situations that precipitate the attacks such as avoiding smoking or caffeinated behaviors. However, other avoidances, such as refusing to ride in a car or go shopping, may severely affect their ability to identify the behavioral patterns that might interfere with treatment, such as ability to get to the clinic for therapy sessions.

2. 心理评估 除了评估患者焦虑的表现外，更为综合广泛的评估还应包括患者对于焦虑的反应、自杀的倾向及想法、认知方式、回避行为方式等。

（1）精神状态的评估：对于惊恐障碍的患者，即使没有出现惊恐发作，也会表现出一些焦虑症状，如坐立不安、易怒、表情焦虑和警觉性增加、注意力下降、忧虑行为或无助感。在惊恐发作时，患者可能表现出思维紊乱，不合理的恐惧，语言交流能力下降。有的焦虑患者可能存在自杀危险，护士须认真评估患者的自杀危险性，并向患者家属及其他相关人员了解情况。

（2）认知方式：虽然灾难性想法单独不会引起惊恐发作，但是，对灾难不恰当的认知可加重惊恐发作的症状及焦虑症状。这些不恰当的认知包括“我将有不幸发生”“我快要死了”等。

（3）回避行为：惊恐障碍患者可能学会回避那些可能引起惊恐发作的场所或活动，如避免咖啡、吸烟等。然而有些回避行为如拒绝乘坐汽车、去商场等将会严重影响那些可能与治疗相关的行为能力，如到医院参加治疗课程的能力。

3. Social Assessment Marital and parental function is adversely affected in clients with anxiety disorder. During the assessment, the nurse should ascertain the clients' understanding of the symptoms and how the disease has affected the client's life and family. There are some questions that may help the nurse assess how this disorder affects the client's life.

(1) To what degree is the client's mobility limited?

(2) Is the client unable to work, use public transportation, or go shopping? Or is the client immobilized?

(3) What coping strategies has the client used to manage symptoms?

3. 社会评估 焦虑障碍对患者的婚姻、家庭功能影响很大，评估时，护士应注意了解患者对于疾病症状的理解以及疾病对患者生活及家庭的影响。下面这些问题可帮助护士了解疾病对患者生活的影响：① 患者因为疾病受限制的程度如何；② 患者是否不能去工作、去商场或乘坐交通工具，或患者是否完全不能活动；③ 患者采取了哪些方法去应对症状；④ 症状对患者的配偶、孩子、父母及其重要相关人员的影响如何？此外，在评估时，护士须考虑社会文化因素对患者的影

(4) How do these symptoms affect the spouse, children, parent, or significant others?

Furthermore, nurses should consider the cultural factors of clients. Differences exist between cultures in terms of how individuals express both physical sensations and feelings.

响，不同社会文化背景的患者在症状和感受上存在差异性。

ii. Nursing Diagnosis

1. Anxiety Related to anxiety and physical symptoms, worries about panic attacks.

2. Powerlessness Related to impaired cognition.

3. Disturbed Sleep Pattern Related to anxiety symptoms.

4. Risk for Suicide Related to anxiety symptoms or violent behaviors caused by anxiety.

5. Ineffective Coping Related to cognitive thought patterns and deficient knowledge.

6. Impaired Social Interaction Related to avoidance behavior patterns.

7. Deficient Knowledge Related to lack of knowledge associated with the disorder and coping skills.

（二）主要护理诊断

1. **焦虑** 与焦虑症状、躯体症状及担心惊恐发作有关。

2. **无能为力** 与不恰当的认知方式有关。

3. **睡眠型态紊乱** 与焦虑症状有关。

4. **有自杀的危险** 与焦虑症状或症状所致可能采取的过激行为有关。

5. **应对无效** 与个体的认知方式及知识缺乏有关。

6. **社会交往障碍** 与担心疾病发作的回避行为有关。

7. **知识缺乏** 与缺乏疾病相关知识、应对方法等有关。

iii. Nursing Planning

1. Nursing Outcome

(1) Shows no signs or symptoms of anxiety or reduced degree of anxiety.

(2) Recognize signs of escalating anxiety and be able to intervene so that anxiety does not reach the panic level.

(3) Has not experienced persistent and aggravated sleep problems.

(4) Has not experienced physical injury or caused harm to self.

(5) Practices techniques of relaxation daily and be able to maintain anxiety at manageable level without use of medication. Discuss long-term plan to prevent panic anxiety when stress situation occurs.

(6) Performs activities of daily living independently and expresses satisfaction for independent functioning.

(7) Acknowledges association between the disorder and internal conflicts, verbalizes relationship among psychological factors, social factors and the disorder.

2. Nursing Intervention These interventions deal chiefly with helping the client attend to and react to input other than the subjective experience of anxiety. These interventions are aimed at helping the client learn to focus on other stimuli and cope with anxiety disorders, so they will not be reiterated in subsequent sections. The

（三）护理计划

1. **护理目标**

（1）患者焦虑症状减轻或消失。

（2）患者能够认识不断增加的焦虑症状，并能主动调整焦虑，避免焦虑的不断升级。

（3）患者睡眠得到改善。

（4）患者住院期间未发生自我伤害事件。

（5）患者能每天进行松弛训练，能不借助药物将焦虑控制在一定水平，当产生压力时，患者能够讨论如何避免焦虑的长期计划。

（6）患者能显示出独立进行日常生活的能力，并表达对独立能力的满意，社会功能基本恢复正常。

（7）患者能正确认识疾病，以及与内心冲突的关系，正确认识心理、社会因素与疾病的关系。

2. **护理措施** 针对焦虑障碍的干预措施主要是帮助患者认识焦虑，协助患者发展应对压力和焦虑的能力。当患者急性焦虑发作时，处于一种危急状态，护士应采用多种方法帮助患者减轻症状。以下列出焦虑障碍患

client experiencing a panic attack is in crisis. The nurse can take several measures to help alleviate symptoms.

(1) Ensure the safety of clients and improve the comfort

1) Stay with the client and offer reassurance of safety and security. Client may fear for life, and the presence of a trusted individual provides a feeling of security and assurance of personal safety.

2) Anxiety produces more anxiety. Understanding this concept is essential in caring for the client with anxiety disorder. It is important for client and nurse to participate in monitoring and managing environmental stress levels. For clients to relax and reduce stress they need a relaxed environment and those around them should be relaxed. Assist the client to an environment with minimal stimulation (reduction of noise, dim lighting, and simple décor). A calm environment will may decrease level of anxiety. The nurse also should consider such factors as time management skills to avoid rushing, decreased clutter, and increased personal space.

3) Administer tranquilizing medication, as ordered by physician. Assess for effectiveness and for side effects. Anti-anxiety medication provides relief from the immobilizing effects of anxiety.

4) Observe clients' feelings closely, for clients with self-injury and suicide risk, nurses should pay attention to eliminate possible dangerous materials and other unsafe factors in the environment to prevent the occurrence of unexpected events.

(2) Sleep management

1) Sleep disturbance is also a common symptom for individuals with anxiety disorder. Therefore, close assessment of the client's sleep pattern and assistance with implementing sleep hygiene measures is important.

2) Evidence exists that clients with anxiety disorder are abnormally sensitive to caffeine. Client with anxiety disorder can take to reduce anxiety when eliminate caffeine from their diets. Thus, nurse can help clients keep away from coffee, tea, chocolate, and other central nervous excited drink or drugs through education and dietary management.

3) Nurses should monitor and manage environmental stress levels, and offer a relaxed environment for clients. The nurse should also teach clients with anxiety disorder some anxiety management skills to reduce levels of anxiety to improve the sleep quality.

4) Teach various measures for self treatment of insomnia, including regular daily life, fixed sleep time,

者的常见护理措施。

（1）保障患者安全，提高舒适度

1）陪伴患者，提供支持和保证安全，当患者处于焦虑状态时，会感到紧张、恐惧，陪伴可减轻患者的恐惧，使患者感到安全。

2）焦虑是一个恶性循环，护士应重视对环境中压力的监督和管理。护士应为患者提供一个放松的治疗环境，减轻环境中的刺激，如安静的环境、柔和的灯光、较少的人员、简单的装饰等；指导患者学习时间管理方法等以避免仓促，减少混乱，增加患者的私人空间等，以帮助减轻焦虑。

3）指导和督促患者进行抗焦虑药物治疗，并评估药物疗效及副作用。

4）密切观察患者情绪变化，对有自伤、自杀危险的患者，应注意防范，排除环境中可能的危险物品及其他不安全因素，防止患者出现意外情况。

（2）睡眠管理

1）睡眠评估：睡眠障碍是焦虑障碍患者常见的问题，应仔细评估患者睡眠型态，帮助患者养成良好的睡眠习惯。

2）饮食管理：焦虑障碍患者常对咖啡等异常敏感，当把咖啡从患者的日常饮食中去除时，患者的焦虑水平就下降，进而睡眠得到改善。因此，护士应指导患者避免使用咖啡、浓茶、巧克力及其他中枢神经兴奋的饮料或药物。

3）减轻焦虑：护士应重视对环境中压力的监督和管理，为患者提供一个放松的治疗环境，并指导患者学习一些控制焦虑的方法，帮助减轻焦虑反应，进而改善睡眠。

4）教会患者自我处理失眠的各种措施，包括生活规律、睡眠时间尽量固定、睡前两

avoiding excitable activity two hours before sleep, and sleep with familiar objects or habits such as listening to music, using familiar blanket. Instruct the client to use relaxation methods, such as abdominal breath, muscle relaxation. A relaxed environment is most important, including soft light, proper temperature and humidity, air circulation, and reduced noise.

5) If necessary, administer sedative hypnotic medication as prescribed by physician. Evaluate for effectiveness and for side effects.

(3) Psychological care

1) Establish trust with clients. The nurse must be aware of own level of anxiety and use appropriate strategies to decrease anxiety to a tolerable level prior to approaching client. Anxiety is readily transferred from person to person.

2) Maintain a calm, non-threatening, matter-of-fact approach. Approach the client in a direct, non-authoritative manner. In a state of panic, the client's ability to think and process complex information is limited. A calm presence will help calm the client. Client develops a feeling of security in the presence of a calm staff person.

3) When level of anxiety has been reduced, explore possible reasons for occurrence. Recognition of precipitating factors is the first step in teaching client to interrupt escalation of anxiety.

4) Encourage clients to express their emotions and unpleasant feelings. Teach cognitive restructuring to stop negative thoughts of powerlessness and substitute reality-based thoughts of hope and control. Self-talk reinforces a sense of realistic ability to master problems.

5) Teach signs and symptoms of escalating anxiety and ways to interrupt its progression (relaxation techniques, breathing control exercises, progressive muscle relaxation, and meditation, or physical exercise, brisk walks, and jogging).

(4) Improve the ability of self-control and social functions

1) Assess for feeling of powerlessness when anxiety attacks. Explore client's reasons or experiences that underlie powerlessness and provide information about available choices and techniques to achieve greater control.

2) Help identify areas of life situation that client can control and that are not within his or her ability to control. Encourage verbalization of feelings related to this inability. This will assist the client to deal with unresolved issues and learn to accept what cannot be changed.

3) Assist client to set realistic goals and carefully/gradually increase goals and skill training to maximize opportunities for success. Unrealistic goals set the client up for failure and reinforce feelings of powerlessness.

小时避免易兴奋的活动，用熟悉的物品或习惯帮助入睡，如听音乐、用习惯的被褥等。指导患者使用睡眠诱导放松的方法，包括腹式呼吸、肌肉放松等。营造最佳的睡眠环境，避免光线过亮，维持适当的温度和湿度，保持空气流通，避免噪音干扰等。

5）必要时遵医嘱指导和督促患者正确应用镇静催眠药物，并评估药物疗效及副作用。

（3）心理护理

1）取得患者的信任，建立良好的护患关系。护士在接触患者前应将自己的焦虑调整至恰当水平，避免护士自身的焦虑影响到患者。

2）保持平静、温和的态度与患者接触，不带命令或权威，语言表达清楚。在极度焦虑状态时，患者的理解和思维能力会受到影响，态度沉着、平静、温和能使患者感到安全，帮助患者恢复平静。

3）当患者的焦虑水平减轻后，探讨焦虑发生的有关因素，帮助患者认识焦虑发生的诱发因素。

4）鼓励患者表达自己的情绪和不愉快的感受，帮助患者矫正扭曲的认知，或终止负性想法，重建基于事实的认知，自我对话能强化患者的现实检验能力进而更好地解决问题。

5）教会患者识别焦虑加重时的症状和体征，并指导患者学习一些控制焦虑的方法，如放松技巧、呼吸控制锻炼、渐进式肌肉放松练习、冥想、体育锻炼如慢跑、散步等。

（4）提高自我控制能力和社会功能

1）评估患者焦虑发作时无能为力的感知程度，寻找导致患者无能为力的原因或经历，提供可选择的解决问题的方法，增强患者的控制能力。

2）帮助患者认识哪些是他能够控制的情境、哪些是他无法控制的情境，鼓励患者用言语表达自己的感受，帮助患者处理那些未能解决的问题和接受不能改变的现实。

3）帮助患者制订恰当的、实际的目标，并且逐步地增加目标的难度和技能训练来增加成功的机会。不实际的目标会使患者感到失

Success experiences will promote and reinforce feelings of self-efficacy and control.

4) Allow client to take as much responsibility as possible for self-care practices. Examples include: allow client to establish own schedule for self-care activities; include client in setting goals of care; provide client with privacy as need is determined; provide positive feedback for decisions made; respect client's right to make those decisions independently, and refrain from attempting to influence him or her toward those may seem more logical. Providing choices, decision-making and positive feedback will increase client's feelings of control.

败，强化患者无能为力的感受，而成功的经验能提高和加强自我效能和自我控制的感受。

4）允许患者尽可能地进行自我照顾，帮助患者改善自我照顾能力，如允许患者制订自我照顾活动内容及目标；尽可能让患者自己作决定，并为患者提供保密和不受干扰的环境；及时提供正性反馈；尊重患者自己做决定的权利，不要试图影响患者自己的逻辑。提供选择、让患者自己做决定、正性的反馈等能够增加患者自我控制的感受，进而促进其社会功能的提高。

iv. Nursing Evaluation

1. Has symptoms of anxiety reduced or disappeared?
2. Can the client recognize signs and symptoms of escalating anxiety and demonstrate the activities most appropriate for him or her that can be used to maintain anxiety at a manageable level?
3. Has sleep problem been improved?
4. Does the client do no harm to self?
5. Can the client use skills learned in order to interrupt the escalating anxiety before it reaches the panic level and maintain anxiety at a manageable level without medication? Can the client verbalize a long-term plan for preventing panic anxiety in the face of a stressful situation?
6. Does the client perform activities of daily living independently, participate in the decision-making process, and has social function been recovered?
7. Is the client able to verbalize influencing factors of the disorder, and associations with anxiety?

（四）护理评价

1. 患者的焦虑症状是否减轻或消失？
2. 患者是否能够认识焦虑逐步升级的症状和体征，并能够采取恰当的方式把焦虑控制在其可耐受的程度？
3. 患者的睡眠问题是否得到改善？
4. 患者住院期间有无出现伤害自己的行为？
5. 患者是否能够运用所学的控制焦虑的方法来控制焦虑，是否能够不使用药物就把焦虑控制在可耐受的程度？患者是否能够陈述面对压力情景时避免焦虑发作的长远计划？
6. 患者能否独立完成日常生活的自我照顾、能够自己做出决定，社会功能是否恢复正常？
7. 患者是否能够说出疾病的相关影响因素以及与焦虑发作之间的关系？

Section 2 Nursing Management for Clients with Phobic Anxiety Disorder

第二节　恐惧性焦虑障碍患者的护理

Phobic anxiety disorders are a type of neurosis predominated by excessive, unreasonable panic over external objects or situations; the clients are fully aware of unnecessary but cannot prevent panic attacks. Panic attacks are usually accompanied by prominent autonomic symptoms; the client tries to avoid phobic objects or situations, or endures with dread. According

恐惧性焦虑障碍是指患者对某种客观事物或情境产生异乎寻常的恐惧和紧张，患者明知这种恐惧反应是过分的或不合理的，但难以控制。恐惧发作时常伴有明显的自主神经症状，以至于患者极力回避所恐惧的客观事物或情境，或是带着恐惧去忍受。据美国

to the National Institute of Mental Health, between 5.1% and 12.5% of Americans suffer from phobias. In the investigation of mental illness in China's four provinces (2001-2005), the prevalence rate of phobic anxiety disorder was 0.74%.

国家心理健康机构估计，约 5.1% ~ 12.5% 的人患有恐惧性焦虑障碍，而中国四省（2001—2005 年）精神疾病调查结果显示恐惧性焦虑障碍的月患病率为 0.74%。

I. Etiology and Mechanism

一、病因及发病机制

i. Biological Theories

Family and twin studies suggest that phobias also can be accounted for by genetic factors. Some studies found that the first-degree relatives of clients with specific phobia had a higher concordance rate of phobic anxiety disorder. The first-degree relatives of clients with social phobia had a higher concordance rate also.

Neurochemical studies of social phobia have to date implicated a number of neurotransmitter systems, including the noradrenergic, GABAergic, dopaminergic, and serotonergic systems. Provocation paradigms that evoke social anxiety have consistently highlighted dysfunctional brain circuits in social phobia. Several imaging studies have demonstrated heightened brain activation in social phobia in brain regions associated with emotional processing. Moreover, there is increasing evidence that the brain circuits mediating conditioned fear responses also applies to specific phobias.

（一）生物学理论

家庭与双生子研究提示恐惧障碍具有一定的遗传学基础。一些研究结果显示特殊恐惧障碍患者的一级亲属较对照组患病率高，社交恐惧障碍患者的一级亲属患病率也较高。

有关社交恐惧症的神经化学研究涉及一系列的神经递质系统，包括去甲肾上腺素能、γ-氨基丁酸能、多巴胺能和 5-羟色胺能系统。此外，引发社交焦虑的激发形式一直强调社交恐惧症中大脑通路的功能失调，一些研究显示社交恐惧症中情感过程相关脑区的脑激活增高。有越来越多的证据表明大脑回路介导的条件恐惧反应也适用于特殊恐惧症。

ii. Psychosocial Theories

From of the perspective of psychoanalytical theory, Freud presented a formulation of phobic neurosis that has remained the analytic explanation of specific phobia and social phobia. Freud hypothesized that the major function of anxiety is to signal the ego that a forbidden unconscious drive is pushing for conscious expression, thus altering the ego to strengthen and mobilize its defenses against the threatening instinctual force. Freud viewed the phobia as a result of conflicts centered on an unresolved childhood oedipal situation. Although theorists originally thought that phobia resulted from castration anxiety, recent psychoanalytic theorists have suggested that other types of anxiety may be involved. For example, in agoraphobia and in erythrophobia, the element of shame implies the involvement of superego anxiety.

Learning theories propose that phobias result from a conditioned response; the person learns to associate the phobic object with a noxious or uncomfortable feeling. Avoidance of the phobia leads to the reduced anxiety and reinforces the fear. At times, phobias may arise in response to a traumatic incident.

（二）心理社会学理论

弗洛伊德明确地提出了有关特殊恐惧症和社交恐惧症的分析解释。他认为焦虑的功能是向自我发出警觉信号，提示被禁止的无意识的冲动可能进入意识的表达，使自我加强和调动防御机制以对抗这种本能驱力的威胁。弗洛伊德认为恐惧性焦虑障碍是童年时期恋母情结冲突未得到解决的结果。尽管理论家们最初认为恐惧来源于阉割焦虑，但最近心理分析学家认为其来源或许也包括其他类型的焦虑，例如，在场所恐惧和红色恐惧中，害羞成分可能涉及超我焦虑。

学习理论认为恐惧症状的发生是由条件反射形成的，个体学着将恐惧的客观事物或场景与不舒服的体验联系在一起，而回避这些害怕的客观事物或情景，则可减轻焦虑，但同时也强化了恐惧。有时，个体的恐惧源于对意外受伤的反应。

II. Clinical Manifestation

Phobias are categorized as specific phobia, social phobia, and agoraphobia.

i. Specific Phobia

Specific phobia is also called simple phobia. It is a persistent fear of a specific object or situation, such as enclosed spaces (claustrophobia), flying, animals, or heights. Anxiety is usually felt immediately on exposure to the phobia object, and the level of anxiety is usually related to the proximity of the object and to the degree to which escape is possible. The farther away and the easier it is to escape the feared stimulus, the more manageable the anxiety. The syndrome has three components: an anticipatory anxiety that is brought on by the possibility of confrontation with the phobic stimulus, the central fear itself, and the avoidance behavior by which the individual minimizes anxiety. In specific phobia, the fear is usually not of the object itself but of some dire outcome that the individual believes may result from contact with that object. For example, persons with driving phobia are afraid of accidents; those with snake phobia, that they will be bitten. The symptoms of specific phobia are constant, restricted to a specific object mainly, neither change nor generalize.

Fewer individuals seek treatment for specific phobia than for agoraphobia and social phobia, both because many specific phobias remit spontaneously and because it is easier to avoid a specific phobic situation than the multiple situations often associated with agoraphobia and social phobia. Specific phobias have been classified according to the phobic stimulus. *The DSM-5* identifies subtypes of the most common specific phobias. They include the following: animal (e.g., spiders, insects, dogs); natural environment (e.g., heights, storms, water); blood-injection-injury (e.g., needles, invasive medical procedures); situational (e.g., airplanes, elevators, enclosed places); other (e.g., situations that may lead to choking or vomiting: in children, e.g., loud sounds or costumed characters).

Specific phobias are the most common anxiety disorders. The 12-month community prevalence estimate for specific phobia is approximately 7%-9% in the United States, and the rates in European countries are similar to those in the United States (about 6%), but rates are lower in Asian, African, and Latin American countries (2%-4%).

二、临床表现

恐惧性焦虑障碍分为特殊恐惧障碍、社交恐惧障碍和广场恐惧障碍。

（一）特殊恐惧障碍

特殊恐惧障碍又称为单一恐惧障碍，是指对某一特定物体或情境强烈的、不合理的恐惧，如害怕封闭的空间（幽闭恐惧症）、害怕飞行、害怕动物、害怕高处等。当患者被置于所害怕的环境或物体面前，焦虑立即发作，其焦虑的程度与接近所害怕物体的距离及逃离这个物体或情境的可能性有关。离所害怕的物体或情境越远、越容易逃离，患者越能控制自己的焦虑。特殊恐惧障碍的症状包括三个部分：可能要面对恐惧刺激所带来的预期焦虑；恐惧本身；以及患者为减少焦虑的回避行为。特殊恐惧障碍患者恐惧的对象通常不是事物本身，而是患者所相信的与物体接触后可能产生的可怕后果，例如，有驾驶恐惧症的人害怕交通事故，有蛇恐惧症的人害怕被蛇咬。特殊恐惧障碍的症状恒定，多只限于某一特殊对象，既不改变，也不泛化。

寻求治疗的特殊恐惧障碍患者比广场、社交恐惧症要少，因为许多特殊恐惧障碍的患者比广场、社交恐惧的患者更易避开所害怕的特定事物或情境。特殊恐惧障碍根据其所恐惧的对象分为许多亚型，根据《美国精神障碍诊断和统计手册（第5版）》可分为：① 动物型（例如，蜘蛛、昆虫、狗）；② 自然环境型（例如，高处、暴风雨、水）；③ 血液－注射－损伤型（例如，针头、侵入性医疗操作）；④ 情境型（例如，飞机、电梯、封闭空间）；⑤ 其他（例如，可能导致哽噎或呕吐的情况，儿童则可能表现为对巨响或化妆人物的恐惧）。

特殊恐惧障碍是一种常见的焦虑障碍。在美国，特殊恐惧障碍的12个月社区患病率约为7%～9%，欧洲国家的患病率与美国大致相同（约为6%），但亚洲、非洲和拉丁美洲通常较低（2%～4%）。女性比男性更易受到影

Females are more frequently affected than males, at a rate of approximately 2:1. Peak onset is in childhood, and a rapid and spontaneous resolution of most of these phobias is the rule, probably because of developmental maturation and natural exposure.

响，比例约为2：1。特殊恐惧障碍的发病高峰期为儿童时期，许多特殊恐惧障碍能自发快速地缓解，可能与自我成长及自然暴露有关。

ii. Social Phobia

（二）社交恐惧障碍

Clients with social phobia have a persistent and recognizably irrational fear of performing in social situations, believing that their performance will be found wanting in some way and lead to embarrassment or humiliation. Individuals asked to face their particular type of social phobia describe anticipatory anxiety and may experience situational panic attacks. Usually, the individual with phobia avoids the situations as much as possible.

社交恐惧障碍的特点是对社交情景持续的、不合理的害怕和恐惧，患者相信他们在公众面前的表现可能导致尴尬或羞辱。社交恐惧障碍的患者在面临社交情境时通常出现预期性焦虑，并可能经历惊恐发作，患者因害怕出丑、尴尬而尽可能回避社交场所或行为。

Typical social phobias are of speaking, eating, or writing in public; using public lavatories; and attending parties or interviews. In addition, a common fear of socially phobic individuals is that other people will detect and ridicule their anxiety in social situations. When forced or surprised into the social situation, the individual experiences profound anxiety accompanied by a variety of somatic symptoms, such as sweating, blushing, and dry mouth. Actual panic attacks may also occur in individuals with social phobia in response to feared social situations.

典型的社交恐惧障碍包括在公共场合谈话、进食或写字，使用公共洗衣间，以及参加派对或面试。此外，社交恐惧障碍的患者通常害怕其他人会发现并嘲笑他们在社交场合中的焦虑。当患者被暴露在社交情景中，几乎不可控制地诱发焦虑发作，并伴随一些躯体症状，如出汗、脸红和口干等，也有部分患者可能出现惊恐发作。

Onset of symptoms of this disorder is usually around puberty, the mean age being 15 years. It appears equally common among men and women. A 1-year and lifetime prevalence of social anxiety disorder is 2.8% and 5.0% respectively. The individual with social phobia may appear impaired in social or occupational functioning, or as having marked distress. Avoidance often is obvious, and can lead to social isolation in extreme cases.

社交恐惧障碍多在青春期起病，平均发病年龄为15岁，男性与女性发病率没有明显差异。社交恐惧障碍的一年和终身患病率分别为2.8%和5.0%。社交恐惧障碍患者多表现出明显的社会功能、职业功能受损，或表现出明显的痛苦。回避往往十分明显，在极端的情况下，可能引起完全的社会隔离。

iii. Agoraphobia

（三）广场恐惧障碍

Agoraphobia is a fear of being caught in a situation from which a graceful and speedy escape to safety would be difficult or embarrassing if the client felt discomfort. The essential feature of agoraphobia is marked, or intense fear or anxiety triggered by the real or anticipated exposure to a wide range of situations. Situations likely to induce fear and avoidance include attendance at auditoriums, eating out (especially at formal sit down restaurants), shopping in supermarket, driving under conditions in which opportunities to pull over, stop, or get off the highway quickly may be restricted. Agoraphobic clients lament their inability to face everyday situations and often become discouraged, depressed, and demoralized by the restrictions in their lives caused by agoraphobia. Agoraphobia is one of the most common phobias accounted for about 60%, and has the greatest impact on

广场恐惧障碍主要表现为对某些特定环境的恐惧，包括难以迅速逃回安全处所的其他场所，或可能使患者感到不适或尴尬的情境。典型表现为实际或预期暴露于各种情境中所引发的明显的或强烈的恐惧或焦虑，这些情景可能引起恐惧及回避，例如就坐观众席、外出就餐（特别是正式餐厅）、超市购物、在限制停止或能迅速离开高速公路的路况驾驶等。患者非常烦恼自己不能面对每天的场景，常常会感到灰心、抑郁，缺乏勇气，日常生活也因此而受到限制。广场恐惧症是恐惧症中最常见的一种，对患者功能影响最大，约占60%，发病高峰年龄约在20岁左右，

clients' function. The age at onset of agoraphobia peaks in the early 20s. Women are more affected than men.

女性多于男性。

III. Treatment

三、治　疗

The treatment of phobic disorder uses both psychotherapy and pharmacotherapy. Some studies indicate that the use of both pharmacotherapy and psychotherapy produces better results than either therapy alone.

恐惧障碍的治疗包括药物治疗和精神心理治疗，有研究报道，两者联合治疗的效果优于任何一种单独的治疗。

i. Pharmacotherapy

The benzodiazepines have been the most widely prescribed drugs for the relief of phobic disorder, with mixed results. Alprazolam and clonazepam appear to be successful in reducing the symptoms of agoraphobia associated with panic disorder. The tricyclic imipramine and the monoamine oxidase inhibitor (MAOIs) phenelzine have been shown to be effective in diminishing symptoms of agoraphobia and social phobias. Selective serotonin reuptake inhibitors (SSRIs) have also been positive in treatment, and they have become first-line treatment for social phobia. For generalized social phobia, SSRIs, MAOIs and benzodiazepines are pharmacological treatments of choice. Gabapentin has also been found effective in treating generalized social phobia and does not cause physical dependency as benzodiazepines.

（一）药物治疗

苯二氮䓬类药物广泛地应用于恐惧性焦虑障碍的治疗，在一定程度上能减轻恐惧障碍引起的焦虑，例如，阿普唑仑和氯硝西泮能有效缓解广场恐惧障碍相关的惊恐发作。三环类抗抑郁药物丙咪嗪和单胺氧化酶抑制剂苯乙肼有助于治疗广场恐惧障碍和社交恐惧障碍。选择性5-羟色胺再摄取抑制剂也显示了治疗的有效性，并成为社交恐惧障碍的一线治疗药物。对于一般的社交恐惧障碍，选择性5-羟色胺再摄取抑制剂、单胺氧化酶抑制剂和苯二氮䓬类药物都是治疗用药的选择，加巴喷丁也能有效治疗社交恐惧障碍且不会发生苯二氮䓬类药物的依赖性。

β-adrenergic blocking drugs are often helpful in decreasing peripheral symptoms of anxiety such as tremor, tachycardia, and sweating. A combination of exposure therapy and β-blocking drugs works well for specific social phobia. Benzodiazepine anti-anxiety drugs are sometimes used in combination with β-blockers as well as alone.

β受体阻滞剂常有助于减轻焦虑的躯体症状，如震颤、心动过速和出汗等。β受体阻滞剂与暴露疗法合并能有效治疗特殊恐惧障碍。苯二氮类药物抗焦虑药有时单独使用，也常常与β-受体阻滞剂联合使用。

ii. Psychotherapy

The psychotherapy for generalized type of social phobia usually involves a combination of behavioral and cognitive methods, including cognitive retraining, desensitization, rehearsal during sessions, and a range of homework assignments.

（二）心理治疗

恐惧障碍的心理治疗通常联合使用认知和行为治疗，包括认知重建、脱敏疗法、角色扮演和家庭作业等。

1. Cognitive-behavior Therapy　Cognitive-restructuring techniques are also used to help phobic clients confront their fears by changing their negative thoughts and substituting healthier ones.

1. 认知行为治疗　主要目的是帮助恐惧症患者改变不正确的想法以及重构正确的认知，以促使患者面对自己的恐惧。

2. Exposure Therapy and Systematic Desensitization　They are commonly used to treat clients with phobic disorder. The therapist first asks the client to create a hierarchy of stressful situations, and then applies exposure or desensitization. For example, for

2. 暴露治疗和系统脱敏疗法　恐惧症最常用的两种治疗方法。通常治疗师首先要求患者把那些能产生压力的情景划分为不同的等级，再进行暴露或脱敏治疗。例如患者害

individuals with a fear of flying, the following hierarchy might be used: seeing a picture of a plane; hearing planes overhead; driving past an airport; entering an airport; walking onto a plane; actually flying. At each step, the individual practices relaxation techniques and continues them at home for mastery. As the relaxation response is paired with the stressful trigger, that is, each step in the hierarchy the client gradually masters and tolerates each step until eventually he or she is able to fly.

怕飞行，其暴露治疗和系统脱敏治疗的压力情境等级划分可能为：① 让患者看飞机照片；② 倾听飞机飞过头顶的声音；③ 坐汽车通过飞机场；④ 进入飞机场；⑤ 从飞机旁边走过；⑥ 实际飞行。在暴露治疗的每一步中都应指导患者进行放松练习，并指导患者在家中坚持训练直至掌握。随着压力触发事件与放松反应的配对，患者逐渐耐受不同等级的压力事件并最终实现飞行。

Other psychotherapies include relaxation training, breath training, and supportive psychotherapies.

其他心理治疗方法包括放松训练、呼吸训练及支持性心理治疗等。

IV. Application of the Nursing Process

四、护理程序的应用

i. Nursing Assessment

Nursing assessment for individuals with phobic anxiety disorder include many of the same considerations as discussed with anxiety disorder. In addition, nurses can obtain more information from the diagnostic characteristics of phobic anxiety disorder described above.

（一）护理评估

恐惧性焦虑障碍患者的护理评估内容请参照焦虑障碍患者的护理评估。另外，在评估时，护士可以从各类型恐惧性焦虑障碍的临床表现中获得一些有用的信息。

ii. Nursing Diagnosis

1. Fear Related to an intense, unreasonable panic of a specifics situation or object.

2. Ineffective Coping Related to phobic response, fear of subsequent phobic responses, lifestyle of avoidant behaviors secondary to fear of phobic stimulus.

Other nursing diagnosis that apply to phobic anxiety disorder are the same as for anxiety disorder such as anxiety, powerlessness, sleep pattern disturbance, and impaired social interaction.

（二）主要护理诊断

1. 恐惧 与对某物体或情境不合理的害怕有关。

2. 应对无效 与恐惧反应、害怕惊恐发作而采用一些不适应行为等有关。

其他相关护理诊断与焦虑障碍患者的护理诊断相同，如焦虑、无能为力、睡眠型态紊乱、社会交往障碍等。

iii. Nursing Planning

1. Nursing Outcome

(1) Discuss the phobic object or situation without becoming anxious.

(2) Demonstrate significant decrease in phobic response and avoidance behaviors during progressive exposure to feared objects, events, or situations.

(3) Verbalize the signs and symptoms of escalating anxiety.

(4) Relate increase in understanding of phobic disorder and behaviors needed to manage phobic response.

(5) Verbalize the thinking process that promotes the irrational fear.

(6) Participate actively in prescribed treatment

（三）护理计划

1. 护理目标

（1）患者能够讨论所恐惧的物体或场所而无焦虑反应。

（2）患者能够面对所恐惧的物体或场所，恐惧反应有明显减轻，回避行为明显减轻。

（3）患者能够描述焦虑水平增加时的信号或症状。

（4）患者对恐惧障碍及控制恐惧反应的行为的理解增加。

（5）患者能够说出哪些认知可能提高不合理的恐惧或害怕。

（6）患者能够积极参与治疗计划，学习降

plan and learned therapeutic strategies to reduce phobic responses; demonstrate techniques that he or she may use to prevent the anxiety from escalating to the panic level.

(7) Leave the room or home to attend group activities voluntarily.

(8) Can create change in his or her life to confront the phobic situation.

2. Nursing Intervention Nursing interventions for clients with phobic anxiety disorder are similar with anxiety disorder. The primary nursing diagnosis fear and ineffective coping will be discussed.

(1) Nursing of fear

1) Assess degree of interference with normal functioning, presence of depression, and substance use. Depression and substance abuse may coexist.

2) At panic level of anxiety, client may fear for his or her own life. Reassure client that he or she is safe to reduce the anxiety.

3) Explore client's perception of the threat to physical integrity or threat to self-concept. It is important to understand client's perception of the phobic object or situation to assist with the desensitization process.

4) Discuss reality of the situation with client to recognize aspects that can be changed and those that cannot. If the client accepts the reality of the situation, the work of reducing the fear can progress.

5) Teach techniques of relaxation and process of desensitization. Understanding and participation of client is elicited.

6) Practice confrontation with stimulus in conditions of relaxation, monitor and reinforce client progress. Reinforces promote hope and behavior change, as does the increased sense of behavior control.

(2) Improve coping capacity

1) Approach the client in a calm, direct manner using soft voice tone, establish trust with clients. Listen actively to the client's fears and concerns no matter how irrational they may seem. Acknowledge the client's feelings, concerns, and limitations in a simple, matter-of-fact manner. Active listening signifies unconditional respect and acceptance for the client as a worthwhile individual.

低恐惧反应的方法，并使用所学习的应对技巧或方法避免焦虑水平升级。

（7）患者能够主动离开家或房间去参加集体活动。

（8）患者能够改变自己的生活从而去面对令其恐惧的场所或情境。

2. **护理措施** 恐惧性焦虑障碍患者的护理措施与焦虑障碍患者类似，下列仅讨论有关恐惧症状及提高应对能力方面的护理措施。

（1）恐惧症状的护理

1）评估恐惧障碍对患者正常生活和社会功能影响的程度，评估患者的抑郁程度及有无物质滥用的情况。

2）在惊恐状态时，患者常常感到不安全，护士应向患者保证他或她是安全的，有助于减轻患者的焦虑反应。

3）与患者讨论关于身体威胁或自我概念威胁的感受，了解患者关于其所恐惧物体或场所的看法，帮助患者进行脱敏，逐渐耐受其恐惧的物体或场所。

4）与患者共同讨论其所恐惧的物体或场所的真实情况，使患者能够认识到哪些是可改变的、哪些是不能改变的，一旦患者能够认识和接受这些真实的物体或情境，患者的恐惧就会逐渐减轻。

5）指导患者学习放松技术和脱敏疗法，引导患者理解及积极参与。

6）指导患者在放松的条件下对抗所恐惧的物体或场所，监督和强化患者的进步。强化和鼓励能够提高患者的希望和促进患者行为发生改变，增加患者对其行为控制的感受。

（2）提高患者的应对能力

1）以平静、温和的态度接触患者，与患者建立信任关系。耐心倾听患者对害怕和恐惧的诉说，不管患者的害怕或恐惧是如何的不合理或过分，都不能嘲笑患者或表现出不耐烦，承认患者的感受和担心，理解患者的恐惧，有效的倾听能够显示护士对患者的尊重和接受。

2) Refrain from exposing the client to identified feared object or situation. Exposure to feared stimuli without adaptive coping strategies could escalate the client's anxiety to a panic state. Forced compliance increases powerlessness and loss of control and decreases the client's trust in staff and treatment regimen. Inform the client that staff understands that refusal to attend the group outing is not attributable to resistance to treatment, but rather to client's phobic disorder.

3) When the client is able to discuss phobic responses without experiencing incapacitating anxiety, assist the client to describe physiologic responses to identified feared objects, situations, or events. Teaching the client to identify autonomic nervous system response to anxiety that will help the client to acknowledge the feelings rather than to deny or avoid them.

4) Assist the client to identify factors that increase or decrease phobic responses. Help the client to differentiate between most and least feared objects. Assist the client to determine other factors associated with feared stimuli that may precipitate a phobic response. The client recognition that factors such as increased noise or fatigue may contribute to his or her vulnerability may encourage the client to modify those situations or elements that can be controlled. Teach the client about the effects of caffeine, nicotine, and other central nervous system stimulants. Caffeine and nicotine stimulate the central nervous system to produce physiologic effects of anxiety.

5) Explore with the client previously successful coping methods. Use of previously successful coping strategies, in conjunction with newly learned skills, better prepares the client to deal with the anxiety of the phobic disorder and promotes more control over the feared situation, objects, or events. Help the client identify alternative adaptive coping techniques to manage the anxiety that emanates from excessive or irrational fears, rather than use avoidance behaviors. The following therapies are useful to help the client to manage the anxiety: relaxation exercises, deep breathing, visual imagery, and cognitive techniques.

6) For the client who is able to use cognitive-perceptual skills: utilize relabeling or reframing techniques to change the client's perceptions of feared objects, situations, or events; reframing or relabeling volatile words with less threatening terms helps the client place thought and feeling in a different perspective and tends to decrease anxiety. Teach the client to combine reframing techniques with another learned strategy when necessary. Combining a newly learned skill with a previously learned strategy provides the client with more than one technique to cope

2）在患者对其所恐惧的对象没有相应的应对技巧之前，应限制患者接触令其恐惧的场所或物体，避免导致焦虑升级，甚至惊恐发作，避免增加患者的无能力感和失控感，影响治疗。让患者知晓护士了解他们拒绝参加集体活动的原因不是对治疗的抵触，而是因为恐惧障碍疾病本身。

3）当患者能够讨论恐惧反应而没有体验到对焦虑的无能为力时，应帮助患者描述其在面对危险物体、场所或事件时产生的生理反应，帮助患者认识和接受这种感受，而不是否认和回避。

4）帮助患者认识哪些因素可引起或降低恐惧反应，让患者认识和区分最大恐惧和最小恐惧的物体或场所。当患者能认识哪些是恐惧的促发因素，如疲劳、噪音等时，可帮助他们减轻或避免这些场所或因素。指导患者认识酒精、咖啡等中枢神经兴奋物质对其的影响，避免使用该类物质引起焦虑反应。

5）与患者共同探索过去成功的应对方法或技巧，将过去成功的应对技巧和新学习的应对技巧联合使用更能有效应对焦虑或恐惧，协助患者认识和选择适应性的应对技巧和方法来控制和管理焦虑反应，减少或消除回避行为，如放松技术、呼吸控制技术、冥想放松和认知技术等。

6）当患者能够运用认知感知技术时，可运用重建技术改变患者对所恐惧的物体或场所的反应，如指导患者用危险性小的词替代危险性强的词，可帮助患者从另外一种观点去了解这些感受或想法。指导患者把重建技术与其他技巧联合使用，将更有效地控制焦虑和恐惧。

adaptively with anxiety.

7) For the client who has successfully practiced the preceding strategies, assist the client to confront the feared object under safe conditions. Confronting the feared object in a familiar setting diminishes the phobic response and the anticipatory anxiety that precedes it. Expose the client progressively to feared stimuli. Continue exposing the client to feared objects or situations with more frequency until the client can tolerate exposure to them with a significant reduction in phobic responses. Offer positive reinforcement whenever the client demonstrates a decrease in avoidance behaviors or an increase in socialization skills and other milieu activities. Positive statements convey confidence and hope and reinforce the client's adaptive coping skills.

7）当患者已成功地进行了上述的治疗过程，在保证安全的情况下，帮助患者面对所恐惧的场所或物体，在熟悉的环境中接触所恐惧的物体，可使患者的恐惧反应较小。逐渐将患者暴露于所恐惧的物体或场所，患者通过多次面对所恐惧的物体或情境，可逐渐减轻其恐惧反应。对患者的进步及时给予表扬和鼓励，增加患者的自信心并强化患者的适应性行为。

iv. Nursing Evaluation

（四）护理评价

1. Can the client discuss the phobic object or situation without becoming anxious?
2. Does the client demonstrate significant decrease in phobic response and avoidance behaviors during progressive exposure to feared objects, events, or situations?
3. Is the client able to verbalize the signs and symptoms of escalating anxiety?
4. Can the client relate increase in understanding of phobic disorder and behaviors needed to manage phobic response?
5. Can the client verbalize the thinking process that promotes the irrational fears?
6. Does the client participate actively in treatment, and is the client able to demonstrate techniques that he or she may use to prevent the anxiety from escalating to the panic level?
7. Does the client voluntarily leave the room or home to attend group activities?
8. Is the client capable of creating change in his or her life to confront the phobic situation?

1. 患者是否能够讨论所恐惧的物体或场所而无焦虑反应？
2. 患者能否面对其所恐惧的物体或场所，恐惧反应和回避行为明显减轻？
3. 患者是否能够表述出焦虑水平增加时的信号或症状？
4. 患者是否能够理解恐惧障碍及控制恐惧反应的行为？
5. 患者是否能表述哪些认知可能提高不合理的恐惧或害怕？
6. 患者是否积极参与治疗学习计划，是否能够使用所学习新的应对技巧或方法避免焦虑水平升级？
7. 患者是否能主动离开家或房间去参加集体活动？
8. 患者是否有能力改变自己的生活从而去面对令其恐惧的场所或情境？

Section 3 Nursing Management for Clients with Obsessive Compulsive Disorder

第三节　强迫性障碍患者的护理

Obsessive-compulsive disorder (OCD) is a type of neurosis predominated by obsessions and compulsions symptoms. The feature of OCD is coexistence of conscious self-obsession and anti-obsession, the sharp conflicts of the two give clients anxiety and affliction. The

强迫障碍（obsessive-compulsive disorder，OCD）是以强迫观念和强迫行为为主要表现的一种神经症，其特点是有意识的自我强迫和反强迫并存，二者的强烈冲突使患者感到焦虑和

clients have the experience of ideas or impulses stemming from ego, but against their own will; they try to resist but unable to control; they are aware of abnormality of obsessive symptoms, but are unable to break away. The clients with delayed duration may be predominated by ceremony acts, and their mental affliction decreases, but social function is severely impaired.

痛苦。患者体验到观念或冲动来自自我，但违反自己的意愿，虽极力抵抗，却无法控制。患者意识到强迫症状的异常，但无法摆脱。病程迁延者，可以仪式动作为主，从而使其精神痛苦减轻，但社会功能严重受损。

The peak age of occurrence of OCD is in adolescence and in early adults, and the symptoms of OCD were predominated by repetitive depravation or alleviation. Between ages 10 and 15 years, 31% of first episodes occur, with 75% developing OCD by age 30. Therefore, the clients with OCD maybe feel extreme affliction and their social function was severely impaired. The lifetime prevalence of obsessive-compulsive disorder in the general population is an estimated 2 to 3 percent. In the investigation of 12 areas of China (1982), the lifetime prevalence rate of OCD was 0.3‰. A study on mental illness survey in China's four provinces (2001-2005) revealed that the prevalence rate of OCD is 0.84‰ . With new developments in behavioral and pharmacological treatments the prognosis of OCD is now considerably improved. As the disorder usually has a major impact on daily functioning, clients are often socially isolated. Predictors of worse outcome were earlier onset, a more chronic course at baseline, poorer social functioning at baseline, having both obsessions and compulsions, and having magical symptoms.

强迫障碍通常起病于青春期和成年早期，具有反复恶化或缓解的慢性病程。31%的强迫症患者首次发病在10～15岁，75%在30岁之前就形成了强迫障碍。一般人群中强迫症患者的终生患病率为2%～3%。我国12个地区（1982年）神经症流行病学调查资料显示，强迫障碍的患病率为0.3‰，2001—2005年中国四省精神疾病调查结果显示强迫障碍的月患病率为0.84‰。随着行为治疗和药物治疗的发展，强迫障碍的预后已有很大程度的改善，但因其对患者日常生活功能有很大的影响，患者常常被社交隔离，预后较差的指征为发病较早、原先病程较长、原先社会功能较差，既有强迫观念又有强迫动作，并且有怪异的症状。

I. Etiology and Mechanism

一、病因及发病机制

i. Neurobiological Factors

A number of biological findings have rendered OCD one of the most elegantly elaborated psychiatric disorders from a biological standpoint. There are many theories put forward with some viewpoints that may be related to the following factors: serotonergic dysregulation; dopaminergic dysregulation; other dysfunctional neurotransmitter systems or neuromodulators (e.g., CSF vasopressin, CSF somatostatin, CSF oxytocin); hyperactivity of orbitofrontal–limbic–basal ganglia circuits; autoimmune process secondary to streptococcal infection; a moderate effect on risk for OCD from homozygosity for the long allele L(A) of the serotonin transporter gene.

（一）神经生物学因素

大量的生物学研究结果从生物学角度阐述了强迫症这一精神障碍，相关理论包括5-羟色胺能的调节异常；多巴胺能的调节异常；其他神经递质系统或神经调节异常（如催产素、加压素、生长抑素）；眶额－边缘系统－基底节区神经节环路活动亢进；某些个体中链球菌感染所导致的自身免疫过程；5-羟色胺转运基因的长等位基因L（A）的同合子性对OCD患病风险的影响等。

Family studies of obsessive-compulsive disorder clients have found that 35 percent of the first-degree relatives of obsessive-compulsive disorder clients are also afflicted with the disorder. The studies of concordance in twins for obsessive-compulsive disorder have consistently

对强迫障碍的家系遗传研究发现，其一级亲属中患病率达35%，单卵双生子研究发现同病率为65%～85%，而双卵双生子同病率为15%～45%。

found a significantly higher concordance rate for monozygotic twins (65%-85%) than for dizygotic twins (15%-45%).

ii. Psychosocial Factors

1. Psychoanalytical Theories Psychoanalytical theorists propose that individuals with obsessive-compulsive disorder have weak, underdeveloped egos (for any of a variety of reasons: unsatisfactory parent-child relationship, conditional love, or provisional gratification). Psychodynamic theory suggests that OCD develops when defense mechanisms fail to contain the obsessional character's anxiety. The clinical symptoms of obsessions and compulsions of OCD clients are thought to utilize the defense mechanisms of isolation, undoing, reaction formation, regression, and ambivalence to control unacceptable sexual and aggressive impulses. These defense mechanisms are unconscious and thus not readily apparent to the client.

2. Cognitive and Behavioral Theories Obsessive-compulsive behavior is a conditioned response to a traumatic event. The traumatic event produces anxiety and discomfort, and the person then engages in compulsive rituals (escape/avoidance responses) in order to decrease anxiety. If the individual is successful in reducing anxiety, the compulsive behavior is more likely to occur in the future. Likewise, anxiety reduction after the ritual preserves the compulsive behavior. Three main types of dysfunctional beliefs have been identified in OCD: responsibility and overestimation of threat, perfectionism and intolerance of uncertainty, and importance and control of thoughts.

II. Clinical Manifestation

Obsessions and compulsions are the two major manifestations of OCD. Clients with both obsessions and compulsions constitute at least 70 percent of the affected clients. Some researchers and clinicians believe that the number may be much closer to 100 percent if clients are carefully assessed for the presence of mental compulsions in addition to behavioral compulsions. However, some researchers and clinicians believe that some clients do have only obsessive thoughts and do not have compulsions.

Obsessions are defined as unwanted, intrusive, persistent ideas, thoughts, impulses, or images that cause marked anxiety or distress. The most common ones include repeated thoughts about contamination, repeated doubts, a need to have things in a particular order, aggressive or horrific impulses, and sexual imagery. The individual often tries to ignore or suppress the obsessive

（二）心理社会因素

1. 心理动力学理论 心理动力学家认为强迫障碍的个体存在自我发展障碍，如与父母关系的不满意、缺乏关爱、暂时满意等，并提出在防御机制无法承受强迫性格的焦虑时则形成强迫症。强迫症患者被认为是利用隔离、抵消、反向形成、推行以及控制不被接受的性冲动和攻击性冲动的矛盾心理的防御机制。这些防御机制是潜意识的，对于患者来说不是显而易见的。

2. 认知行为理论 强迫行为是对创伤事件的条件反应。创伤事件引起焦虑和不舒适，患者为了减少焦虑开始出现强迫性仪式（逃避 / 回避反应），如果患者成功地减轻了焦虑，强迫行为在将来更可能发生。因此，在强迫仪式后焦虑减轻则维持了强迫行为。此外，强迫症患者中存在三个主要的功能失调性信念：责任感和对威胁的过度估计；完美主义和对不确定的无法容忍；重要性和对想法的控制。

二、临床表现

强迫观念和强迫行为是强迫障碍的主要症状，有报道 70% 的患者两者都存在，有的报道更高，甚至接近 100%。但是，有些研究者发现某些患者确实只有强迫观念，而无强迫行为。

强迫观念是指违背自己意志，反复出现的思维、联想、冲动或意念，使个体感到焦虑和痛苦。最常见的一些强迫观念，如对脏的强迫观念、强迫性怀疑、过于条理性、攻击性冲动及与性有关的强迫观念等。患者经常试图忽略或压制这种产生过度焦虑的强迫

thoughts, which creates a great deal of anxiety, and thus the individual attempts to neutralize the thoughts by repeating behaviors, so-called compulsions.

Compulsions denote unwanted repetitive behavior patterns or mental acts (e.g., praying, counting, repeating words silently) that are intended to reduce anxiety, not to provide pleasure or gratification. They may be performed in response to an obsession or in a stereotyped fashion. The individual recognizes that the behavior is excessive or unreasonable but is compelled to continue the act. The most common compulsions involve washing and cleaning, counting, checking, requesting or demanding assurances, repeating actions, and ordering.

Obsessions and compulsions have certain features in common: (a) An idea or an impulse intrudes itself insistently and persistently into the person's conscious awareness. (b) A feeling of anxious dread accompanies the central manifestation and frequently leads the person to take countermeasures against the initial idea or impulse. (c) The obsession or the compulsion is ego-alien, that is, it is experienced as being foreign to the person's experience of himself or herself as a psychological being. (d) No matter how vivid and compelling the obsession or the compulsion is, the person usually recognizes it as absurd and irrational. (e) The person suffering from obsessions and compulsions usually feels a strong desire to resist them. However, about half of all clients offer little resistance to the compulsion. About 80 percent of all clients believe that the compulsion is irrational.

Although distinct symptom clusters of OCD exist (washers, checkers, those who are purely obsessional, hoarders, and those with primary slowness), these symptoms may overlap or develop sequentially. Studies identified four symptom dimensions of OCD: symmetry/ordering hoarding contamination/cleaning, and obsessions/checking. These four syndromes can coexist in any one client and be continuous with more normative obsessive-compulsive phenomena.

III. Treatment

i. Pharmacotherapy

The efficacy of pharmacotherapy in obsessive-compulsive disorder has been proved in many clinical trials.

1. Serotonin Reuptake Inhibitors A series of clinical trials supported the efficacy of clomipramine in reducing OCD symptoms. Numerous controlled trials have documented the efficacy of all serotonin-specific

观念，并且企图通过反复的行为，即强迫行为来抵消此类思想。

强迫行为是指为了减轻焦虑而出现的违背自己意志、不能提供愉悦和满足、反复出现的行为模式或思想行为，如祈祷、计数、复述等。强迫行为可能是对强迫观念的应对或是一种刻板的形式，患者明知这个行为多余、没必要，但是却强迫自己实施。最常见的强迫行为包括反复洗手和清洁、反复计数、反复检查、要求保证、反复动作及命令等。

强迫观念和强迫行为有以下共同特征：①强迫思想和冲动是有意识的强加于患者的思维，违背了其意愿；②担忧恐惧的感受常导致患者采取相反的措施，来抵制内心的想法和冲动；③症状源于自我，并非外力所致；④无论强迫观念和强迫行为如何生动、强制，患者通常能意识到这是荒诞和不合理的；⑤强迫观念和强迫行为使患者感到痛苦并力图摆脱它。然而，大约有一半的患者对强迫行为采取较小的抵抗，约80%的患者相信强迫行为不合理。

虽然强迫症有明显的症状群，包括清洗者、检查者、单纯强迫观念者、储藏者、和原始迟缓者，但这些症状可以相互交叠或继续发展。有研究报道强迫症有四个一致的“综合征”，包括强迫对称 / 计数、强迫储藏、强迫污染 / 清洁和强迫观念 / 检查，这四个综合征可以同时存在于一个患者，并且发展出更多标准化的强迫现象。

三、治 疗

（一）药物治疗

1. 5-羟色胺再摄取抑制剂 大量的研究已证明氯丙咪嗪对减轻OCD症状的有效性。此外，也有许多对照试验证明了所有选择性

reuptake inhibitors (SSRIs) for OCD, which are fluoxetine, sertraline, paroxetine and citalopram. The serotonin and noradrenaline reuptake inhibitor (SNRI) venlafaxine also appears effective in treating OCD. The SSRIs are better tolerated than clomipramine by most clients, and have therefore become the well-established first line of treatment for OCD. If clients do not have a good response to an adequate trial of at least two SSRIs, augmentation with clomipramine or switching to clomipramine alone should be undertaken; the reverse is also true.

5-羟色胺再摄取抑制剂对OCD的有效性，包括氟西汀、舍曲林、帕罗西汀和西酞普兰，5-羟色胺和去甲肾上腺素再摄取抑制剂类药物文拉法辛也对治疗OCD有效。因大多数患者对选择性5-羟色胺再摄取抑制剂的耐受性比对氯丙咪嗪好，所以选择性5-羟色胺再摄取抑制剂成为主要治疗OCD的一线药物。但是如果患者对至少两种选择性5-羟色胺再摄取抑制剂药物足疗程的治疗没有很好的效果，则应该加入氯丙咪嗪或换成氯丙咪嗪单独治疗，反过来也是一样。

2. Medication Combination and Augmentation Various combination and augmentation strategies are often needed to attain a satisfactory response. The most commonly used augmenting agents in OCD are buspirone, clonazepam, atypical antipsychotics, inositol, and glutamatergic agents. The combination of clomipramine with an SSRI is also a commonly used strategy for treating refractory clients and is generally well tolerated.

2. 药物联合与增效剂治疗 强迫症治疗中常常需要不同药物联合治疗的策略来获得满意的疗效，最常使用的添加药物是丁螺环酮、氯硝西泮、非典型抗精神病药、肌醇和谷氨酸盐剂。此外，氯丙咪嗪与一种5-羟色胺再摄取抑制剂类药物合用也是治疗难治性强迫症患者的常用策略。

ii. Psychotherapy

Behavioral treatments of OCD mainly involve two components: exposure procedures that aim to decrease the anxiety associated with obsessions, and response prevention techniques that aim to decrease the frequency of rituals or obsessive thoughts.

（二）心理治疗

OCD的行为治疗包括两个主要组成部分：①以减轻与强迫观念有关的焦虑为目的的暴露法；②以减轻强迫性仪式动作或强迫想法为目的的反应预防法。

1. Exposure Techniques Exposure techniques range from systematic desensitization with brief imaginal exposure to flooding, in which prolonged exposure to the real-life ritual-evoking stimuli causes profound discomfort. Combined behavioral techniques, exposure and response prevention (ERP) can be highly effective for clients with OCD.

1. 暴露治疗 暴露技术包括使用简单想象暴露的系统脱敏疗法，以及延迟暴露于现实中唤起仪式性动作的刺激而引起不适的冲击疗法。联合行为技术，即暴露和反应预防法（ERP）能最大程度改善OCD的症状。

2. Response Prevention This technique is used for OCD clients with rituals (with or without obsessive thoughts). One goal of this procedure is to help the client understand that willingness to be exposed to the feared object while resisting the accompanying rituals is less time consuming and less stressful than the obsessive compulsive behaviors previously used. Another goal is to disconfirm the expectation of the compulsive outcomes and eventually extinguish the compulsive behaviors.

2. 反应预防法 这种方法主要用于有强迫行为的患者（不管有无强迫性观念），其目的是帮助患者认识到强迫行为只是为了减轻焦虑和不愉快情绪的手段，实际上患者是可以逐渐抵抗这种行为的，学习以非强迫行为的方式来逐渐减轻焦虑反应。另一个目的是帮助患者驳斥对强迫的期望结果并逐渐消除强迫行为。

3. Thought Stopping Thought stopping is used with clients who have obsessive thoughts. Clients are taught to interrupt obsessive thoughts by say "stop!" either

3. 思想停止法 思想停止法适用于有强迫想法的患者，当强迫想法出现时，通过对自己说"停止"来打断这种思想。这种方式

aloud or subvocally. This activity interrupts and delays the uncontrollable spiral of obsessive thoughts.

可以打断和拖延强迫观念的再次出现。

4. Relaxation Techniques Relaxation exercise (progressive muscle relaxation and breathing control exercises) do not affect OCD symptoms, but they may be used to decrease anxiety associated with the disorder.

5. Cognitive Restructuring Cognitive therapy has also been proved to be efficacious, centering on cognitive reformulation of related themes. It is a method of teaching the client to restructure dysfunctional thought processes through a system of defining and testing the client's distorted thought patterns. The client is taught to monitor automatic thoughts, then to recognize the connection between thoughts, emotional response, and their behavior. The distorted thoughts are examined and tested by for, or against evidence presented by the therapist. In this way, the therapist helps the client doubt the real likelihood that the feared event will happen. Finally, the client learns to identify and question dysfunctional beliefs that predispose the individual to distort reality.

6. Cue Cards It is a tool used to help the client restructure thought patterns and contain statements that are positively oriented and pertain to the client's specific obsessions and compulsions. Cue cards use information from the client's symptom hierarchy, an organizational system that breaks down the obsessions and compulsions from least to most anxiety provoking. These cards can help reinforce in clients the belief that they are safe and can tolerate the anxiety caused by delaying or controlling compulsive rituals. Following are examples of cue cards statements:

(1) It's the OCD, not me;

(2) They are only obsessive thoughts, thoughts don't mean action. I will not act on the thoughts;

(3) My anxiety level goes up but will always go down, I never sat with the anxiety long enough to see that it would not harm me;

(4) Trust myself;

(5) I did it right the first time;

(6) Checking the locks again won't keep me safe, I really am safe in the world.

iii. Other Therapies

1. Family therapy is often useful in supporting the family, helping reduce marital discord resulting from the disorder, and building a treatment alliance with the family members for the good of the client. Group therapy is useful as a support system for some clients.

2. Electroconvulsive therapy is sometimes helpful in individual with severe primary depression and secondary

4. 放松技术 虽然放松训练如渐进式肌肉放松、呼吸训练等方法对缓解强迫症状没有效果，但是可以减轻患者的焦虑症状。

5. 认知重建 认知疗法用于治疗 OCD 主要集中于有关主题的认知重建上，是一种通过对患者歪曲的思维模式系统进行定义和检测来重建患者正确认知系统的方法。它以改变患者对情境的错误认知为目标，指导患者监控自己的强迫思想，教导患者认识到思想、情绪及行为之间的关系。治疗者通过呈现某些“赞同–反对”的证据来检查患者歪曲的思想，通过这种方式，治疗者可帮助患者认识并怀疑将要发生的、令人害怕事件的真实性，患者学会如何识别使其思想歪曲的错误认识。

6. 提示卡 用于帮助患者重建认知方式和内容的一种治疗工具，主要针对患者的强迫观念及行为。提示卡使用一些从患者症状中提炼的信息，组成一个组织系统，此系统主要根据诱发焦虑的程度分解强迫观念及行为，这些卡片可以帮助患者强化自身是安全的信念，并可以逐渐耐受延迟或控制强迫动作所引起的焦虑。下面是提示卡的步骤：① 这是强迫症状，不是我；② 这只是强迫思维，并不意味着我要这么做，我不会这么做的；③ 我的焦虑水平在上升，但它会自动缓解的，事实上它从来没有持续到伤害我的时间；④ 相信我自己；⑤ 我第一次做对了；⑥ 反复检查不能确保我的安全，我一直很安全。

（三）其他治疗

1. 主要是帮助家庭成员减轻因此障碍所致的不协调，并与家庭成员建立治疗联盟以促进患者康复。此外，小组治疗对一些患者也非常有效。

2. 主要用于强迫障碍合并严重抑郁，继发性的强迫观念和强迫行为，但在单独强迫

obsessions and rituals, but has not been shown to be beneficial for OCD alone.

3. In extreme cases of severely impaired clients with refractory OCD, neurosurgery can be considered. Recently, a new development is deep-brain stimulation, which may gradually replace neurosurgery for refractory OCD.

症的治疗中还未发现有效。

3. 严重功能受损的难治性OCD患者的极端病例可考虑选择神经外科治疗。近年来，深部脑刺激治疗是难治性OCD的新发展，并逐渐替代神经外科治疗。

IV. Application of the Nursing Process

四、护理程序的应用

i. Nursing Assessment

1. Biologic Assessment Clients with OCD do not often have physical abnormalities. However, they may complain of multiple physical symptoms. Clients must be carefully evaluated and not merely dismissed. Dermatologic lesions should be assessed in each client with OCD, because of symptoms such as repeated hand-washing, excessive cleaning with caustic agents, or bathing. In addition, nurse should observe client's osteoarthrosis secondary to cleaning rituals. Cerebral pathology should be excluded in client with OCD which has a febrile illness.

2. Psychological Assessment

(1) Obsessions and compulsions: Nurse should assess the type and severity of the client's obsessions and compulsions. But in most instances direct questions must be asked to reveal symptoms of the disorder. Nurse should ask the individual how long it takes to dress in the morning or leave the house, but usually follow-up questions such as: "Do you find yourself frequently returning to the house or the stove, even when you know that you have already checked this? Does this happen every day?"

(2) Mental status examination: Orientation, insight, memory, judgment and psychiatric symptoms of clients should be assessed. Orientation and memory of clients with OCD are not usually impaired, but at times they may be distracted by obsession thoughts. Some obsessions may appear out of touch with reality and extremely eccentric, but frank psychosis is not part of OCD. Delusion and hallucinations will not be present unless there is another psychiatric disorder involved. Most often the individual will be able to state that the obsessions are unreasonable, but they will not be able to control them, which cause them to sometimes doubt this as certain. Judgment and insight are not usually impaired except as they relate to their obsessions or compulsions.

(3) Thought patterns: Individual with obsessive style of thinking will exhibit circumstantial speech. This is speech that is difficult to follow, loaded with irrelevant

（一）护理评估

1. 生理评估 强迫障碍患者常不伴有躯体异常症状，然而，他们关于躯体异常的主诉较多，护士应认真进行评估检查。强迫障碍患者因症状原因常反复洗手、洗澡或过度清洁等，护士应仔细评估患者的皮肤完整性及受损情况，此外，也应评估因强迫清洁可能导致的骨关节受损情况。对于伴有发热症状的强迫障碍患者，应排除脑器质性问题。

2. 心理评估

（1）强迫观念与强迫行为：评估患者强迫观念、强迫行为的类型及严重程度。护士须仔细询问疾病的实际症状，如询问患者“每天需要用多长时间完成穿衣和洗脸等行为？什么时候能离开家？即使知道自己刚检查过，是否经常要回去检查？这样的情况每天要发生多少次？”等。

（2）精神状态评估：评估患者的定向力、自知力、记忆力、判断力及有无精神症状等。强迫症患者的定向力和记忆力一般不会受影响，但会因强迫观念而受到干扰。强迫症状患者的有些强迫观念可能脱离现实和十分古怪，但是确没有明显的精神病性症状，患者一般不会出现妄想和幻觉，除非患者还存在其他精神疾病。多数患者能够认识到强迫观念和症状不合理，自己却不能控制，这使患者容易怀疑其合理性。当不涉及强迫观念和行为时，患者的判断能力和自知力完好。

（3）思维方式：强迫症患者的思维方式很难理解，多为一种环形的方式，并有很多不相关的内容，但还能清楚描述问题，护士

details, but eventually addresses the question. Nurse should remember that it is part of the disorder and may be beyond the client's awareness.

(4) Risk factors: Nurse must assess the suicidal risk and correlated influence factors of the client with OCD. This disorder causes great distress to the client who realizes the futility and unreasonableness of the behavior. The client may feel a sense of hopelessness and helplessness and may contemplate suicide to end the suffering. An additional risk for suicide is comorbidity OCD with depression.

(5) Scale assessment: Several rating scales can be used to identify symptoms and monitor the degree, such as Yale-Brown obsessive compulsive scale (YBOCS), Maudsley obsessive- compulsive inventory.

3. Social Assessment Nurse must consider sociocultural factors when evaluating OCD. At times, cultural or religious beliefs may be misunderstood and mistaken for obsessions. These beliefs must be evaluated in the context of the individual's life. Moreover, marital status appears to be affected by OCD. Clients with OCD are able to gradually draw their families into accommodating abnormal behavior, which can lead to serious family dysfunction. Client with OCD tend to remain single more often than persons without the disorder. Family assessment will reveal the amount of education and support needed, as well as begin the partnership among the client, family, and treatment team. At times, obsessions and compulsions make it difficult for the individual to leave the home or function at work. Financial difficulties may result and add to the stress or the concerns of the family. These factors should be assessed and appropriate assistance obtained through social services when necessary.

ii. Nursing Diagnosis

1. Anxiety Related to conflicts between conscious self-obsession and anti-obsession.

2. Powerlessness Related to uncontrolled ritualistic behavior and/or obsessive thoughts.

3. Impaired Skin Integrity Related to excessive washing or bathing.

4. Ineffective Coping Related to ritualistic behavior and/or obsessive thoughts.

5. Impaired Social Interaction Related to obsessions and/or compulsions.

6. Ineffective Role Performance Related to need to perform rituals and inability to fulfill usual patterns.

应了解患者不是有意识的，而是疾病的一种表现。

（4）危险因素评估：评估患者有关自杀的危险性和相关因素。因强迫障碍可引起患者极大的痛苦，使患者感到无助和没有希望，可能会产生一些自杀或自伤的行为。另外一个自杀的危险因素则是强迫症患者同时患有抑郁症。

（5）量表评估：强迫症相关评估量表有助于识别强迫症状及严重程度，如 Yale−Brown 强迫症状量表、Maudsley 强迫观念与行为量表等。

3. 社会评估 在评估中护士需考虑患者的社会文化因素，如宗教信仰、社会文化等，这些因素可能影响患者的强迫观念和强迫症状。此外，患者的婚姻状况可能受强迫障碍的影响，患者常常使其家庭卷入不正常的状态，使家庭功能失调，强迫障碍患者单身者居多，通过对患者家庭的评估将帮助护士制订有关家庭教育和支持的措施。有时候，强迫观念和强迫行为常使患者离家出走或者不想工作，经济的困难也将导致和加重患者的压力及家庭的关注，在评估时护士应考虑到这些因素。

（二）主要护理诊断

1. 焦虑 与有意识的自我强迫与反强迫之间的冲突有关。

2. 无能为力 与不能控制的仪式性动作和 / 或强迫观念有关。

3. 皮肤完整性受损 与过度清洗有关。

4. 应对无效 与仪式性动作和 / 或强迫观念有关。

5. 社会交往障碍 与强迫观念和 / 或强迫行为有关。

6. 无效性角色行为 与执行仪式动作但不能完成日常行为有关。

iii. Nursing Planning

1. Nursing Outcome

(1) The client is able to maintain anxiety at a manageable level without resorting to the use of ritualistic behavior.

(2) The client understands relationship between anxiety and ritualistic behavior, verbalizes specific situations that in the past have provoked anxiety and resulted in seeking relief through rituals.

(3) The client doesn't appear new skin damage due to compulsive behaviors, and the defect of skin has been repaired.

(4) The client demonstrates more adaptive coping strategies to deal with obsessions and/or compulsions, such as thought stopping, response prevention, and relaxation techniques.

(5) The client can perform activities of daily living independently.

(6) The client is able to resume role-related responsibilities.

(7) The family understands the disorder and the treatment, and willing to help the client practicing cognitive and behavioral techniques.

2. Nursing Intervention

(1) Skin care

1) For the client with cleaning or hand-washing compulsions, pay attention to skin condition is necessary. Nurses should evaluate impaired skin of hand and redness, and also should assess the whole body skin conditions of clients with compulsive cleaning.

2) Initially, before the client begins to experience relief from obsessions, it may be necessary to work with her or him to protect the skin during hand-washing or cleaning, rather than eliminate the behavior. Encourage the client to use hand cream after washing, to decrease the frequency of washing, or to decrease the length of time spent in washing.

3) For clients with severe impaired skin caused by compulsive cleaning, when necessary, behavioral therapy and appropriate restraints can be taken to reduce the frequency and duration of time of ritualistic behaviors, so as not to aggravate the defect of skin. Give medications under the orders by physicians.

(2) Improve the coping capacity of clients

1) Help the client to identify situations that increase anxiety and result in ritualistic behaviors. Recognition of precipitating factors is the first step in teaching the client to interrupt the escalating anxiety.

2) Initially meet the client's dependency needs as required. Allow plenty of time for rituals. Do not be

（三）护理计划

1. 护理目标

（1）患者能把焦虑控制在适当水平而不会采用仪式行为去缓解焦虑。

（2）患者认识到焦虑与仪式性动作之间的联系，能描述出过去引起焦虑并通过强迫行为减轻焦虑的特定情境。

（3）患者皮肤受损情况得到明显改善，未因强迫行为出现新的皮肤损伤。

（4）患者能应用应对技巧应对强迫观念和/或行为，如思想停止法、反应性预防技术和放松技巧等。

（5）患者能独立完成自我生活照顾。

（6）患者重新显示出相关角色的能力。

（7）患者家属理解该疾病及其治疗并乐意帮助患者参与认知和行为治疗的活动。

2. 护理措施

（1）皮肤护理

1）对于强迫清洗的患者，护士应仔细评估患者的皮肤状况，如强迫洗手的患者手部皮肤有无破损、发红等，强迫清洗的患者全身皮肤有无异常等。

2）在患者未能消除强迫观念和强迫行为的影响时，护士应与患者一起，提供支持和帮助，如指导患者减少清洗的次数和时间，对于强迫洗手的患者在每次洗手后使用护手霜等，以降低因反复洗手导致的皮肤受损。

3）因强迫清洗行为致皮肤受损较严重的患者，必要时可采取行为治疗适当约束患者以减少强迫行为的频率及时间，以免加重皮肤受损情况，并遵医嘱给予相应的治疗药物。

（2）提高患者的应对能力

1）帮助患者识别哪些是可能导致焦虑进而引起仪式性行为的情境，识别诱发因素是教会患者中断不断升级的焦虑的第一步。

2）刚开始应满足患者的需求，允许患者有足够的时间去完成自己的仪式行为，并对

judgmental or verbalize disapproval of the behavior. Sudden and complete elimination of all dependency requires would create intense anxiety.

3) Support client's efforts to explore the meaning and purpose of the behavior. Help client to understand the irrational thoughts and behaviors as a disease process not a personal identity. Client should be instructed about the biologic components of OCD.

4) Provide structured schedule of activities for client, including adequate time for completion of rituals. Structure provides a feeling of security for the anxious client.

5) After the client becomes more involved in other activities, gradually begin to decrease amount of time assigned for compulsive behaviors to minimize anxiety. Behavioral treatment may be initiated. Nurse may help the client arrange a schedule of activities that allows for some private time but that integrates the client into normal activities of daily living.

6) Give positive reinforcement for non-ritualistic behaviors and independent behaviors to enhance self-esteem and encourage repetition of desired behaviors.

7) Help client learn methods of interrupting obsessive thoughts and ritualistic behavior with techniques such as response prevention, thought stopping, relaxation, and physical exercise. Knowledge and practice of coping techniques that are more adaptive will help client change and let go of maladaptive responses to anxiety.

(3) Help clients restore roles, and strengthen support function of family.

1) Nurses must control their own anxiety, interact with the client with a calm, no authoritarian fashion while demonstrating empathy. It is important that the client know that the nurse understands the life distress that the disorder has caused and that he or she does not "disapprove" of the client or the client's behaviors.

2) Identify client's previous role within the family and present role altered by the illness. Identify roles of other family members.

3) Work with clients to discuss their perception of role expectations, and to evaluate if the role expectations are realistic.

4) Encourage client to discuss conflicts evident within the family system. Identify specific stressors, as well as adaptive and maladaptive responses from the client and other family members within the system.

5) Explore available options for changes or adjustments in role, and practice those options through role-play. Planning and rehearsal of potential role

此不进行批判或表示反对，因突然完全中断患者的需求可能引发强烈的焦虑。

3）帮助患者理解强迫行为的意义及目的，帮助患者认识和理解他们的这些不合理的想法和行为是疾病，而与患者的人格无关，应向患者讲解有关强迫障碍的生物学理论。

4）为患者提供结构化的活动安排，包括完成仪式性动作的足够时间，活动安排可以为焦虑的患者提供安全的感觉。

5）当患者开始参与其他活动时，应逐渐减少对强迫行为的时间分配以减少焦虑，此时可以开始行为治疗，护士可以帮助患者进行活动安排以促使患者回到日常生活活动中，但允许患者有一些私人时间。

6）对患者的非仪式行为及独立行为及时给予表扬和鼓励，增加患者的自信心并强化患者的适应性行为。

7）帮助患者学习中断强迫想法和行为的方法，包括反应预防法、思想停止法、放松技术及体育锻炼等。应对技巧的学习及实践可以帮助患者更好地适应并改变对焦虑的适应不良。

（3）协助患者重塑角色行为，增强家庭支持功能

1）与患者接触时护士须显示出平静、稳重和温和的态度，让患者了解护士理解其不恰当的观念和行为及生活压力，且愿意帮助他们。

2）识别患者以前在家庭中的角色以及患病后的角色，识别患者其他家庭成员的角色。

3）与患者一起讨论他们对于角色期待的认知，并评估这些角色期待是否现实。

4）鼓励患者讨论家庭中的冲突，识别特定的压力，包括患者和家庭成员的适应和不适应的反应。

5）探讨角色改变或角色调整的其他可用方式，并通过角色扮演实践这些方式，潜在角色转变的策划与排练可以帮助减少焦虑。

transitions can reduce anxiety.

6) Encourage family members' participation in resolving the cause of the anxiety from which the client resorts to the use of ritualistic behaviors. Educating families of clients with OCD the information of the etiology of the disorder may decrease some of the stigma and embarrassment they may feel related to the client's obsessions and compulsions.

7) Give positive reinforcement for capability to resume role responsibilities by decreasing need for ritualistic behaviors. Positive reinforcement enhances self-esteem and promotes repetition of desired behaviors.

iv. Nursing Evaluation

1. Can the client demonstrate substitute behaviors to maintain anxiety at a manageable level?

2. Does the client recognize the relationship between escalating anxiety and the dependence on ritualistic behaviors for relief? Can the client verbalize specific situations that in the past have provoked anxiety and resulted in seeking relief through rituals?

3. Does the client have new skin damage, or has defect of skin been repaired?

4. Can the client demonstrate more adaptive coping strategies to deal with obsessions and/or compulsions?

5. Can the client perform self-care activities independently?

6. Can the client verbalize a plan of action for dealing with these stressful situations in the future, and demonstrate an ability to fulfill role-related responsibilities?

7. Does the family understand the disorder and the treatment, and is the family able and willing to help the client practice cognitive and behavioral techniques?

6）鼓励患者的家庭成员参与减少促使患者实施强迫行为的焦虑。向强迫障碍患者的家属提供有关疾病的病因等信息，以降低患者家属对疾病的担忧和由此引起的困扰。

7）对患者减少对仪式行为的需求并恢复角色职责的能力进行及时的鼓励，正强化可以增强患者的自信心并增加期待行为。

（四）护理评价

1. 患者是否采用替代行为将焦虑保持在可控制的水平？

2. 患者是否认识到焦虑与仪式行为之间的关系？能否描述引起焦虑并通过强迫行为减轻焦虑的特定情境？

3. 患者有无出现新的皮肤受损，或已受损皮肤状况是否得到改善？

4. 患者能够运用所学的应对技巧应对强迫观念和/或行为？

5. 患者是否表现出能够独立完成自我生活的照顾？

6. 患者是否有计划来应对未来生活中的压力，是否表现出有能力完成自己的应该承担的责任？

7. 患者家属是否理解该疾病及其治疗，是否乐意帮助患者参与认知和行为治疗的活动？

Section 4 Nursing Management for Clients with Somatoform Disorders

Somatoform is defined as the use of physical symptoms to express emotional problems and psychosocial stress. The character of somatoform disorders is that physical symptoms are suggested medical disease, but without demonstrable organic pathology or known pathophysiological mechanism to account for them. They are classified as mental disorders because

第四节 躯体形式障碍患者的护理

躯体形式障碍是一种以躯体症状来表达其情绪和内心冲突的精神障碍。其特点是躯体症状类似于躯体疾病，但没有可证实的器质性病变或者病理性改变，实验室检查也不能发现阳性结果。其被归类于精神障碍，是因为通过现存的实验室检查手段和方法，没

pathophysiological processes are not demonstrable or understandable by existing laboratory procedures, and there is either evidence or strong presumption that psychological factors are the major cause of the symptoms.

It is now well documented that a large proportion of client in general medical outpatient clinics and private medical offices do not have organic disease requiring medical treatment. It is likely that many of these clients have somatoform disorder, but they do not perceive themselves as having a psychiatric problem and thus do not seek treatment from psychiatrists.

有发现明显的证据能解释其病理生理过程。在ICD-10中，躯体形式障碍主要包括躯体化障碍和疑病障碍。

现已证实，在医院的门诊或私人诊所接受治疗的很多患者并没有器质性的疾病。这可能与患者有躯体方面的症状，但却没有感觉到自己具有精神方面的问题，因此，通常不去看精神科医生而去到别的科室就诊。

I. Somatization Disorder

Somatization disorder is characterized by many somatic symptoms that cannot be explained adequately on the basis of physical and laboratory examination. Somatization disorder is distinguished from other somatoform disorders because of the multiplicity of the complaints and the multiple organ systems that are affected. The disorder is chronic (with symptoms present for several years and beginning before age 30) and is associated with significant psychological distress, impairment in social and occupational function, and excessive medical help-seeking behavior.The lifetime prevalence of somatization disorder in the general population is estimated to be 0.1 to 0.2 percent. Somatization disorder occurs primary in women, it outnumber men by 5 to 20 times. This disorder seems to be inversely related to social position, occurring most often among little-educated and poor patients.

一、躯体化障碍

躯体化障碍是一种表现为多种躯体症状的，但是却不能用体格检查或实验室检查来解释这种症状为特征的精神障碍。其症状可涉及身体的任何系统或器官，因此与其他躯体形式的疾病区别开来。多在30岁之前发病并持续多年，患者往往有明显的心理压力、社会功能受损、工作能力下降及频繁就医行为。该病在一般人群中的发病率估计为0.1%～0.2%，女性的患病率远高于男性，发病率是男性的5～20倍。该病的发生与社会地位负相关，在教育程度低和贫穷的人中发病率较高。

i. Etiology

The cause of somatization disorder is unknown, but there are several theories reviewed the causes of somatization.

1. Biological Theories Some studies point to a neuropsychological basis for somatization disorder. Those studies propose that the clients have characteristic attention and cognitive impairments that result in the faulty perception and assessment of somatosensory input. A limited number of brain-imaging studies have reported decreased metabolism in the frontal lobes and in the nondominant hemisphere. Another theory holds that some individuals may have deficient communication between brain hemispheres and thus are unable to express their emotions directly; they therefore present physical instead of emotional symptoms.

2. Psychological and Psychosocial Theories Personality and psychological factors have been

（一）病因

躯体化障碍的病因并不完全清楚，但有许多理论对其相关因素进行了讨论。

1. 生物学因素 神经心理方面的研究提出神经心理是该障碍的发病基础，躯体化障碍患者在注意和认知上常有某些损害，从而导致对输入的躯体感知信息不能进行正确评估和感受。有关脑影像研究报告，可能与额叶和非优势大脑半球的新陈代谢降低有关。另外一些理论提出一些人可能存在大脑半球之间信息的沟通障碍，从而导致不能直接的表达他们的情绪，因此以躯体症状替代情绪症状。

2. 社会心理因素 躯体化障碍的发生有一定的人格基础和心理因素。社会心理学家

implicated. Psychosocial theories viewed that somatization may be a way of experiencing and communicating somatic distress in response to psychosocial stress, which cause the client to seek medical help.

认为躯体化障碍是表达和传递心理社会压力的一种方式，这种方式使患者寻求医学帮助。

3. Sociocultural The ories Even though somatization disorders occur cross-culturally, the symptoms may vary from culture to culture. Also, the conceptualization of somatization disorder in Western society and Non-Western societies have different meanings and explanations. In some Asian cultures, symptoms of depression or anxiety are believed to be caused by a weakness in some parts of the body such as the kidney, heart, bones, lung, or nerve or as having a vitamin deficiency (Ganesan, 1989).

3. **社会文化因素** 虽然躯体化障碍发生在不同文化和地域，但其症状却与其文化背景有关，症状可能因文化变化而不同，西方国家和亚洲国家对此疾病的定义和解释也存在差异。一些亚洲国家认为抑郁或焦虑的症状常常是某些器官如肾脏、心脏、骨骼、肺脏或神经功能的衰弱，或是维生素的缺乏（Ganesan，1989）。

ii. Clinical Manifestation

（二）临床表现

The main features of somatization disorder are multiple, frequently changing physical symptoms. Symptoms may be referred to any part or system of the body, but gastrointestinal sensation (pain, belching, regurgitation, vomiting, nausea, etc.) and blotchiness are among the commonest. Sexual and menstrual complaints are also common. Marked depression and anxiety are frequently present. The course of the disorder is chronic and fluctuating, and is often associated with long-standing disruption of social, interpersonal and family behavior. The disorder is for more common in women than in men, and usually onsets in early adult life. Suicide threats are common, but actual suicide is rare. If suicide does occur, it is often associated with substance abuse. The client's medical histories are often circumstantial, vague, imprecise, inconsistent, and disorganized. Clients classically but not always describe their complaints in a dramatic, emotional, and exaggerated fashion, with vivid and colorful language. Such clients may confuse temporal sequences and cannot clearly distinguish current symptoms from past symptoms. The clients may be perceived as dependent, self-centered, hungry for admiration or praise, and manipulative. Many somatic symptoms of somatization disorder cannot be explained adequately on the basis of physical and laboratory examination.

躯体化障碍的患者表现多种多样，以经常变化的躯体症状为主要特征。症状可涉及身体的任何系统或器官，最常见的是胃肠道不适（如疼痛、打嗝、返酸、呕吐、恶心等），异常的皮肤感觉（如瘙痒、烧伤感、刺痛、麻木感、酸痛等），皮肤斑点、性及月经方面的主诉也较常见。其常为慢性波动性病程，伴有社会、人际及家庭行为方面长期存在的严重障碍。女性远多于男性，多在成年早期发病。常存在明显的焦虑和抑郁，自杀的威胁也很常见，但是很少发生自杀行为。如果发生了自杀行为，则往往伴有物质滥用。患者通常描述不清楚病史，并夸大疾病的严重程度。体格检查和实验室检查不能解释躯体化障碍的症状。患者也不总是用夸张、生动、丰富的语言抱怨，可能他们只是混淆了时间，分不清现在的和以前的症状有什么区别。患者也可表现为依赖、以自我为中心、渴望被赞美、崇拜或是有控制欲。

iii. Treatment

（三）治疗

The treatment of somatization disorder and the other somatoform disorder is complicated because the etiology is unknown and few treatment studies have been done. The general consensus is providing long-term general management of clients with these disorders.

躯体化障碍的发病原因尚不清楚，对其治疗的研究较少，因此，治疗起来比较困难。一般从对疾病的长期综合管理来着手，包括躯体症状的治疗、心理治疗和药物治疗。

1. Treatment of Somatic Symptoms Somatization disorder is a long-term chronic condition with multiple unexplained physical symptoms. The cornerstone of management is the establishment of

1. **躯体症状的治疗** 躯体化障碍的患者认为自己的疾病是躯体上的疾病而非精神上的疾病，往往不愿意到精神科就医。因此，

trusting relationship. The clients with somatization usually resist psychiatric ill for their disorder because they regard themselves physically rather than mentally ill. Once somatization has been diagnosed, a reasonable long-range strategy for a primary care physician who is treating a client with somatization disorder is to increase the client's awareness of the possibility that psychological factors are involved in the symptoms until the client is willing to see a mental health clinician, probably a psychiatrist, on a regular basis.

一旦被诊断为躯体化障碍，治疗的基础就是与患者建立互信。医生可采用一种长期的、合理的方法来提高患者对该病的心理学因素的认识（该病是由于心理因素引起的），直到患者自己愿意去看精神科医生为止。

2. Psychotherapy Psychotherapy is useful to the client with somatization disorder. It may decrease client's personal health expenditures by 50 percent, largely by decreasing their rates of hospitalization. In psychotherapy settings, clients are helped to cope with their symptoms, to express underlying emotions, and to develop alternative strategies for expressing their feelings.

2. 心理治疗 心理治疗对躯体化障碍患者非常有效，它能减少患者就医开支的50%，且大大减少患者住院治疗的几率。心理治疗的主要目的是帮助患者应对这些躯体症状，表达隐藏在症状之后的情绪问题，帮助患者发展适应性行为。

(1) Individual psychotherapy: The goal of psychotherapy is to help client develop healthy and adaptive behaviors, encourage them to move beyond their somatization, and manage their lives more effectively (Barsky, 1989). The focus is on personal and social difficulties that the client is experiencing in daily life and the achievement of practical solutions for these difficulties. Treatment is initiated with a complete physical examination to rule out organic pathology. Once this has been ensured, the physician turns his or her attention to the client's social and personal problems and away from the somatic complaints.

（1）个体心理治疗：其目的是帮助患者发展健康的适应性行为。鼓励患者转移对症状的关注，更有效地完成自我生活的照顾（Barsky，1989）。治疗的焦点是帮助患者解决个人的和社会交往方面所存在的困难。在治疗之初，应注意排除躯体器质性疾病，而一旦被确诊，治疗者就应注意将患者的注意力转向患者的社会和个人的问题，避免讨论身体的症状。

(2) Group psychotherapy: Group therapy may be helpful to somatization disorder because it provides a setting where clients can share their experiences of illness, learn to verbalize thoughts and feelings, and be confronted by group members and leaders when they reject responsibility for maladaptive behaviors (McCracken, 1985).

（2）团体心理治疗：团体心理治疗为躯体化障碍患者提供表达其疾病体验的帮助，患者学习通过言语表达情绪和感受。当患者因为适应不良行为而拒绝承担责任时，必须面对来自小组成员和领导的压力，从而可以使其更好地履行责任（McCracken，1985）。

(3) Behavior therapy: Behavior therapy focuses on teaching these individuals to reward the client's autonomy, self-sufficiency, and independence. This may involve working with the client's family or other significant others who may be perpetuating the physical symptoms by rewarding passivity and dependency and by being overly solicitous and helpful.

（3）行为治疗：行为治疗的重心是指导患者学会欣赏自己、肯定自己和帮助患者自理和独立。行为治疗还涉及与患者家属和与其有紧密关系的人员。

3. Psychopharmacology Treatment The clients with somatization disorder often have marked depression and anxiety. The physician can prescribe antidepressants and anxiolytics in order to relieve symptoms.

3. 药物治疗 躯体化障碍患者常常继发抑郁、焦虑以及药物依赖，因此，可对症给予抗抑郁和抗焦虑药物治疗。

II. Hypochondriasis

Hypochondriasis can be defined as a kind of neurosis whose essential feature is a persistent preoccupation with worry or a belief in having serious physical disease. The clients repeatedly seek medical advice for physical symptoms that they themselves think they have, and negative medical investigations and doctor's explanation cannot dismiss their doubt. Even though the clients sometimes have some physical disorder, this disorder cannot explain the quality, degree of symptoms told, and their affliction, preoccupation. Anxiety and depression are often present. Hypochondriasis is common in general medical practice and seems to occur with equal frequency in men and woman.

i. Etiology

There are many theories about hypochondriasis as following:

1. Firstly, because hypochondriacal persons have lower thresholds than usual for physical discomfort, they augment and amplify their somatic sensations so that the symptoms reflect a misinterpretation of bodily symptoms.

2. A second theory is that hypochondriasis is understandable on the basis of a social learning model. The symptoms of hypochondriasis are viewed as a request for admission to the sick role made by a person who is facing seemingly insurmountable and insolvable problems. The sick role offers a way out, because the sick client is allowed to avoid noxious obligations and to postpone unwelcome challenges and is excused from usually expected duties.

3. A third theory regarding the cause of hypochondriasis is that it is a variant form of other mental disorders. The disorders most frequently related to hypochondriasis are depressive disorder and anxiety disorder. An estimated 80 percent of clients with hypochondriasis may have coexisting depressive disorder and anxiety disorders.

4. A fourth school of thought regarding hypochondriasis is the psychodynamic school, which posits that aggressive and hostile wishes toward others are transferred (through repression and displacement) into physical complaints.

Hypochondriasis is also viewed as a defense against guilt, a sense of innate badness, an expression of low self-esteem, and a sign of excessive self-concern. Pain and somatic suffering thus becomes a means of atonement and expiation and can be experienced as deserved punishment for past wrongdoing (either real or imaginary) and the sense that one is wicked and sinful.

二、疑病障碍

疑病障碍是一种以担心或相信患严重躯体疾病的优势观念为主要特征的神经症。患者因为这种症状反复就医，各种医学检查阴性和医生的解释均不能打消其疑虑。即使患者有时存在某种躯体障碍，也不能解释所述症状的性质与程度，常伴有焦虑或抑郁。男女患病率无明显差异。

（一）病因

关于疑病障碍的病因目前有多种观点和理论：

1. 与一般人相比，疑病障碍的患者对躯体不适的耐受性较低，他们过度夸大自己的躯体感觉，以致将身体的一些自然征象误解为疾病症状。

2. 社会学习模式认为，当疑病障碍患者遇到不能克服的困难或不能解决的问题时，迫切需要进入患者角色，因为患病或身体不适可以使患者免除应尽的义务，于是认为自己身体的正常征象是疾病症状。

3. 有理论认为疑病是其他精神疾病的表现形式，常常与抑郁和焦虑有关。据估计80%的疑病障碍患者可能共存抑郁和焦虑障碍。

4. 精神动力学派认为，疑病障碍是一种将对他人的攻击、敌意心理转换为躯体症状的表现，也有理论认为疑病是一种对罪恶、人性本恶感的心理防卫，是一种低自尊、过度关注自己的表现，患者将躯体痛苦作为对不道德行为的惩罚和赎罪。

ii. Clinical Manifestation

The chief manifestation of hypochondriasis is fear of having (or the belief that one has) a serious physical disease. This fear is based on individual misinterpretation of bodily symptoms. Despite tests and reassurances, hypochondriacal client's fear is not allayed.

The preoccupation in hypochondriasis may be with small physical problems such as a cough or cut; with unusual physical functioning such as heartbeat, peristalsis, or sweating; or with vague physical complaints such as "burning feet" or "weak heart". The symptoms may involve one or several body systems, one or several organs. These symptoms are then attributed to some suspected disease such as cancer or AIDS, and the client becomes very concerned and focuses on them. Hypochondriasis is often accompanied by symptoms of depression and anxiety, and it commonly coexists with a depressive or anxiety disorder.

（二）临床表现

疑病障碍主要表现为患者担心自己患有严重的躯体疾病。这种恐惧由其对某些正常的身体感觉的错误理解造成。尽管各项医学检查结果阴性，患者对疾病的担心和恐惧仍然不能减轻。

患者在早期可能表现为一些小的躯体问题，如咳嗽、割伤等；有些患者感觉自己的心跳、肠蠕动或出汗异常；或患者述说一些含糊的不适，如“手脚心发热”或“心里不舒服”等。症状可涉及躯体各个系统和器官。患者把这些症状与一些严重的躯体疾病如癌症和艾滋病等进行联系，并且整日关注这些症状和疾病。另外，疑病障碍患者常常伴有抑郁和焦虑障碍。

iii. Treatment

Hypochondriacal clients are usually resistant to psychiatric treatment. Some hypochondriacal clients accept psychiatric treatment if it takes place in a medical setting and focuses on stress reduction and education in coping with chronic illness. The treatment includes psychological therapy and medications.

1. Psychotherapy Among such clients, group psychotherapy is the modality of choice, in part because it provides the social support and social interaction that seem to reduce their anxiety. Individual insight-oriented psychotherapy may be useful, but it is generally not successful. When hypochondriasis is a transient situational reaction, the clinician must help clients cop with the stress without reinforcing their illness behavior and their use of the sick role as a solution to the problem.

2. Pharmacotherapy Pharmacotherapy alleviates hypochondriacal symptoms only when the client has an underlying drug-responsive condition, such as an anxiety disorder or major depressive disorder.

（三）治疗

尽管疑病障碍的患者往往不愿进行精神病学治疗，但多数患者愿意在医院接受有关减轻压力和应对慢性疾病方面的心理治疗。疑病障碍的治疗包括心理治疗和药物治疗。

1. 心理治疗 小组心理治疗通过提供社会支持和社会干预帮助患者减轻焦虑。同时，个别的认知心理治疗通过提供信息、探讨分析，帮助患者逐渐认识其问题，改变患者对症状性质的看法。当患者处于应激状态时，要帮助患者学会如何去应对。

2. 药物治疗 当患者伴随抑郁、焦虑等问题时，应根据患者情况，采取抗抑郁和焦虑药物治疗。

III. Application of the Nursing Process

Caring for individual with somatization disorder is challenge. Caring means that the nurse will try to understand the client as she is, accept her personality, her complaints, and her need for care. Often, the clients with somatization disorder have low self-esteem, repressed hostility, and guilt derived from a dysfunctional family background. A nurse must see through the presenting symptoms in order to begin caring for the person behind the presenting illness.

三、护理程序的应用

护理躯体形式障碍患者对有些护士而言是项挑战，护士需努力去了解患者，接受其个性，理解其痛苦。躯体形式障碍患者常存在着低自尊、压抑、敌意和不良的家庭背景，护士需要通过患者的表面症状来认识患者真正的问题。

i. Assessing Human Response to Somatization Disorder

1. Biologic Assessment Nursing assessment of this client begins with reviewing the client's current complaints and history of illness. If the client has not already been diagnosed with somatization disorder, the nurse should screen for it by determining the presence of the most commonly reported problems associated with this disorder, which include dysmenorrhea, lump in throat, vomiting, shortness of breath, burning in sex organs, painful extremities, and amnesia. During the assessment interview, the nurse needs to allow enough time for the client to explain all the medical problems because a rushed assessment interview will block communication. In addition, a careful review of systems is important because the appearance of physical problems is usually related to psychosocial problems.

2. Psychological Assessment The mental status of individuals with somatization disorder usually is within normal limits. What is most noticeable is the flamboyant appearance and exaggerated speech. Their language is colorful and can be entertaining. Generally, cognition is not impaired. Individuals with somatization disorder usually have intense emotional reactions to life stressors. It is critical that the physical assessment data be linked to psychological and social event that are occurring in the client's life. There are some questions will help nurse to assess for recent life stressors.

(1) Have you been under stress recently?

(2) Has anyone close to you been ill or died?

(3) Have you ever lost a child?

(4) Tell me about your job.

The individual's mood is usually labile, often shifting from extremely excited to depress. There are some questions will help nurse to assess for coexisting depression and suicide ideation.

(1) Have you felt down or sad lately?

(2) Is it harder to do your usual activities?

(3) Do you ever feel hopeless?

3. Social Assessment People with this disorder spend excessive time seeking medical care and treating their multiple illnesses. They believe themselves to be very sick, disabled and cannot work. Most of them are unemployed. Nurse should identify the client's support network. Family members become weary of the individual's constant complaints of physical problems. These individuals live in chaotic families with multiple problems. In assessing the family structure, other members with psychiatric disorders need to be identified. It is important to identify the positive and negative

（一）护理评估

1. 生理评估 护士应系统评估患者的身体状况，注意了解患者当前抱怨的躯体不适和疾病历史。如果患者过去未被诊断为躯体形式障碍，护士应注意评估患者所抱怨的主要的躯体不适，如月经期疼痛、吞咽困难、呕吐、呼吸急促、性器官烧灼感、肢端疼痛及健忘等。在进行护理评估时，护士应允许患者有足够的时间来讲述他们的身体不适，因为一次匆忙的评估或打断患者的谈话将会阻断沟通。同时，系统的仔细评估可帮助护士排除患者真正存在的躯体疾病。

2. 心理评估 躯体形式障碍患者常常表现出一些特殊的人格特征，如歇斯底里的人格特征、好表现自己、喜欢引人注意、情感丰富、情绪不稳、依赖性强、喜欢操纵别人等。通常，患者的认知没有受损。患者有明显的情绪反应或应激事件，在评估时应注意了解患者心理社会因素。下列一些问题可帮助护士进行评估：① 你最近是否存在很大的压力？② 你生活中亲密的人是否生病或死亡？③ 在你生活中有没有重大的丧失事情发生，如小孩的丢失？④ 你最近工作情况怎么样？

另外，患者的情绪常不稳定，可以从极度的兴奋到抑郁。护士应注意评估患者的情绪问题，如问：① 你近来是否感到悲伤或痛苦？② 你完成日常活动是否感到困难？③ 你是否感到毫无希望，甚至有过死亡的念头？

3. 社会评估 躯体形式障碍患者常常花很多时间寻求治疗，他们相信自己生病了，没有工作能力，许多患者失业，护士应注意评估患者的支持系统。家庭成员对患者的抱怨非常苦恼，护士应注意评估患者的家庭结构、功能和家庭成员之间的关系等问题。

relationships within the family.

4. Pharmacologic Assessment A psychopharmacologic assessment of these clients is challenging. Clients with somatization disorder frequently move from one provider to another or "provider shop". They are usually taking a large number of medications. They will often protect their sources and may not be truthful in identifying the actual number of medications they are ingesting. A pharmacologic assessment is needed not only because of the number of medications, but also because of these individuals have many unusual side effects.

4. 药物治疗评估 对躯体形式障碍的患者进行药物治疗方面的评估具有挑战性。多数患者有比较复杂的用药史和就诊史，患者常常会说出很多药物的名称。因此，护士应仔细评估患者的用药史和有关药物的反应。

ii. Nursing Diagnosis

Nursing diagnoses targeting responses to somatization disorder include:

1. Anxiety Related to nervous and unpleasant body experience.

2. Ineffective Coping Related to narcissism personality and deficient knowledge.

3. Impaired Social Interaction Related to dependence psychology and avoidance behavior patterns.

（二）护理诊断

躯体形式障碍患者的护理诊断包括：

1. 焦虑 与紧张担心、不愉快的身体体验有关。

2. 个体应对无效 与自恋型性格与缺乏相关知识有关。

3. 社会交往障碍 与依赖心理、回避行为有关。

iii. Nursing Objectives

The following criteria may be used for measurement of outcomes in the care of the client with somatization disorder. The client:

1. Identifies stressors that cause anxiety level to rise. Verbalizes understanding of correlation between times of increased anxiety and onset of physical symptoms.

2. Demonstrates adaptive coping strategies. Effectively uses adaptive coping strategies during stressful situations without resorting to physical symptoms.

3. Demonstrates control over life situation by meeting needs in an assertive manner.

（三）护理目标

躯体形式障碍患者的护理目标包括：

1. 能认识目前存在的压力因素和焦虑水平；能认识不良情绪与躯体症状之间的关系。

2. 能显示出适应性的行为；能有效地应用应对技巧，避免用身体症状替代情绪问题。

3. 能与家庭成员建立亲密关系；能与他人建立信任关系。

iv. Planning and Implementing Nursing Interventions

Developing a positive nurse-client relationship is important in the care for client with Somatoform disorder Without the relationship, the nurse will be just one more provider who fails to meet the client's expectations. Developing a relationship will require time and patience. Therapeutic communication techniques should be used to redirect the client to psychosocial problems that are related to the physical manifestations.

（四）护理措施

建立信任的护患关系是护理躯体形式障碍患者的基础，如果护患缺乏信任，护士就没有办法理解患者的感受、满足患者的期待。建立信任的护患关系需要护士的耐心和时间，同时需要应用治疗性沟通技巧。

1. Biologic Interventions Several biologic interventions may be useful in caring for clients with somatization disorder. The biologic interventions as following: continuously monitor medical assessments, lab findings, and other reports to assure absence of organic

1. 生理方面 首先，护士要了解患者身体不适的症状表现，提供恰当的方法满足其情绪需要。其次，护士要与患者商议护理计划，包括减轻身体疼痛、不适的措施。帮助

illness. Recognize that physical symptoms are real to the client, and provide a means for meeting emotional needs. Establishing pain management program; it includes nonpharmacologic pain relief measures. Setting up daily routine for client. Helping the client establish a daily routine may help alleviate some of the clients with sleeping disturbance. Encouraging regular exercise. Regular exercise will improve their overall physical state. Administering medications. The nurse should monitor the response to medication. Monitor appropriate use of medical and occurrence of side effects. Monitoring nutritional intake. Emphasizing positive health care practice.

患者制订日常作息时间表，鼓励患者建立良好的作息习惯，减轻睡眠方面的问题。鼓励患者进行规律的锻炼，改善身体状况。注意患者的饮食，保证充足的营养摄入。同时，还要监测患者药物治疗的情况，包括药物的治疗效果和副作用。

2. Psychological Interventions Psychological interventions are key in helping a client with somatization disorder. Counseling with a focus on problem-solving is needed. These clients have chaotic lives and need support through the multitude of crises. The psychological interventions include:

2. 心理护理 心理护理是最重要的，因患者常存在一定的危机，需要护士的支持和帮助，所以心理护理的要点是帮助患者如何解决问题。具体措施包括：

(1) Establish an ongoing, trusting relationship with the client. The nurses concern with the client as an individual rather than symptoms allows formation of trust.

(2) Avoid focusing on the physical symptoms, disabilities, or impairment unless the client needs assistance. Because focusing on somatic complaints reinforces and interferes with relating them to psychological cause.

(3) Focus on problem-solving strategies. The nurse should assist the client to identify stressors and positive coping strategies and improve client's problem-solving and decision-making skills. Identifying stresses and strengthening positive coping responses will help the client deal with her chaotic life.

(4) Teach client about the relationship of mind and body, anxiety and stressor, and basic body function. It will increase client's awareness of link between physical symptoms and emotional stressors.

(5) Reinforce anxiety reduction strategies, the nurse should teach the client about the coping skills such as relaxation techniques. Teaching relaxation techniques may alleviate stress. The nurse should consider a variety of techniques including simple relaxation techniques, distraction, and guided imagery. It will provide reduction in anxiety and physical symptoms. If depress occurs, additional supportive or cognitive approaches may be needed.

（1）建立一个连续的、信任的护患关系，护士应把患者视为一个独立的人而非只是某些症状。

（2）尽量不要关注患者的躯体症状和无能为力的主诉，除非患者确实需要帮助。因为过分关注患者的躯体症状反而会强化患者的躯体不适。

（3）着重于解决患者的问题。护士应帮助患者认识其存在的压力，采用有效的应对方法，提高患者解决问题的能力。帮助患者认识生活中的应激以及学会积极应对 的方法，帮助患者耐受疾病带来的困扰。

（4）帮助患者了解认知、焦虑、压力和身体功能之间的关系，提高患者对身体症状和情绪之间关系的认识。如果患者存在抑郁，应注意加强支持性的心理护理。

（5）指导患者学习放松技术，如肌肉放松、精神想象放松等技术来减轻压力。帮助患者建立良好的生活方式和习惯，弱化疾病的影响。

3. Social Interventions These individuals respond to group interventions. Even though they are not candidates for insight group psychotherapy, they

3. 社会功能 在集体活动中，帮助患者学习和应用解决问题的技巧与方法，并要关注他人的反应。躯体形式障碍集体治疗小组

do benefit from problem-solving groups that focus on developing coping skills for everyday life. Because most of the clients are women, participation in groups that address feminist issues should be encouraged to strengthen their assertiveness skills and improve their generally low self-esteem. Social interventions include involving in problem-solving groups, assisting with developing skills for everyday life, encouraging use of resources for support and information, and promoting social interaction outside the home.

中以女性为主，在集体活动中，她们可以分享信息，相互鼓励，有助于提高自尊。采用的干预措施包括：① 以解决问题为主要目的的集体活动；② 帮助患者发展自我照顾能力；③ 鼓励患者利用有关资源，包括支持和信息；④ 鼓励患者参与户外活动，促进患者的社会交往。

v. Evaluation

Reassessment is conducted to determine if the nursing actions have been successful in achieving the objects of care. Evaluation of the nursing actions for the client with somatization disorder may be facilitated by gathering information using the following types of questions:

1. Can the client recognize signs and symptoms of escalating anxiety?

2. Can the client intervene with adaptive coping strategies to interrupt the escalating anxiety before physical symptoms are exacerbated?

3. Can the client verbalize an understanding of the correlation between physical symptoms and times of escalating anxiety?

4. Does the client have a plan for dealing with increased stress to prevent exacerbation of physical symptoms?

5. Can the client demonstrate assertiveness skills?

6. Does the client exercise control over life situation by participating in the decision-making process?

7. Can the client verbalize resources outside the hospital from which he or she may seek assistance during times of extreme stress?

（五）护理评价

判断护理措施是否有效，是否达到预定的护理目标，可通过询问下列一些问题来帮助护士评价护理效果：① 患者是否能够认识到焦虑水平增加时的症状？② 患者是否能在躯体症状加重之前采取恰当的应对策略，来防止焦虑加重？③ 患者是否能够认识焦虑增加与躯体症状之间的关系？④ 患者是否有计划地应对生活中的压力以防止躯体症状加重？⑤ 患者是否能显示出积极的应对技巧？⑥ 患者是否能积极参与学习如何应对自己生活中困境的训练？⑦ 当患者处于困境时，是否能够利用医院以外的资源来寻求帮助？

Section 5 Nursing Management for Clients with Dissociative Disorder

第五节　分离性障碍患者的护理

The term of hysteria is still used in *CCMD-3* instead of the dissociative (conversion) disorder of the *ICD-10*. The dissociative symptoms are a group of psychiatric syndromes characterized by partial or complete disruption of some aspect of consciousness, identity, memory, motor behavior, or awareness of the environment. Conversion symptoms are referred as the unpleasant affect caused by stresses and conflicts that the individual cannot

在*ICD-10*中，癔症（*CCMD-3*仍沿用）的概念已被废弃，取而代之的是分离（转换）性障碍。分离症状系指过去经历与当今环境、记忆、运动行为和自我身份的认知完全或部分不相符合。转换症状则指由精神刺激引起情绪反应，接着出现躯体症状，一旦躯体症状出现，情绪反应便褪色或消失，这时的躯体症状便称为转换症状，转换症状无法用躯

resolve that is somatazied transformed into physical symptoms. Conversion symptoms cannot be explained by any physical disorder or known pathophysiological mechanism.

体障碍或已知的病理生理机制来解释，其确诊必须排除器质性病变。

It is no longer used in *DSM-V*, which categorizes various features of hysteria under dissociative disorders and somatoform disorders. The *DSM-V* (2015), published by the American Psychiatric Association, lists five dissociative disorders (dissociative identity disorder, dissociative amnesia, depersonalization/derealization disorder, other specified dissociative disorder, unspecified dissociative disorder).

DSM-V 中也不再使用癔症一词，而用分离性障碍和躯体形式障碍的名称。由美国精神病学会 2015 年出版的 *DSM-V* 列出了五种分离性障碍，即分离性身份识别障碍、分离性遗忘、人格解体障碍、其他特定的分离性障碍和未特定的分离性障碍。

BOX 10-2 Learning More

Historical Aspects of Hysteria

Hysteria is one of the oldest diagnostic terminologies in psychiatry, and has been recorded as early as 1900 BC in Egypt. It was believed to result from the "wandering uterus" moving from its normal anatomical position into various other parts of the body.

There was a great deal of interest in the dissociative processes during the nineteenth century, when the concept of dissociation was first formulated by the French physician, Pierre Janet. He used it to explain the myriad bizarre symptoms of hysteria, which he described as "a form of mental disintegration characterized by a tendency toward the permanent and complete undoubling of consciousness". By the late nineteenth century, conversion symptoms had become a legitimate focus of medical and scientific investigation. Charcot suggested that a degeneration of the nervous system was the underlying cause of hysteria.

Now in the West the contemporary practice is to refer to Dissociative and Somatoform Disorders, rather than "hysteria", because "hysteria" is perceived as a "negative" quality that might reflect personal failure or unreasonable behavior rather than a clinical/medical diagnosis.

BOX 10-2 知识拓展

癔症概念的历史演变

癔症是精神病学诊断术语中最为古老的病名之一。本症在公元前 1900 年埃及即有记载。当时认为本病是子宫在妇女体内游走所致。

十九世纪以来，法国医生 Pierre Janet 首次采用“分离”这一概念来解释癔症的种种表现，引起了人们对“分离”现象的广泛兴趣。Pierre 认为“分离”的本质是人意识的彻底瓦解。同时期对转换症状的研究甚多，例如 Charcot 认为在诱发因素的作用下，个体神经系统的器质性缺陷导致转换症状。

目前，西方趋向于使用“解离性障碍”和“躯体形式障碍”，而不再使用“癔症”这一诊断名词。原因是“癔症”一词在西方语言中常用于描述个体失败或无理行为的贬义词，而非临床或医学诊断术语。

In China, according to the epidemiological statistics in 1980s, the prevalence rate of the dissociative (conversion) disorder was about 3.55‰ in general population. Hysteria may begin at any age, but is most likely to make its first appearance in adolescence or young adults. The morbidity rates in different age groups are: before the age of 20, 14%; age 20-30 years, 49%; age 31-40, 37%; age 41 or older, quite rare. It appears to be more common in women than in men with the ratio of 8:1. The morbidity rate among the illiterate and lower educational level population is much higher than

国内 20 世纪 80 年代的流行病学调查资料中，本病在普通人群中的患病率约 3.55‰。各地的调查均证实：① 年轻人的患病率显著高于年长者。首次发病年龄在 20 岁以前者占 14%，20～30 岁者占 49%，31～40 岁者占 37%，41 岁及以上初发者少见。② 女性患病率明显高于男性，女性与男性之比约为 8∶1。③ 文盲及文化程度低的人群患病率显著高于高文化人群。④ 农村患病率（5‰）明显高于城市

that of high education. Furthermore, the morbidity in rural area (5‰) is higher than that in the city with the morbidity rate of 2.09‰. There may be only one episode, or episodes may recur over a lifetime. Therefore, the onset of the dissociative (conversion) disorder is influenced by the factors of geography, gender, age, social culture and economy.

(2.09‰)。⑤ 疾病可仅发作 1 次，或终身反复发作。由此可见，本病的发病受城乡、性别、年龄和社会文化经济因素等各方面的影响。

I. Etiology

一、病　因

1. Genetics The Ljungberg study indicated that the dissociative (conversion) disorder is more common in first-degree relatives of people with the disorder than in the general population. The morbidity is 2.4% in men and 6.4% in women. The disorder is often seen in more than one generation of a family.

1. 遗传因素 Ljungberg 的研究证实一级亲属发病率为男性 2.4%，女性 6.4%，明显高于一般人群的患病率。分离（转换）性障碍常在一个家庭中的几代人中发生，说明其发病与遗传有关。

2. Psychological Trauma A growing body of evidence points to the etiology of the dissociative (conversion) disorder as a set of traumatic experiences that overwhelm the individual's capacity to cope by any means other than dissociation. These experiences usually take the form of severe physical, sexual, or psychological abuse by a parent or significant other in the child's life. Hysterical identify disorder is thought to serve as a survival strategy for the child in this traumatic environment, enabling him/her to create a new personality or self that is capable of dealing with the trauma without being overwhelmed and allowing the primary self to escape any awareness of the trauma. Kluft (1984) suggests that the number of an individual's alternate personalities is related to the number of different types of abuse he or she suffered as a child.

2. 心理创伤 越来越多的研究证实，童年时期的创伤经历，如遭受躯体或性摧残、精神虐待等，是后来发病的重要原因。分离性身份识别障碍的发生被认为是儿童在这种创伤环境中的一种生存策略。他（她）所产生的新的身份能够面对现实中巨大的痛苦和创伤，而其原本的身份则可逃避这种痛苦。Kluft（1984）认为一个人出现的多重人格也与其在童年时期所经历的摧残和虐待有关。

3. Neurobiological Factors Some clinicians have suggested a possible correlation between neurological alterations and hysterical disorders. Although available information is inadequate, it is possible that hysterical amnesia and hysterical fugue may be related to alterations in the ascending reticular activating system and thalamocortical projections. Some studies have suggested a possible link between hysterical identity disorder and certain neurological conditions, including temporal lobe epilepsy, severe migraine headaches, cerebral cortical damage, and visual alterations. Electroencephalographic abnormalities have been observed in some clients with hysteria. However, it has not been determined that these abnormalities are causative or the result of the behaviors in questions; nor has it yet been determined to what degree there exists some correlation between such abnormalities and "hysterical" disorders.

3. 神经生物因素 有学者认为分离（转换）性障碍的发生与某些神经系统异常有关。例如分离性遗忘患者与其上行网状激活系统和丘脑皮层的异常放射有关；分离性身份识别障碍与神经系统的异常有关，如患者常伴有癫痫、严重的偏头痛、大脑皮质的损伤以及视觉改变等；有些患者可见脑电图的异常。然而，尚不能证明这些异常是导致分离性障碍的原因还是后果，也无法说明这些异常与分离性障碍存在多大程度的关联。

4. Psychodynamic Theory Freud (1962) believed that dissociative behaviors occurred when

4. 精神动力理论 Freud（1962）认为当个体有意识地压抑其痛苦时，心理就会发生分

individuals repressed distressing mental content from conscious awareness. He believed that the unconscious was a dynamic entity in which repressed mental content was kept unavailable to conscious recall. Some current psychodynamic explanations of dissociation reflect Freud's concepts- behaviors such as amnesia, fugue, and depersonalization are defenses against unresolved and painful issues. The emotional pain and associated anxiety are repressed and the individual is incapable of recall; or, in the case of depersonalization, pain and anxiety expressed as feelings of unreality or detachment from the environment of the painful situation.

离反应，被压抑的心理内容储存在潜意识中，且不能被重新唤回至意识。现代精神动力学对分离的解释就是基于Freud的这一观点，即一些行为如失忆、神游及人格解体行为是对不能解决的痛苦的一种防御。情感上的痛苦和与之相关的焦虑被压抑，并且个体没有唤醒的能力，或在人格解体的情况下，就表现为不现实或与痛苦的状态相分离的情感。

II. Clinical Manifestation

二、临床表现

The onset is generally in adolescence and early adulthood, and is often rapid. A number of psychosocial factors are believed to predispose to the development of the dissociative (conversion) disorder. The clinical manifestations of each sub-type of the dissociative (conversion) disorder are presented as the following:

本病多起病于青年期，起病急骤，在起病前多有心理社会因素。现将各型临床表现分述如下：

i. Dissociative Disorders

（一）分离性障碍

1. Dissociative Amnesia The onset of dissociative amnesia is normally rapid, and is an inability to recall important personal information, usually of a traumatic or stressful nature, that is too extensive to be explained by ordinary forgetfulness and is not due to the direct effects of substance use or general medical condition. The client with amnesia usually appears alert and may give no indication to observers that anything is wrong, although at the onset of the episode there may be a brief period of disorganization. Onset of an amnesic episode usually follows severe psychosocial stress. The inability to recall all incidents associated with the life event for a specific time period following the event (usually a few hours to a few days) is called "localized amnesia" or "selective amnesia". Generalized amnesia is a more unusual phenomenon and is characterized by the inability to recall anything that has happened during the client's entire lifetime, including his or her name, age, and other significant information.

1. 分离性遗忘 多急性发病，患者突然对自己经历的重大事件失去记忆，通常是一个创伤或压力事件，这种失忆很难用一般的忘记、应用某些物质或疾病来解释。患者往往很清醒，很难让人发现他有什么问题，且被遗忘的事件往往与精神创伤有关。患者的记忆缺失并非器质性损害引起。如果只对生活事件中某一段时期内（常常为几个小时到几天）发生的事件不能回忆，称为局限性和选择性遗忘。若对全部生活已经失去记忆，甚至包括自己的姓名、年龄等，称为广泛性遗忘。

2. Dissociative Fugue The hysterical fugue is characterized by sudden, unexpected travel away from home or customary place of daily activities-and an inability to recall some or all of one's past. An individual in a fugue state cannot recall personal identity and often assumes a new identity. He or she does not appear to be behaving in any way out of the ordinary. He or she can assume responsibility for simple self-care, including eating, drinking, and personal hygiene. Contacts with

2. 分离性漫游 表现为患者突然从家中或工作场所出走，外出漫游，所去地点可能是以往熟悉的地方，或是对患者有意义的场所。患者常常不能回忆起自己的身份，而赋予自己一个全新的身份。此时患者仍能保持基本的日常生活能力（如饮食起居等），并能进行简单的社会交往（如购票、乘车等）。患者的新身份可能是简单或不完整的，也可能

other people are minimal and simple, such as buying ticket or taking bus. The assumed identity may be simple and incomplete or complex and elaborate. If a complex identity is established, the individual engages in intricate interpersonal and occupational activities and is often more socially gregarious and uninhibited than was his or her previous style. The duration of such fugue states is usually brief-hours or days, and rarely months- and recovery is rapid and complete. If the client later regains his or her memory, he or she remembers nothing of what happened while he or she was in the fugue state.

是复杂而精细的。如果患者的新身份是复杂的，则可以从事复杂的社交和职业，并且常常比以前的身份更善于交际和放荡不羁。此种漫游事先无任何目的和构想，突然开始，历时数小时至数天后，又突然结束，清醒后患者对发病经历不能完全回忆。

3. Dissociative Identity Disorder Dissociative identity disorder is also called double or multiple personality disorder. It is characterized by a division of the person's identity into two or more distinct personalities, each clearly defined and different from the others. Each personality is unique and is complete with its own memory, behavior, preferences, and social relationships that surface during the dominant interval. Only one of the personalities is evident at any given moment and exercises control over behavior when that personality is manifest. One of them is dominant most of the time over the course of the disorder. The transition from one personality to another is usually sudden, often dramatic, and usually precipitated by stress. Individuals with this disorder may suddenly "wake up" in unfamiliar situations with no idea where they are, how they got there, or who the people around them are. They may frequently be accused of lying when they deny remembering of being responsible for events or actions that occurred while another personality controlled the body. Cases in which only two personalities emerge are referred to as double personality disorder, while cases with more than two personalities are referred to as multiple personality disorder.

3. 分离性身份识别障碍 又称双重或多重人格障碍，主要表现为患者突然分裂为两种或多种人格，各种人格各自独立，互不相同，各有其记忆、行为和爱好，并且有其以不同人格出现时所建立的不同的社会关系。在某段时间仅有一种人格特征表现突出，并在那段时间内完全控制其行为。在整个发病过程中常有一种人格占主导。从一种人格转为另外一种人格往往很突然，且常与压力有关。患者也许会突然在一个陌生的地方清醒，且不知身处何地，如何到这个地方，甚至周围的人也不认识。此时，他们常常因为无法回忆起以另外一种身份控制自己时发生的事情，否认所应承担的责任而受到他人的谴责。以两种人格交替出现者称双重人格，多种人格交替出现者称多重人格。

4. Dissociative Stupor Dissociative stupor is characterized by a long period of stupor. The client can maintain a fixed position without any response to outside stimuli. The onset always follows intense psychosocial stress, and duration is usually only a few minutes to an hour.

4. 分离性木僵 精神创伤后出现较深的意识障碍，可在相当长的一段时间内维持某一固定的姿势，没有言语和随意动作。对外界刺激可没有反应。通常数十分钟后即自行缓解。

5. Dissociative Possession Disorders Dissociative possession disorders are characterized by a perception of the self as being possessed by a deity or a spirit of the dead. This perception may extend to be delusion that the person and his/her body are fully controlled by this spirit or deity. Hysterical possession disorders are often found in combination with increased levels of suggestibility and autosuggestion, and with double and multiple personality disorders.

5. 出神与附体 表现为患者以神鬼、灵魂附体，以死人的口气说话，取代了自己的身份，可达到妄想程度。它常伴有情感爆发、哭笑无常、暗示性明显增高。

ii. Conversion Disorders

Conversion disorders are included under the category of somatoform disorders in *DSM-V*. These include a wide range of physical dysfunctions with no organic bases. The client becomes paralyzed, blind, or deaf, or loses sensation in some part of the body. The symptoms are not under voluntary control and cannot be explained by any physical disorder or known pathophysiological mechanism. Rather, symptoms appear to express psychological conflict. Three types of hysterical somatic disorders are discussed in *CCMD-3*. They are motor disorders, convulsions, and sensory disorders.

1. Motor Disorders The client with motor disorders exhibits somatic akinesia, such as paralysis of limbs and abasia (impaired coordination in walking). There should be no evidence of neurological, anatomical, physiological, or other organic bases for somatic akinesia.

2. Convulsions The characteristic feature of hysterical convulsions is a sudden and unexpected seizure that appears similar to epileptic seizures. The client falls down slowly with body ankylosis (the stiffening and immobility of a joint), tetania (hyperactivity of nerves and muscles), and is unresponsive to shouted commands. But, the client does not demonstrate tongue-biting, serious bruising due to falling, incontinence, or loss of consciousness associated with epileptic seizures. The duration is usually several ten minutes.

3. Sensory Disorders Sensory disorder is also called hysterical anaesthesia or hysterical sensory loss. The client with this disorder demonstrates physical sensory disorders, such as aphonia, deafness, blindness, and partial or complete loss of sensation in specific places on the skin or on the entire body. But, it has no evidence of neurological, anatomical, or physiological bases, basis, and no evidence of organic diseases.

III. Treatment

In the absence of neurological or anatomical causes of symptoms, and because there is no underlying disease process that has caused symptoms, treatment for the dissociative (conversion) disorder focuses on psychotherapy, which may include systematic desensitization and hypnotherapy. In addition, pharmacotherapy and physical therapy may assist in the treatment for client with the dissociative (conversion) disorder.

1. Psychotherapy Because the symptoms

（二）转换性障碍

转换性障碍在DSM-V中被划分为躯体形式障碍，主要指无器质性损害的躯体功能障碍，患者常表现为偏瘫、失明、失聪或身体某部位失去感觉，这些症状并非自己可以控制，且无法用躯体疾病或已知的病理生理机制来解释，相反，却与患者的心理冲突密切相关。

1. 运动障碍 表现为躯体运动障碍，例如肢体瘫痪、站立或行走不能。瘫痪者以单瘫或双下肢瘫痪多见，该类瘫痪不符合神经分布特点。且患者没有可证实的器质性疾病会导致此类瘫痪。

2. 抽搐发作 常在受到精神刺激或暗示时突然发生，与癫痫发作相似，表现为缓慢倒地，全身僵直或肢体抖动，呼之不应，无意识丧失，咬舌、严重摔伤或小便失禁，一般持续数十分钟。

3. 感觉障碍 表现为感觉麻木和感觉丧失，患者可出现各种各样的躯体感觉障碍，如失声、耳聋、失明等感官功能障碍，皮肤或整个躯体部分或全部感觉缺失或异常，但却没有可查证的神经、解剖、生理改变以及器质性疾病。

三、治　疗

分离（转换）性障碍患者并无神经、解剖病变，也无器质性疾病，因此，应以心理治疗为主，合并药物治疗和物理疗法。

1. 心理治疗 主要包括系统脱敏疗法和

demonstrated in the dissociative (conversion) disorder are functional (serve an emotional purpose, e.g. limiting or eliminating a spouse's request for sexual activity or reducing the demands for academic performance), treatment focuses on psychotherapeutic interventions. Therapy may include: systematic desensitization, and hypnotherapy. The dissociative (conversion) disorder client often experiences a wide range of concerns; he/she often believes that he/she is suffering from a serious physical disease or a major psychiatric disorder. The client's family members are experiencing the stress of the client's on-going emotional condition. Therefore, nursing care and the rapport established by the nurse with the client and his/her family enhances the effectiveness of psychotherapy.

催眠疗法，催眠疗法应在合适的临床环境中进行。癔症患者常深信自己患有严重疾病或可怕的精神病，所以顾虑重重。亲属的紧张，常可使患者病情恶化。故护士应关心、同情患者，建立良好的护患关系，取得患者和亲属的信赖，以利于心理治疗的成功。

2. Pharmacotherapy Clients with the dissociative (conversion) disorder may experience a wide range of symptoms, including anxiety, depression, insomnia, and dysphoria, each of which enhances the client's perception of the seriousness of his disorder and, therefore, exacerbates the dissociative (conversion) disorder. Pharmacological interventions can be used to limit the course and severity of symptoms. The client with hysterical disorders always has anxiety, depression, debility and insomnia, which are the basis of self-suggestion caused onset of the dissociative (conversion) disorder. Therefore, using necessary drugs to effectively control theses symptoms is benefit for preventing the onset of the dissociative (conversion) disorder. For example, a small dosage of ataractic can be used for the client with acute emotional and behavioral disorders.

2. 药物治疗 患者常常伴有焦虑、抑郁、衰弱、失眠等症状，且这些症状往往是疾病发生的自我暗示的基础。因此，使用相应的药物有效地控制这些症状，对治疗和预防本病的发作是有益的。如对急性情绪或行为障碍的患者，可给予小剂量镇静药物治疗。

3. Other Treatments Other treatments include Chinese Traditional Medicine, acupuncture and electric acupuncture, especially in the treatment of client with hysterical motor disorder.

3. 其他治疗 中医、中药及针灸或电针等治疗，在患者易接受暗示的基础上，尤其分离性肢体瘫痪患者，可获得较好的疗效。

IV. Application of the Nursing Process

四、护理程序的应用

i. Nursing Assessment

1. Biologic Assessment Assessment should include the client's present and past physical history, disturbances in appetite and nutritional statues, sleep patterns and disturbances, gastrointestinal functioning, and the client's ability to maintain ordinary daily activities. All changes in client functioning should be fully documented in the client records.

（一）护理评估

1. 生理评估 全面评估患者的健康史与既往病史，患者的食欲及营养状况、睡眠情况、饮食情况、大小便情况以及每天的活动等。详细记录患者身体功能状况的改变。

2. Psychological Assessment A full psychological assessment should be a part of the client's nursing record and should include an account of pre-

2. 心理评估 对患者进行全面的心理评估并详细记录，主要包括患者的心理功能、所存在心理问题的既往史，如各种分离性障

morbid psychological functioning, and past history of psychological problems, including occurrences of hysterical disorders. The nurse should carefully question and document significant psychosocial stressors immediately prior to the onset of the present disorder and at earlier stages in the client's life. Psychological assessment should also include any history of psychological disorders among members of the client's family.

碍发生的情况等。护士应认真询问和记录与患者疾病发作有关的心理社会压力事件，或患者早期成长过程中曾出现过的一些生活压力事件。此外，心理评估还应包括患者亲属的心理障碍既往史。

3. Social Assessment The client's ethnic/cultural and educational background should also be examined and noted in the record. The nurse should be familiar with the client's levels of functioning in the family and the community before and after the onset of symptoms, as well as with quality and level of client interaction with family and friends before and after the onset of the present problem. The client's occupational and educational histories and the client's spiritual beliefs and practices should also be questioned and documented.

3. 社会评估 详细评估和记录患者的种族、文化和教育背景，了解患者发病前后在家庭或社区等环境中的社会功能状况如何，以及患者在社会环境中与家人和朋友的交往能力和水平如何。同时，还应了解和记录患者的职业和教育状况以及精神信仰等。

ii. Nursing Diagnoses

（二）护理诊断

Some common symptoms to be noted in the diagnosis of hysteria include:

1. Altered thought processes related to severe psychological stress and repression of anxiety, evidenced by loss of memory.

1. 思维混乱 与患者由于记忆缺失，而致严重的心理压力和极度焦虑有关。

2. Ineffective individual coping styles related to unresolved painful issues and repressed severe anxiety, evidenced by sudden travel away from home with inability to recall previous identity.

2. 个人应对无效 与突然离家并无法回忆从前的身份，而导致痛苦与严重的焦虑有关。

3. Personality identity disturbance related to childhood trauma/abuse evidenced by the presence of more than one personality within the individual.

3. 人格识别障碍 与儿时的创伤或虐待等导致个体目前存在多种人格有关。

4. Risk for violence directed toward others related to fear of unknown circumstances surrounding emergence from fugue state.

4. 受伤的危险 与漫游状态，对周围陌生环境恐惧有关。

5. Sensory-perceptual alteration related to repressed severe anxiety, evidenced by loss or alteration in physical function, without evidence of organic pathology.

5. 感知改变 与极度焦虑导致躯体功能丧失或改变有关，但无器质性改变。

iii. Nursing Outcome

（三）护理目标

The objectives of nursing interventions include:

1. The client will recover deficits in memory and develop more adaptive coping mechanisms to deal with stress.

1. 患者能够恢复记忆，并发展更多的适应性应对措施来解决其心理压力和焦虑。

2. The client will demonstrate more adaptive ways of coping in stressful situations than resorting to dissociation.

2. 患者在压力环境下能运用恰当的应对方法，而没有出现分离症状。

3. The client will verbalize understanding about the existence of multiple personalities within the self, the reason for their existence, and the importance of eventual integration of the personalities.

3. 患者能够表述自身存在多种人格，并知道存在多种人格的原因，以及最终要使其人格统一的重要性。

4. The client will not harm self or others.

4. 患者将不会伤害自己和他人。

5. The client will demonstrate recovery of lost or

5. 患者丧失和改变的躯体功能将得以恢复。

altered function.

iv. Nursing Interventions

1. Biologic Interventions Monitor physician's ongoing assessments, laboratory reports, and other data to ensure that possibility of organic pathology is clearly ruled out. Failure to do so may jeopardize client safety; identify primary or secondary gains that the physical symptoms are providing for the client, such as increased dependency, attention, and protection from experiencing a stressful event. These are considered to be etiological factors and will be used to assist in problem resolution. Do not focus on the disability, and encourage client to be as independent as possible. Intervene only when client requires assistance. Positive reinforcement would encourage continued use of the maladaptive response for secondary gains, such as dependency. Help identify physical symptoms as a coping mechanism that is used in times of extreme stress.

2. Psychological Interventions Encourage client to discuss situations that have been especially stressful and to explore the feelings associated with those times. Verbalization of feelings in a non-threatening environment may help the client come to terms with unresolved issues that may contribute to the dissociative process. As anxiety levels decrease and memory returns, use exploration and an accepting, non-threatening environment to encourage client to identify repressed traumatic experiences that contribute to chronic anxiety. Client must confront and deal with painful issues to achieve resolution. Identify specific conflicts that remain unresolved, and assist client in identifying possible solutions. Unless these underlying conflicts are resolved, any improvement in coping behaviors must be viewed as only temporary. Provide instruction regarding more adaptive ways to respond to anxiety so that dissociative behaviors are no longer needed. Identify specific conflicts that remain unresolved, and assist client in identifying possible solutions.

3. Safety Interventions Reassure client of safety and security through your presence. Once recognized. Dissociative behaviors may be frightening to the client. Use nursing interventions necessary to deal with maladaptive behaviors associated with individual sub-personalities. For example, if one personality is suicidal, precautions must be taken to guard against client's self-harm. If another personality has a tendency toward physical hostility, precautions must be taken to protect others. The safety of client and others is a nursing priority. Administer tranquilizing medication as ordered by physician. Monitor medication for its effectiveness and for any adverse side effects. If the client is not calmed by "talking down"

（四）护理措施

1. 生理方面 护士要随时了解医生对患者所进行的各项检查、患者的实验室报告及其他资料，以确定和排除患者是否存在器质性病理改变。否则，一方面可能使患者的安全受到威胁，另一方面不能正确理解当患者经历压力事件时所出现的躯体症状。护士不应把注意力只放在患者某一躯体功能丧失的方面，而应鼓励患者尽可能自立，只是在患者需要协助时提供帮助。如果护士对患者过于关注，将使患者的依赖性增加。帮助患者认识到其出现的躯体症状是在极度压力下机体做出的应对反应。

2. 心理护理 护士应鼓励患者说出自己感到压力最大时的情景及当时的感受。在与患者谈论其感受时，应注意尽量在一个安静的没有任何恐吓的环境下进行，这有助于患者谈出导致其出现解离症状的原因。同时，帮助患者认识到在严重压力的情况下，其具有的不平衡的感觉是可以存在和接受的，别人在同样情景下，也许会出现相同的行为，这有助于保护患者的自尊。另外，护士应注意确认患者仍存在的一些未被解决的特殊冲突，并协助患者寻求可能的应对方法。

3. 安全护理 患者发生分离性身份识别障碍时，护士应采用不同的应对方法来保证患者和他人的安全。例如，对于具有自杀人格的患者，护士必须采取适当的防范措施，避免患者进行自我伤害。而对于具有伤害他人倾向人格的患者，护士首先要做的是保证患者和他人的安全。护士可遵医嘱给患者镇静剂，注意观察药物的作用和副作用。如果患者在用药后仍不能平静，必要时可给予保护性约束。当患者的狂躁和兴奋减低时，逐步为患者解除约束，并观察和评价患者的反

or by medication, use of mechanical restraints may be necessary. Be sure to have sufficient staff available to assist. Observe client in restraints every 15 minutes. Ensure that circulation is not compromised by checking temperature, color, and pulse. Assist client with needs related to nutrition, hydration, and elimination. Position client so that comfort is facilitated and aspiration can be prevented. As agitation decreases, assess client's readiness for restraint removal or reduction. Remove one restraint at a time, while assessing client's response.

应，从而使对患者和医护人员的伤害减少到最低。

4. Social Interventions Identify community resources to which the individual may go for support if past maladaptive coping patterns return.

4. 社会功能 护士应注意协助患者认识和选择有效的社区资源，尤其当患者出院后，在压力存在时又选择了不适当的应对方式，如何寻求社区服务。

v. Evaluation

Reassessment is conducted in order to determine if the nursing actions have been successful in achieving the objectives of care. Gathering information using the following types of questions may facilitate evaluation of the nursing actions for the client with a dissociative-conversion disorder:

1. Has the client's memory been restored?

2. Can the client connect occurrence of psychological stress to loss of memory?

3. Does the client discuss fears and anxieties with members of the staff in an effort toward resolution?

4. Can the client recognize and discuss the presence of various personalities within the self?

5. Can he or she verbalize why these personalities exist?

6. Can the client verbalize situations that precipitate transition from one personality to another?

7. Can the client maintain a sense of reality during stressful situations?

8. Can the client demonstrate more adaptive coping strategies for dealing with stress without resorting to dissociation?

9. Does the client demonstrate full recovery from previous loss or alteration of physical function?

(Chen Juan Zhao Wei)

（五）护理评价

对患者的重新评价可以帮助护士确认所采取的护理措施是否对达到护理目标有效。在对分离（转换）性障碍患者进行护理评价时，护士常常通过如下问题来获得对有关护理措施实施效果的信息，从而判定患者的护理效果：① 患者的记忆是否恢复了？② 患者是否能将其经历的心理压力的事件与记忆丢失联系起来？③ 患者是否与医护人员讨论其恐惧和焦虑，以寻找解决的办法？④ 患者是否能够和护士讨论其存在的不同人格？⑤ 他（她）是否能口述为什么会存在这些人格？⑥ 患者是否能口述其突然从一种人格转变为另外一种人格的情形？⑦ 患者是否能在压力情形下保持一种真实的感觉？⑧ 患者能否采取适当的应对技巧来解决压力，而不是转变人格。⑨患者以前丧失的机体功能是否完全恢复？

（陈　娟　赵　伟）

Key Points

1. Neurosis is a group of mental disorders, without any demonstrable organic basis, usually onset after psychosocial factors and last for a long time. The main manifestations are anxiety, depression, phobia, obsession-compulsion, hypochondriasis, somatic systems, or

内容摘要

1. 神经症是一组精神障碍的总称，起病常与社会心理因素有关，症状主要表现为焦虑、抑郁、恐惧、强迫、疑病症状、各种躯体不适感等，症状没有任何可证实的器质性病变，与患者的现实处境不相称，但患者的疾

neurasthenic symptoms, which are disproportional to the client's actual situation. The clients have insight of the illness, but feels affliction and no significance.

2. Anxiety is considered abnormal or pathological if: the response is greatly disproportionate to the risk and severity of the danger or threat; the response continues beyond the existence of a potential danger or threat; intellectual, social, or occupational functioning is impaired; the individual suffers from a psychosomatic effect (e.g., colitis or dermatitis).

3. Panic disorder refers to recurrent unexpected panic attacks. In panic disorder, people experience panic in situations that do not pose any real danger or alter the person's general behavior. The major mental symptoms are extreme fear and a sense of impending death and doom; feelings of going crazy or losing control and desperation are common. The frequency with which clients with panic disorder experience panic attacks varies from multiple attacks during a single day to only a few attacks during the course of a year.

4. Generalized anxiety disorder is defined as a kind of anxiety disorder predominated by breathlessness with anxiety and nervousness which are not restricted to clear objects and concrete content, and accompanied by autonomic symptoms, muscular tension, and motor intranquility. The symptoms of this type of anxiety fall within two broad categories: apprehensive expectation and worry, and physical symptoms.

5. Phobic anxiety disorders are a type of neurosis predominated by excessive, unreasonable panic over external objects or situations; the clients are fully aware of unnecessary but cannot prevent panic attacks. Phobias are categorized as specific phobia, social phobia, and agoraphobia.

6. Obsessive-compulsive disorder (OCD) is a type of neurosis predominated by obsessions and compulsions symptoms. The feature of OCD is coexistence of conscious self-obsession and anti-obsession, the sharp conflicts of the two give clients anxiety and affliction. Obsessions are defined as unwanted, intrusive, persistent ideas, thoughts, impulses, or images that cause marked anxiety or distress. Compulsions denote unwanted repetitive behavior patterns or mental acts (e.g., praying, counting, repeating words silently) that are intended to reduce anxiety, not to provide pleasure or gratification.

7. The treatment of phobic anxiety disorders and other anxiety disorders includes cognitive-behavior therapy, expose therapy, systematic desensitization, relaxation training, and group therapy. Psychotherapy applied

病痛苦感明显并对此感到无能为力，病程大多持续迁延。

2. 正常的焦虑和病理性的焦虑的区别在于：① 情绪反应的强度与实际危险是不相称的，大大地超过实际的危险或威胁；② 持续的焦虑反应，远远超过其可能的或潜在的威胁或威胁；③ 智力的、社会的或职业的功能常常有受损或削弱；④ 个体身心受到影响（如肠炎、皮炎等）。

3. 惊恐障碍的基本特征是严重焦虑的反复发作，具有不可预测性，惊恐障碍患者发生惊恐时所处的场景并非能构成真正的威胁或改变个体的行为。患者惊恐发作时常突然感到一种突如其来的恐惧体验，觉得死亡将至，并伴有濒死感或失控感，以及绝望感。惊恐发作的频率可一日发作多次或一年仅发作几次。

4. 广泛性焦虑障碍又称慢性焦虑症，其特征是对没有明确的客观对象和固定内容的过分担心、紧张不安等，常伴随自主神经功能紊乱症状、肌肉紧张、运动性不安等。其临床症状主要包括两大类：焦虑性期待与担心，躯体症状。

5. 恐惧性焦虑障碍是指患者对某种客观事物或情境产生异乎寻常的恐惧和紧张，患者明知这种恐惧反应是过分的或不合理的，但难以控制。恐惧性焦虑障碍包括特殊恐惧障碍、社交恐惧障碍和广场恐惧障碍。

6. 强迫性障碍是以强迫观念和强迫行为为主要表现的一种神经症，其特点是有意识的自我强迫和反强迫并存，二者的强烈冲突使患者感到焦虑和痛苦。强迫观念是指违背自己意志，反复出现的思维、联想、冲动或意念，使个体感到焦虑和痛苦。强迫行为是指为了减轻焦虑而出现的违背自己意志、不能提供愉悦和满足、反复出现的行为模式或思想行为，如祈祷、计数、复述等。

7. 焦虑障碍的心理干预方法包括认知行为治疗、暴露疗法、系统脱敏疗法、放松训练、团体治疗等，而强迫性障碍的心理干预方法则包括暴露疗法、反应预防技术、思想停止

to OCD may include exposure techniques, response prevention, thought stopping, cognitive restructuring, and family therapy.

8. The person with somatization disorder has physical symptoms that may be vague, dramatized, or exaggerated in their presentation. No evidence of organic pathology can be identified.

9. Hypochondriasis is an unrealistic preoccupation with fear of having a serious illness. This disorder may follow a personal experience, or the experience of a close family member, with serious or life-threatening illness.

10. Various modalities have been implemented in the treatment of somatization disorder and hypochondriasis. It is same to the treatment of anxiety disorder. Nurses can assist client with these disorders by helping them to understand their problem and identify and establish new, more adaptive behavior patterns.

11. The term hysteria is still used in *CCMD-3* instead of the dissociative (conversion) disorder used in *ICD-10*. Hysteria is a group of mental disorders associated with some traits of hysterical personality. Onset is generally associated with increases in psychosocial stressors. The main manifestations are dissociative and/or conversion (somatoform) symptoms.

12. The treatment for the dissociative (conversion) disorder is focused on psychotherapy, as the signs and symptoms of each type of the dissociative (conversion) disorder are functional.

13. Nurses can assist clients with the dissociative (conversion) disorder by helping them to understand their problem and identify and establish new, more adaptive behavior patterns.

Exercises

(Questions 1 to 2 share the same question stem)

A client with OCD, who was admitted early yesterday morning, must make his bed 22 times before he can have breakfast. Because of his behavior, the client missed having breakfast yesterday with the other clients.

1. Which nursing actions would the nurse institute to help the client reducing ritualistic behavior?
2. Which psychotherapies could be applied in this client?

(Questions 3 to 4 share the same question stem)

A client is brought to the hospital emergency room by his brother. The client is perspiring profusely, breathing rapidly, and complaining of dizziness and palpitations.

法、认知重建、家庭治疗等。

8. 躯体化障碍的患者在陈述其躯体症状时往往模糊并夸大其症状，现在没有证据显示躯体化障碍的患者有器质性的改变。

9. 疑病障碍主要表现为患者担心自己患有严重的躯体疾病，常在个人或者是其亲密的家庭成员患有严重疾病或死亡威胁的体验之后出现。

10. 在护理躯体形式障碍患者时，护士通过帮助患者建立新型的、适应性的行为模式来帮助他们理解疾病。

11. *CCMD-3* 中应用的癔症这一诊断名词在 *ICD-10* 中已不再使用，*ICD-10* 称为分离（转换）性障碍。起病常与心理社会压力因素有关，主要表现有分离症状和转换（躯体形式）症状两种。

12. 分离（转换）性障碍患者的症状是功能性的，并无器质性疾病，因此应以心理治疗为主。

13. 护士在应用护理程序对分离（转换）性障碍患者进行护理时，应协助患者认识他们存在的问题，并帮助患者明确和建立新的应对行为方式。

思考题

（1～2 题共用题干）

一名强迫性障碍患者，于昨日早晨住院，该患者在每次进早餐之前，必须要整理他的床 22 次。因此，他昨天错过了和其他患者一起用早餐的时间。

1. 护士可以采取哪些干预措施以帮助患者减少强迫行为？
2. 适用于该患者的心理干预技术有哪些？

（3～4 题共用题干）

一位患者被他的哥哥送到医院急诊科，患者大汗淋漓，呼吸急促，主诉眩晕和心悸。排除心血管系统疾病后，患者诊断为惊恐发作。患者症状消失后，他对护士说：“我以为

Problems of a cardiovascular nature are ruled out, and the client's diagnosis is tentatively listed as panic attack. After the symptoms pass, the client states, "I thought I was going to die."

3. Which nursing interventions would be appropriate for the client when panic attacks?

4. Which method could be used to change the client's false beliefs about this disease?

(Questions 5 to 6 share the same question stem)

The physician refers a client with somatization disorder to the outpatient clinic because of problems with nausea.The client's past symptoms involved back pain,chest pain,and problems with urination. The client tells the nurse that the nausea began when his wife asked him for a divorce. The next day, the client is talking with the nurse about fishing when he suddenly revers to talking about the pain in his arm.

5. Which nursing actions would the nurse institute to help the client dealing with the pain in his arm?

6. Which psychotherapies method could be used to reduce the client's somatization?

我就要死了"。

3. 该患者惊恐发作时的护理干预措施包括哪些?

4. 有哪些方法可以帮助患者改变对疾病不恰当的认知?

(5~6题共用题干)

一名躯体化障碍的患者表现为恶心,医生建议其到门诊接受治疗。患者过去有背痛、胸痛和排尿困难。患者告诉护士在其妻子要求和他离婚时,开始出现了恶心症状。第二天,患者正在和护士谈论钓鱼的事情,患者突然又转移到他的胳膊疼痛的话题上。

5. 此时,护士对患者的胳膊疼痛可以怎样处理?

6. 护士可以采用哪些心理干预技术来减轻患者的躯体症状?

Chapter 11 Nursing Management for Clients with Substance-related Disorders

第十一章 精神活性物质所致精神障碍患者的护理

Learning Objectives

Memorization

1. Define concepts of abuse, dependence, intoxication, and withdrawal.
2. Describe classification of psychoactive substances.

Comprehension

1. Discuss etiological implications for substance-related disorders.
2. Identify symptomatology of intoxication and withdrawal related to various substance-related disorders.
3. Explain various modalities relevant to treatment of clients with substance-related disorders.

Application

1. Formulate nursing diagnoses and relevant outcome criteria common to clients with substance-related disorders.
2. Apply appropriate nursing intervention in the care of individuals with substance-related disorders.

学习目标

识记

1. 能准确描述滥用、依赖、中毒及戒断的概念。
2. 能正确概述精神活性物质的分类。

理解

1. 能归纳精神活性物质所致精神障碍病因学方面的影响因素。
2. 能识别不同类型物质相关障碍中毒及戒断的主要临床表现。
3. 能具体说明不同类型精神活性物质所致精神障碍的主要治疗方式。

运用

1. 能提出精神活性物质所致精神障碍患者的常用护理诊断及相应的护理目标。
2. 能为精神活性物质所致精神障碍患者提供恰当的护理干预措施。

John, male, age 56 and married, was admitted for inpatient treatment of alcoholism. He began drinking when he was 25 years old because of insomnia. Since then, his consumption of alcohol has increased gradually. He often drinks white wine (52°) and consumed at least 250 g per day for the last 5 years. He used to drink wine only after dinner, but recently he started to drink in the morning as well. When he attempted to stay clean under the requirement of family members, he experienced tachycardia, sweating, craving, tremor.etc. His wife reports that he becomes irritable after drinking and tends to quarrel with family members over insignificant issues, and even throwing things. Since a month ago, he constantly told his wife that someone had been calling him downstairs, while no one was there when his wife went downstairs. He has been sneaking drinks at work, and his effectiveness has started to decline. The last time he drank was one day ago, consuming about 200 g of white wine (52°).

约翰，男，56岁，已婚，因饮酒问题入院。患者25岁时因失眠开始饮酒，随后饮酒量逐渐增加，其主要饮用52度白酒，近5年平均每日饮酒量约250g，饮酒习惯为晚餐后饮酒，但早晨也逐渐开始饮酒。曾因家人要求戒酒一次，出现心慌、出汗、手抖等症状。其妻子提供患者饮酒后容易发脾气，常因小事与家人吵架，甚至摔东西。1个月前，家属发现患者经常说有人在楼下喊自己，但当妻子下楼时却发现没有人。患者在工作期间也偷偷饮酒，工作效率明显下降。末次饮酒时间为1天前，饮52度白酒约200g。

Please think about the following questions based on the case:

1. What symptoms of withdrawal may this client present?
2. How do nurses assess this client comprehensively, and provide effective nursing care for him?

请思考：

1. 患者可能出现的戒断症状有哪些？
2. 护士如何对患者进行全面评估并实施有效的护理干预？

Drugs are a pervasive part of our society. Throughout history, members of almost every society have used indigenous psychoactive substances for widely accepted medical, religious, or recreational purposes. A wide variety of drugs have been produced for medicinal purposes such as relieving pain and reducing anxiety. Society has even developed a relative indifference to an occasional abuse of these substances, including alcohol, caffeine, and nicotine, despite documentation of their negative impact on health.

现代社会中药物及相关化学物质普遍存在。纵观历史，精神活性物质在每个社会中均被广泛用于医疗、宗教和娱乐领域，而且医疗性使用某些精神活性物质用于缓解疼痛、减少紧张焦虑的做法非常普遍。尽管这些物质的使用对健康有负面影响，但某些精神活性物质的使用甚至被社会认为是正常的，如饮酒、咖啡以及烟草等。

However, the abuse of drug and chemical substance has resulted in severe social problems. According to the World Drug Report 2012, about 230 million people, or 5 percent of the world's adult population, are estimated to have used an illicit drug at least once in 2010. Problem drug users number about 27 million, which is 0.6 percent of the world adult population. China has also become a victimized country of drugs. Opioids, mainly heroin, are the primary drug of concern, followed by Amphetamine-type Stimulants (ATS) and tranquillizers. Drug abuse leads to labour force shortage, human immunodeficiency virus (HIV) infection and fast spread of other infectious diseases, which has endangered people's physical and mental health, and social stability in our country. In addition, from the perspective of public health, the health

药物和相关化学物质的滥用已导致严重的社会问题。根据2012年世界毒品报告，2010年大约有2.3亿人至少使用过一次非法药物，占世界成人人口的5%，问题吸毒者的数量约为2 700万人，占世界成人人口的0.6%。中国已成为毒品受害国，阿片类物质，主要是海洛因，仍然是主要的滥用物质，其次是苯丙胺类兴奋剂及镇静剂。毒品滥用所导致的劳动力丧失、HIV感染以及其他传染性疾病的传播等已严重威胁到我国人民的身心健康及家庭社会稳定。此外，从公共卫生角度出发，由于我国吸烟及饮酒人群基数较大，其

effect caused by the large amount of drinking and smoking population in China should not be ignored. This chapter will discuss the clinical manifestation, therapy and nursing intervention of substance-related disorders such as alcohol, opioids, central nervous system (CNS) stimulants, hallucinogens and others.

所造成的健康影响更不容忽视。本章主要介绍酒精、阿片类物质、中枢神经系统兴奋剂、致幻剂等物质相关障碍的临床表现、治疗方法及护理干预。

Section 1 Introduction

第一节　概　述

Psychoactive substances are also called addictive substances, which can influence mood, emotion, behavior, consciousness, and cause dependence. People use these substances to get or keep some special psychological and physiological state.

精神活性物质又称成瘾物质，指能够影响人类心境、情绪、行为、意识状态，并有致依赖作用的一类化学物质，人们使用这些物质的目的在于获得或保持某些特殊的心理、生理状态。

I. Definitions and Terms

一、相关概念

The substance-related disorders are categorized as substance use disorders and substance-induced disorders. The following conditions may be classified as substance-induced: intoxication, withdrawal, and other substance/medication-induced mental disorders. Different terms are used to describe behavior patterns regarding substance use.

物质相关障碍包括物质使用障碍及物质所致的障碍两个类别，后者又包括中毒、戒断及其他物质或药物所致的精神障碍，以下介绍描述物质使用行为方式的相关概念。

i. Abuse

Abuse is to use wrongfully or in a harmful way, and is described as a maladaptive pattern of substance use manifested by recurrent and significant adverse consequences related to repeated use of the substance.

（一）滥用

滥用是指错误或有害的使用方法，一种适应不良的方式，指由于反复使用物质导致了明显的不良后果。

ii. Dependence

Dependence, composed of physical dependence and psychological dependence, is a compulsive or chronic requirement despite adverse consequences on physical, social, and psychological well-being. Physical dependence on a substance is evidenced by a cluster of cognitive, behavioral, and physiological symptoms indicating that the individual continues use of the substance despite significant substance-related problems. Psychological dependence is described as psychologically dependent on a substance when there is an overwhelming desire to repeat the use of a particular drug in order to produce pleasure or avoid discomfort.

（二）依赖

依赖包括躯体依赖和精神依赖，是指个体对物质的强迫性或慢性需求，尽管该物质会导致明显的身体、心理和社会问题。物质的躯体依赖主要表现为躯体和精神出现一系列特有的症状促使个体继续使用该物质，尽管会导致严重的物质相关问题。精神依赖指为了使用物质后产生一种愉快或欣快的感觉或避免不舒服感觉的发生，驱使个体具有周期性地或反复连续性使用该物质的强烈渴求。

iii. Addiction

Addiction describes a physical and mental state in which individuals have so strong desire for certain drugs that these drugs will be used repeatedly to achieve pleasure or avoid suffering.

（三）成瘾

成瘾是指对物质有一种强烈的渴求，并反复地应用，以获得快感或避免停用后产生痛苦为特点的一种精神和躯体性病理状态。

iv. Tolerence

Tolerance is defined as the need for increasingly larger or more frequent doses of a substance in order to obtain the desired effects originally produced by a lower dose, even to a toxic dosage.

(四)耐受性

耐受性是指反复使用某种物质后，个体需要增加物质使用频率或使用比初始剂量大得多的剂量以获得最初低剂量使用该物质所产生的快感，甚至会使用可能导致中毒的剂量。

v. Intoxication

Intoxication is a physical and mental state of exhilaration and emotional frenzy or lethargy and stupor. Substance intoxication is defined as the development of a reversible substance-specific syndrome caused by the recent ingestion of (or exposure to) a substance.

(五)中毒

中毒是指一种身心状态的紊乱、情绪激惹或昏睡、昏迷。物质中毒主要表现为近期使用或暴露于某种物质后所出现的可逆的与物质相关的特有的综合征。

vi. Withdrawal

Withdrawal is the physiological and mental readjustment that accompanies the discontinuation of an addictive substance. Substance withdrawal is the development of a substance specific maladaptive behavioral change, with physiological and cognitive concomitants, that is due to the cessation of or reduction in, heavy and prolonged substance use.

(六)戒断

戒断是指停用某种物质后所出现的躯体和心理的不适应状态。物质戒断主要为绝对或相对戒断某种长期大剂量使用的物质后所出现的一组与物质相关的、特有的、不适应的躯体和精神症状。

II. Classification of Psychoactive Substances

The *DSM-5* classifies substance-related disorders as disorders related to 10 separate classes of drugs: alcohol; caffeine; cannabis; hallucinogens (with separate categories for phencyclidine [or similarly acting arylcyclohexylamines] and other hallucinogens); inhalants; opioids; sedatives, hypnotics, and anxiolytics; stimulants (amphetamine-type substances, cocaine, and other stimulants); tobacco; and other (or unknown) substances. Psychoactive substances can be classified into four groups according to their pharmacological features.

1. CNS Depressants　CNS depressants include opioids (e.g., heroin, morphine, dolantin, methadone, buprenorphine) ,alcohol, barbiturates, benzodiazepines.

2. CNS Stimulants　CNS stimulants include amphetamines (methamphetamine, 3,4-methylenedioxy-methamphetamine), cocaine, tobacco, drink with caffeine.

3. Hallucinogens　Hallucinogens include cannabinoids, lysergic acid diethylanide, phencyclidine.

4. Volatile Inhalants　Volatile inhalants include acetone, tetrachloromethane, and some menstruum.

二、精神活性物质的分类

根据《美国精神障碍诊断和统计手册（第5版）》，物质相关障碍主要包括10种不同类别的药物：酒精、咖啡因、大麻、致幻剂[包括分属于不同类别的苯环利定（或类似活性芳基环已胺）和其他致幻剂]、吸入剂、阿片类物质、镇静剂、催眠药和抗焦虑药、兴奋剂（苯丙胺类物质、可卡因及其他兴奋剂）、烟草及其他（或未知）物质。而精神活性物质按药理学特性可分为四类。

1. 中枢神经抑制剂　中枢神经抑制剂包括阿片类（如海洛因、吗啡、杜冷丁、美沙酮、丁丙诺啡）、酒类、巴比妥类、苯二氮䓬类。

2. 中枢神经兴奋剂　中枢神经兴奋剂包括安非他明类（如冰毒、摇头丸）、可卡因、烟草、含咖啡因饮料。

3. 致幻剂　致幻剂包括大麻、麦角酸二乙胺（LSD），苯环已哌啶（PCP）等。

4. 挥发性溶剂　挥发性溶剂包括丙酮、四氯化碳、某些溶媒等。

III. Epidemiology

i. Epidemiological Status in the World

A wide variety of chemical substances and drug abuse has resulted in severe social problems. According to the United Nations Office on Drugs and Crime (UNODC) data in 2012, the extent of global illicit drug use remained stable in the five years up to and including 2010, at between 3.4 and 6.6 per cent of the adult population (persons aged 15-64). About 10-13 percent of drug users continue to be problem users with drug dependence and/or drug-use disorders. Approximately 1 in every 100 deaths among adults is attributed to illicit drug use. Opioids is the dominant drug type in Asia and Europe, while cocaine is the most common in America. Cannabis is the main drug causing treatment demand in Africa, and the use of ATS is most common in Asia. The two most widely used drugs remain cannabis (global annual prevalence ranging from 2.6 to 5.0 percent) and ATS, excluding "ecstasy" (0.3-1.2 percent) in the world.

ii. Epidemiological Status in China

In China, the proportion of registered drug users who use heroin as a primary drug decreased from 83 percent in 2001 to 69.2 percent in 2011. However, the total number of heroin users in the registry has continued to increase. Along with this, the proportion of registered synthetic drug users in China increased from 19 percent of total drug users in the country in 2008 to 28 percent in 2010. According to the 2015 Chinese drug situation reports of the China National Narcotics Control Commission, the number of drug abusers was 2.345 million by the end of 2015, of which heroin and other opioids abusers were 980 000 (41.8%); synthetic drug abusers were 1 340 000 (57.1%); and other was 25 000 (1.1%). About 43 000 drug abusers are under the age of 18, accounting for 1.8%. There are 1.422 million drug users between 18 to 35 years old, accounting for 60.6%; 870 000, between 36 to 59, accounting for 37.1%; 11 000, over the age of 60, accounting for 0.5%. Intravenous drug abuse is the most common source of HIV transmission in the country, causing 72.4% of the HIV/AIDS transmission.

IV. Etiology and Mechanism

Many factors influence dependence on or abuse of substances, including biological, psychological, and

三、流行病学

（一）世界范围内流行状况

当今社会中药物和有关化学物质滥用已成为极其严重的社会问题。根据2012年联合国毒品和犯罪问题办公室报告，在2010年（含）之前的5年里，全球非法药物使用范围保持稳定，占成人（15～64岁）总人口的3.4%至6.6%，然而，大约10%～13%的吸毒者仍然是有药物依赖和/或药物滥用症的问题吸毒者。每100例成人死亡中就有将近1例死于非法药物的使用。类阿片依然是亚洲和欧洲占主导地位的毒品类别，而可卡因的使用主要涉及美洲，大麻是造成非洲治疗需求的主要毒品，而使用苯丙胺类兴奋剂在亚洲最为常见。从全球来看，使用最为广泛的两种非法药物依然是大麻（全球年度流行率从2.6%到5.0%不等）和苯丙胺类兴奋剂（不包括"摇头丸"）（0.3%～1.2%）。

（二）我国的流行状况

在中国，吸毒人员中滥用海洛因人员所占比例由2001年的83%下降至2011年的69.2%，然而滥用海洛因人员总数仍在增加，此外，合成毒品滥用人员比例由2008年的19%上升至2010年的28%。根据2015年中国国家禁毒委员会办公室发布的2015年中国毒品形势报告，截至2015年底，全国现有吸毒人员234.5万名，其中，滥用海洛因等阿片类毒品人员98万名，占41.8%，滥用合成毒品人员134万名，占57.1%，滥用其他毒品人员2.5万名，占1.1%。在全国现有吸毒人员中，不满18岁的有4.3万名，占1.8%；18岁到35岁的有142.2万名，占60.6%；36岁到59岁的有87万名，占37.1%；60岁以上的有1.1万名，占0.5%。静脉注射毒品是我国传染HIV的主要途径，占72.4%。

四、病因及发病机制

物质依赖、滥用与许多因素相关，包括

sociocultural factors. Interaction among various elements forms a complex collection of determinants that influence a person's vulnerability to abuse substances (figure 11-1).

生理、心理及社会文化等方面，各因素之间的相互作用形成了影响个体物质滥用易感性的复杂的综合因素（图 11-1）。

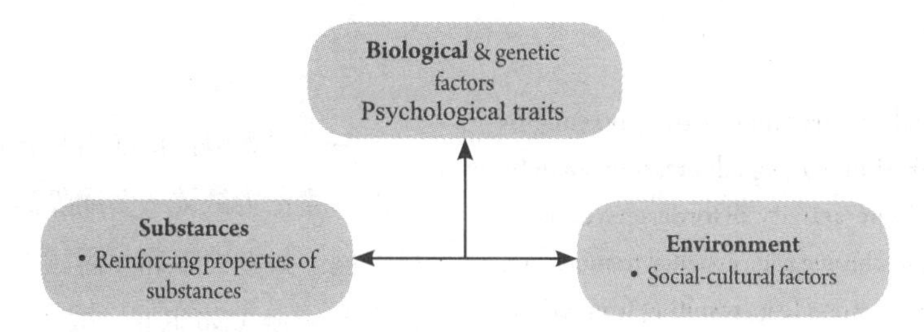

Figure 11-1 Factors and determinants of substance abuse

i. Biological Factors

1. Neurobiological Mechanisms Drugs that are taken in excess have in common direct activation of the brain reward system, which is involved in the reinforcement of behaviors and the production of memories. They produce such an intense activation of the reward system that normal activities may be neglected. Instead of achieving reward system activation through adaptive behaviors, drugs of abuse directly activate the reward pathways. Furthermore, individuals with lower levels of self-control, which may reflect impairments of brain inhibitory mechanisms, may be particularly predisposed to develop substance use disorders.

Another biological aspect relates to neuroadaptation. This refers to the neuronal changes and consequent clinical signs and symptoms that result from repeated drug application. It encompasses biological substrata of tolerance and physical (as opposed to psychological) dependence. Changes in synaptic membrane composition, receptor function, and post receptor intracellular events have all been proposed as the basis of neuroadaptation to psychoactive drug abuse.

2. Genetic Factors A heuristically useful paradigm for understanding the genetic factors that can contribute to the development of most substance use disorders is alcohol dependence. Findings from twin and adoption studies demonstrate the relative contributions of genetic and environmental factors in predisposition to alcohol dependence. The concordance rate for alcohol dependence is substantially higher in monozygotic than dizygotic twins, whereas concordance rates are no different for less severe forms of alcohol abuse. Adoption studies show that adopted-away men with alcoholic biological parents have an increased likelihood of developing

（一）生物学因素

1. 神经生物学机制 药物摄入过量的共同点是直接激活大脑的犒赏系统，此系统能强化这些行为，产生记忆。药物使用对大脑犒赏系统的强烈激活作用以至于正常活动可以被忽略。药物滥用直接激活犒赏路径，而非通过适应性行为达到犒赏系统的激活。此外，自我控制水平较低的个体，它反映了大脑抑制机制的损害，可能特别倾向于产生物质使用障碍。

神经生物学因素的另外一方面主要是神经适应性，神经适应性是指因神经元改变而出现相应的临床体征和症状，其形成主要来源于药物的重复使用，它包括生理耐受和躯体依赖（相对于精神依赖）。突触膜上成分的改变、受体功能和受体后细胞内活动都被认为是滥用精神活动物质导致神经适应现象的基础。

2. 遗传因素 关于遗传因素对形成物质使用障碍的影响的研究中最具有代表性的是酒精依赖。双生子和寄养子的研究证明，环境和遗传因素均可影响酒精依赖。虽然轻度酒精使用障碍的同期患病率相同，但酒精依赖的同期患病率单卵双生子明显高于双卵双生子。而对寄养子的研究表明，酗酒的父母，无论其子女是否被寄养在酗酒的环境中，其子女嗜酒的可能性较高。一般来说，父母酗酒的严重程度会影响寄养子酗酒的发生率，

alcoholism regardless of whether they are raised in an alcoholic environment. In general, the severity of parental alcoholism tends to influence the prevalence of alcoholism in adopted-away sons; patients with the most severe alcoholism have the highest rates of alcohol dependence in their offspring.

父母酗酒越严重，其后代发生酒精依赖的比率越高。

ii. Psychological Factors

Psychological factors such as the presence of comorbid psychopathology (e.g., depression, anxiety, attention-deficit/hyperactivity disorder, psychosis), medical illnesses (e.g., chronic pain, essential tremor); and past or present severe stress (e.g., resulting from crime, battle exposure, sexual trauma, or economic difficulties) have received considerable attention, being regarded as potential causes for "self-medication". There is a probability that susceptibility to psychological stressors and substance use disorders may have similar etiologies. For example, some of the etiologic factors that predispose an individual to depression following major losses (e.g., dysregulation of noradrenergic neurotransmission or the hypothalamic-pituitary-adrenal axis) may also contribute to the development of substance use disorders.

（二）心理因素

一些因素包括伴随有精神症状（如抑郁、焦虑、注意力缺陷/多动障碍、精神病）、内科疾病（如慢性疼痛、震颤）、过去或现在有较强的应激（如犯罪、战争、性创伤、经济困难），均是可能导致个体使用药物的潜在因素。心理压力的易感性与物质使用障碍可能存在相似的病因。例如，个体面临重大丧失后导致其易患抑郁的一些病因（例如，去甲肾上腺素神经传递或下丘脑－垂体－肾上腺轴功能紊乱）也可能引起个体出现物质使用障碍。

Individuals who abuse substances have some common personality traits. These personality traits have been associated with a tendency toward addictive behavior, which include low self-esteem, frequent depression, passivity, the inability to relax or to defer gratification, and the inability to communicate effectively. Substance abuse has also been associated with antisocial personality and depressive response styles.

物质滥用个体可能存在一些共同的个性特征，其与成瘾行为倾向有关，包括低自尊、频繁的抑郁、被动、无法放松或延迟的满足感以及无法进行有效的沟通，物质滥用也与反社会人格及抑郁反应模式有关。

iii. Social-cultural Factors

Social factors also contribute to the initiation of drug use and progression of substance use disorders. Such social factors include peer group attitudes toward, shared expectations of the benefits, purpose of drug use (such as enhanced pleasurable activities with drug use), the availability of competing reinforcers in the form of educational, recreational, and occupational alternatives to substance use, and the availability of drugs during particular developmental stages. Moreover, because of effects of modeling, imitation, and identification on behavior, family and peers appear to be important influences on substance use. An individual's culture and availability of the substance also help to establish patterns of substance use. For example, the French and Italians have considered wine an essential part of the family meal, even for the children, and the English pub is known for its attraction as a social meeting place.

（三）社会文化因素

一些社会因素同样会导致物质使用并促进物质使用障碍的形成，这些社会因素包括同一集体的态度、共同的利益期待、药物使用的目的（比如使用药物以促进娱乐活动）、社会竞争增强、在特定发育阶段有获得药物的可能性等。此外，由于榜样、模仿及行为识别的影响，家庭和同伴似乎成为影响物质使用的重要因素。个人所处的社会文化、物质的易获得性也会影响物质使用。例如，法国和意大利人认为葡萄酒是家庭聚会的一个重要组成部分，甚至小孩子也可以使用，而英国酒吧则闻名于其为重要的社交场所。

iv. Dependence of Substances

Generally, the addictive degree of psychoactive

（四）物质的依赖性

一般认为，精神活性物质的成瘾强度可

substances can be regarded as a continuous spectrum, one end is more addictive drug, such as heroin, on the other side is less addictive chemicals, such as caffeine, and most of psychoactive substances are in between. Strongly addictive psychoactive substances, such as heroin, can generate physical dependence and/or impulsive drug-craving when individuals have enough dosage and using time. This is more prominent in vulnerable population.

以看成是连续谱，一端是成瘾性很强的毒品，如海洛因，而另一端是成瘾性较低的化学物质，如咖啡因，多数精神活动物质介于两者之间。成瘾性较强的精神活性物质如海洛因只要具备足够的剂量和使用时间，多能产生躯体依赖和/或冲动性的用药渴求，在易感人群中则更为突出。

V. Diagnosis and Prognosis

五、诊断与预后

The diagnostic criteria of substance-related disorders can be based on *International Classification of Diseases Tenth Revision (ICD-10)*, *Diagnostic and Statistical Manual of Mental Disorders Fifth Edition (DSM-5)*, and *Chinese Classification and Diagnostic Criteria of Mental Disorders Third Edition (CCMD-3)*. It is advisable to seek corroboration from more than one source of evidence relating to substance use to identify the psychoactive substance use. The diagnosis may be made on the basis of self-report data, objective analysis of specimens of urine, blood, etc, or other evidence (presence of drug samples in the client's possession, clinical signs and symptoms, or reports from informed third parties). The diagnosis criteria of a substance use disorder can be considered to fit within overall groupings of impaired control, social impairment, risky use, and pharmacological criteria. As to substance intoxication, diagnostic criterias include recent ingestion of a substance; significant problematic behavioral or psychological changes associated with intoxication; symptoms not attributable to another medical condition and not better explained by another mental disorder. The essential feature of criteria for substance withdrawal includes the cessation of, or reduction in heavy and prolonged substance use; significant distress or impairment in social, occupational, or other important areas of functioning; symptoms not due to another medical condition and not better explained by another mental disorder.

精神活性物质所致精神障碍的诊断可参考《国际疾病分类系统（第10版）》、《美国精神障碍诊断和统计手册（第5版）》及《中国精神疾病分类方案与诊断标准（第3版）》，诊断时建议参考多个来源的与物质使用相关的证据。诊断的依据可能来源于自我报告、尿液或血液等标本分析或其他（患者持有药物、临床症状和体征或第三方报告）。物质使用障碍的诊断标准需满足控制力受损、社会障碍、危险使用及药理标准，而对于物质中毒，诊断标准则包括最近物质的摄入、与中毒相关的重大的问题行为与心理改变、症状与其他疾病无关也不能由另外的精神障碍更好地解释。物质戒断的重要特征则包括减少或停止长期大量使用的物质；社会、职业或其他重要领域功能受损；症状与其他疾病无关也不能由另外的精神障碍更好地解释。

The prognosis in substance abuse disorders depends on numerous factors involving a complex interaction of biological, psychological, and environmental elements. Problems of low socioeconomic status, comorbid psychiatric conditions, and lack of family and social supports are among the most important predictors of poor adherence during addiction treatment and of relapse following treatment. The prognosis for individuals who abuse drugs other than alcohol is complicated by a lifestyle in conflict with the legal system. Treatment of comorbid

精神活性物质所致精神障碍患者的预后与多种因素有关，是生理、心理及社会因素共同作用的结果。社会经济地位低下、伴有精神疾病及缺乏家庭社会支持是成瘾治疗依从性差和治疗复发的重要预测因素。除酒精滥用以外，个人物质滥用预后的复杂性也与生活方式与法律制度之间的冲突相关，其次，对精神疾病的共病治疗有利于改善预后。大

psychiatric illnesses may be important in improving prognosis. The majority of alcoholic clients also have another psychiatric illness, including affective and anxiety disorders and personality disorders, which can worsen the prognosis if not addressed. A 1-year postdischarge follow-up studies (of substance abuse treatment show that) 40% to 60% of discharged clients are continuously abstinent, although an additional 15% to 30% have not resumed dependent use during this period.

多数酒精依赖患者伴有另一种精神疾病，包括情绪和焦虑障碍、人格障碍，如果不能得到治疗将使其预后恶化。一项有关物质滥用患者出院一年后的随访研究显示，40% 到 60% 的患者不再复吸，另外有 15% 到 30% 的患者在此阶段没有再次形成物质依赖。

Section 2 Alcohol-related Disorders

第二节　酒精相关障碍

Alcohol is known scientifically as ethyl alcohol. It can induce a general, nonselective, reversible depression of the CNS, resulting in behavioral and mood changes. The use of alcohol is legal in most countries. The effects of alcohol on the CNS are proportional to the alcohol concentration in the blood. At low doses, alcohol produces relaxation, loss of inhibitions, lack of concentration, drowsiness, slurred speech, and sleep, but chronic abuse of alcohol results in multisystem physiological impairments. Alcohol is one of the most commonly used psychoactive substances. Based on combined data from the 2002-2004 National Surveys on Drug Use and Health in America, it is estimated that 7.6% of persons age 12 years or older met the criteria for alcohol dependence or abuse in the past year. According to the survey of alcohol consumption status of residents aged 15 and above in China, the drinking rate in the group of people was 34.3%, of which, drinking rate of men (54.6%) were higher than women (13.3%). The drinking rate of people aged 45-49 was highest (38.6%).

酒精，又称乙醇，其可以引起一般的、非选择性的、可逆的中枢神经系统抑制，主要表现为行为和情绪的变化。酒精使用在大多数国家合法。酒精对中枢神经系统的影响与血液中酒精的浓度成正比，酒精低剂量使用时，其主要作用包括松弛、自控力丧失、注意力不能集中、困倦、口齿不清以及嗜睡等，而慢性酒精滥用常导致多系统器官功能障碍。酒精是最常使用的精神活性物质之一。2002～2004 年美国全国药物使用和健康状况调查显示，既往一年，12 岁以上的人群中有 7.6% 满足酒精依赖或者酒精滥用诊断标准。而 2010～2012 年中国 15 岁及以上居民饮酒状况调查显示饮酒率为 34.3%，男性（54.6%）高于女性（13.3%），45～59 岁人群饮酒率最高（38.6%）。

I. Clinical Manifestation

一、临床表现

i. Alcohol Intoxication

Alcohol intoxication proceeds in stages that depend on dosage and time following administration. Apparent CNS stimulation, which occurs early in alcohol or at low dosage, results from depression of inhibitory control mechanisms. Excitation resulting from intoxication is characterized by increased activity, verbal communication, and often aggression. Higher blood concentrations of alcohol cause mild impairment of motor skills and slowing of reaction time, followed by sedation, decreased motor

（一）酒精中毒

酒精中毒的表现与使用剂量及服用时间密切相关。早期或小剂量服用时，由于大脑的抑制机能受到抑制，患者出现明显的中枢神经系统兴奋症状，其主要表现为活动增多、多语和易激惹。酒精的血液浓度过高会导致行动迟缓、反应迟钝，进而出现镇静、行动协调性降低、判断力下降、记忆力受损及其

coordination, impaired judgment, diminished memory and other cognitive deficits, and eventually diminished psychomotor activity and sleep. If blood concentration of alcohol gets much higher, midbrain functions will gradually be hindered, resulting in dysfunction of spinal reflexes, temperature regulation, and medullary centers controlling cardiorespiratory function. Alcohol intoxication usually occurs at blood alcohol levels between 100 and 200 mg/dl. Table 11-1 summarizes the signs of alcohol intoxication correlated with progressive blood alcohol levels.

他认知障碍，最终引起精神活动的减少及嗜睡。若浓度更高，可因进行性的中脑功能障碍，引起脊髓反射、温度调节及心血管和呼吸中枢失调，患者出现昏睡、昏迷，甚至死亡。酒精中毒的乙醇血液浓度通常在 100 mg/dl 到 200 mg/dl 之间。表 11-1 总结了各乙醇血液浓度水平所对应酒精中毒的临床表现。

Table 11-1　Signs of intoxication correlated with blood alcohol levels

Blood Alcohol Level(mg/dL)	Signs of Intoxication
20-99	Muscular incoordination Impaired sensory function Changes in mood, personality, and behavior
100-199	Marked mental impairment Incoordination Prolonged reaction time Ataxia
200-299	Nausea and vomiting Diplopia Marked ataxia
300-399	Hypothermia Severe dysarthria Amnesia Anesthesia
400-700	Coma Respiratory failure Death

表 11-1　乙醇血液浓度水平及对应的酒精中毒临床表现

乙醇血液浓度 (mg/dl)	中毒表现
20 ~ 99	肌肉运动不协调 感觉器官受损 情绪、人格及行为改变
100 ~ 199	明显心理障碍 不协调 反应时间延长 共济失调
200 ~ 299	恶心和呕吐 复视 显著的共济失调
300 ~ 399	体温过低 严重的构音障碍 失忆 麻木
400 ~ 700	昏迷 呼吸衰竭 死亡

ii. Alcohol Withdrawal

The onset, severity, and duration of the withdrawal syndrome in a given class of CNS depressants are determined by the rate of elimination of the drug and metabolites from the body. Among the CNS depressants, alcohol withdrawal is of intermediate severity.

1. Uncomplicated Alcohol Withdrawal Cessation of alcohol or CNS depressant intake after prolonged use is associated with a syndrome of neuronal hyperexcitability with increased noradrenergic and adrenocortical activity. Alcohol withdrawal typically begins at 6-12hours after the last drink; this syndrome is initially characterized by anxiety, impaired appetite, nausea, apprehension, restlessness, irritability, and insomnia with clinically apparent hand tremors and hyperreflexia. Clients have a strong alcohol craving. At 24-36 hours after cessation of alcohol, moderately severe cases progress to visible tremors, anxiety, agitation, and signs of autonomic hyperactivity with tachycardia, hypertension, diaphoresis, hyperthermia, and muscle fasciculations. Often clients experience anorexia, nausea, or vomiting with subsequent dehydration and electrolyte disturbances. At this stage, clients also have intermittent confusion, transient visual and auditory hallucinations and illusions mostly at night. The withdrawal symptoms peaks at 48-72 hours after the last drink, and generally abate by 4-5 days. Severe symptoms include marked disorientation, confusion, hallucinations, delusions related to the hallucinations, delirium, and uncontrollable tremors.

2. Alcohol Epilepsy Seizures, another complication of alcohol withdrawal, estimated to occur in 5%-15% of patients, usually happen in the first 24 hours from last drink, but they can happen any time in the first 5 days. Alcohol withdrawal seizures are usually grand mal in type. Paroxysmal EEG discharges may precede generalized tonic-clonic seizure activity. Those with a past history of alcohol withdrawal seizures are at increased risk for seizures in subsequent episodes of alcohol withdrawal.

3. Alcohol Withdrawal Delirium In the alcohol withdrawal syndrome, delirium tremens begins at 48-72 hours after the last drink. Typical signs of delirium are agitation, disorientation, muscle fasciculations, fluctuating level of consciousness, visual and auditory hallucinations, and intense autonomic arousal. If treated improperly, patients also die due to high fever, dehydration, infection.etc. The death rate is about 5%.

（二）酒精戒断

酒精戒断症状的严重程度和持续时间取决于酒精在体内的代谢和清除率。在中枢神经系统抑制剂中，酒精戒断是相对很危险的。

1. 单纯性戒断反应 长期使用酒精或其他中枢神经抑制剂如突然停用，会伴发去甲肾上腺素和肾上腺皮质活性增加的神经元高度兴奋。酒精戒断症状通常在停用后6～12小时出现，主要症状有焦虑、食欲下降、恶心、恐惧、坐立不安、易激惹、失眠，并伴有明显的手部震颤和反射亢进。患者有强烈的饮酒渴求。停止饮酒后24～36小时，可能出现中度戒断症状，患者具有明显的震颤、焦虑、易激惹，可出现自主神经活动增强，表现为心动过速、血压增高、出汗、发热和肌肉抽搐，并伴有厌食、恶心、呕吐、脱水和电解质紊乱。在这个阶段，患者可能出现间歇性的意识障碍，在晚上出现大量的幻觉。戒断症状在停止饮酒后48～72小时达到高峰，然后在4～5天后逐渐缓解，严重的戒断症状包括定向力障碍、意识模糊、视幻觉或听幻觉、与幻觉相关的妄想、谵妄以及全身肌肉的粗大震颤。

2. 酒精性癫痫 酒精戒断的另一个严重的并发症是癫痫，约5%～15%的患者在酒精戒断中曾发生癫痫，其通常在戒断后的24小时内发生，但也可出现在戒断后的5天内。酒精戒断所致癫痫通常为癫痫大发作类型，阵发的脑电图可表现为普遍的强直痉挛样癫痫发作。那些具有癫痫发作史的酒精戒断患者在之后的酒精戒断中癫痫发作风险增高。

3. 酒精戒断性谵妄 在酒精戒断时，震颤性谵妄一般发生于停止饮酒后的48～72小时内。谵妄的典型表现为激越、定向力障碍、肌肉的粗大震颤、意识模糊、视幻觉和听幻觉以及强烈的自主神经唤醒状态。如果处理不当，患者常因高热、脱水、感染等死亡，死亡率大概在5%左右。

iii. Other Alcohol-Induced Disorders

1. Abuse of alcohol It usually causes multisystem physiological complications, including peripheral neuropathy, alcoholic myopathy, alcoholic cardiomyopathy, esophagitis, gastritis, pancreatitis, alcoholic hepatitis, cirrhosis, etc.

2. Wernicke's Encephalopathy The main symptoms of Wernicke's encephalopathy include paralysis of the ocular muscles, diplopia, ataxia, somnolence, and stupor. It is the most serious form of alcoholics. The primary cause of Wernicke's encephalopathy is thiamine deficiency.

3. Korsakoff's Psychosis Korsakoff's psychosis, identified by a syndrome of confusion, loss of recent memory, and confabulation, is frequently encountered in patients recovering from Wernicke's encephalopathy.

（三）其他酒精相关障碍

1. 酒精滥用 通常会导致多器官系统并发症，包括周围神经病变、酒精性肌病、酒精性心肌病、食道炎、胃炎、胰腺炎、酒精性肝病、肝硬化等。

2. 韦尼克脑病 主要症状包括眼肌麻痹、复视、共济失调及嗜睡。韦尼克脑病是最严重的酒精中毒性精神病，其原因主要为B族维生素的缺乏。

3. 科萨科夫综合征 主要表现为定向力障碍、近记忆损害、错构、虚构等，常见于韦尼克脑病恢复期患者。

II. Treatment

The general approach is to administer a CNS depressant that has a longer elimination half-life than the drug from which the client is being withdrawn once obvious clinical signs of withdrawal are apparent. A long-acting benzodiazepine, such as diazepam, has historically been considered the gold standard for the treatment of alcohol withdrawal. Other treatment strategies in alcohol detoxification include adjunctive treatment of comorbid medical problems, rehydration, correction of electrolyte abnormalities, and oral multivitamin preparations containing folic acid. The replacement of thiamine, particularly before giving glucose, is especially important to prevent Wernicke's encephalopathy, precipitated by depletion of thiamine reserves.

All drugs currently used for the treatment of CNS depressant withdrawal have dependence liability. When prescribing these medications, careful client education is needed concerning the balance between risks and benefits, particularly with regard to the potential for dependence.

It is very difficult to achieve the maintenance of abstinence for clients with alcohol use disorders. Psychosocial support and recent advances in pharmacotherapy (disulfiram, naltrexone, a long-acting intramuscular formulation of naltrexone, and acamprosate) have been a valuable addition. Psychosocial support, cognitive-behavioral, motivational enhancement, and 12-Step facilitation individual behavioral treatment contribute to sustained abstinence and reduced drinking.

二、治　疗

酒精戒断常采用的药物治疗方法是中枢神经抑制剂，但治疗药物的半衰期需比患者已用的中枢神经抑制剂要长。例如，长效苯二氮䓬类药物（如地西泮）被认为是酒精戒断治疗的金标准。酒精解毒治疗的方法包括补液、纠正电解质异常以及口服含有叶酸的复合维生素制剂等。需要注意的是，在给予葡萄糖之前补充维生素 B_1 对于预防韦尼克脑病非常重要，其可减少维生素 B_1 储存的消耗。此外，现有的治疗中枢神经抑制剂戒断反应的药物均有一定的成瘾性，在使用这些药物时，需向患者说明利弊，特别应讲明其可能的成瘾性。

帮助酒精相关障碍患者预防复饮非常困难，可以使用一些辅助治疗措施，如心理社会支持治疗、认知行为治疗、动机强化治疗以及12步戒酒法等。其次，一些新的药物治疗方法，如戒酒硫、纳曲酮、纳曲酮长效肌内注射剂以及阿坎酸等也有助于减少复饮。

Section 3 Opioid-related Disorders

第三节 阿片类物质相关障碍

Opioids, capable of inducing tolerance, physiological, and psychological dependence, refers to a group of compounds that includes opium, opium derivatives, and synthetic substitutes. They desensitize an individual to both psychological and physiological pain and induce a sense of euphoria. Lethargy and indifference to the environment are common manifestations of opioid-related disorders. Opioids abuse is public health and social problem in the world.

阿片类物质包括鸦片、鸦片类衍生物及合成替代品，其能够导致耐受及躯体和精神依赖。阿片类物质可以降低个体的生理和心理痛苦并引起欣快感，阿片类物质相关障碍的常见表现为嗜睡及对外界环境的反应降低。阿片类物质滥用是世界范围内的公共卫生和社会问题。

I. Clinical Manifestation

一、临床表现

i. Opioid Intoxication

The pharmacologic feature of opioids is analgesia. Major features of opioid intoxication are initial euphoria followed by apathy, dysphoria, psychomotor agitation or retardation, impaired judgment, and physical symptoms including pupillary constriction (or dilation due to anoxia from severe overdose), drowsiness, facial flushing, itchy face, dry mouth, slurred speech, and impairment in attention or memory. Intravenous use can cause lower abdominal sensations described as an orgasm-like "rush". This is followed by a feeling of sedation (called the "nod") and dreaming. Severe intoxication may cause respiratory suppression, coma, areflexia, hypotension, tachycardia, apnea, cyanosis, and even death.

（一）阿片类物质中毒

阿片的药理学特性是镇痛，其中毒的主要特点为最初欣快感后的冷漠、烦躁不安、精神运动性兴奋或抑制、判断力受损，以及一些躯体症状包括瞳孔缩小（或严重中毒导致缺氧后引起的瞳孔扩大）、嗜睡、面部潮红、面部皮肤发痒、口干、口齿不清、注意力及记忆力下降。静脉使用者可出现下腹部的痉挛“冲击”感，伴随镇静感（称为“点头”）和做梦。严重的中毒反应可导致呼吸抑制、昏迷、反射消失、血压降低、心动过速、呼吸暂停、发绀，甚至死亡。

ii. Opioid Withdrawal

Opioid withdrawal is characterized by a pattern of signs and symptoms that are opposite to the acute agonist effects. Withdrawal of opioids is characterized by hyperalgesia, dysphoric mood, photophobia, lacrimation or rhinorrhea, pupillary dilation, goose flesh, piloerection, or increased sweating, yawning, fever, and insomnia, diarrhea, tachycardia, increased blood pressure, gastrointestinal cramps, joint and muscle aches. Spontaneous withdrawal results in intense craving.

（二）阿片类物质戒断

阿片类物质戒断的症状和体征与其急性兴奋作用完全相反，其戒断症状的特征性表现包括痛觉过敏、烦躁不安、畏光、流泪或流鼻涕、瞳孔扩大、皮肤起鸡皮疙瘩、汗毛竖立、出汗增多、哈欠、发热，以及失眠、腹泻、心动过速、血压增高、胃肠绞痛、关节和肌肉痛等。阿片类物质的自行戒断可能会导致强烈的渴求。

The occurence and severity of withdrawal associated with opioids depend on the half-life of the opioid used. With short-acting drugs such as heroin, withdrawal symptoms occur within 6 to 12 hours after the last dose, peak within 1 to 3 days, and gradually subside over a period of 5 to 7 days. Less acute withdrawal symptoms, including anxiety, dysphoria, anhedonia, and insomnia, can last for weeks to months. With longer-acting drugs

阿片类物质戒断的严重程度与所使用阿片类物质的半衰期有关，短效阿片类物质如海洛因，其戒断症状在中断用药后6~12小时出现，1~3天内达到高峰，一般在5~7天内逐渐减轻，一些较轻的戒断症状如焦虑、烦躁不安、快感缺失和失眠可以持续数周至数

such as methadone, L-alpha-acetylmethadol (LAAM), or buprenorphine, withdrawal symptoms may take 2-4 days to emerge after the last dose and gradually vanish in 10 to 14 days. Withdrawal from the ultra-short-acting meperidine begins quickly, reaches a peak in 8 to 12 hours, and vanishes in 4 to 5 days.

月。长效阿片类物质如美沙酮、乙酰美沙酮、丁丙诺啡，其戒断症状可以在中断用药后 2～4 天才出现，10～14 天后逐渐消失。超短效阿片类物质如哌替啶的戒断症状出现非常迅速，8～12 小时可达到戒断高峰，4～5 天后逐渐消失。

II. Treatment

二、治 疗

Opioid withdrawal and dependence can be treated in several ways. The first option is to convert the client to an equivalent dose of a longer-acting opioid and gradually taper the dose to minimize withdrawal. Methadone and buprenorphine are frequently used in this manner. Often a slow taper of methadone is given at approved facilities. In other circumstances, a 5-10 day taper of the abused opioid or clonidine is used to reduce withdrawal symptoms. Another option includes the use of a clonidine taper for amelioration of tremor, diaphoresis, and agitation. Adjuvant medications may be used, such as nonsteroidal anti-inflammatory drugs for myalgias, benzodiazepines or other hypnotics for short-term management of insomnia.

阿片类物质依赖及戒断有多种治疗方法，首选的治疗方法是将患者所用阿片类物质的剂量转变成等效剂量的长效阿片类物质，并逐渐减少使用剂量以控制戒断症状，最终撤药，这种治疗方法的常用药物为美沙酮和丁丙诺啡。通常缓慢递减美沙酮治疗只能在政府批准的机构中实施。在某些情况下，也可用阿片类物质或可乐定 5～10 天逐步减量法来减少戒断症状。其他治疗方法包括使用可乐定递减法缓解震颤、出汗及激越等戒断症状，也使用辅助药物帮助改善一些戒断症状，如非甾体类抗炎药物用于肌肉疼痛，苯二氮䓬类药物或其他安眠药用于睡眠的短期管理。

Maintenance treatment with agonist therapy provides relief from opioid withdrawal symptoms and thereby allows psychosocial stabilization. Methadone maintenance programs (for 1-2 years or longer) are used in some locations to help reduce the client's risk of reentering the drug and crime cultures. In late 2002 the Food and Drug Administration (FDA) also approved buprenorphine for both detoxification and maintenance treatment of opioid dependence. In the treatment of chronic pain, nonaddicting medications (e.g., carbamazepine and certain antidepressants) and other modalities (e.g., physical therapy, nerve blocks) should be used in appropriate clients to minimize the likelihood of relapse to opioid use. Furthermore, psychosocial intervention is an essential part in the treatment of opioid-related disorders to prevent relapse, such as cognitive-behavioral therapy, supportive group, and family therapy.

此外，维持兴奋剂疗法能减轻阿片类物质的戒断症状并促进心理社会的稳定，一些地区美沙酮维持治疗的应用（1～2 年或更长时间）有助于降低患者的复吸率及暴力的发生。2002 年末，美国食品药品监督管理局批准了丁丙诺啡可用于阿片类物质依赖的解毒和维持治疗。在治疗慢性疼痛时，使用非成瘾药物（如卡马西平及一些抗抑郁药）及理疗、神经阻滞等治疗方法，可大大降低复吸的可能性。心理社会干预治疗包括认知行为治疗、支持团体及家庭治疗等也有助于帮助预防物质相关障碍患者的复吸，是重要的治疗组成部分。

Section 4 Stimulant-related Disorders

The CNS stimulants are identified by the behavioral stimulation and psychomotor agitation that they induce, usually including amphetamine and amphetamine-type stimulants (ATS) (such as amphetamine, dextroamphetamine, methamphetamine, and methylenedioxymethamphetamine), cocaine, caffeine, and tobacco, etc.

I. Clinical Manifestation

i. Stimulant Intoxication

Amphetamine and cocaine intoxication usually begins with a "high" feeling and accompanied by one or more of the following symptoms: euphoria with enhanced vigor, gregariousness, hyperactivity, restlessness, hypervigilance, interpersonal sensitivity, talkativeness, anxiety, tension, grandiosity, stereotyped and repetitive behavior, anger, impaired judgment, and, in the case of chronic intoxication, affective blunting with fatigue or sadness and social withdrawal. These behavioral and psychological changes are accompanied by two or more of the following signs and symptoms that develop during or shortly after stimulant use: tachycardia or bradycardia; pupillary dilation; elevated or lowered blood pressure; perspiration or chills; nausea or vomiting; evidence of weight loss; psychomotor agitation or retardation; muscular weakness, respiratory depression, chest pain, or cardiac arrhythmias; and confusion, seizures, dyskinesias, dystonias, or coma. Severe intoxication can lead to convulsions, cardiac arrhythmias, hyperpyrexia, and death.

ii. Stimulant Withdrawal

Withdrawal syndrome from stimulants such as amphetamines and cocaine is characterized by dysphoric mood, fatigue, vivid and unpleasant dreams, insomnia or hypersomnia, increased appetite, and psychomotor retardation or agitation. Bradycardia is often present and is a reliable measure of stimulant withdrawal.

II. Treatment

The treatment of stimulant intoxication is usually supportive care. Psychosocial and behavioral approaches, including cognitive-behavioral therapy and supportive-expressive psychotherapy, are the mainstays of treatment, and have been shown to help retain people in treatment

第四节 兴奋剂相关障碍

中枢神经系统兴奋剂主要引起兴奋行为及精神运动性兴奋，通常包括苯丙胺及苯丙胺类兴奋剂（如苯丙胺、右旋苯丙胺、甲基苯丙胺、亚甲基二氧基甲基苯丙胺）、可卡因、咖啡因及烟草等。

一、临床表现

（一）兴奋剂中毒

可卡因和苯丙胺类兴奋剂中毒通常由特殊的快感开始并包括以下一种及以上症状：兴奋及活动增强、群集性、活动增多、坐立不安、过度警觉、人际敏感性、说话增多、焦虑、紧张、警觉性、夸大、刻板重复行为、愤怒、判断力缺失。如果是慢性中毒，则主要表现为情感迟钝、疲劳或悲伤以及不合群。这些行为和心理变化通常在中断药物使用后出现，伴随着以下 2 种或以上的症状和体征，包括心动过速或过缓、瞳孔扩张、血压升高或降低、出汗或寒战、呕心或呕吐、体重下降、精神运动性兴奋或抑制、肌无力、呼吸抑制、胸痛、心律失常，以及精神错乱、癫痫、运动障碍、肌张力障碍或昏迷。严重中毒可导致抽搐、心律失常、高热和死亡。

（二）兴奋剂戒断

苯丙胺类物质和可卡因等兴奋剂物质的戒断症状主要包括烦躁不安、疲劳、不愉快的梦、失眠或嗜睡、食欲增加，以及精神运动性兴奋或抑制。心动过速是常见的戒断症状，并可将其作为兴奋剂戒断的判断依据。

二、治 疗

兴奋剂中毒的治疗原则主要是支持治疗。行为治疗，包括认知行为治疗和支持性心理治疗都可以增加患者的治疗依从性，帮助患者保持戒断。此外，近来 Matix 模式也成为

and can lead to abstinence. Moreover, the Matrix model, a 16-week manualized outpatient treatment is also an effective treatment for stimulant disorders. It combines cognitive-behavioral therapy materials and techniques, educational materials for client and family on the effects of stimulants, 12-step program participation, and positive reinforcement for behavior change and treatment compliance. Psychostimulants can be highly addicting, and chronic users must address causes of relapse and strategies for relapse prevention. Therefore, treatment should address conditions that lead to relapse, that is, reducing the effects of conditioned cues that trigger craving (such as persons with whom, or situations in which, the individual has used cocaine and the availability of cocaine in one's neighborhood).

一种有效的药物依赖干预方式，该模式是一种为期16周的院外治疗模式，其将认知行为治疗、患者及家庭健康教育、12步治疗及正性奖励等干预方式综合运用以改变成瘾行为。精神兴奋剂常是高度成瘾的，成瘾者必须清楚和理解复发的原因，掌握防止复发的策略。因此，治疗的关键在于排除引起复发的环境，减少可能引起复吸的触发因素，如与吸毒人群的交往、邻近社区中可获得可卡因等，从而彻底摆脱成瘾。

Anxiolytics or neuroleptics may be needed for agitation. But if an overdose of these medications occurs, further treatment may be needed. An α-adrenergic antagonist can be used to decrease elevated blood pressure, and antipsychotics may be needed to diminish CNS overstimulation. Cocaine overdoses can be more complicated because of the greater potential for cardiac arrhythmia, respiratory failure, and seizures. Chlorpromazine may be useful in reducing CNS and cardiovascular problems (as it has some α-adrenergic-inhibiting action). Artificial respiration or cardiac life support may be needed.

此外，可使用抗焦虑药或安定类药物来缓解兴奋，但若此类药物使用过量，需要紧急处理。例如可使用α肾上腺素拮抗剂降低血压，并可使用抗精神病药物减少中枢神经系统的过度兴奋。在可卡因过量使用时，因患者可能并发心律不齐、呼吸衰竭及肌肉阵挛，使该情况处理更加复杂。临床上可用氯丙嗪减轻中枢神经系统及心血管系统并发症，必要时采用呼吸支持或生命支持。

Section 5 Other Substance-related Disorders

第五节　其他物质相关障碍

I. Cannabis-Related Disorders

一、大麻相关障碍

Cannabis is the world's most widely used illicit substance. There are between 119 million and 224 million cannabisusers worldwide. Cannabis intoxication typically begins with a "high" feeling followed by symptoms that include euphoria, sedation, anxiety, a sensation of slowed time, lethargy, impairment in short-term memory, difficulty in implementing complex mental processes, impaired judgment, distorted sensory perceptions, and impaired motor performance. These psychoactive effects are accompanied by two or more of the following signs, developing within 2 hours of cannabis use: conjunctival injection, increased appetite, dry mouth, and tachycardia. Regarding cannabis withdrawal, the essential features may include irritability, anxiety, sleep difficulty, decreased

大麻是世界上使用最广泛的非法药物，全世界大麻使用者在1.19亿至2.24亿之间。大麻中毒的典型特征通常以"高亢"感开始，随后出现以下症状：不恰当的笑和夸张的欣快感、镇静、焦虑、感到时间变慢、昏睡、短期记忆损害、难以执行复杂的精神过程、判断力受损、感知觉扭曲及动作表现受损。这些精神效应通常伴有2个或更多以下的体征，通常发生在大麻使用后2小时以内：眼结膜充血、食欲增加、口干、心动过速。大麻戒断综合征的典型表现包括易激惹、焦虑、

appetite or weight loss, restlessness, or depressed mood. Physical symptoms comprise abdominal pain, shakiness or tremors, sweating, fever, chills, or headache.

睡眠困难、食欲下降或体重减轻、焦躁不安、心境抑郁，躯体症状包括腹痛、震颤、出汗、发热、寒战或头痛。

The treatment of cannabinoid intoxication usually requires only a safe, calm environment. Anxiolytic medications are used only in acute cases of severe agitation or anxiety. Studies support the use of brief intervention for problematic use or abuse of cannabis for instance, cognitive-behavioral, motivational enhancement, and contingency management approaches for the treatment of dependence. Educational programs are important parts of cannabis treatment, particularly among younger populations.

对大麻戒断的治疗通常需要为患者提供一个安全、安静的治疗环境，必要时，可应用抗焦虑药物以防止患者出现严重的激越或焦虑。目前研究支持对于大麻使用障碍可以采用简短认知行为干预、动机增强治疗、行为奖励、情境管理方法等心理行为干预方式。此外，健康教育对大麻戒断的治疗非常重要，尤其针对年轻人的教育。

II. Hallucinogen-Related Disorders

二、致幻剂相关障碍

Hallucinogens includes drugs that induce a distortion of reality in the user, including alterations of sensory perceptions of sight and sounds as well as changes in emotions. Lysergic acid diethylamide (LSD) is the prototypical hallucinogen. For hallucinogen intoxication, maladaptive behavioral or psychological changes include marked anxiety or depression, ideas of reference, fear of losing one's mind, paranoid ideation, and impaired judgment. Perceptual changes occur when individuals are fully aware and vigilant, including intensification of perceptions, depersonalization, derealization, illusions, hallucinations, and synesthesias. Physical symptoms include pupillary dilation, tachycardia, sweating, palpitations, blurring of vision, tremors, and incoordination. Hallucinogen withdrawal is not a recognized disorder, about 10% of hallucinogen users experience withdrawal symptoms, including fatigue, irritability, and anhedonia.

致幻剂是指可以使滥用者产生现实扭曲感的一类药物，包括对声、光感知障碍，以及相应的情绪改变。麦角酸二乙酰胺是最常见的致幻剂。致幻剂中毒主要表现为一系列不适应的行为或心理改变，包括显著的焦虑或抑郁、牵连观念、害怕“失去控制”、偏执观念及判断力受损。知觉的变化通常出现在完全清醒和警觉的状态下，如主观知觉的强化、人格解体、现实解体、错觉、幻觉以及联觉。躯体症状包括瞳孔扩大、心动过速、出汗、心悸、视物模糊、震颤及共济失调。通常致幻剂所致的戒断症状不被称为精神障碍，致幻剂使用者中通常有10%曾经历过戒断症状，包括疲乏、易激惹和快感丧失。

Detoxification from low dosages of hallucinogens can often be achieved with a safe, structured environment and emotional support. Anxiolytics and possibly neuroleptics may be needed. If respiratory suppression occurs, emergency oxygen may be required.

致幻剂中毒后的治疗主要为对症支持治疗，为患者提供一个安全、舒适的环境并提供心理支持是治疗的关键，对于有惊恐和紧张感的患者可以给予少量抗焦虑药和镇静药物。若发生呼吸抑制，则需要紧急给氧。

III. Inhalant-Related Disorders

三、吸入剂相关障碍

The National Institute on Drug Abuse has specified inhalant into four categories: volatile solvents, nitrites, gases, and aerosols. Inhalant intoxication is an inhalant-related, clinically significant mental disorder that develops during, or immediately after, intended or

美国药物滥用研究所将吸入剂主要分为四类：挥发溶剂、亚硝酸盐、笑气、气雾剂。吸入剂中毒是一种与吸入剂相关的，有临床意义的精神障碍，其发生在有意或无意的挥

unintended inhalation of a volatile hydrocarbon substance. Intoxication by volatile inhalants clears within a few minutes to a few hours after the exposure ends. Confusion, sedation, and possible euphoria often may result from use. Physical effects include analgesia, respiratory depression, hypotension, and ataxia. Withdrawal symptoms are not common with these drugs, however, the anticholinergic substances may cause tachycardia, sweating, depression, anxiety, or psychomotor agitation after use has been discontinued.

发性烃类物质吸入过程中或不久后。吸入剂中毒症状通常在终止接触后的数分钟或数小时内消失。在接触吸入剂后可能出现意识模糊、镇静、欣快感等，躯体反应包括痛觉丧失、呼吸抑制、血压降低和共济失调等。吸入剂使用后的戒断症状较少，然而抗胆碱能物质停止使用后可能会引起心动过速、出汗、抑郁、焦虑或精神激越。

Treatment of inhalant related disorders is supportive and addresses the acute medical complications resulting from inhalant use. Death can result from anoxia, aspiration, asphyxia, cardiac arrhythmias, respiratory depression, and sudden trauma.

吸入剂相关障碍的治疗主要是支持治疗以及吸入后的紧急处理，吸入剂使用后引发的不良反应包括缺氧、窒息、心律失常、呼吸抑制和意外损伤等均可能导致死亡。

IV. Sedative, Hypnotic, or Anxiolytic-Related Disorders

四、镇静、催眠药及抗焦虑药相关障碍

Benzodiazepines, as well as other sedative-hypnotics, are commonly used in the setting of polysubstance abuse. The essential feature of sedative, hypnotic, or anxiolytic intoxication may include inappropriate sexual or aggressive behavior, mood lability, impaired judgment, or impaired social or occupational functioning. Other symptoms that may develop with excessive use include slurred speech, incoordination, unsteady gait, nystagmus, impairment in attention or memory, and stupor or coma. Withdrawal symptoms associated with sedatives, hypnotics or anxiolytics include autonomic hyperactivity, increased hand tremor, insomnia, nausea or vomiting, hallucinations, illusions, psychomotor agitation, anxiety, or grand mal seizures.

苯二氮䓬类药物以及其他镇静催眠药物是最容易被合并滥用的药物。镇静、催眠药或抗焦虑药中毒的临床表现包括不恰当的性或攻击行为、情绪不稳定、判断力受损或社会功能及职业能力受损。其他的一些中毒症状或体征包括口齿不清、不协调、步态不稳、眼球震颤、认知损害、意识模糊或昏迷。戒断症状包括自主神经活动亢进、手部震颤、失眠、恶心或呕吐、幻觉、精神运动性激越、焦虑或癫痫大发作。

General strategies for the management of sedative-hypnotic withdrawal usually include gradually reducing the dosage of the sedative-hypnotic on which the client is dependent; substituting with a long-acting benzodiazepine and tapers off; substituting with a long-acting barbiturate (usually phenobarbital) and then tapers that; using valproate or carbamazepine. Management of severe benzodiazepine overdose includes careful monitoring of the patient's airway and ventilatory support when necessary. Repeated doses of activated charcoal may be particularly helpful in barbiturate or other non-benzodiazepine ingestions.

镇静催眠药物戒断症状的治疗通常包括以下措施：逐渐减少镇静催眠药物的使用剂量；选择长效的苯二氮䓬类药物替代并逐渐减量；使用长效巴比妥类药物（如苯巴比妥）替代并逐渐递减；使用丙戊酸钠或卡马西平。苯二氮䓬类药物过量使用的首要措施应保持呼吸通畅，必要时给予呼吸支持。巴比妥类药物或其他苯二氮䓬类药物过量使用后可使用活性炭进行吸附。

V. Tobacco-Related Disorders

五、烟草相关障碍

Tobacco use disorder is common among individuals who use cigarettes and smokeless tobacco daily. Cessation

烟草使用障碍常见于天天使用香烟和无

of tobacco use can produce withdrawal syndrome. Nicotine is thought to be the primary substance in tobacco that causes neuroadaptation, but nicotine intoxication is very rare. Withdrawal symptoms of tobacco often occur with abrupt discontinuation of nicotine intake. Symptoms include craving, anxiety, depression, irritability, headaches, poor concentration, sleep disturbances, enhanced blood pressure, appetite or weight gain and decreased heart rate. Tobacco withdrawal can produce clinically significant mood changes and functional impairment.

烟烟草的个体。烟草停用后的戒断症状多是由于尼古丁缺乏所致，但是尼古丁中毒非常少见。尼古丁摄入突然中断后通常出现戒断症状，包括渴求、焦虑、抑郁、激越、头痛、注意力不集中、睡眠障碍、血压升高、食欲或体重增加以及心率减慢。烟草戒断会产生有临床意义的心理变化及功能受损。

Non-pharmacologic approaches are frequently used to help tobacco users quit smoking. Issues such as weight gain and mood liability may need to be addressed, and strategies may need to be developed to help users get through the day without the need for tobacco use. Clonidine can help reduce withdrawal symptoms. Nicotine-containing products such as dermal patches and gum can be used to help titrate smokers off the nicotine. Antidepressants and limited anxiolytic drug therapy have also been helpful in some clients.

常用非药物治疗方法帮助烟草使用者戒烟。医护人员应向抽烟者说明增加体重及保持心境稳定的重要性，并协助抽烟者在戒烟阶段采用其他方式替代烟草，以逐渐戒断烟草。可乐定可用于缓解烟草戒断症状，也可用含尼古丁的产品如尼古丁贴片、尼古丁口香糖等帮助其戒烟，抗抑郁药及某些抗焦虑药也有一定的效果。

Section 6 Application of the Nursing Process

第六节　护理程序的应用

The nursing process is presented as the vehicle for delivery of care to the client with a substance-related disorder. Nurses must first examine his or her own feelings about working with clients who abuses substances. Only the nurse who can be accepting and nonjudgmental of substance-abuse behaviors will be effectively working with these clients.

应用护理程序对精神活性物质所致精神障碍患者进行护理至关重要。护士应首先明确自己对物质滥用的认识，只有充分且不带偏见地认识物质滥用的行为，才能对患者进行有效地干预和护理。

I. Nursing Assessment

一、护理评估

In psychiatric and substance abuse treatment programs, the assessment process is, in part, a treatment intervention. Clients are often in denial of the severity of the problem and the emotional, social, legal, vocational, or other consequences of it. Therefore, the assessment is crucial to understanding level of use, abuse, or dependence and determining the client's denial or acceptance of treatment. Assessment is often detailed and may involve family members and loved ones. Assessment often involves substance use assessment, physiological, psychological and social assessment.

对患者的全面评估是精神活性物质所致精神障碍治疗的一部分，患者常否认自己问题的严重性，且不承认因滥用物质所带来的情感、社会、法律及职业等一系列问题。因此，护士在评估时，评估对象应包括患者的家属，并尽可能获得有关患者物质使用的所有详细信息，了解患者物质的使用情况是使用、滥用还是依赖，患者是接受还是拒绝接受治疗，从而帮助明确患者物质使用或滥用的严重程度。评估的内容包括用药史、生理、心理及社会评估。

1. Substance Use Assessment Substance history assessment usually include type of substance, first use, pattern of use (amount, route, frequence, and length of use), last use, tolerance, problems caused by substance use, and withdrawal symptoms. Moreover, previous drug abuse treatment, desire or efforts to decrease use or control use, and social, vocational, recreational activities affected by use should be evaluated.

1. 用药史评估 内容通常包括患者用药的种类、首次使用时间、用药方式（药量、途径、频率以及用药持续时间）、末次使用时间及使用量、耐受性、物质使用所致的相关问题以及戒断症状等。此外，患者既往治疗情况、减少或控制物质使用的渴望以及因物质使用所引起的社会、职业及娱乐问题等也应该进行评价。

2. Physiological Assessment Contents are as follows: general condition of clients (vital signs, skin integrity, nutritional status, etc.); neurological status (reflex, peripheral nerve injury, etc.); physical withdrawal symptoms (tremors, hyperreflexia, insomnia, ataxia, etc.); complications (peripheral neuropathy, cardiovascular disorder, hepatic disfunction, gastritis, etc.); and laboratory examination, such as γ-Glutamyltransferase (GGT) and carbohydrate-deficient transferrin (%CDT), which can be clues to an alcohol use disorder.

2. 生理评估 包括患者的一般情况（生命体征、皮肤完整性及营养状态等）、神经系统状况（反射情况、周围神经损伤情况等）、躯体戒断症状（震颤、恶心呕吐、失眠、共济失调等）、并发症（神经系统疾病、心血管系统疾病、肝肾功能损害、消化道疾病等）、实验室及其他辅助检查，如γ-谷氨酰转移酶、糖缺乏转铁蛋白可作为酒精相关障碍的评估依据。

3. Psychological Assessment Psychological assessment comprises several aspects: cognition (such as consciousness, thought, intelligence, memory, attention, orientation, etc.), emotion (such as anxiety, depression, agitation, etc.), activities (drug use motivation, ways of coping, drug-seeking behavior, etc.), and personality characteristics of clients.

3. 心理评估 内容包括认知活动（例如意识、思维、智力、记忆力、注意力及定向力等）、情感活动（例如焦虑、抑郁、激越等）、意志行为活动（例如用药动机、应对方式、觅药行为等）、患者的人格特征。

4. Social Assessment In terms of social assessment, work or learning status, interpersonal skills, activities of daily living, bad behavior, relationship with families, and social support system should be contained.

4. 社会评估 评估内容包括工作或学习状态、人际交往能力、日常活动能力、不良行为、患者与家庭成员的关系以及社会支持系统等。

5. Evaluation Tools Some evaluation tools could be used for assessment, such as the clinical institute withdrawal assessment of alcohol scale, revised (CIWA-Ar), used to assess risk and severity of withdrawal from alcohol; penn alcohol craving scale (PACA), measurement of alcohol craving. Moreover, other screening tools exist for determining whether an individual has a problem with substances, such as alcohol use disorders identification test (AUDIT) used to help determine if clients have alcoholism problems.

5. 评估工具 评估过程中可以借鉴一些评估工具，如用于评估酒精戒断症状及严重程度的临床机构用酒精戒断状态评定量表、用于评估酒精渴求程度的宾夕法尼亚酒精渴求量表，也有一些用于评估个体是否存在物质使用障碍的筛查量表，如用于筛查酒精使用障碍者的酒精使用障碍筛查评估问卷。

II. Nursing Diagnosis

二、护理诊断

1. Acute Confusion Related to substance intoxication and withdrawal symptoms.

1. 急性意识障碍 与物质使用过量中毒、戒断反应有关。

2. Disturbed Sensory Perception Rrelated to substance use and physiologic changes secondary to substance withdrawal.

3. Risk for Injury Related to CNS agitation (tremors, hallucinations, seizures, etc.).

4. Imbalanced Nutrition Less than body requirements related to use of substances evidenced by loss of weight, electrolyte imbalance, anemias and/or other signs and symptoms of malnutrition.

5. Ineffective Denial Related to weak, underdeveloped ego evidenced by statements indicating no problem with substance use.

6. Ineffective Coping Related to inadequate coping skills and weak ego evidenced by use of substance as a coping mechanism.

7. Chronic Low Self-esteem Related to weak ego, lack of positive feedback and use of substances as coping mechanism.

8. Deficient Knowledge Related to denial of problems with substance abuse.

2. 感知觉紊乱 与物质使用、物质戒断所引起的生理改变有关。

3. 有受伤害的危险 与中枢神经系统兴奋如震颤、幻觉及癫痫发作等有关。

4. 营养失调：低于机体需要 与物质使用所致体重下降、电解质失衡、贫血和/或其他营养不良等有关。

5. 无效否认 与自我价值感降低、认知歪曲有关。

6. 应对无效 与应对技巧不足、将物质使用作为应对机制有关。

7. 长期性低自尊 与低自尊、缺乏正性反馈、滥用物质行为有关。

8. 知识缺乏 与否认物质滥用的危害性有关。

III. Nursing planning

i. Nursing Outcome

The following criteria may be used for measurement of outcomes in the care of the client with substance-related disorders.

The client:

1. The client has not experienced persistent and aggravated withdrawal symptoms, keeps stable vital signs.
2. The client has not experienced physical injury or caused harm to self or others.
3. The client shows no signs or symptoms of infection or malnutrition.
4. The client follows the plan to substance cessation and controls the drug-seeking behavior.
5. The client accepts responsibility for own behavior, and acknowledges association between personal problems and use of substance.
6. The client demonstrates more adaptive coping mechanisms that can be used in stressful situations instead of taking substances.
7. The client exhibits evidence of increased self-worth by attempting new projects and demonstrating less defensive behavior toward others.
8. The client verbalizes importance of abstaining from use of substances.

三、护理计划

（一）护理目标

精神活性物质所致精神障碍患者的护理目标一般包括以下内容：

1. 患者的戒断症状得到控制，生命体征保持平稳，并逐渐恢复正常。
2. 患者没有躯体伤害或未对自己或他人造成伤害。
3. 患者的营养状态得到改善，未发生感染性疾病。
4. 患者能按计划进行物质戒断，并控制物质觅取行为。
5. 患者能够承认自己行为的责任，承认自己的问题和物质使用之间的关系。
6. 患者能够逐渐建立积极的应对机制并代替物质使用将其运用于压力处理过程。
7. 患者能够逐渐建立正向的自我概念，并有效控制对他人的防御行为。
8. 患者能够表明物质戒断对维持躯体健康的重要性。

ii. Nursing Intervention

Implementation of clients with substance-related disorders is a long-term process. Nurses should formulate nursing interventions based on comprehensive analysis of assessment information.

1. Diet Management

(1) If clients can consume oral diet, appropriate number of calories required to provide adequate nutrition and realistic weight gain should be determined. While if clients are unable to maintain an adequate oral intake, liquid diet may be administered via nasogastric tube. Parenteral support may be required initially to correct fluid and electrolyte imbalance, hypoglycemia, and some vitamin deficiencies.

(2) Document intake and output and keep strict record of calorie count. Weigh client daily to maintain ongoing nutritional assessment. Assess skin turgor and integrity regularly.

(3) Provide small frequent feeding of client's favorite foods. Supplement nutritious meals with multiple vitamin and mineral. Ensure that the amount of protein in the diet is correct for the individual client's condition. Protein intake should be adequate to maintain nitrogen equilibrium, but should be drastically decreased or eliminated if there is potential for hepatic coma. Sodium may need to be restricted if fluid retention (e.g., ascites and edema) is a problem. Provide foods that are nonirritating to clients with esophageal varices, to avoid irritation and bleeding of these swollen blood vessels. Encourage cessation of smoking.

2. Safety Care

(1) Assess client's level of disorientation to determine specific requirements for safety. Identify severity of withdrawal symptoms, and monitor gait and motor coordination, presence of tremors, mental status, electrolyte balance, etc. Obtain a drug history, if possible, to determine the type of substances used, time of last ingestion and amount consumed, length and frequency of consumption, and amount consumed on a daily basis.

(2) Obtain urine or blood sample for laboratory analysis of substance content. Subjective history is often not accurate. Knowledge regarding substance ingestion is important for accurate assessment of client's condition.

(3) Vital signs provide the most reliable information regarding client's condition, monitor vital signs every 15 minutes initially and less frequently as acute symptoms subside. Follow the medication prescription as ordered.

（二）护理措施

精神活性物质所致精神障碍患者的护理干预是一个长期的过程，护士需在全面分析评估资料的基础上，制订相应的护理措施。

1. 饮食管理

（1）患者能够经口进食时，应根据患者的实际体重、活动量等提供足够的营养物质及热能，患者不能经口进食时则需要安置胃管以提供足够的营养需求，必要时建立静脉通路，给予静脉营养支持以纠正水电解质失衡、血糖过低以及一些维生素缺乏等。

（2）观察患者每餐进食情况，记录每日的出入量及所需热量，每日记录患者的体重以进行持续的营养评估，定期评估患者的皮肤水肿情况及完整性等。

（3）给予少量多餐易消化饮食，食物富含维生素和矿物质，确保患者每天足够的蛋白摄入量，以维持机体的正氮平衡，但当患者有肝昏迷的危险时，注意禁用或限用蛋白质，当患者有腹水或水肿时，应限制钠的入量，对有食管静脉曲张的患者，避免粗硬及刺激性食物，以免引起消化道出血。针对吸烟的患者应鼓励患者戒烟。

2. 安全护理

（1）评估患者的意识水平、精神状态、戒断症状的严重程度、共济失调、震颤、电解质平衡等，详细询问患者的用药史，包括服用药物的种类、量、时间和频率，最后一次服用的药物总量、时间及每天服用量等，确定患者是否有安全隐患。

（2）获取患者的尿样进行分析，以确定患者服用药物的浓度和量，从而获得有关患者状况的准确资料。

（3）监测患者的生命体征，尤其是在急性脱毒期，必要时每15分钟一次或根据患者病情进一步缩短监测间隔时间，遵医嘱给予必要的药物支持。

(4) Place client in a quiet and private room. Avoid sudden moves, loud noises, discussion of client at bedside. Excessive stimuli may increase client's agitation. Institute necessary safety precautions: (a) observe client's behaviors frequently, assign staff on one-to-one basis if condition is warranted; (b) aAccompany and assist client when he or she is ambulating, use wheelchair for transporting long distances; (c) be sure that side rails are up when client is in bed; (d) pad headboard and side rails of bed with thick towels to protect client in case of seizure; (e) use mechanical restraints as necessary to protect client if excessive hyperactivity accompanies the disorientation.

（4）保持病房环境安静，避免外界刺激引起或加重患者的激惹，如突然移动患者、噪音、床旁讨论患者病情等。护士应注意对患者实施必要的安全防护措施，例如：密切观察患者的病情变化，必要时安排1名护士床旁护理；长距离转运时使用轮椅；当患者卧床时确保床护栏立起；用厚毛巾保护床头板和床栏以避免患者癫痫发作时受伤；必要时使用制动装置如保护性约束以确保患者的安全等。

(5) Ensure that smoking materials and other potentially harmful objects are stored away from client's access. Client may harm self or others in disoriented, confused state. Suicide precautions may be needed.

（5）确保患者远离可能导致伤害的物品，如利器等，以免患者在意识模糊时伤害他人和自己，必要时应采取自杀预防措施。

(6) Frequently orient client to reality and surroundings. Disorientation may endanger client safety if he or she unknowingly wanders away from safe environment.

（6）引导患者适应现实及周围环境，因定向力障碍可能危及患者安全。

3. Special Nursing

3. 特殊护理

(1) Acute intoxication nursing: Reduce environmental stimuli. Keep the environment safe and quiet, and bed comfortable and clean. Firstly, confirm what kind of drug, observe symptoms of acute intoxication closely, for example, the symptoms of clients with acute alcohol intoxication often include unsteady gait, disorientation, and confusion, etc. Focus on laboratory test results, such as blood alcohol level, evaluate the clinical manifestations that clients may present and take preventive measures. Prescribed for intravenous rehydration therapy and medication such as naloxone, benzodiazepines drugs, etc. if necessary, vomiting and gastrolavage will be used. Monitor vital signs closely, keep respiratory tract unobstructed, maintain fluid and electrolyte balance. Sputum suction and oxygen inhalation may be required when necessary.

（1）急性中毒的护理：保持病房环境安全、安静，患者床单位舒适整洁，减少环境刺激。首先确认是何种药物中毒，密切观察患者急性中毒的表现，如急性酒精中毒时患者常表现为步态不稳、定向力障碍、意识模糊等。关注患者实验室检查结果，如血乙醇浓度检查结果，判断患者可能出现的临床表现并采取预防性措施。遵医嘱予以静脉补液治疗及对症药物治疗如纳洛酮、苯二氮䓬类药物等，必要时给予催吐、洗胃。严密监测生命体征，保持呼吸道通畅，维持水电解质及酸碱平衡，必要时吸痰、吸氧。

(2) Nursing of withdrawal symptoms: Assess whether clients ever experienced withdrawal symptoms and its severity, and closely observe withdrawal symptoms, such as palpitation, sweating, etc. Symptomatic treatment and medication will be needed follow the prescription to control withdrawal symptoms of clients. According to the type of substances used, time of last used and amount consumed, etc., combining with the scale evaluation and laboratory test results, estimate the possible withdrawal symptoms that clients may present and give preventive measures in advance. Clients with alcohol dependence may appear severe withdrawal symptoms such as tremor, delirium and grand mal, nurses should closely observe

（2）戒断症状的护理：评估患者以往是否出现过戒断症状及其严重程度，密切观察目前戒断症状的出现，如心慌、出汗等，遵医嘱给予对症处理及药物治疗，控制患者出现的戒断症状。根据患者的末次物质使用时间、类型及使用量等，结合量表评定及实验室检查结果，评估患者可能出现的戒断症状，提前给予预防措施。酒依赖患者可能出现震颤、谵妄及癫痫大发作等严重戒断症状，应密切观察其病情变化，尽量让患者卧床休息，确保其安全，保持呼吸道通畅，防止出现舌咬

clients' conditions, let clients rest in bed as far as possible to ensure safety, keep respiratory tract unobstructed, and prevent tongue bite and trauma. Moreover, nurses should assess orientations and the state of consciousness of clients, and give corresponding medication treatment by doctor's orders to maintain fluid and electrolyte balance and nutrition supply.

4. Psychological Nursing

(1) Develop trust. Convey an attitude of acceptance. Be honest and keep all promises. Ensure that client understands it is not the person but the behavior that is unacceptable. Unconditional acceptance promotes dignity and self-worth that individual has been trying to achieve with substances.

(2) Establish therapeutic relationship. Usually nurses encounter individuals during crisis when they seek professional help. These situations offer an opportunity to explore the denial that keeps their addiction thriving. Approaches that are punitive or attempt to elicit feelings of guilt or shame are destructive to the therapeutic relationship. There are several general guidelines for establishing therapeutic interactions with clients: encourage honest expression of feelings; listen to what the individual is really saying; express caring for the individual; hold the individual responsible for behavior; provide consequences for negative behavior that are fair and consistent; talk about specific actions that are objectionable; do not compromise your own values or nursing practice; communicate the treatment plan to the client and to others on the treatment team; monitor your own reactions to the client.

(3) Correct any misconceptions about substance abuse, such as "I don't have a drinking problem. I can quit at any time I want to." Do this in a matter-of-fact, nonjudgmental manner. Explain the pharmacological effects of substances to the clients and emphasize the relationship between prognosis and abstinence. Answer any questions the clients may have regarding the disorder. These interventions help the client see the condition as an illness that requires help.

(4) Identify recent maladaptive behaviors or situations that have occurred in the client's life, and discuss use of substances may be a contribution factors. Let the client know the relationship between substance use and personal problems.

伤及外伤，及时评估患者的定向力及意识状态，遵医嘱给予相应的药物治疗，保持水电解质平衡及营养供给。

4. 心理护理

（1）获得患者的信任。护士应以接受的态度面对患者，并保持诚信，要让患者明白是行为本身不能被接受而非其本人。护士无条件地接受患者可以增加患者的自尊和自我价值感，而这些感觉也许是患者以前只能在服用药物时才可获得。

（2）建立良好的治疗性护患关系。通常护士所面对的是处于危机状况下寻求医疗帮助的个体，治疗性关系的建立为防止患者进一步使用物质提供了机会，而惩罚或试图唤起负罪感和羞耻都可能破坏治疗性关系的建立。在治疗性护患关系的建立中，护士可以遵从以下原则：① 鼓励患者诚实地表达自己的感情；② 认真倾听患者的陈述；③ 对患者表示关怀；④ 保留患者对自己行为的责任；⑤ 对负面行为进行公平、一致的处理；⑥ 与患者交谈某些会引起反对的行为；⑦ 坚持自己的价值观和护理措施；⑧ 与患者和其他医护人员交流有关患者的治疗计划；⑨ 监督自己对患者的反应。

（3）纠正患者对物质滥用的错误认知，弥补患者对物质滥用危害相关知识的缺乏。比如患者会说："我没有酗酒，只要我想，我可以随时戒掉"，但也许事实并非如此。因此，护士应以实事求是、无偏见的态度帮助患者纠正错误认知，向患者讲解滥用物质的药理作用及危害，并向患者强调物质使用与疾病预后之间的关系，尽可能解答患者关于物质相关障碍疾病的疑问，让患者意识到目前的状况是一种疾病状态，并应积极寻求专业帮助。

（4）帮助患者识别生活中最近发生的不良事件，并与其讨论物质使用可能是导致这些事件发生的原因，帮助患者认识物质使用和个人问题之间的关系。

(5) Do not allow client to rationalize or blame others for behaviors associated with substance use. This only serves to prolong the denial. When clients express insight gained regarding illness and acceptance of responsibility for own behavior, immediate positive recognition should be offered to enhance self-esteem and repetition of desirable behaviors. Moreover, nurses should help the client to set limits on behaviors and let the client know what is acceptable and the consequences for violating the limits. Make sure all staff know the limits and keep consistency with it.

（5）阻止患者合理化物质使用的相关行为或指责他人，因患者的这些行为只会延长患者的否认，但当患者表现出对疾病有所认识以及愿意对自己行为负责时，护士应立即予以积极回应以提高患者的自尊并促进期望行为的重复发生。此外，护士应帮助患者能够约束和管理自己的行为，让患者清楚哪些行为是可以接受的，并共同制订违反行为规定的后果，护士应确保所有医务人员都知道该患者的约束行为规定并保持一致的态度。

(6) Enhance the coping skills. Help the clients exploring the options available to cope with stressful situations rather than resorting to substance use and instructing knowledge of adaptive responses to stress. Encourage the clients to verbalize feelings, fears, and anxieties, which may help them come to terms with long-unresolved issues. Encourage the clients to be as independent as possible in performing his or her self-care. Provide positive feedback for independent decision-making and effective use of problem-solving skills.

（6）提高患者的应对技巧。护士应帮助患者分析、识别及运用更有效地正确应对方式来对待和处理压力问题，从而避免采用服用药物的方式减轻压力。此外，护士应向患者讲解有关压力适应反应的相关知识帮助患者有效识别压力；鼓励患者用言语表达感受、恐惧和焦虑等，这可能会帮助患者正面面对长期未解决的问题；鼓励患者尽可能独立地进行自我照顾，当患者能独立决策和有效运用问题解决技巧时应及时给予积极反馈。

(7) Encourage clients to participate in group therapy, such as recreation therapy, music activities, self-help groups, etc. This can help clients dealing with drug cravings. Moreover, more accepted peer feedback and peer pressure can strongly influence individuals who are experiencing or who have experienced similar problems.

（7）鼓励患者参与团体治疗，例如工娱治疗、音乐治疗、压力管理等，其有助于患者应对物质渴求。此外，患者更愿意接受来自同伴的反馈，而团体治疗中来自同伴的压力对于那些正在经历或已经经历同样问题的个体有很大影响。

5. Health Education and Social Support

5. 健康教育与社会支持

(1) Strengthen health education about substance related disorders aiming at the client and families to improve the understanding of the harm caused by substance use, including the damage of substance use to the body, the influence of substance use for life, and so on. In addition, knowledges about disease management such as stress coping skills, relaxation techniques, problem solving skills, nutrition related knowledge explained in health education, and instruction of social support services resources, also can promote the health of client.

（1）加强对患者及家属物质相关障碍的健康教育，提高其对物质危害性的认识，内容包括物质对躯体的危害、物质使用对生活的影响等。此外，关于疾病管理方面的知识如压力应对技巧、放松技术、问题解决技巧、营养相关知识等的健康教育，以及社会支持服务资源的相关宣教，也可为患者的健康促进及维持提供支持。

(2) Assist to establish family social support system. It is very important for clients' rehabilitation that family members provide reliable support for clients with substance related disorders. Clients should be encouraged to participate in family therapy to help their families to know substance abuse related knowledge, strengthen

（2）协助建立家庭社会支持系统。家庭成员提供可靠支持对物质相关障碍患者的康复非常重要，应鼓励患者参与家庭治疗，协助患者家属了解物质滥用相关知识，强化家庭功能，提高患者的家庭支持，其有助于患者

family function and improve family support. It can help clients coping with substance desires. In addition, introducing substance related disorders in community is significant to improve relevant knowledge about the disease in community residents. Community stations can be established to encourage clients to participate in community activities. This intervention may create a good environment for the community rehabilitation of clients.

应对物质渴求。此外，加强对物质使用相关障碍的社区宣传，提高社区居民对疾病的相关认识，可以建立社区活动站，鼓励患者参与社区活动，有利于为患者创造良好的社区康复环境。

(3) Encourage participation in self-help groups. Self-help groups are organized by clients with substance use disorders spontaneously. The purpose is helping substance withdrawal mutually and back to a normal life. All the members will remain external anonymous. In the group, members share their experiences, confidence and hope, to achieve the purpose of withdrawal. The core of self-help group is combination of self-help and mutual assistance, and to solve problem by the power of all members. Current mode of self-help groups mainly develop from 12 steps of Alcoholic Anonymous (AA), including alcohol dependent anonymous group, nicotine dependent anonymous group, and methamphetamine dependent anonymous group, etc.

（3）鼓励参与自助团体。自助团体是物质使用障碍者自行组织的团体，活动宗旨是成员之间互助戒断物质，重新过正常的生活，所有成员对外都保持匿名。在活动中物质依赖者互相分享各自的经历、自信和希望，以达到戒断的目的。自助团体的核心是自助与互助相结合，依靠物质使用障碍者集体的力量共同解决问题。目前的自助团体模式主要是在酒依赖匿名协会（Alcoholic Anonymous，AA）12 步策略上发展起来的互助者小组，包括酒精依赖者匿名小组、尼古丁依赖者匿名小组、冰毒依赖者匿名小组等。

IV. Nursing Evaluation

四、护理评价

To determine if the nursing interventions have been effective in achieving the intended goals of care, the client with a substance-related disorder may be evaluated by the following reassessment questions.

1. Has detoxification or withdrawal occurred without complications?

2. Does the client cooperate with treatment and do no harm to self or others?

3. Has nutritional status been restored? Does the client consume adequate diet according to his or her own needs? Has the client remained free of infection during hospitalization?

4. Has the client remained substance-free during hospitalization?

5. Does the client accept responsibility for his or her own behavior? Has the client acknowledged a personal problem with substances? Has a correlation been made between personal problems and the use of substances?

6. Is the client able to verbalize alternative adaptive coping strategies instead of substance use? Has these strategies been used? Does positive reinforcement encourage repetition of these adaptive behaviors?

7. Does the client still make excuses or blame others for use of substances? Does the client refrain from

通过护理计划的实施，护士可以通过以下问题，对精神活性物质所致精神障碍患者进行评价。

1. 患者脱毒或戒断过程中有无发生并发症。

2. 患者是否配合治疗，有无出现伤害自己或他人的行为。

3. 患者营养状态是否得到改善，其饮食摄入能否满足机体和活动需要，有无发生躯体感染性疾病。

4. 患者住院期间是否不再服用精神活性物质，能否控制药物觅取行为。

5. 患者能否为其行为承担责任，是否承认物质使用所带来的个人问题，并认识到物质使用与个人问题之间的联系。

6. 患者能否说出一些替代物质使用的其他应对方法，是否已采用这些方法，正面强化是否促进了这些方法的重复应用。

7. 患者是否仍为自己使用物质寻找借口或归咎于他人，是否能控制和约束自己。

manipulative behavior and violation of limits?

8. Is the client able to verbalize the effects of substance abuse on the body? Does the client express that he or she wants to recover and abstain from use of substances?

(Chen Juan)

8. 患者是否能够说出物质滥用对机体的损害，是否表达他/她希望康复并拥有一个远离物质使用的生活。

（陈 娟）

Key Points

1. Psychoactive substances can be classified into four groups according to their pharmacological features. These include central nervous system (CNS) depressants, CNS stimulants, hallucinogens, and volatile inhalants.

2. The etiology of substance use disorders has been conceptualized in terms of an integration of biological, psychological, social-cultural theories, and dependence of substances, such as genetics, biochemical changes, personality factors, social learning, and cultural and ethnic influences.

3. Inappropriate medical prescription or repeated self-administration of psychoactive drugs may cause dependence syndrome and/or other mental disorders, such as intoxication, withdrawal syndrome, psychotic symptoms, affective disorders, and residual or delayed-onset mental disorders.

4. Substance abuse is to use wrongfully or in a harmful way, described as a maladaptive pattern of substance use manifested by recurrent and significant adverse consequences related to repeated use of the substance.

5. Substance intoxication is defined as the development of a reversible substance-specific syndrome caused by the recent ingestion of (or exposure to) a substance.

6. Substance withdrawal is the development of a substance specific maladaptive behavioral change, with physiological and cognitive concomitants, that is due to the cessation of or reduction in, heavy and prolonged substance use.

7. Treatment of substance abuse requires a multistage process. Generally, clients must go through detoxification, rehabilitation, and then relapse prevention (aftercare). The biopsychosocial model is a useful guide to the treatment of substance use disorders. As a result, both pharmacologic and non-pharmacologic approaches are important in the treatment of substance abuse.

8. Treatment modalities for substance-related disorders include self-help groups, individual counseling, group therapy, and family therapy. Substitution pharmacotherapy is frequently implemented with clients experiencing substance intoxication or substance withdrawal.

内容摘要

1. 精神活性物质按药理学特性可分为四类，包括中枢神经抑制剂、中枢神经兴奋剂、致幻剂和挥发性溶剂。

2. 精神活性物质所致精神障碍的病因是生物、心理、社会文化因素及精神活性物质的依赖性几方面共同作用的结果，包括遗传因素、生物化学因素、个人因素、社会学习因素以及文化影响等。

3. 精神活性物质可由医生处方不当或个人擅自反复使用导致依赖综合征和其他精神障碍，如中毒、戒断综合征、精神病性症状、情感障碍，残留性或迟发性精神障碍等。

4. 物质滥用是指错误或有害的使用方法，一种适应不良方式，由于反复使用物质导致了明显的不良后果。

5. 物质中毒主要表现为近期使用或暴露于某种物质后所出现的可逆的与物质相关的特有的综合征。

6. 物质戒断主要为绝对或相对戒断某种长期大剂量使用的物质后所出现的一组与物质相关的特有的不适应的躯体和精神症状。

7. 精神活性物质所致精神障碍的治疗是一个长期的过程。一般来说患者要经过脱毒、康复和复吸的预防（治疗后）三个阶段的治疗。治疗应以生理、心理、社会医学模式为指导，采用药物和非药物治疗方法进行综合治疗，以提高治疗效果。

8. 精神活性物质所致精神障碍的治疗方法包括自助团体、个人咨询、团体治疗和家庭治疗等。替代药物疗法通常运用于物质中毒或物质戒断，其治疗方法取决于损害的严重

Treatment modalities are implemented depending on the severity of the impairment.

9. The nursing process is presented as the vehicle for delivery of care of the client with a substance-related disorder. The nurse must first examine his or her own feelings regarding personal and others' substance use. Only the nurse who can be accepting and nonjudgmental of substance-abuse behaviors will be effective in working with these clients.

程度。

9. 应用护理程序对精神活性物质所致精神障碍患者进行护理至关重要。护士应首先明确自己对物质滥用的认识，只有充分认识物质滥用的行为，才能有效对患者进行干预和护理。

Exercises

(Questions 1 to 2 share the same question stem)

While admitting a client to the alcohol treatment program, the nurse asks the client how long she's been drinking this time, how much she's been drinking and when she had her last drink. The client replies that she has been drinking about a liter of vodka a day for the past week and her last drink was about an hour ago.

1. What should the nurse expect as a result of this statement?

2. Which nursing interventions would be appropriate for the client?

(Questions 3 to 4 share the same question stem)

A client who is brought to the emergency room by ambulance begins to thrash about on the stretcher, slapping the sheets and yelling, "Go away, bugs, go away!" Assessment reveals disorientation, a blood pressure of 189/75 mmHg, and a pulse of 86 bpm. The friend who accompanied the client to the hospital states, "He was drinking a lot when I saw him 4 days ago and asked me for money to get more liquor, but I didn't have any cash to give him."

3. Based on an analysis of these findings, the nurse suspects that the client is experiencing which conditions?

4. Which nursing actions would the nurse institute to help the client to relieve the symptoms?

(Questions 5 to 6 share the same question stem)

During an interaction with the nurse, the client states that her "life has gone down the tubes" since her divorce 6 months ago. Afterwards, she lost her job and apartment and then she "took those pills to sleep and not wake up."

5. From this data, the nurse would identify which nursing diagnoses for the client?

6. Which psychological interventions could be applied in this client?

思考题

（1～2题共用题干）

在戒酒治疗中心为患者办理入院手续时，护士询问患者这次饮酒持续了多长时间，饮酒量是多少，以及最后一次饮酒的时间。患者回答在过去的一周内，她每天大约饮用伏特加1L，她最后一次饮酒是在1小时前。

1. 患者提供的这些信息，护士可以做出哪些判断？

2. 针对该患者可以提供的护理措施有哪些？

（3～4题共用题干）

一位患者被救护车送到急救病房，他在担架上翻腾着，拍打着被单大声喊叫："滚开，家伙们，滚开"，评估显示：患者定向力障碍，血压189/75 mmHg，脉搏86次/min。陪同患者来的朋友陈述："我4天前见他时，他喝了很多酒，并且向我借钱要买更多的烈性酒喝，但是我没有现金给他。"

3. 分析以上信息，护士应该怀疑患者正处于哪种状态？

4. 护士可以采取哪些护理措施以帮助患者缓解症状？

（5～6题共用题干）

在与护士交流的过程中，一名患者说自从6个月前离婚后，她的生活就被彻底毁坏了。后来，她失去了工作和公寓，然后她吃了那些药使自己沉睡不醒。

5. 从这些信息中，护士应优先考虑护理诊断有哪些？

6. 针对该患者可以采取的心理干预措施有哪些？

(Questions 7 to 8 share the same question stem)

The friend of a client brought to the hospital's emergency room states, "I guess she had some bad junk (heroin) today." The client is drowsy and verbally non-responsive.

7. Based on the information, which assessment findings would be of immediate concern to the nurse?

8. Which nursing interventions would be appropriate for the client when she is in stable condition?

（7～8题共用题干）

一位在医院急诊室住院的患者的朋友说："我猜想她今天吸了海洛因"。患者处于昏昏欲睡的状态且没有口头回应。

7. 根据以上信息，哪些评估内容是需要护士立即关注的？

8. 哪些心理治疗方法适合对该患者进行干预？

Chapter 12 Nursing Care of Clients with Organic Mental Disorders

第十二章 器质性精神障碍患者的护理

Learning Objectives

Memorization

1. Describe the terms of organic mental disorder, delirium, dementia, Alzheimer's disease and vascular dementia.
2. Describe clinical manifestations of delirium and dementia.
3. Describe treatment modalities relevant to care of clients with delirium, dementia, Alzheimer's disease or vascular dementia.

Comprehension

1. Explain predisposing and precipitating factors to delirium.
2. Discuss characteristic neuropathological changes of Alzheimer's disease and the predisposing factors to vascular dementia.
3. Identify nursing diagnoses common to clients with delirium, dementia, Alzheimer's disease or vascular dementia.

Application

1. Assess clients with delirium or dementia based on the clinical manifestations.
2. Plan the principles of nursing interventions to clients with common neurocognitive disorders based on the corresponding nursing diagnoses.
3. Implement care plan for clients with delirium or dementia based on their nursing diagnoses and nursing plan.

学习目标

识记

1. 能描述器质性精神障碍、谵妄、痴呆、阿尔茨海默病和血管性痴呆的概念。
2. 能描述谵妄和痴呆的临床表现。
3. 能描述谵妄、痴呆、阿尔茨海默病和血管性痴呆的治疗方式 。

理解

1. 能解释谵妄的易感因素和诱发因素。
2. 能讨论阿尔茨海默病的神经病理学特征和血管性痴呆的易感因素。
3. 能识别谵妄、痴呆、阿尔茨海默病和血管性痴呆患者的常见护理诊断。

运用

1. 基于临床表现评估谵妄或痴呆患者。
2. 能在护理诊断的基础上制订常见神经认知功能障碍患者的护理措施。
3. 能在护理诊断和护理计划的基础上实施对谵妄或痴呆患者的护理措施。

Mr. Chen is accompanied by his wife to the outpatient department. He is a 67-year-old man who has lived with his wife in Shanghai. The couples reared two sons who are married and have been living in the districts nearly an hour's bus from their home. Mrs. Chen found her husband's memory became poor which is different from the decline of normal memory with his age. For example, he always forgot quickly the words she told him and she had to repeat several times. One month ago, Mrs. Chen found her husband's motion of dialing mobile phone numbers was very slow and uncoordinated. She felt his condition was abnormal, but she did not know which department she should take him to see a doctor. Last week, Mrs. Chen watched a TV program introducing Alzheimer's disease. She doubted that her husband might suffer from this illness because his symptoms are very similar to what introduced in the program, such as poor memory, repeating words, and slow movement, etc.

Please think about the following questions based on the case:

1. What are the core symptoms of Alzheimer's disease?
2. What are the roles of psychiatric mental health nurses in care for persons with Alzheimer's disease and other types of neurocognitive disorders?

陈先生由他的太太陪同到门诊部。他是一个67岁的男子，和他的妻子住在上海。夫妇俩养育了两个儿子，均已婚、居住的小区到他们家要坐将近一小时的公交车。陈太太发现她丈夫的记忆力变差了，且记忆下降的程度与他的年龄不符。比如，他总是很快就忘记了她告诉他的话，她不得不重复几次。一个月前，陈太太发现他用手机拨号的动作非常缓慢、不协调。她觉得他的情况不正常，但又不知道她应该带他去看哪科的医生。上周，陈女士观看了一个介绍阿尔茨海默病的电视节目。她觉得她丈夫可能患了这个病，因为他的症状和电视节目里介绍的很相似，如记忆力差、话不断重复、行动迟缓等。

请思考：

1. 阿尔茨海默病的核心症状有哪些？
2. 精神科护士在照护阿尔茨海默病和其他神经认知障碍患者中的角色及作用？

Organic mental disorder is a form of mental disorder due to cerebral or systemic diseases. Mental disorders due to cerebral organic diseases refer to a series of psychotics resulted from known biological causes and pathophysiological mechanisms in brain. They can be differentiated from so-called "functional disorders", such as schizophrenia to mood disorders. The disorders due to cerebral diseases include degenerative diseases, cerebrovascular diseases, intracranial infection, cerebral trauma, encephalomas and epilepsy. The term "symptomatic" is used for those organic mental disorders in which cerebral involvement is secondary to a systemic extracerebral disease.

Organic mental disorders can be categorized into three groups: mental disorders due to cerebral organic diseases, mental disorders due to physical illness, and mental disorders due to substance abuse. Mental disorders due to physical illness are introduced in the *Medical Nursing*. This chapter will introduce mental disorders due to cerebral organic diseases, including major brain syndromes and the most common cerebral organic diseases.

器质性精神障碍是一组由脑部疾病或躯体疾病导致的精神障碍。脑器质性疾病所致精神障碍是指大脑发生组织形态改变所致的精神障碍，应与功能性精神障碍，如精神分裂症、心境障碍等相鉴别。由脑部疾病导致的精神障碍包括脑神经退行性病变、脑血管病、颅内感染、脑外伤、脑瘤等所致精神障碍；躯体疾病导致的精神障碍只是原发躯体疾病症状的组成部分。

器质性疾病所致精神障碍可以分为三大类：脑器质性疾病所致精神障碍；躯体疾病所致精神障碍；物质滥用所致精神障碍。躯体疾病所致精神障碍的内容请参阅《内科护理学》中相关章节。本章主要阐述脑器质性精神障碍的常见综合征、及常见脑器质性精神障碍的临床特点、治疗与护理。

Section 1 Mental Disorder Due to Cerebral Organic Disease

第一节 脑器质性精神障碍的常见综合征

Mental disorders due to cerebral organic diseases can be divided into two subgroups: acute (delirium) and chronic (dementia). This section will introduce delirium and dementia. In addition, delirium and dementia are subsumed under neurocognitive disorder (NCD) in the DSM-5.

脑器质性疾病所致精神障碍主要包括两类综合征，第一类的主要临床表现是明显的认知功能或意识减退，例如痴呆、谵妄和遗忘。第二类的临床表现与功能性精神障碍的临床表现相似。本节主要讨论谵妄和痴呆两种综合征。在 DSM-5 中，谵妄和痴呆被归为神经认知障碍。

I. Delirium

一、谵 妄

Delirium is a mental state usually caused by an underlying somatic illness and characterized disturbance in attention and awareness and a change in cognition that develop rapidly over a short period of time (usually hours to a few days). Delirium is the most common acute cognitive impairments among clients in general hospitals, particularly in those aged 65 years and older. Majority of delirious cases are reversible, and 30%-40% of all delirious cases are preventable.

谵妄是由躯体因素所致的脑功能障碍，表现为短时间内快速发展的注意障碍、意识障碍和认知改变。在综合医院里，谵妄是最常见的精神病性综合征，尤其多见于老年患者。大多数谵妄是可逆的，其中 30%～40% 的病例是可以预防的。

i. Epidemiological Data

（一）流行病学资料

1. Delirium can occur at any age. Children and elderly people are most vulnerable. The occurrence is low among young and middle-aged inpatients and when present, it is often associated with alcohol or illicit drug use.

2. The occurrence (prevalence and incidence rates) of delirium varies in different care settings. The overall occurrence of delirium in general medical and geriatric wards is 18%-35%, and in emergency departments is 8%-17% of all elderly clients. The highest incidences are noted in ICU and palliative care settings, with 31% of clients in ICU, while the figure soars to 82% when mechanical ventilation and intubation are required. The prevalence in the community care settings is only 1%-2%, but onset usually brings the client to emergency department.

3. Delirium has been associated with some adverse patient outcomes such as increased mortality and length of stay, and impaired physical function for 30 days or more after discharge.

1. 谵妄可发生于任何年龄段，多见于儿童和老年患者。中青年患者较少出现谵妄，若是出现，则多与酗酒或使用成瘾物质有关。

2. 不同护理场所中谵妄的发生率（包括患病率和发病率）各异。在内科和老年病房中谵妄的发生率（包括患病率和发病率）可达 18%～35%。在急诊科的老年患者中谵妄的发病率为 8%～17%。重症监护室和舒缓病房中谵妄的发生率最高。在重症监护室，机械通气和气管插管患者中谵妄的发病率可高达 82%。在社区照顾机构中谵妄的患病率仅为 1%～2%，一旦发生常导致患者被送入急诊。

3. 谵妄可导致一些不良的患者结局。如死亡率的上升、住院时间延长、出院 30 天后躯体功能的残障。

ii. Etiology and Mechanism

（二）病因及发病机制

The etiology of delirium is usually multifactorial, determined by a complex interaction between

谵妄的病因常与患者本身的易感性、所患疾病的种类和数量以及严重程度等因素相关。

vulnerability of clients and the number and severity of conditions. Based on the etiology, categories of delirium include substance intoxication delirium, substance withdrawal delirium, medication-induced delirium, delirium due to another medical condition, and delirium due to multiple etiologies.

其病因可分为五类，主要包括：① 物质过量或中毒；② 物质的戒断；③ 药物过量或中毒；④ 由其他躯体疾病所致谵妄；⑤ 由于多种病因所致的谵妄。

Based on the multifactorial interaction model, individuals with serious medical, surgical, or neurological conditions are most vulnerable; and of all conditions, abnormal laboratory examination value is the factor precipitating delirium in all clients.

根据上述多因素相互作用的模型，有严重内外科或神经系统问题的患者是谵妄易感人群；在不同病情的患者中，异常的实验室指标为谵妄的诱发因素。

Clients might overcome a delirious state without any residual effects, or develop neurological sequelae. Those most likely to fully recover are clients with identifiable and completely treated medical conditions such as an infection and those with drug-induced delirium. Researches find that length of delirium episode (e.g., over 2-3 days) is associated with a worse prognosis particularly among elderly clients.

患者发生谵妄后可能痊愈，也可能出现神经系统的后遗症。大多数患者可以恢复到发病前的功能状态，尤其是那些病因明确且得到及时恰当处理的患者，如感染或成瘾物质戒断的患者。研究发现老年患者中，谵妄持续时间长短（如2~3天以上）与预后不良相关。

iii. Clinical Manifestations

（三）临床表现

Delirium is associated with acute failure of the brain, and is often under-recognized and overlooked. Attention deficits along with acute onset, fluctuating course of symptoms (waxing and waning course) and overall disturbance of consciousness are the core features of delirium. Inattention is usually related to disturbed consciousness and cognition.

谵妄是易被忽视的急性脑病综合征。其基本特征包括急性发作的注意障碍、意识障碍，症状呈波动性。注意力改变常与患者的意识障碍或认知功能障碍相关。

Common symptoms of cognitive disturbances include alteration in awareness (reduced orientation to the environment), disorientation to time and place, impaired reasoning ability and goal-directed behavior, impairment of recent memory, and incoherent speech.

认知功能障碍表现为意识改变、时间和地点的定向力障碍，推理能力和目标导向行为受损，近记忆障碍和语言逻辑障碍。

Changes in arousal and disturbance in sleep-wake cycle, and misperceptions of the environment such as visual and auditory hallucinations and illusions, are common. The clients may exhibit emotional disturbance such as fear, anxiety, depression, irritability, anger, euphoria, and apathy. Clients may shift from one emotional state to another rapidly and unpredictably. Autonomic manifestations are also common, such as tachycardia, sweating, flushed face, dilated pupils, and elevated blood pressure.

常见睡眠－觉醒周期紊乱和幻视、幻听。患者可伴情感障碍，表现为恐惧、焦虑、抑郁、易激惹、愤怒、欣快和淡漠。谵妄患者的情感变化快、难以预测。患者还可表现为心动过速、出汗、脸色潮红、瞳孔扩大和血压升高等自主神经功能紊乱症状。

Duration of delirium is brief (e.g., 1 week, rarely more than 1 month), and the disorder subsides completely on recovery from the underlying determinant. If the underlying conditions persist, the delirium may gradually progress to stupor, coma, seizures, or death.

谵妄持续时间较短，原发疾病治愈后谵妄症状可迅速消失。如患者的原发疾病持续存在，症状可发展为木僵、昏迷、惊厥甚至死亡。

iv. Treatment

（四）治疗

While majority of clients with delirium are reversible, early recognition and intervention usually

大多数患者的谵妄是可逆的，早识别、早干预常可缩短谵妄的持续时间。初步的处

shorten the duration of delirium. Principles of the initial management include identification and correction of the underlying medical issues, maintenance of client's safety, and symptom management.

理原则包括早期确诊和纠正病因、保证患者安全和对症治疗。

1. Management of Medical Issues Since delirium can be the marker of serious medical issues, all clients should be screened for acute physiological disorders.

1．病因治疗 首先是查找病因、积极治疗原发病。

2. Maintenance of Client's Safety Safety efforts should focus on airway protection and aspiration prevention, maintenance of the balance of fluid and electrolyte status, maintenance of nutrition, prevention of skin breakdown, and maintenance of safety mobility.

2．保证患者安全的措施 包括保持呼吸道通畅、纠正水电解质紊乱，补充营养，预防皮肤破损和跌倒。

3. Symptom Management Evidence-based recommendations suggest that non-pharmacological interventions are the first-line strategy of symptom management, including discontinuation or reduction of psychoactive drugs, monitoring behavior, providing reorientation and assurance, creating a quiet and warm environment, promoting relaxation and enhancing sleep. However, clients in hallucinations and delusions, or in severe agitation and aggression, may require chemical and/or physical restraint for his or her personal safety. Low-dose antipsychotics are the pharmacological treatment of choice in most cases.

3．对症治疗 循证建议指出应将非药物干预作为对症治疗的一线措施，包括停用或减少精神活性药物剂量，监测患者精神行为，为患者提供一个安全、放松的环境，减轻患者定向障碍，促进睡眠。低剂量的抗精神病药主要针对幻觉、妄想、和有严重激惹与攻击性行为的患者。

II. Dementia

二、痴　呆

i. Introduction

According to the *ICD-10*, dementia is defined as "a syndrome due to disease of the brain, usually of a chronic or progressive nature, in which there is disturbance of multiple higher cortical functions, including memory, thinking, orientation, comprehension, calculation, learning capacity, language, and judgment. Consciousness is not clouded. The impairments of cognitive functions are commonly accompanied, and occasionally preceded, by deterioration in emotional control, social behavior or motivation." Dementia is also subsumed under major neurocognitive disorder in the DSM-5. Approximately 5%-15% of all dementias can be reversed if the cause is identified and treated appropriately and in time.

Alzheimer's disease (AD), vascular dementia (VaD), dementia with Lewy bodies (DLB) and frontotemporal dementia (FTD) are commonest subtypes of dementia, accounting for approximately 60%, 15%, 15% and 5% of all cases, respectively. Prevalence of dementia increases exponentially with increasing age, although certain etiological factors may cause dementia at any age. Longer life expectancy is the strongest risk factor for higher prevalence. Lower educational level is also one of the main risk factors for dementia.

（一）概述

根据*ICD-10*的定义，痴呆是“一种慢性脑病综合征，病程通常为慢性或进展性的，其临床基本特征是出现记忆、思维、定向、理解、计算、学习能力、语言和判断力等多种认知功能障碍。意识障碍尚不存在。情绪控制能力、社交行为或动机的衰退常与认知损害相伴随，偶尔会早于认知损害”。在DSM-5中，痴呆也被归入重度神经认知障碍。大约5%～15%的痴呆是可逆的。如果病因明确、治疗恰当及时，则预后较好。

阿尔茨海默病（Alzheimer's disease，AD）、血管性痴呆（Vascular dementia，VaD）、路易体痴呆（dementia with Lewy body，DLB）和额颞叶痴呆（frontotemporal dementia，FTD）是最常见的痴呆类型，分别占痴呆总数的60%，15%，15%和5%。虽然痴呆可发生于任何年龄，但其患病率随年龄显著上升。预期寿命延长和受教育程度低是主要危险因素。

BOX 12-1 Scientific Data

Global Burden of Dementia Care

It is estimated 35.6 million people with dementia worldwide in 2010, almost doubling every 20 years, to 65.7 million in 2030. Nearly 60% of dementia cases lived in low- and middle- income countries in 2010, with the proportion expected to 63% in 2030. By 2025, the absolute number of dementia cases in China will be higher than in other countries, and the figure is predicted to be around 11% of the aging population.

Worldwide costs of dementia care are enormous, including direct cost (paid care provided by medical and social care) and indirect cost (unpaid care provided by families and friends). In 2010, the total costs of care were $ 604 billion, almost equivalent to the GDP of the world's 21st largest economy. In low-and-middle-income countries, the cost of unpaid care accounted for approximately two thirds of total costs, compared with 40% in high-income countries. The rapid growth of dementia cases and a predominant proportion of unpaid care in total cost indicate an insufficient support system to the clients and families and a tremendous caregiver burden in low-and-middle-income countries.

ii. Etiology and Mechanism

The pathogenesis of dementia depends largely on the etiology, although they share common symptom presentation. The following are the major categories classified by *DSM-5*: NCD due to Alzheimer's disease, vascular NCD, frontotemporal NCD, NCD due to traumatic brain injury, NCD with Lewy bodies, NCD due to Parkinson's disease, NCD due to HIV infection, substance-induced NCD, NCD due to Huntington's disease, NCD due to Prion disease, NCD due to another medical condition, NCD due to multiple etiologies, and unspecified NCD.

The reversibility of dementia is determined by the basic etiology of the disorder. In most cases, the course is irreversible. Reversible cases may be found in clients with cerebral lesions, depression, side effects of certain medications, normal pressure hydrocephalus, vitamin or nutritional deficiencies (especially B_{12} or folate), central nervous system infections, and metabolic disorders. For example, some studies reported that people with depression are at increased risk of developing dementia, and severe depression can cause dementia, but can be

BOX 12-1 科学数据

全球痴呆照料负担

预计全球的痴呆患者总数将由2010年的3千5百多万上升至2030年的6千5百多万，几乎每20年翻一倍。在2010年，近60%的患者住在中低收入国家，预计到2030年这一比例将升至63%。到2025年，中国的痴呆患者将占老年人口的11%，成为患者绝对数量最多的国家。

全球在痴呆照料上的花费巨大，这些费用包含了医疗和社会支出的直接照料费用以及由患者家庭和朋友提供的间接照料费用。2010年，全球总照料费用为604亿美元，相当于全球排名第21位的经济体的国民生产总值。在中低收入国家，痴呆照料的间接照料费用大致占总费用的三分之二，而在高收入国家，这一比率为40%。中低收入国家中痴呆患者数量的快速增长和照料花费中高比率的间接照料费用数据提示了对患者及其家庭的支持系统的不足和其家庭巨大的照料负担。

（二）病因及发病机制

痴呆患者的临床表现有相似处，但其病理改变很大程度上取决于引起痴呆的病因。根据*DSM-5*的分类，痴呆病因包括阿尔茨海默病、血管病、额颞叶变性、创伤性脑损伤、路易体病、帕金森氏病、HIV、物质/药物使用、亨廷顿病、朊病毒病，其他躯体疾病、多种病因和未特定的病因所致疾病。

大多数痴呆的病程是不可逆的，但也有可逆的案例，多见于脑损伤、抑郁、某些药物副作用、正常颅压脑积水、维生素B_{12}或叶酸缺乏、中枢神经系统感染、代谢障碍等。研究报道，抑郁症患者发生痴呆的风险增高，且严重抑郁可导致痴呆，但抑郁治愈后痴呆也可痊愈。而AD等神经退行性痴呆是不可逆的，其病程为渐进性发展，导致不可逆的神

treated. On the other hand, neurodegenerative dementias such as AD are incurable and fatal because these diseases result in a progressive and irreversible loss of neurons and brain functions.

经元脱失和脑功能受损。

iii. Clinical Manifestation

（三）临床表现

The manifestation of dementia includes three domains: impairment of cognition, impairment of functioning, and non-cognitive psychic symptoms. Impairment in memory is a prime symptom in Alzheimer's disease, but memory loss is not necessarily characterized in vascular dementia or frontotemporal dementia.

痴呆的临床表现包括三方面：认知功能缺损、社会生活功能减退和非认知性精神症状。记忆障碍是AD的特征，但不一定是血管性痴呆和额颞叶痴呆的早期表现。

Staging of dementia can provide health professionals and caregivers an overview of the dementia process. Defining a person's dementia stage also helps health professionals evaluate the therapeutic efficacy and aids communication with caregivers. The global deterioration scale (GDS) is the most common used scales to assess global severity of dementia, and has been proven to be sensitive in response to treatment among clients with mild and moderate dementia. The GDS divides the process of cognitive decline into seven stages from "no cognitive decline" to "very severe cognitive decline" (severe dementia). Among the seven stages, Stag 3 (GDS 3) to Stage 7 (GDS 7) present clinical characteristics of dementia progression from mild cognitive decline (but without diagnosed dementia), to mild, moderate, moderately severe and severe stage of dementia, respectively.

痴呆分期有助于医护人员和照料者了解痴呆的病程，也可帮助医护人员评估治疗的效果、与照顾者沟通。《整体退化量表》（global deterioration scale，GDS）是最常用评估痴呆严重程度的工具，其对轻中度痴呆的治疗反应的敏感性已被证实。GDS根据AD的认知退化过程分为“无认知退化”至“重度痴呆”七期。其中第三期（GDS 3）至第七期（GDS 7）分别为轻度认知功能下降（但确诊无痴呆）、轻度、中度、中重度及重度痴呆。

GDS 3 (Mild cognitive decline). In this stage, there is clear-cut evidence that the person's impairment of memory and function exceed the norm for his or her age. The objective evidences of deficits can be observed with an intensive clinical interview, but these evidences are not sufficient to be given to a diagnosis of dementia. This stage can last for 7 years. Clients at this stage may demonstrate decreased ability to remember names upon introduction to new people, or may read a passage or a book and retain relatively little material. Concentration may be interrupted. The person may have lost or misplaced an important item, or may have lost when traveling to an unfamiliar location. The person may demonstrate decreased performance in demanding employment and social settings. Co-workers may become aware of the person's relatively poor performance. Denial begins to manifest in the person, and mild to moderate anxiety accompanies symptoms.

GDS 3 轻度认知功能下降。此期患者表现为记忆和功能下降程度超出其实际年龄应有的水平，但客观检查结果还未达到痴呆的诊断标准。此期表现可长达7年。患者可能记不起刚认识的人的名字或几乎记不得刚看的一段文字或书的内容。工作和注意力也会受到干扰，可能会遗失或放错重要物品，到不熟悉的地方去会迷路。面对有难度的工作时表现不佳，同事也会注意到这些情况。伴随着上述症状，患者开始表现出否认、轻中度的焦虑。

GDS 4 (Mild dementia). GDS 4 is the first stage of cognitive decline at which an individual can definitively be diagnosed with dementia. This stage generally lasts about 2 years. In a careful clinical interview, the individual may forget major events in personal history; experience

GDS 4 轻度痴呆。患者的认知功能下降程度已达到痴呆的诊断标准。此期表现大约持续2年。患者可能会忘记日常生活中重要的事情，购物、处理财务等处事能力下降，或不

declining ability to perform tasks such as shopping, handle finances, etc.; or be unable to understand current news events. Clients may deny that a problem exists by covering up memory loss with confabulation. Depression and social withdrawal are common. Generally, there is no deficit in orientation to time and place, recognition of familiar persons and faces, or ability to travel to familiar locations.

能理解近期发生的新闻事件。患者可能用虚构的方式来掩盖其记忆力丧失的事实，患者可表现出抑郁和社交退缩。通常对时间、熟悉的人物或地点无定向障碍。

GDS 5 (moderate dementia). This stage typically lasts about one year and a half. The individuals lose some basic activities of daily living (ADLs) such as choosing the proper clothing to wear. They are unable survive without some assistance. During interview, they are unable to recall their addresses, phone numbers, and names of close relatives. Disorientation to time or place is common, but they still retain major knowledge about themselves.

GDS 5 中度痴呆。此期表现大约持续 1 年半。患者会丧失一些基本的日常生活能力、如不能正确地穿衣，没有帮助患者无法独立生活；常常忘记地址、电话号码或亲人的名字，常见时间、地点定向障碍。

GDS 6 (moderately severe dementia). This stage lasts approximately two and a half years. At this stage, the individual may recall their own name, but unable to recall recent major life events or occasionally forget the name of his or her spouse. Disorientation to surroundings and time is common. They are impaired in ADLs, and incontinence is common. Sleeping becomes a problem. Personality and emotional changes occur, and symptoms are quite variable including wandering, delusion, obsessiveness, agitation and aggression. Symptoms seem to worsen in the late afternoon and evening, a phenomenon termed sundowning. Communication becomes more difficult due to progressive loss of language skills. Institutional care is usually required at this stage.

GDS 6 中重度痴呆。此期表现大约持续 2 年半。此期患者可记得自己的名字，但无法回忆最近生活中发生过的主要事情，偶尔记不住其配偶的名字。常见时间地点定向障碍。日常生活能力明显受损，常发生大小便失禁和睡眠紊乱。有睡眠障碍、人格改变、情绪障碍，如徘徊、妄想、强迫行为、易激惹和攻击性等。黄昏时症状加重，故又称“落日现象”。患者丧失语言技巧，与人沟通困难。此期患者往往需要由机构照料。

GDS 7 (severe dementia). The duration of this stage depends on patient's etiology of dementia, age and physical condition.In this stage, the individual is aphasia, apraxia and agnosia. In the end stage, the client is commonly chairbound or bedbound. Problems associated with immobility, such as pressure ulcer and muscle contractures, may occur. Generalized rigidity and developmental neurologic reflexes are frequently present.

GDS 7 重度痴呆。此期表现持续时间取决于患者的痴呆病因、年龄、躯体状况等。此期患者出现失语、失用、失认。晚期患者常依靠轮椅或卧床不起，可出现压疮或肌肉挛缩等并发症。

iv. Treatment

The main goals of treatment are: to optimize function, to slow the progression of the dementia, and to improve quality of life of the clients. Currently there is no cure for common neurodegenerative disorders such as AD, FTD and DLB. However, symptom management and supportive interventions are usually of value.

（四）治疗

痴呆治疗的主要目标是维持患者的最佳功能状态，延缓疾病的进展，提高患者的生活质量。痴呆的治疗包括改善认知功能的药物治疗、非药物干预、和针对非认知性精神症状的治疗三方面。对于神经退行性变引起的痴呆如 AD、FTD 和 DLB，目前尚无有效的治疗手段，较为有效的措施包括对症处理和支持性干预。

The core symptoms are treated with acetylcholinesterase inhibitors and memantine. Cholinesterase inhibitors are commonly used in symptomatic treatment in mild-to-moderate AD, but in FTD, no convincing evidence shows the benefits of these drugs. Memantine, the N-Methyl-D-aspartate receptor (NMDA receptor) antagonist, is commonly used in moderate-to-severe AD. Other drugs are used in treatments for neuropsychiatric symptoms. The atypical antipsychotics (risperidone, quetiapine, olanzapine and aripiprazole) are used to control agitation, aggression, hallucinations, thought disturbances, and wandering. The selective serotonin reuptake inhibitors (SSRIs) are the first-line antidepressants to treat depression in elderly people with dementia. Benzodiazepines, the antianxiety medications, are used to control anxiety of the clients.

痴呆的药物治疗效果主要包括两方面：一是改善认知功能的药物治疗，如乙酰胆碱酯酶抑制剂（如多奈哌齐、卡巴拉汀、加兰他敏）可用于轻、中度AD，但对FTD效果不明显；NMDA受体拮抗剂（盐酸美金刚）多用于中、重度AD。二是缓解非认知性精神病性症状，非典型性抗精神病药物（如利培酮、喹硫平、奥氮平和阿立哌唑）多用于控制激惹、攻击行为、幻觉、思维障碍、徘徊症等症状。SSRI类药物是治疗痴呆患者抑郁症状的首选药物。抗焦虑药如苯二氮䓬类，可用于控制患者的焦虑症状。

Although pharmacotherapies appear to slow symptom progression, the long-term effects of these drugs are mixed. Moreover, the effects of some drugs are overwhelmed by the co-occurrence of cerebrovascular and neurodegenerative diseases. Instead, non-pharmacological therapies such as psychosocial and environmental management emerge as versatile and potentially effective and cost-effective approaches to symptom relief of the clients and to improvement of quality of life in clients and family caregivers.

虽然药物治疗可能减轻症状，但药物干预的长期疗效还有待观察，特别是一些药物还有引起脑血管和神经退行性疾病的风险。而非药物干预如心理社会干预、环境干预等，形式多样，有助于改善患者症状，提高患者及其家庭的生活质量，且带来的经济负担较低。

Section 2 Alzheimer's Disease and Vascular Dementia

第二节 阿尔茨海默病和血管性痴呆

I. Alzheimer's Disease

一、阿尔茨海默病

i. Introduction

（一）概述

Alzheimer's disease (AD) is a neurodegenerative disorder characterized by insidious and gradual onset of dementia. Progressive memory loss is the characteristic of AD. Onset of AD is commonly after the age of 60 years, although in some cases as early as 40 years of age. The average course of AD is about 10 years. The course of AD is irreversible, and the clients are in a progressively dementing condition till death.

阿尔茨海默病是一种脑神经退行性病变，起病缓慢而隐匿，呈进行性发展的痴呆综合征。记忆障碍是AD的特征性表现。患者大多在60岁后发病，少数病例可在40岁左右发病。AD是不可逆性病变，其病程约为10年，呈渐进性，最终导致死亡。

AD accounts for 60% to 80% of dementia cases across different countries. Clients with AD are more frequently seen in women than in men. The high prevalence may be associated with longer life expectancy

阿尔茨海默病是最常见的痴呆类型，占所有痴呆患者的60%～80%。女性患病率高于男性，可能与女性的预期寿命较长有关。其他可修正的风险因素包括认知储备如智力、

in women. The modifiable risk factors for AD include cognitive reserve (intelligence, education and occupation), physical activity and exercise, midlife obesity, alcohol intake and tobacco use.

教育和职业，身体活动与锻炼，中年肥胖，酒精摄入以及吸烟。

ii. Etiology and Mechanism

The characteristic neuropathological changes include generalized cerebral atrophy, enlarged ventricles (color figure 12-1), marked neurone loss, and the presence of numerous amyloid plaques and neurofibrillary tangles (color figure 12-2). The exact cause of AD is unknown, but several hypotheses have been proposed, such as reduction in acetylcholine transferase and acetylcholine levels of brain, the formation of amyloid plaques and neurofibrillary tangles, serious head trauma, and genetic factors.

（二）病因及发病机制

AD 特征性的病理改变包括广泛性脑萎缩、脑室扩大（文末彩图 12-1）、神经元显著性脱失、神经纤维缠结和神经斑（文末彩图 12-2），伴有明显的乙酰胆碱转移酶和乙酰胆碱水平降。AD 的病因和发病机制尚不清楚。可能的发病原因与中枢神经系统中胆碱乙酰基转移酶和乙酰胆碱水平下降、神经斑与神经纤维缠结（NTF）、脑外伤、遗传因素有关。

1. Acetylcholine Alterations Research found that in AD clients, production of acetylcholine decreases, which in turn reduce the level of neurotransmitter released to cells in the cortex and hippocampus. This reduction can render the cognitive processes disrupted.

1. 乙酰胆碱转移酶和乙酰胆碱水平降低 研究发现 AD 患者中枢神经系统中乙酰胆碱水平下降，使得皮质和海马回的神经细胞中神经递质水平下降，导致认知过程受到影响。

2. Plaques and Tangles According to amyloid cascade hypothesis, the plaques are formed due to accumulation of amyloid beta (Aβ). Aβ deposits are toxic and can trigger synaptic dysfunction and neuronal cell death in the brain. Tau is a microtubule-associated protein and normally soluble, but the tau in neurofibrillary tangles is hyperphosphorylated and insoluble. The amyloid cascade hypothesis proposes that changes in tau and consequent tangle formation are triggered by toxic concentrations of Aβ. However, the exact pathways linking Aβ and tau have not been elucidated.

2. 神经斑与神经纤维缠结 根据β淀粉样蛋白级联学说，β淀粉样蛋白（Aβ）低聚物的产生是形成神经斑（老年斑）的始动环节，也是老年斑的核心成分。Aβ 在脑内蓄积，进而形成具神经毒性的 Aβ 可溶性低聚物，导致突触功能障碍和神经细胞的死亡。tau 蛋白是可溶性的神经元特异性蛋白，主要分布于神经元轴突，起稳定微管的作用。NTF 的主要成分是不溶性的、过度磷酸化的 tau 蛋白。Aβ 可溶性低聚物触发了 NTF 的形成，导致神经元结构和功能障碍，引起神经元变性。但是，Aβ 与 tau 蛋白间的确切路径目前还未阐明。

iii. Clinical Manifestations

The main clinical feature is cognitive decline in one or more area of cognitive domains including learning and memory, language, complex attention, executive function, perceptual-motor or social cognition.

（三）临床表现

AD 患者主要表现为一个或多个认知维度的功能进行性退化，如学习、记忆、语言、复杂注意、执行功能、知觉动作、及社会认知。

1. Early Stage The first appeared symptom is a subjective sense of memory loss, such as difficulty remembering newly learned information. Client often repeats self within the same conversation, or cannot keep track of short list of items when shopping. But in the early stage of AD, it is very difficult to distinguish a subjective memory deficit from benign forgetfulness which are

1. 早期表现 患者最早表现的症状是主诉记忆力下降。如容易遗忘近期信息，反复重复谈话内容或遗忘购物内容。但在疾病早期很难区分主观感觉记忆障碍与良性遗忘，因良性遗忘通常是由家人而不是患者发现的。有些 AD 患者可呈现轻微的人格改变，表现为

usually first noticed by the family rather than the client. Subtle personality changes can be seen in clients with AD. Those clients often become passive, coarse and less spontaneous, and some even become depressed.

生活懒散、行为粗鲁、缺乏主动性，甚至出现抑郁。

2. Progressive Stage As the disease progresses, clients enter a state of global cognitive impairment, which can be noticed by family and friends. Clients need to rely on others to plan instrumental (complex) and basic ADLs because of impaired executive function (such as thinking, planning, problem-solving and weighing up long-term consequences). Apraxia may progress gradually or change abruptly in persons with dementia. It is difficult to distinguish memory impairment (can the person remember what he is supposed to do?) from problem of apraxia (can the person make his muscles to do what they are supposed to do?) because both impairments occur in the person with dementia. The client may also show insensitivity to social standards because of deficit in social cognition, such as making decisions without regard to safety. The client usually has little insight into these changes. Anxiety is replaced by denial.

2. 进展期表现 随着疾病的进展，患者出现广泛的认知功能障碍，并且为家人或朋友察觉。患者的思考、计划、解决问题和权衡长期结果等执行功能受损，日常生活能力下降、需依赖他人照料。失用症的严重程度可呈渐进性或突然的变化。往往很难区分患者执行功能受损是由于失用还是记忆障碍所致。社会认知的下降以及自知力缺乏，导致患者对自身行为安全性的判断能力受损。患者在认知功能减退的基础上至少合并一种精神症状。患者自己感到焦虑，但通常予以否认。

3. Terminal Stage The typical features of dementia (such as disturbance of orientation, memory, calculation and judgment) finally appear. The clients become aimless, abulic, aphasic, and restless, abnormal neurologic reflection (such as the snout, palmomental reflex, and grasp reflexes).

3. 晚期表现 患者可表现出典型的痴呆症状，如定向力、记忆、计算与判断能力障碍等。患者变得毫无目的性，意志缺乏，失语，激越，出现病理性反射，如强握、掌颏反射、吸吮反射等。

iv. Treatment

Treatments of AD that use an approach based on etiology are not available. The therapeutic principles include pharmacological and non-pharmacological interventions.

（四）治疗

本病病因不明，目前尚无特效治疗。AD的治疗主要是针对认知、社会生活功能减退和非认知性精神症状的治疗。治疗方法包括药物治疗与非药物干预。

1. Pharmacological Intervention The purposes of pharmacotherapy in AD are to prevent the disease in asymptomatic individuals, to modify the natural course of the disease in those already diagnosed, and to improve clients' cognition and memory. Cholinesterase inhibitors (such as donepezil, rivastigmine, and galantamine) are reported to have modest and short-term (3-6 months) improvements in the clients' cognitive function, indirect improvement in ADLs, and moderate improvement in mood particularly apathy and social interaction. Memantine is reported to have a significant improvement in cognition, function and neuropsychiatric symptoms particularly agitation and aggression.

1. 药物治疗 AD药物治疗的目的包括：① 对无症状的患者起预防作用；② 对已经确诊的患者延缓其自然病程；③ 增强患者的认知功能和记忆力。研究报道乙酰胆碱酯酶抑制剂在3~6个月内对患者的认知功能有中度的改善，并间接改善患者的日常生活能力。NMDA受体拮抗剂能明显改善患者的认知功能、躯体功能以及易激惹、攻击行为等神经精神症状。

2. Non-pharmacological Interventions Non-pharmacological interventions mainly include functional intervention, environment intervention and psychosocial

2. 非药物治疗 常见非药物治疗包括日常生活能力干预、环境干预和社会心理干预。日常生活能力的干预有助于维持患者的躯体

therapy. Physical or functional interventions and environmental and behavioral interventions have proven to be beneficial to the clients. Physical or functional interventions help to maintain the clients' health status, facilitate independence and also reduce caregiver burden. Environment interventions provide a home-like environment and facilitate interaction between the clients and environment. Behavioral interventions help clients and caregivers to minimize potentially triggering reaction. The purposes of psychosocial interventions are to maintain the clients' cognitive functioning and social functioning, and to make sure of the clients' safety and comfort as well. In order to develop psychosocial therapy well, the clients and their family members or caregivers should be involved and nursing care principles of AD should be provided for family members or caregivers. Strategies of psychosocial intervention such as support group, education and counseling are essential for clients at mild stage and their family caregivers. For serious AD clients, emphasis should be put on nursing care.

功能，减轻照料者负担。环境干预旨在为患者创造居家的照顾环境、促进患者适应环境。在此基础上，通过行为干预，帮助患者及其家属减少触发患者精神行为症状的因素。社会心理干预的目的主要是尽可能维持患者的认知和社会生活功能，保证患者的安全与舒适。开展社会心理治疗，须与患者和家属建立良好的合作关系，告诉家属或照料者护理的基本原则。对症状轻微的患者可采用支持小组、健康教育与咨询等社会心理干预策略，对病情较重的患者应加强护理。

II. Vascular Dementia

i. Introduction

Vascular dementia (VaD) is a clinical syndrome mainly due to significant cerebrovascular disease. Compared to AD, VaD is characterized by an abrupt onset and stepwise decline of dementing process. In clients with early VaD, memory is often preserved, and impaired attention and executive function are common.

VaD accounts for approximately 15% of all the dementia and is thought to be the second most common cause of dementia. VaD is more common in men than in women. VaD and AD are also co-existed in 50% of VaD cases. Therefore, increasing number of specialists prefers using the term "vascular cognitive impairment (VCI)" to "vascular dementia" because VCI is an umbrella term which can comprise VCI-no dementia, vascular dementia, and mixed primary neurodegenerative dementia (usually AD) with vascular dementia. In *DSM-5*, VCI is categorized as mild and major vascular neurocognitive disorders.

The major risk and prognostic factors for VaD are the same as those for cerebrovascular disease, such as hypertension, diabetes, smoking, obesity, hypercholesterolaemia, hyperhomocysteinemia, etc. The prognosis for clients with VaD is worse than that for AD. Life expectancy was shortened for clients with VaD. The five-year survival rate is 39% for VaD clients compared with 75% for age-matched controls. About one-third of VaD clients died from dementia itself, the remaining died

二、血管性痴呆

（一）概述

血管性痴呆是由脑血管病变而引起的一组临床综合征。患者表现为急性起病和阶梯式恶化的痴呆。早期的VaD患者往往存在注意障碍和执行功能障碍，而未出现记忆障碍。

VaD约占所有痴呆患者的15%，是痴呆的第二大原因。男性多于女性。VaD患者中半数合并AD，因此，越来越多的学者倾向于用“血管性认知损害”取代VaD，因为血管性认知损害涵盖了有血管性认知损害而无痴呆、VaD、以及同时存在神经退行性痴呆与VaD的混合性痴呆。在*DSM-5*中，血管性认知损害又分为轻度和重度血管性神经认知损害。

VaD的风险因素及预后相关因素与心血管疾病的非常相似，包括高血压、糖尿病、吸烟、肥胖、高胆固醇血症和高同型半胱氨酸血症等。VaD患者的预后较差，预期寿命比AD患者短。五年生存率为39%，约为同年龄对照组的一半。VaD患者的3年死亡率几乎比同年龄对照组高出3倍。1/3的患者死于痴呆本身，其余的死因则可能与脑血管疾病、心

from cerebral vascular disease, cardiac disease, or other unrelated conditions.

脏疾病或其他因素有关。

ii. Etiology and Mechanism

（二）病因及发病机制

Subtype of VaD includes poststroke dementia, multi-infarct dementia, subcortical dementia, and leukoaraiosis (white matter lesions). The vascular etiologies range from large vessel disease (leading to poststroke dementia) to small vessel diseases (including subcortical infarcts and leukoaraiosis).

VaD包括卒中后痴呆、多发梗死性痴呆、皮质下痴呆以及脑白质疏松症（脑白质损伤）。VaD的病因包括导致卒中后痴呆的大血管疾病，小血管疾病如皮质下痴呆和脑白质疏松症等。

The progression and presentation of VaD are determined by types of vascular lesions, location, number (focal or multifocal) and volume of lesions, co-occurrence of vascular disease and AD or another dementing process.

下列因素与VaD的病程和表现有关：①血管损伤的类型、损伤的部位、数量（局灶性或多灶性）与体积；②血管性疾病合并AD或其他痴呆类型。

Abrupt onset of VaD is directly related to interruption or reduced perfusion of major cerebral vessels. Symptoms of VaD result from the death of nerve cells in areas nourished by diseased vessels. Multiple minor strokes affecting small cerebral vessels may lead to cumulative brain damage, and the client's symptoms worsen gradually. There is also robust evidence regarding the association with cognitive and functional decline in VaD. VaD and AD share common pathogenetic mechanisms. Cerebrovascular pathologies also interact with pathologies related to other types of dementia (such as AD), accelerating dementing process.

急性起病的VaD与脑血流中断或低氧－低灌注损伤有关，症状的发生与病变血管灌注部位的神经细胞坏死有关。多发性中风如影响小血管，则导致脑损伤程度的逐步累积，症状可呈进行性恶化。VaD患者的认知功能损害还与躯体功能障碍有关，且VaD和AD的发病机制重叠，因而患者脑血管的病理表现与其他类型痴呆的病理表现相互作用，加速了痴呆的病程。

iii. Clinical Manifestations

（三）临床表现

The pattern of deficits of vascular dementia is variable up to which regions of the brain have been affected. Many clients with VaD as a result of multiple infarctions present an abrupt onset with partial improvement to "stepwise" decline. For example, sometimes the dementia seems clear up and the client presents fairly lucid thinking. Others with small vessel disease leading to lesions in the white matter, basal ganglia and/or thalamus generally present a gradual onset and progressive decline in cognition.

VaD的临床表现差异较大，与血管病变的部位和类型有关。多发性梗阻所致的VaD患者往往起病较急，病程多呈阶梯式加重。VaD患者的认知功能损害程度常有波动，有时患者病情似乎好转，思维清晰，记忆力有所增强。小血管疾病导致的脑白质损伤、基底节和/或丘脑损伤的患者常表现为逐渐发病和认知功能的进行性下降。

Certain focal neurological signs such as problems with reflexes, small-stepped gait, muscle weaknesses of the limbs, and difficulty with speech, occur first in people with VaD. Memory loss often occurs later. Early impairment of attention and alterations in behavior and/or difficulties with executive functions are common manifestations in people with VaD, particularly those with sub-cortical ischaemic vascular disease.

本病的临床特征为伴局灶性神经损害的缓慢性发展的痴呆，这类神经损害包括步行障碍、共济失调、言语障碍等。记忆障碍多见于进展期患者。注意障碍和执行功能受损尤其多见于皮质下缺血性脑血管疾病患者。

Since people with VaD often have more insight into their condition, they are prone to depression and mood instability. Client may become optimistic that the improvement is occurring before experiencing

VaD患者对自己的疾病状况比较了解，因而容易出现抑郁和情绪不稳，症状时好时坏，这种波动的方式使得患者的焦虑情绪加重。

further decline of functioning in a fluctuating pattern of progression. The irregular pattern of decline appears to be an intense source of anxiety for the client with this disorder.

iv. Treatment

Assessing and controlling major vascular risk factors are the mainstay of primary preventive strategies. The target in primary preventive strategies should be based on knowledge of pathophysiological mechanisms. Since prestroke hypertension is associated with poststroke dementia, treatment of hypertension is perhaps the single most important preventive measure. But the blood pressure could not be lowered too much to cause hypoperfusion. Importance also should be attached to the control of diabetes and to smoking cessation. Prevention of stroke recurrence is the most import intervention in management of VaD. Medication is primarily used to prevent further worsening of VaD by treating the underlying disease such as hypertension, hyperlipidemia, and diabetes. Antiplatelet agents such as aspirin have been found to slow the progression of VaD.

（四）治疗

评估和控制重要的血管风险因素是一级预防的重点。一级预防的目标还应根据相应的病理生理机制。卒中前高血压与卒中后痴呆有关，因而控制高血压可能是最有效的预防措施。但血压不能降得太低，以免引起低灌注，同时也要注意控制糖尿病和戒烟。此外，预防中风的复发是最关键的干预措施。积极治疗高血压、高脂血症和糖尿病有助于防止 VaD 的恶化。抗血小板药如阿司匹林有助于延缓 VaD 的病程。

BOX 12-2 Experience Sharing

The Most Burdensome Caregiving Task: Responding to Behavior Disturbances

Almost all the participants (family caregivers) stated that the most difficult caregiving task was responding to the constant behavior disturbances of their care recipients. These behavior symptoms included passive (such as withdrawal) and active symptoms (such as aggression, sleep disturbance, restlessness, mood swings, continually changing clothes, pulling the drawers and searching for something, losing control of spending money, or wandering). Sometimes they responded to care recipient behavior with patience (such as reassurance or adherence) or distraction. For example, a wife commented: "I have to answer him several times." A son of the care recipient complained: "Whenever she told me that her sheet was stolen, I had to buy a new one for her."

The caregivers also reported that they responded with impatience (anger or ignoring) because of the difficulty of controlling their distress (or resentment) concerning the behaviors. The following comment from a son reflected their distress: "Sometimes I was very angry and raised my voice when she refused to do these (washing face or taking bath)." A husband of a patient also complained: "She quarreled with me very loudly when the neighbors were still sleeping ... I feel so resentful and shameful. I can't control myself, and also quarrel with her loudly. I even hit her several times."

BOX 12-2 经验分享

负担最重的照料任务：回应患者的行为障碍

几乎所有受访的家属照料者都表示应对（痴呆）患者不断出现的精神行为问题是照料中最困难的事情，这些行为包括淡漠或攻击行为、睡眠障碍、坐立不安、情绪不稳、不停地更衣或拉抽屉找东西、乱花钱、徘徊症等。有时照料者予以耐心地回应或转移患者的注意力。例如，一位患者的妻子说道："我不得不回答（我丈夫）好几遍。" 另一位患者的儿子也说："当她（我母亲）告诉我她的床单被偷了，我就不得不给她买新的。"

面对这些行为，照料者也很难控制恼怒或愤恨，会对患者不耐烦，如生气或充耳不闻。有两位照料者这么描述这些情境。其中一位患者的儿子说："有时当她（我母亲）又拒绝洗脸或洗澡时，我非常生气，忍不住提高嗓门。" 另一位患者的丈夫抱怨道："（半夜里）当邻居还在睡觉时，她（我妻子）和我吵得很大声……我觉得非常愤怒和难堪。我实在控制不住，也和她大声吵起来，有几次我甚至还打了她。"

Section 3 Application of the Nursing Process for Clients with Cognitive Impairment

I. Nursing Assessment

i. History

One important role of nurses' care is obtaining the client's history, particularly the occurrence and duration of the specific mental and physical changes. If the clients have difficulty describing the information accurately and adequately, the data should be acquired from the persons be aware of physical and psychosocial histories of the clients, in most cases, from their family members or friends.

When collecting history information, the following areas should be concerned by the nurses:

1. Frequency and severity of emotional lability (mood swings);

2. Personality and behavioral changes;

3. Catastrophic emotional reactions;

4. Changes in cognitive domains, such as problems related to learning, recent and remote memory, language difficulties, attention span, thinking process, executive functioning, orientation to person and surrounding, perceptual-motor, and social cognition;

5. Relationship of the principal caregiver to the client, caregiver knowledge and perception of the client's illness and behavior, impacts of caregiving on families, and amount and quality of available social support;

6. Current and past drug usage, alcohol use and possible exposure to toxins should also be collected. Furthermore positive family history of related symptoms or specific illness will be important.

ii. Physical Assessment

Physical assessment should note both the signs of impairment in nervous system and the evidence of somatic disorders which may affect mental function.

The neurological examinations focus on an individual's mental status and alertness, language skills, sensory perception, muscle strength, reflexes and coordination.

Confusion, memory impairment and behavior disturbance can be induced by diseases of other organ systems. These causes must be taken into account when diagnosing cognitive disorders. Since depression is common among aged people, diagnostic examinations

第三节　认知功能障碍患者的护理

一、护理评估

（一）病史

病史包括特定的精神及生理变化。如患者无法准确、充分地提供信息，还应重视其家人或知情者提供的信息。

在收集病史时，应考虑以下几方面：① 情绪波动的发生频率、严重程度；② 患者人格和行为的改变；③ 对重大事件的情感反应；④ 认知功能改变的情况如学习，远期、近期记忆，语言功能受损情况，注意力改变情况，思维过程，执行功能，人、物、时间、地点的定向力，知觉动作以及社会行为的恰当性等；⑤ 以及患者与主要照顾者的关系，照顾者对有关患者所患疾病和行为的知识与看法，照料过程对患者家庭的影响，可及的社会支持的质量；⑥ 同时还应注意以下问题，包括药物使用史、酒精和其他药品的使用情况、毒物接触史以及阳性家族史。

（二）体格检查

体格检查重点包括：① 神经系统损害的体征；② 其他可能影响精神状态的器质性疾病的证据。

神经系统检查应注意患者的精神症状、意识、语言能力、感知觉、肌力、反射、动作协调性。

许多器官系统的疾病均可出现意识障碍、记忆损害和行为改变等症状，故在诊断认知功能障碍时应慎重考虑。由于抑郁症在老年人群中常见，抑郁症患者在认知功能方面的

should also comprise a battery of neuropsychological assessment. The results of the assessment will help to make a differential diagnosis between dementia and depression (pseudodementia).

症状可能会与痴呆相混淆，为了区分痴呆和假性痴呆（尤其是抑郁患者）还需做一系列诊断性的神经心理测验。

iii. Laboratory Evaluations and Neuroimaging Examination

（三）实验室评估和影像学检查

1. Laboratory Test Nurses are required to assist the client to fulfill some routine laboratory evaluations, such as collecting blood and urine samples to screen infectious diseases, diabetes or hypoglycemia, hepatic and renal dysfunction, metabolic and endocrine disorders, electrolyte imbalances, nutritional deficiencies, and presence of toxic substances. There are no laboratory tests available that will positively diagnose AD during life. A range of laboratory tests are used to screen for thyroid function, vitamin B_{12} and folate, syphilis or HIV. The purpose of these tests is to differentiate between suspected AD and other forms of dementia. Other laboratory tests are to check for genetic risk factors, such as amyloid beta 42 peptide and Tau protein correlation (Tau/Aβ42), apolipoprotein E genotype (ApoE), amyloid precursor protein (APP).

1. **实验室检查** 护士有时需要协助患者完成诊断性实验室检查，包括筛查感染性疾病、糖尿病或低血糖、肝肾功能、内分泌和代谢性疾病、电解质、营养缺陷、毒性物质。实验室检查可用于诊断疑似AD病例和鉴别其他导致痴呆的疾病，包括甲状腺功能、维生素B_{12}和叶酸，以及遗传学检查，如β淀粉样蛋白42肽和tau蛋白，载脂蛋白E基因型淀粉样前体蛋白（APP）。

2. Neuroimaging Examination Neuroimaging examination is preferred to rule out other causes of dementia. CT scan or MRI reveals a degenerative pathology of the brain, including atrophy, widened cortical sulci, and enlarged cerebral ventricles. MRI revealed reduced volume of brain structure and higher CFS volume in AD clients. Hippocampal atrophy may be relatively specific to AD and may eventually be useful for early detection and differential diagnosis. Etiological certainty also requires neuroimaging evidences, otherwise white matter lesions or some "silent" cerebral infarction may be overlooked.

2. **影像学检查** 诊断神经认知障碍还需ECG、CT、MRI、PET等影像学检查。神经影像学检查有助于鉴别AD与他导致痴呆的疾病。AD患者脑CT和磁共振检查的突出表现是脑皮质萎缩、脑沟增宽、脑室扩大，但脑萎缩并不意味着可以诊断为AD。磁共振显示AD患者脑血流量减少，脑脊液量增加。颞叶特别是海马结构萎缩是AD的重要病理变化，在AD的早期诊断和鉴别诊断中有重要作用。影像学证据有助于确诊脑白质损害或一些症状不明显的脑梗塞。

II. Nursing Diagnosis

二、护理诊断

Appropriate nursing diagnoses are determined according to information collected during the assessment. Possible nursing diagnoses for clients with cognitive disorders include:

应根据评估阶段收集到的信息做出恰当的护理诊断。认知功能障碍的患者常见的护理诊断有：

1. Risk for trauma related to impairments in cognitive and psychomotor functioning.

1. **受伤的危险** 与患者的认知和精神运动功能下降有关。

2. Altered thought processes related to cerebral degeneration evidenced by disorientation, confusion, memory deficits, and hallucinations.

2. **思维过程改变** 与脑的退行性变有关，表现为定向力障碍、神志不清、记忆障碍、幻觉。

3. Risk for other-directed violence related to aggressiveness and/or assaultiveness.

4. Impaired verbal communication related to impairments in memory, aphasia, agnosia.

5. Self-care deficit related to inability to fulfill activities of daily living.

6. Situational low self-esteem related to expressions of shame and self-degradation, progressive social isolation, apathy and withdrawal, depressed mood caused by loss of independent functioning.

3. **伤人的危险** 与攻击行为有关。

4. **语言交流障碍** 与记忆受损、失语、失认有关。

5. **自理缺陷** 与不能完成日常活动有关。

6. **自尊紊乱** 与丧失独立能力所致的病耻感和自责感、进行性社交孤立、淡漠与回避、抑郁情绪有关。

III. Nursing Objectives

For clients with cognitive disorders， there are some proposed objectives in the following:

1. The clients have not experienced physical injury;

2. The clients have maintained reality orientation to the best of their capability;

3. The clients have not harmed self and others;

4. The clients are able to communicate with consistent caregivers;

5. The clients fulfill activities of daily life with assistance;

6. The clients would like to discuss positive aspects about self and life.

三、护理目标

针对存在认知功能受损的患者。

1. 患者未出现外伤；

2. 患者最大限度地保持目前的定向力；

3. 患者没有伤害自己和他人；

4. 患者能与照顾者交流；

5. 患者在他人帮助下能完成日常生活；

6. 患者愿意与人讨论有关自己和生活中的积极方面。

IV. Nursing Intervention

i. Physiological Domain

1. It is very important for clients with cognitive impairment to establish a regular, predictable and simple routine of activities (such as meals, medication, exercising and bedtime) and to avoid changes day to day. If possible, keep the client's daily life similar to his family life.

2. Clients with self-care deficit need necessary assistance with ADLs. If possible, avoid changing caregivers frequently.

3. Modify and simplify tasks for clients with deficit in ADLs. For instance, wearing shoes that just slip on are easier than wearing ones with laces.

4. Take things one step at a time, and give client directions step by step to promote independent actions, and give the client plenty of time to perform a task.

5. Accept client's change of ADLs level when offering assistance. For example, if the client can eat successfully with his fingers but cannot appropriately use chopsticks or

四、护理措施

（一）生理方面

1. 为患者制订明确、清晰、规律的活动计划，含就餐、服药、锻炼、休息等活动，避免变化。日常作息尽可能与其居家时作息一致。

2. 给予自理能力缺陷的患者必要的辅助，尽可能安排固定的照顾者。

3. 尽量简化患者的日常活动，如避免穿要系鞋带的鞋。

4. 鼓励患者的独立行为；耐心指导患者按步骤、独立完成动作。

5. 对患者日常生活能力的变化应保持灵活应对，如患者不能正确使用调羹时，则可

spoon, serve as many finger foods as possible and do not fight for the problem.

ii. Psychological Domain

Avoid excess stimulation or pressure that may trigger the client's catastrophic reactions.

1. Frequently reorientation to the clients. Clients going to a strange situation (such as hospital) will benefit from frequent orientation to reality, such as using clocks and calendars with large numbers that are easy to read.

2. Plan demanding tasks for the client's best time of day, and avoid asking the client to do things when he or she is tired.

3. There are several ways to reduce the number and frequency of outbursts, such as keeping the room tidy and simple, controlling the noise level, allowing clients to keep personal belongings, involving family caregivers in care and providing support to them.

4. If a client seems more irritable than usual, check carefully for signs of illness or pain. Even minor illness or discomfort can cause the outbursts. Monitor side effects of medication as reaction to medication also can cause these outbursts.

5. Assess and report client's hallucinations, and never argue with the client that his or her hallucination is not real. Avoid increasing the client's anxiety and agitation related to rumination of delusional thinking.

6. Provide soft restrains if client is very hyperactive and disoriented.

iii. Social Domain

1. Keep interactions with the client with calm and reassuring, and identify yourself to the clients.

2. Keep face-to-face contact with the client. Avoid unexpected approach or touch from behind since it may trigger aggressive behavior.

3. Use short and simple sentence, or simple words. Speak slowly and wait for the client to respond.

4. Nonverbal gestures are also used to help the client understand what you want him or her to complete.

5. When instructing the client to perform a task, watch for signs of increasing stress, such as refusing to follow the instruction, stubbornness, flushing, or irritability. Stop doing the task and let the client calm down.

6. Communication with the wandering client.

多提供可以用手取食的食物。

（二）心理方面

心理护理的目标是减少环境刺激源、减轻患者心理压力、避免触发其情绪的爆发。

1. 经常对患者进行定向能力的训练。使用数字大且易辨的日历或时钟，必要时使用显著的标志。

2. 复杂的活动应选择在患者状态最佳的时间段，避免在患者疲劳时。

3. 保持房间布置简洁、降低噪音，允许患者自己保存个人物品、让家属照料者共同参与护理并提供照料支持。这些措施可有助于减少和减轻患者情绪的爆发。

4. 如患者比平时易怒，应检查是否是因病或身体不适所致。药物的副作用也可引起患者情绪的爆发。

5. 对患者的幻觉、妄想症状进行评估，避免与患者争论是否其妄想内容真实存在之类的内容。与患者讨论真实的事和人，尽量避免患者陷入妄想之中，增加患者的焦虑和激惹。

6. 对定向力严重受损或呈极度活跃状态的患者进行适当约束。

（三）社交方面

1. 与患者交流时态度平和、亲切，并做自我介绍。

2. 与患者面对面的交流。交流起始时，避免从背后碰触患者，以免引起患者的攻击行为。

3. 交流时尽量使用简洁的语言，放慢语速，给予患者足够时间理解和反应。

4. 必要时，运用肢体动作帮助患者理解需要其完成的动作和步骤。

5. 在指导患者做动作时，应观察患者是否感到困难和压力。如拒绝按照指导，表现出固执、面红耳赤或易怒。如出现这些表现，则停止动作，让患者平静下来。

6. 与徘徊症患者的沟通。徘徊症是常见

Wandering is a common and serious behavioral symptom that usually makes it impossible for care settings to care for the clients. Wandering can have various causes, such as simple disorientation, a need to use the toilet, stress of changing a new environment, or expression of feelings such as boredom. Communicating with the client to identify the causes of wandering is essential to plan strategies to manage it.

的严重行为障碍。常见引起徘徊症的原因有定向力障碍、如厕的需求、对陌生的环境感到压力、觉得无聊等。应与患者进行沟通，了解其徘徊的原因，进行针对性的干预。

iv. Safety Domain

1. Independent Manage It is important to help the clients manage as independently as possible.

2. Prevention of Fall Loss of coordination due to apraxia, memory loss or physical conditions leads to risk of fall. Clients may benefit from the following preventive strategies, including:

(1) assigning room near nurse station and observing frequently;

(2) providing an area within which wandering can be done safely if the client is going to wander;

(3) arranging furniture (such as a higher chair with armrests and a firm seat), handrail, or other devices which are specifically helpful to accommodate client's disabilities;

(4) keeping bedrails up when client is in bed and assisting with ambulation;

(5) storing frequently used items within easy access.

3. Prevention of Other Hazards In addition to falls, attention should also be paid to other hazards including burn, cut and even poisons. The bathroom can be the most dangerous place for the client with impaired social cognition. Lower temperature on the water heater and keep adequate night lights in and on the way to bathroom at night. Make sure there are also handrails and slip mat in the bathroom. Items such as shampoo are stored in a cabinet with childproof lock.

（四）安全方面

1. **独立活动** 应帮助和鼓励患者的独立活动行为。

2. **跌倒的预防** 失用、记忆障碍或躯体疾病的患者容易发生跌倒，可采取一些预防措施：① 患者的房间应靠近护士站，以便加强巡视；② 为徘徊症的患者提供安全的走动环境；③ 重新布置房间物品，适应患者的残疾；④ 床位不要过高，患者卧床时加上护栏，协助患者移动；⑤ 经常使用的物品放在容易拿到的位置。

3. 其他受伤风险的预防 应防止患者被烫伤、锋利物品割伤、误饮液体中毒。对无法判断自己行为的安全性的患者来说，卫生间往往是这些伤害的高发地点。因此可采取以下措施避免这些伤害，包括降低热水器的水温设置、通往卫生间的过道和卫生间内设置夜灯、设置扶手和防滑垫、洗发水等应放置在有锁的橱内。

v. Specific Domain

The principles of discharge plan for clients with self-care deficit are:

1. To submit the client to medication regimen;

2. To assess the client's competency to meet his or her nutritional needs; to ensure personal safety;

3. To assess the caregiver's ability to fulfill client's unmet need;

4. To give informational support for caregivers such as available community services.

（五）其他

针对自理能力缺陷的患者的出院计划应包括：① 确保患者坚持用药；② 继续评估患者满足其自身营养需要的能力和确保自身安全的能力；③ 评估照顾者的能力能否满足患者的需要；④ 为照顾者提供信息支持，如社区服务等。

V. Nursing Evaluation

It is hard to resolve the clients' all problems

五、护理评价

评价的目的是检验护理措施是否达到既

completely. Evaluation should be based on both short-term and long-term goals. Evaluation should determine if the nursing interventions have been effective in achieving the intended goals of care, and emphasis should be put on slowing down the process rather than striving for resolution of the problem.

定的目标。因不可能一次解决患者的所有问题，所以评价应建立在短期和长期目标的基础之上，重点应放在减缓痴呆病程上。

(Zhang Shuying)

（张曙映）

Key Points

1. Organic mental disorders comprise a range of mental disorder due to cerebral or systemic diseases. The disorder due to cerebral diseases includes degenerative diseases, cerebrovascular diseases, intracranial infection, cerebral trauma, encephalomas and epilepsy.

2. Delirium is a mental state usually caused by an underlying somatic illness and characterized disturbance in attention and awareness, and a change in cognition that develop rapidly over a short period of time (usually hours to a few days). Majority of delirious cases are reversible and 30-40% of them are preventable. The treatment of delirium involves correction of the primary causative condition, maintenance of client's safety and symptom management.

3. Dementia is a syndrome manifested by cognitive deficits in memory, thinking, orientation, comprehension, calculation, learning capacity, language, and judgment. The manifestation of dementia includes three aspects: impairment of cognition, impairment of functioning and non-cognitive psychic symptoms.

4. Alzheimer's disease is a neurodegenerative disorder characterized by insidious and gradual onset of dementia. The etiology is uncertain. Treatments of AD that use an approach based on etiology are not available. The therapeutic strategies include psychosocial therapy and somatic therapy.

5. Vascular dementia is a clinical syndrome mainly caused by significant cerebrovascular disease. Vascular dementia is characterized by an abrupt onset and stepwise deterioration of dementia.

6. Possible nursing diagnoses for clients with cognitive disorders include risk for trauma, altered thought processes, risk for self-directed violence, risk for other-directed violence, impaired verbal communication, self-care deficit, and situational low self-esteem.

内容摘要

1. 器质性精神障碍是一组由脑部或躯体疾病导致的精神障碍。脑器质性精神障碍是器质性精神障碍的一种，是由脑神经退行性病变、脑血管病、颅内感染、脑外伤等脑部疾病所致的精神障碍。

2. 谵妄是多由躯体因素所致的脑功能障碍，表现为短时间内快速发展的注意障碍、意识障碍和认知改变。大多数谵妄是可逆的，其中30%～40%的病例是可以预防的。其治疗包括病因治疗、保证患者安全和对症状治疗。

3. 痴呆是一种慢性脑病综合征，表现为记忆、思维、定向、理解、计算、学习能力、语言和判断力等多种认知功能障碍。痴呆的临床表现包括三方面：认知功能缺损、社会生活功能减退和非认知性精神症状。

4. 阿尔茨海默病是一种脑神经退行性病变，表现为起病缓慢而隐匿、呈进行性发展的痴呆综合征。治疗方法包括社会心理治疗和药物治疗。

5. 血管性痴呆是由脑血管病变而引起的一组临床综合征，表现为急性起病和阶梯式恶化的痴呆。

6. 认知功能障碍常见的护理诊断有有受外伤的危险；思维过程改变；有自伤的危险；有伤人的危险；语言交流受损；自理缺陷；自尊紊乱。

Exercises

(Questions 1 to 2 share the same question stem)

A client with uremia, admitted to a medical unit, is

思考题

（1～2题共用题干）

一名入院的尿毒症患者突然出现睡眠紊乱、

suddenly experiencing sleep disturbances, inability to focus, memory deficits, altered perceptions, and disorientation to time and place.

1. The psychiatric liaison nurse conducts an evaluation of the client. Based on an analysis of the findings, the psychiatric liaison nurse suspects which possible diagnosis?

2. Which treatment strategy would be *most* critical when caring for a client who is experiencing the above condition?

(Questions 3 to 4 share the same question stem)

The client in the early stage of Alzheimer's disease (AD) and his adult son attend appointment at the community mental health center. While conversing with the nurse, the son states, "I'm tired of hearing about how things were 30 years ago. Why does Dad always talk about the past?"

3. The nurse interprets the son's statement to indicate which main problem?

4. When providing family education with those who have a relative with AD about minimizing stress, which suggestion would be most relevant?

注意力障碍、记忆缺损、知觉改变及对时间和地点的定向力障碍。

1. 精神科的联络护士对患者进行了评估。基于以上情况，该护士应初步评估哪项内容？

2. 护理上述情况的患者时，最关键的措施是什么？

（3～4题共用题干）

一名患阿尔茨海默病尚属早期的患者和已成年的儿子参加社区精神健康中心的活动。在与护士交谈时，儿子说：“我很厌烦听30年前的事情，为什么爸爸总是谈论过去的事情？”

3. 护士认为儿子的话表明他存在哪个主要问题？

4. 患者的家属提供关于减小压力的家庭教育时，护士认为与减压关系最为密切的建议是什么？

Chapter 13 Nursing Management for Children and Adolescents with Psychiatric Disorders

第十三章 儿童及青少年精神障碍患者的护理

Learning Objectives

Memorization
1. Define mental retardation.
2. Describe common child and adolescent behavioral disorders.

Comprehension
1. Discuss the impact of early childhood trauma on a child's mental health.
2. Identify four factors that can contribute to a child developing emotional problems or mental problems.
3. Identify general guidelines and considerations for working with clients with intellectual and developmental disabilities.

Application
1. Develop a nursing care plan for a child or adolescent with a psychiatric or behavioral disorder.
2. Identify nursing interventions in assisting clients and their families to cope with tic disorders.
3. Identify nursing interventions in assisting children and their families to cope with attention deficit and hyperactivity disorder.

学习目标

识记
1. 能准确描述精神发育迟滞的定义。
2. 能描述常见的儿童和青少年品行障碍临床表现。

理解
1. 能探讨早期童年创伤对孩子精神健康的影响。
2. 能识别导致儿童情绪障碍的四个因素。
3. 明确工作中对待精神发育迟滞儿童、青少年的一般准则和注意事项。

运用
1. 为精神或行为障碍儿童或青少年制订一份护理计划。
2. 制订护理措施帮助患儿和他们的家庭应对抽动症。
3. 制订护理措施帮助患儿和他们的家庭应对注意缺陷与多动障碍。

Jesse, a boy, had always been a troublesome child. Even in the preschool period, he would destroy the house like a tornado, shouting, and climbing the furniture. Not any toy or activity ever attracted his attention for more than a few minutes. He would often run in a busy street or a crowded market without warning, seemingly unaware of the dangers in these places.

杰西一直是一个会制造麻烦的男孩。甚至到了学龄前期，他还像龙卷风一样破坏房子，大吼大叫，踩踏家具。没有任何玩具或活动能吸引他注意超过几分钟，经常在繁忙的街道或拥挤的市场飞奔，毫无戒备，也意识不到危险。

He often made his parents exhausted, but his parents hadn't been too concerned the deep reasons. Boys will be boys, they thought so. But at age 7, Jesse was no easier to handle. He can not settle down long enough to complete even the simplest tasks, from chores to homework. His teacher gave comments that he often can't concentrate in class and have destructive behaviors, these troubles became too frequent to ignore.

他常常让父母筋疲力尽，但是他父母一直没有考虑深层原因。男孩就是男孩，本性难移，他们这样认为。但是在他7岁的时候，问题不再容易处理了。很难让杰西安静下来完成任何简单任务，从家务活到家庭作业。老师评价他在课堂上经常不能集中注意力并且有破坏性行为，已经不容忽视。

Please think about the following questions based on the case:

1. What is the most likely medical diagnosis for Jesse?
2. What is the major nursing diagnosis for Jesse?

请思考：

1. 最可能的医疗诊断是什么？
2. 主要的护理诊断是什么？

The psychiatric care of children has become a growing worldwide crisis. Almost 21% of U.S. children and adolescents ages 9 to 17 years have a diagnosable mental or addictive disorder associated with at least minimum impairment. Nearly four million (11%) suffer from a major mental illness that results in significant impairments at home, at school, and with peers; 5% have extreme functional impairment with their wellness. Approximately 70% of children and adolescents in need of psychiatric services do not receive treatment. In much of the world, the problems normally associated with these disorders of infants and children are exacerbated by a dearth of clinicians specifically trained to work with infants and children, including psychiatrists, psychologists, and mental health counsellors, as well as specifically trained nurses, advanced nurse practitioners, and social workers. The same situation is also happened in China with psychiatric disorders in childhood now receiving much more attention. This chapter will focus on the most common problems experienced by infants, children and adolescents: mental retardation, autism, attention deficit/hyperactivity disorder, tic disorders, conduct disorders, and emotional disorder.

婴儿、儿童和青少年的精神科护理工作越来越受到世界范围的重视。以美国为例，9~17岁的儿童和青少年中，约21%曾患过精神障碍。近400万（11%）儿童和青少年患有严重精神疾病，导致其家庭、学校以及社会功能的严重损害，5%的儿童和青少年因严重的功能损害而影响其自身健康。然而，令人遗憾的是，需要治疗的儿童和青少年中，约70%未能得到应有的治疗和护理。由于缺乏受过训练的儿童精神科临床专家，包括精神病专家、心理学家、精神健康咨询工作者、精神科护士及社会工作者等，婴儿、儿童及青少年的精神障碍问题变得更为复杂和棘手。本章将主要介绍婴儿、儿童及青少年精神障碍中最常见问题：精神发育迟滞、儿童孤独症、注意缺陷和多动障碍、抽动障碍、品行障碍和情绪障碍等患者的护理。

Section 1 Nursing Management for Children and Adolescents with Mental Retardation

I. Introduction

i. Definition

Mental retardation is a disorder characterized by a. significantly subaverage intellectual functioning (an IQ of approximately 70 or below); b. onset before 18 years of age; c. and concurrent deficits or impairments in adaptive functioning including at least two of the following: communication, self-care, home living, social/interpersonal skills, use of community resources, self-direction, functional academic skills, work, leisure, health, and safety.

ii. Epidemiology

The World Health Organization reports that mental retardation is one of the most common disorders with prevalence rates ranging from 3% for mild retardation to 3‰ -4‰ for moderate and severe retardation. However, it should be noted that rates of retardation may vary according to the criteria used to determine the existence of the disorder, methods of assessment, and populations studied. In China, approximately 1.07‰ of children and adolescents aged 0 to 14 years have a diagnosable level of mental retardation and estimates range from 0.75‰ among children in urban populations and 1.4‰ in rural communities according to a survey in 1988. Rates for boys are estimated at 1.24‰ , and for girls at 1.06‰ . It should be noted that the prevalence increases with age.

II. Etiology and Mechanism

The etiology of mental retardation may be ascribed to biological (including genetic) and psychosocial factors, or a combination of the two. And, in approximately 30%-40% of individual seen in clinical settings no clearly defined etiology can be determined. However, six major predisposing factors have been identified: heredity; early alterations in embryonic development; pregnancy and perinatal factors; general medical conditions acquired in infancy or childhood, including infections, traumas and poisoning (especially lead and mercury poisoning); other mental disorders, including autistic disorder and pervasive developmental disorder; and environmental influences, including deprivation of nurturance and of social, linguistic, and other stimulation.

第一节 精神发育迟滞患者的护理

一、概　述

（一）概念

精神发育迟滞通常于18岁之前发病，主要表现为智力低下（IQ低于70）和至少以下两种功能适应不良：交流能力、自理能力、日常生活能力、社会/人际间技巧、社区资源利用、自我引导以及学习、工作、娱乐、健康和安全等方面的功能。

（二）流行病学

世界卫生组织报告精神发育迟滞是一种常见的精神障碍，轻度精神发育迟滞的患病率为3%，中度和重度约为3‰~4‰。然而，由于调查方法及诊断标准的不同，各国所报告的患病率差异很大。我国八省市对0~14岁儿童精神发育迟滞流行病学调查表明，患病率为1.07‰，城市为0.75‰，农村为1.40‰，农村患病率明显高于城市。本症男女患病率有差异，男童高于女童，男童患病率为1.24‰，女童为1.06‰。且患病率有随年龄增长而增高的趋势。

二、病因及发病机制

精神发育迟滞为生物（包括基因）和心理社会等因素相互作用的结果。30%~40%的患者发病原因不明确。研究表明以下六种因素是导致精神发育迟滞的主要危险因素：遗传因素；胚胎早期受到干扰；母孕期间及围生期各种不利因素；婴儿及儿童期的疾病，包括感染、创伤及中毒（特别是铅和汞中毒）；其他精神障碍的影响，如儿童孤独症和广泛性发育障碍；环境因素，包括教育、社会交往、语言和其他刺激匮乏。

III. Types and Clinical Manifestation

Although the symptoms of retardation may vary according to the severity of the disorder, in order to meet diagnostic criteria, the onset of retardation must be before 18 years of age. The initial manifestation of symptoms may occur shortly after birth or within the first year of life, as the child fails to meet expected developmental milestones such as rolling over, crawling, sitting, walking, and initiating speech patterns. Some children with moderate mental retardation may not exhibit developmental delays until two to four years of age, while children with mild retardation may not be identified until they have entered school and fail to attain the skills expected of children their age.

Retardation can occur independently of other mental or physical disorders. A determination of mental retardation requires that a child receive a score of approximately 70 or lower of an individually administered intelligence test-the Wechsler intelligence scales for children and social adaptive ability scale.

The *CCMD-3* lists four degrees of severity of mental retardation: mild mental retardation-IQ level 50-69, with a mental age of 9 to 12 years; moderate retardation-IQ level 35-49, with a mental age of 6 to 9 years; severe mental retardation 20-34, with a mental age of 3 to 6 years; and, profound mental retardation-below 20, with a mental age of 0 to 3 years.

The various behavioral manifestations and abilities associated with each of these levels of retardation are outlined in table 13-1.

三、常见类型与临床表现

本症临床表现多与其严重程度有关。根据诊断标准，均于18岁前发病。严重者可于出生时或出生后1年内发病，主要表现为翻身、爬行、坐立、行走及说话延迟；中度者可于2～4岁发病；而轻度者常于入学后由于表现出与同龄儿童有差距才被发现。

本病可伴有或不伴有其他精神或生理疾病。主要表现为智力低下（智商低于70），常用的心理测验为韦氏智力测验和社会适应能力量表。

CCMD-3 将本病分为轻度、中度、重度和极重度四个水平。轻度者智商为50～69，智龄为9～12岁；中度者智商为35～49，智龄为6～9岁；重度者智商为20～34，智龄为3～6岁；极重度者智商低于20，智龄为0～3岁。

各水平行为和能力表现如表13-1所示。

Table 13-1 Characteristics of mental retardation

Subtype	IQ level	Deficits	Comments
Mild	50-69	None apparent in early childhood May need some minimal assistance with self-help and when experiencing social or economic stress	85% of all persons with mental retardation fall into this category Individuals have difficult in adapting to school but may achieve some degree of educational, social and vocational skills The 6th grade can be achieved by late tens "Educable"—can acquire academic skills up to approximately the 6th grade
Moderate	35-49	Poor awareness of needs of others Usually no progression beyond second-grade level Need moderate supervision due to self-care deficits Require supervision and guidance under mild social and economic stress	10% of all persons with mental retardation; May profit from vocational training Can function in sheltered workshops as unskilled or semiskilled persons Previously referred to as "trainable"

continued

Subtype	IQ level	Deficits	Comments
Severe	20-34	Poor motor development and minimal speech Unable to learn academic skills, but may learn to talk and be trained in elementary hygiene skills or activities of daily living Require complete supervision in a controlled environment	3%-4% of all persons with mental retardation; May learn to perform simple work tasks
Profound	below 20	Minimal capacity for sensorimotor function Require total nursing care and highly structured environment with supervision due to self-care deficit	1%-2% of all persons with mental retardation; May learn some productive skills "Custodial"

表 13-1　精神发育迟滞的特点

亚型	智商水平（IQ）	缺陷	评价
轻度	50～69	① 儿童早期不发病 ② 在面临社会或经济应激时需要帮助	① 占全部患者的 85% ② 学校适应困难，经过最小的自我支持，可获得社会和职业技能，10 岁以后可达 6 年级水平 ③ "可教育的"——能获得学校技能，达到大约 6 年级水平
中度	35～49	① 严重缺乏对他人需要的意识 ② 通常低于 2 年级水平 ③ 由于自理能力欠缺，需要中等程度的监督 ④ 在面临轻微的社会或经济应激时需要指导	① 占全部患者的 10% ② 可从职业培训中获益 ③ 在安全工作组中可承担无技术或半技术的工作 ④ "可训练的"
重度	20～34	① 动作技能发展较差，语言发育水平低下 ② 不能学习学校技能，但可学习讲话，可对其进行基本卫生技能和日常活动行为的训练 ③ 在控制的环境中需要完全的监督	① 占全部患者的 3%～4% ② 可以学习完成简单的工作任务
极重度	20 以下	① 感觉运动功能极低 ② 由于自理能力的欠缺需要完全的护理照护，以及监督下的高度结构化环境	① 占全部患者的 1%～2% ② 可学习一些生产性的技巧 ③ "监禁的"

IV. Treatment

i. Principle of Treatment

Treatment should aim to maximize the potential of those with mental retardation, with a particular focus on adaptive skills. Treatment generally includes specialized educational instruction with educational mainstreaming of children in the regular school environment, whenever possible. Families may need help with behavior management. Psychopharmacologic and behavior management may be required for those with severe behavior problems.

四、治　疗

（一）治疗原则

精神发育迟滞患者治疗目的是最大限度发挥患者潜能，尤其是提高适应性技能。治疗包括特殊的教育指导、训练以及其他康复措施。只要可能，应在学校正常学习、生活。患者家庭需要行为治疗的支持。严重者，应配合药物治疗和行为治疗。

ii. Treatment Measures

1. Psychoeducational Intervention Appropriate intervention should be based on the needs of the child as determined by a team of professionals, address the priorities and concern s of the family, and be provided in the least restrictive and most inclusive setting possible.

(1) Infant/Toddler services: Services to infants and toddlers can be home-based, center-based, or some combination of the two. The nature of the services should be based on the results of the child's assessment and family's priorities for the child. These should be used to develop an individual family service plan (IFSD) for the child that includes all parties participating in the intervention and is coordinated by a Services Coordinator (case manager) who is available and acceptable to the family. The services may include assistive technology, intervention for sensory impairments, family counseling, parent training, health services, language services, nursing intervention, nutrition counseling, occupational therapy, physical therapy, and case management.

(2) Preschool and school services: Services to preschool children, ages 3 to 5, and school-aged children, 6 to 12, can be home-based, but are more frequently center-based. As in the case of infants and toddlers, a team evaluation and parent input is used to develop an intervention plan. This plan-the Individualized Education Plan (IEP)-details the objectives for improving the child's skills. Services may include special education provided by a certified teacher and focused on the needs of the child; child counseling; occupational, physical therapy, and language therapy; recreational activities; school health and transportation services; and parent training or counseling. These services should be provided in the most inclusive and "least restrictive setting" available (e.g., a regular preschool program, Headstart Center, or the child's home).

2. Social/Interpersonal Intervention Social and interpersonal interventions can be both preventative and therapeutic. As noted above, children with mental retardation may be at an increased risk for behavioral disorders. Therefore, a variety of group social and recreational activities should be included in the child's educational program. These activities should include non-disabled peers and may include participation in birthday parties, attending recreational activities such as ball games and movies, participating in youth sports activities, and visiting community sites such as the zoo. The goal of the activities should be teaching appropriate social skills relevant to group participation and building self-esteem. Social or parent support groups can also be an outlet for

（二）治疗措施

1. 心理教育干预 由专业人员确定儿童及其家庭需要，在最低限制的环境中为其提供最合适的干预措施，使其有机会得益于同伴的影响，享受和其他儿童一样的社区资源。

（1）针对婴幼儿的服务：对此年龄儿童的教育可以以家庭、保健机构为中心，或二者结合。根据对儿童及其家庭需要的评估，确立个人家庭服务计划，由项目管理者负责参与和协调实施。教育内容包括帮助的技巧、感觉障碍的干预、家庭咨询、父母训练、保健服务、语言服务、护理干预、营养咨询、工作疗法、物理疗法、个案管理等。

（2）针对学龄前以及学龄儿童的服务：学龄前3～5岁，学龄期6～12岁，对此阶段儿童的服务可在家庭，但更多在机构里进行。针对小组评估及父母所提供信息的基础上，制订护理计划，即个体化教育计划。此计划中应详细列出改善儿童技能的目标，服务内容包括由相应资历的教师提供教育，以满足其需要，如儿童咨询、工作疗法、语言治疗、娱乐疗法、学校健康服务，以及父母的训练和咨询。这些训练最好在限制最小的环境下进行，如常规学校、幼儿园、儿童家里等。

2. 社会/人际间干预 社会/人际间干预包括预防和治疗两部分。精神发育迟滞的儿童多有行为障碍，所以，儿童的教育项目中应包括大量的集体活动和娱乐活动，如参加生日宴会、球类比赛、运动会，参观社区设施（如动物园等），以教给儿童社会交往技巧，建立自尊心。另外，有同类问题儿童的家长在活动中还可以讨论各自感受，这对家长来说也有较好的治疗和预防作用。

parents to discuss their feelings with individuals who have similar experiences.

Therapeutic interventions with other children and families may include family therapy, individual child behavior therapy, parent training, and group therapy with mildly mentally disabled children and adolescents focusing on developing appropriate social skills. Child behavioral interventions can be used to teach self-care, leisure, interpersonal, and survival skills. Disruptive behaviors such as throwing tantrums, self-injury, noncompliance, and aggression toward others can also be addressed through behavioral techniques.

儿童和家庭治疗措施主要包括家庭治疗、个体化儿童行为治疗、父母训练、小组训练等。通过对轻度障碍的儿童行为干预，可教会儿童和青少年自理，训练其娱乐、人际和生存的技巧，而通过行为技能的训练可帮助儿童克服发脾气、自伤、不依从、攻击性等社会适应不良行为。

3. Psychopharmacological Intervention Treatment specifying the use of medication should only be considered when a particular psychiatric condition known to benefit from a specific drug coexists with the mental retardation or developmental disability. These conditions may take the form of a severe depression, obsessive-compulsive disorder, attention deficit-hyperactivity disorder, or a variety of other psychiatric disorders. When drug treatment is used, it should only be one component of an overall treatment approach.

3. 药物治疗 应尽量避免应用药物，只有伴严重抑郁、强迫、注意缺陷伴多动等障碍的儿童才考虑用药。药物治疗必须联合其他方法同时进行。

4. Final Comments The following two approaches need to be considered in the treatment of children with mental retardation:

(1) Interdisciplinary approach: Because children with mental retardation often have other problems, it is necessary to involve a team of practitioners from different areas (e.g., child psychiatrists, social workers, child psychologists, special education teachers, speech and language specialists, and community agencies) in the comprehensive diagnosis and treatment of the child. This type of interdisciplinary team approach is considered to be imperative for comprehensive assessment, treatment, and management of children with mental retardation.

4. 注意事项 在对精神发育迟滞儿童的治疗中，应注意以下两个方面：

（1）团队合作：因为此类儿童问题涉及多方面，多方面专家组成的团队治疗非常重要。团队成员包括儿童精神科专家、社会工作者、儿童心理学家、特殊教育者、语音和语言专家、社区机构等。通过团队合作，可达到对儿童全面了解和治疗全面实施。

(2) Family involvement: An invaluable resource in evaluating and treating children with mental retardation is the child's family. Consequently, including the families of children with or at-risk for disabilities in every phase of intervention, from identification and planning through implementation and monitoring should be considered. However, including families making decisions about the treatment or management of their children's problems presents new challenges. Nevertheless, trying to understand and include families in the decision-making process can ultimately be rewarding and beneficial for all involved. The team must consider the level of knowledge and understanding of the family related to the disability of the child and/or the service/treatment options. If families are to participate in the decision-making process

（2）家庭参与：儿童家庭是治疗过程中最重要的资源。从评估到计划、实施、监督的各个阶段，家庭的作用都不容忽视。然而，让家庭参与决定其孩子的治疗和护理也常常给家庭带来新的挑战。无论怎样，鼓励家庭成员参与治疗计划的制订都会收到较好的效果。当然，这应以家庭对相关知识的了解为前提，否则将影响家庭的有效参与。一旦家庭掌握了其孩子的疾病知识，并了解可选择的服务或治疗，家庭成员会更需要通过和医务人员共同的决策过程来充实自己的知识。总之，团队中的工作人员应鼓励家庭的参与，

they must have the knowledge necessary to select appropriate alternatives. Once the family has an adequate understanding of the condition and service/treatment alternatives, they may need to be nurtured through the team decision-making process. Certainly, as a primary care provider the parent or family member has more at stake than the other team members. Over time, however, the cautious or reticent family member may become an active and vital team member.

使之成为团队中主动的、关键的一部分。

V. Application of the Nursing Process

五、护理程序的应用

Often a child's maladaptive responses are expressed differently from those of an adult. Nurses are challenged to develop realistic, well-defined goals, respond to the complex social needs of the child, understand and advocate for the child, and develop a comprehensive treatment plan that identifies and integrates the child's needs and resources.

通常来讲，儿童的适应不良表现与成人不同。对儿童精神科护理工作者来说，应根据儿童复杂的社会需要，确立现实而具体的目标，利用各种有效的资源，制订全面的治疗护理计划。

i. Nursing Assessment

（一）护理评估

The assessment of a young person is often complicated in the developmental process by the interaction of the child's psychopathology and his environment.

由于精神病理改变与儿童环境以及发展水平的相互作用，护理评估较为复杂。

The assessment focuses on the current physical abilities, psychological status, and social functioning. These data are compared with information on normal growth and development expectations. A developmental history is a useful way to gather information about past and current capabilities. The nurse should also assess the support systems (family, school, rehabilitative, and psychiatric) to ensure that the child's special needs have been identified and are being addressed.

护理评估内容：① 主要包括目前身体状况和能力、心理状况以及社会功能等方面，并将所得结果与正常生长、发育指标作对照。② 发展史评估对于评估精神发育迟滞儿童正常的成长和发展能力很有帮助。③ 护理人员还应评估支持系统（家庭、学校、康复、精神），以确认儿童的特殊需要是否被认识到，并努力得以满足。

In any assessment of a child, an interview with at least one parent or adult caregiver is essential; information gathered from teachers will enhance the quality of the assessment. Because mentally retarded children often have limited verbal expressive abilities, play therapy can provide opportunities and means of self-expression and allow children to act-out feelings behaviorally. A wide range of play materials, including dolls of various sizes and both genders can be provided. Among adolescents, privacy has been found to be the single most important criterion by which adolescents judge the value of their interactions with health care providers. It is, therefore, essential that teenagers be assured of the confidentiality of their interactions in order to avoid suspicion and evasiveness. The significance of the nurse's approach during the assessment cannot be overstated. The nurse should be

护理评估过程中，至少应有一名父母或成人照护者在场，一些信息也应征求教师的意见。由于儿童语言表达能力有限，评估中可应用游戏疗法。通过游戏材料，儿童可表达其感觉和行为。能否保护隐私是青少年判断他们与健康照护提供者之间关系的最重要标准。因此护理人员应做好保密的承诺，否则，将导致青少年的怀疑和逃避。在评估过程中，护理人员的方法至关重要。中立性态度，不做假设，耐心地倾听和等待儿童的回答是基本要求。

nonjudgmental, make no assumptions, listen, and wait patiently for responses to open-ended questions.

It is important to:

(1) Explore all of the possibilities that could explain a child's behaviors;

(2) Identify additional problems such as learning disabilities, conduct disorders, or depression;

(3) Identify significant elements of the family structures and classroom situations;

(4) Determine the child's thinking ability and academic skills.

在评估过程中，应重视以下方面：

（1）应努力探索可解释儿童行为的各种可能；

（2）寻找儿童可能存在的其他问题，如学习障碍、行为障碍、抑郁等；

（3）了解家庭结构和班级情况；

（4）了解儿童的思维能力和学习技能等。

ii. Nursing Diagnosis

The nursing diagnosis for children and adolescents is based on the client's problems, strengths, and coping abilities, the child's adaptive capabilities, and possible inferences about the etiology of the specific disorder. There are four reasons why the development of a nursing diagnosis for a child with mental disorder is difficult. They include the following: children can be inconsistent and unpredictable in behavior; the relationship and degree of comfort with the examiner may affect the result of data collected; children are constantly developing; and, children are affected and shaped by their parents, teachers, and others with whom they interact.

The determination of an appropriate nursing diagnosis for the mentally retarded client should reflect the severity of retardation and the client's level of adaptive functioning. The common nursing diagnosis includes the following:

1. Risk for injury related to altered physical mobility or aggressive behaviour.

2. Impaired social interaction related to speech deficiencies or difficulty in adhering to conventional social behaviour.

3. Self-care deficits related to physical mobility or lack of maturity.

4. Defensive coping related to feelings of powerlessness and threats to self-esteem.

5. Ineffective individual coping related to inadequate coping skills as a result of developmental delays.

6. Anxiety (moderate to severe) related to hospitalization and absence of familiar surroundings.

（二）护理诊断

护理诊断应基于服务对象的问题性质和程度、应对能力、适应情况以及可能的病因等评估结果。一般来讲，确立精神障碍儿童的护理诊断比较困难，原因有四点：一是儿童在行为上多表现不一致和不可预测；二是与检查者的关系影响资料的收集；三是儿童处于不断发展中；四是儿童的行为会受其父母、老师及其他所接触的人影响和塑造。

针对精神发育迟滞儿童的护理诊断应反映其疾病的严重程度和适应功能的水平，常见的护理诊断包括：

1. **潜在受伤的可能**　与身体活动能力改变或攻击性行为有关。

2. **社会交往能力受损**　与语言缺陷或遵守常规社会行为困难有关。

3. **自理能力欠缺**　与身体活动能力改变或成熟度不足有关。

4. **防御性应对**　与感到无能为力及自尊受到威胁有关。

5. **个人应对无效**　与缺乏应对技巧有关。

6. **焦虑**　与住院和对周围环境陌生有关。

iii. Nursing Care Planning and Implementation

1. Outcome Identification The established outcomes of intervention generally focus on a reduction of clinical symptoms, decreasing in degrees of stress and identifiable stressors, progressing in the realization of normal developmental stages, and therapeutic changes.

（三）护理计划与措施

1. **护理目标**　针对精神发育迟滞儿童的主要护理目标是减少临床症状、减轻压力、促进正常的生长发育及针对病情及时调整治疗措施。具体护理目标如下：

The following criteria may be used to measure the results of interventions with mentally retarded clients:

(1) Absence or reduction of incidence of physical harm;

(2) Increased levels of socially appropriate interaction with others;

(3) Satisfaction of self-care needs;

(4) Increased ability to accept direction from others without becoming defensive;

(5) Increased use of adaptive coping skills in response to stressful situations;

(6) Increased ability to cope appropriately with anxiety and to maintain manageable levels of anxiety.

儿童能够：

（1）不发生或少发生身体受伤；

（2）用社会可接受的方式与他人进行交往；

（3）满足自理需要；

（4）接受别人的指导和建议；

（5）在压力环境下表现出适应性的应对技巧；

（6）恰当应对焦虑和保持焦虑处于可被控制的水平。

2. Nursing Intervention Many factors, such as the establishment of a therapeutic relationship and effective role modeling, affect the outcome of nursing intervention.

(1) Establishing a therapeutic relationship: As stated earlier, the relationship and degree of comfort the child and adolescent feels with the psychiatric nurse affect the type of data collected. The same can be said for the response of a child or adolescent during the planning and implementing of nursing interventions. The following are a list of ground rules for establishing a therapeutic relationship with children and adolescents while providing therapeutic interventions:

1) Accept the child or adolescent client as an equal when able, keeping in mind the person's age.

2) Do not use baby talk or substandard language or "talk down" while communicating with the child or adolescent. Listen to the emotions expressed and encourage verbalization.

3) Do not force on the client or push him or her to confide in you.

4) Accept the client but discuss any undesirable behavior. Ignoring behavior such as tics also may be necessary in some situations. Each behavior needs to be evaluated to decide the appropriate approach.

5) Be a good role model.

6) Be aware of body language and nonverbal communications. Children and adolescents are quite observant of what adults say and how they communicate feelings-both verbally and nonverbally. They should know that adults have good and bad days that can affect their interpersonal relationships, especially in the area of communication.

(2) Being a good role model: The following rules can apply to nurses who work with children and adolescents in the psychiatric setting:

2. 护理措施 治疗性护患关系的建立、良好角色榜样的塑造等因素影响护理干预的效果。

（1）建立治疗性关系：儿童与护理工作者良好关系的建立直接影响资料收集，护理计划和实施效果。以下为护理工作者在为儿童提供治疗性干预中的普遍原则：

1）接受儿童和青少年，视其为平等的关系，同时应考虑其年龄。

2）不要用儿童语言，不标准语言，或居高临下的交流方式与其交流，仔细倾听其情绪的反映表达，鼓励其运用语言表达自己。

3）不要强迫服务对象完全接受或信任护士。

4）接受儿童本人，但应与其讨论他的不良行为，并确定适当的应对方法。

5）做一个良好的角色榜样。

6）意识到形体语言和非语言沟通。儿童和青少年经常通过观察成人的语言和非语言表达来获得信息，应该让儿童知道，成人的交流会受日常中很多事情的影响。

（2）努力成为良好的角色榜样：成人角色榜样的原则对护理工作者也是有效的。

1) Do not lose control in stressful situations because children are great imitation of adult behaviours.

2) Do not use alcohol or pills as a crutch. Your behaviour tells children that it is okay to do the same.

3) Be an appropriate and consistent disciplinarian. Such an attitude denotes love and provides security. Children do not always want what they ask for; they just test adults.

4) Do not try to imitate children by dressing, talking, or acting younger. Children need good role models, not adults who try to be peers.

5) Be honest and give compliments when they are deserved.

(3) Others: Other aspects of nursing intervention include:

1) Helping the child or adolescent master developmental tasks to overcome regressive, slow, or impaired developmental behaviour.

2) Establishing a method of communication with clients who have difficulty in communicating, such as withdrawn, disoriented, mute, hostile, preoccupied, or autistic children or adolescents.

3) Identifying stimuli that might foster abusive, destructive, or otherwise negative behaviour.

4) Allowing time for the client to respond to therapeutic interventions.

(4) Special nursing intervention: The nurse working in an institutional setting is challenged to provide environmental stimulation, as well as meet the emotional and physical needs of the child, because individuals with mental retardation do not always communicate physical symptoms. Helping the child master activities of daily living may be a slow process involving behavioral therapy. Protective care may be necessary if the client is epileptic, prone to acting-out behavior, disoriented, or self-mutilating (head banging or biting self). The administration of anticonvulsant and psychotropic drugs is also the nurse's responsibility. Education of the family is an important factor not to be overlooked, because many persons who are mentally retarded attend an institution during the week but go home for weekends or holiday visits. Others attend a day hospital, special school, or sheltered workshop, and return home at night as well as on weekends. The nurse is the client's advocate in the institutional setting and when relating to the family. Identifying the family's ability to cope and continue with the therapy at home is important to maintaining and promoting progress and to minimize the stress that can

1）因为儿童多模仿成人的行为，所以在压力情境下，应保持稳定的情绪。

2）不要滥用酒精和药物，因为儿童会认为此行为可接受。

3）做一名恰当而言行一致的教育者，坦率但不妥协，这种态度会传达爱和安全感。因为儿童要求的常常并不是他们真正想要，只是用来考验成人。

4）成人应保持成熟的形象，不要刻意学着儿童的样子打扮和表现得年轻。

5）做一名诚实的人，并适当给予儿童赞赏。

（3）其他：在护理实施中其他应注意的方面包括：

1）帮助儿童、青少年掌握发展的任务，克服退化、缓慢或者受损的发展行为。

2）与沟通困难者建立一种有效的沟通方法。

3）确认可导致一些消极行为的刺激源。

4）不急于求成。

（4）特殊护理措施：对于被收容在医疗机构中进行治疗的精神发育迟滞儿童，由于此类儿童很少报告自身生理症状，所以护理人员在满足其情绪和生理需要的同时，应努力提供环境刺激。帮助儿童掌握日常生活行为是一项需要涉及行为治疗的缓慢过程。如果儿童有癫痫、冲动行为、定向力障碍、自伤等倾向，护理人员应注意提供保护性护理。抗抽搐药物和抗精神病药物的管理也是护理工作者的职责。另外儿童经常会在周末或节假日回到家里，所以对家庭的教育也是不容忽视的重要方面。无论在医疗机构中，还是在家里，护理人员都是服务对象的支持者。确认家庭的应对能力和家庭在持续照护中的能力对于促进治疗效果和最大限度降低环境变化造成的压力非常重要。

occur when changing environments.

iv. Nursing Evaluation

The evaluation of nursing interventions for children and adolescents who are seen in the clinical setting for the treatment of mental disorders is an ongoing process. Consideration is given to the developmental stage of the client and whether any changes in mood or behaviour have occurred since the initial assessment. The efficacy of prescribed medication is reviewed. Family dynamics are reassessed. Socialization and progress in school are discussed. Evaluation of care given to the mentally retarded client should reflect positive behavioural changes. Evaluation is accomplished by determining if the goals of care have been met through implementation of the nursing actions selected. The nurse reassesses the plan and makes changes when required. Reassessment data may include information gathered by asking the following questions:

1. Have nursing actions providing for the client's safety been sufficient to prevent injury?

2. Have all of the client's self-care needs been fulfilled? Can he or she fulfill some of these needs independently?

3. Has the client been able to communicate needs and desires so that he or she can be understood?

4. Has the client learned to interact appropriately with others?

5. When regressive behaviors surface, can the client accept constructive feedback and discontinue the inappropriate behavior?

6. Has anxiety been maintained at a manageable level?

7. Has the client learned new coping skills through behavior modification? Does the client demonstrate evidence of increased self-esteem because of the accomplishment of these new skills and adaptive behaviors?

8. Have primary caregivers been taught realistic expectations of the client's behavior and methods for attempting to modify unacceptable behavior?

9. Have primary caregivers been given information regarding various resources from which they can seek assistance and support within the community.

（四）护理评价

评价过程是一个持续进展的过程。评价过程中应考虑儿童的发展阶段，判断情绪和行为是否发生了变化，药物治疗是否有效，家庭情况是否有变化，社会化情况和学校技能方面是否进步等。护理评估应该反应正向的行为改变。评估要考虑实施护理措施的结果是否完成了护理目标。重新评估护理计划和做相应的改变也是必需的。在重新评估收集资料阶段护理人员应提出以下问题：

1. 护理行为是否足以保护患者不受伤害?

2. 患者的自理需要是否均得到了满足。患者能否独立完成部分或全部的自理需要?

3. 患者能够进行有效地交流以使他人了解他的需要吗?

4. 通过学习，患者是否能与他人进行适当的相处?

5. 当退缩行为出现时，患者能否接受建设性反馈意见并及时终止不合适的行为?

6. 患者的焦虑水平是否被保持在一个可被控制的水平?

7. 在改变患者行为的过程中患者是否学会了新的应对技巧。由于新技巧和适应性行为的获得，患者的自尊水平是否得到了提高?

8. 通过教育，患者的生活照护者是否对患者的期望更现实，同时学会了有效的方法以纠正患者的不良行为?

9. 患者的生活照护者是否被告之社区中的各种资源，以便在需要时可及时获取帮助和支持?

Section 2 Nursing Management for Children and Adolescents with Autistic Disorder

I. Introduction

i. Definition

Autistic disorder is a childhood onset disorder manifested by markedly abnormal or impaired development in social interaction and communication and a markedly restricted repertoire of interests and activities.

ii. Epidemiology

According to DSM-Ⅳ, the rate of occurrence ranges from 2 to 20 per 10 000 individuals, with the median rate of Autistic Disorder in epidemiological studies is 5 per 10 000 individuals. More recent reports, however, place prevalence estimates at 1-2 per 1 000 for autism, and 6-7 per 1 000 for the entire spectrum of autistic disorders. The increase in prevalence estimates over time is generally attributed to the gradual broadening in how we define autism/ASD, and our increased awareness and detection of its diverse manifestations, particularly in the more cognitively or linguistically capable.

It is yet to be determined whether the rate of occurrence reflects differences in the methodologies of studies or actual increases in frequency of the condition. California, for example, has shown close to a 300% increase in the number of autism diagnoses during the last quarter of the 20th Century. However, there is an increased risk of Autistic Disorder among siblings of individuals with the disorder, with approximately 5% of siblings also exhibiting the Autism. While girls with Autistic Disorder are more likely to have more severe Mental Retardation, rates of Autism are four to five time higher in males than in females.

II. Etiology and Mechanism

Although the exact underlying pathology associated with autistic disorder is unknown, several theories have evolved speculating about etiology.

i. Social Environmental Factors

While there are proponents for a number of "social environment" causes there appears to be little scientific background for these theories. Nonetheless, the proponents of these theories have suggested that autistic disorder is caused by the parents and the social environment they provide. Some of the specific causative factors proposed in these theories are parental

第二节 儿童孤独症患者的护理

一、概 述

（一）概念

儿童孤独症是起病于婴幼儿期，以不同程度人际交往障碍、兴趣狭窄和行为方式刻板为主要表现的精神障碍。

（二）流行病学

据DSM-Ⅳ，儿童孤独症的患病率为0.2‰～2‰，中位数为0.5‰。然而近来的研究表明某些地区孤独症的患病率为1‰～2‰，孤独障碍的患病率为6‰～7‰，患病率的增加是由于放宽了孤独症的诊断标准，提高了对孤独症各种症状尤其是认知、语言方面的认识和检测水平。

也有必要确定发生率增加是由于研究方法的不同或实际情况就是如此。例如，加利福尼亚在上世纪后25年孤独症的人数增加了将近3倍。孤独症患者的同胞患有该病的危险性增加，约有5%也患有孤独症。男女之比为4～5∶1，但女孩一般都伴有较严重的精神发育迟滞。

二、病因及发病机制

目前，直接导致儿童孤独症的病理还不确定，根据一些研究，可能的病因如下：

（一）社会环境因素

虽然“社会环境”导致孤独症尚缺乏科学的理论依据，但一些学者认为儿童孤独症与父母及其社会环境有关。主要原因包括被父母遗弃、父母人格异常、家庭破裂、家庭危机、缺乏刺激以及不良的沟通方式等。

rejection, child responses to deviant parental personality characteristics, family break-up, family stress, insufficient stimulation, and faulty communication patterns.

ii. Biological Factors

Biological factors include genetics and neurological factors.

1. Genetics Some studies have shown that siblings of autistic children have a 50 times greater chance of being autistic than the general population, with the morbidity rate of 3%.Studies have also shown that the concordance rate in identical twins is very much higher (60% to 90%) than in fraternal (non-identical) twins (0 to 20%), thereby establishing that genetic factors play a key role. The discovery of the genes-and it seems clear that there are a number of different genes involved-is made more complex by the complex nature of autism and the fact that people with autism vary dramatically in degree and form.

2. Neurological Factors Because of the wide range of factors involved in Autistic Disorders, it has proven extremely difficult to define specific neurological factors involved with the Disorder. Nonetheless, some researchers have identified a number of possible factors, including: postnatal neurological infections, congenital rubella, phenylketonuria, and fragile X syndrome as possible causative agents. Several studies have also implicated various structural and functional abnormalities in the brain. These include ventricular enlargement, left temporal abnormalities, increased glucose metabolism, and an elevated blood serotonin level.

iii. Environmental Factors

The only environmental factors for which we have preliminary evidence of such causation are thalidomide-induced abnormalities produced during the embryonic period and anti-convulsants taken during pregnancy.

III. Types and Clinical Manifestation

Onset of the disorder occurs prior to age 3 and in most cases it runs a chronic course, with symptoms persisting into adulthood. The clinical features include impairment in reciprocal social interactions, restricted repertoire of interests and stereotyped behaviours. In most cases there is some degree of mental retardation. The overall severity of autistic disorder, as well as the specific behavioural manifestation of each characteristic, can vary as a function of age and developmental level.

i. Social Deficits

Deficits in social relating and reciprocity are currently viewed as core characteristics of autistic disorder.

（二）生物学因素

其中包括遗传因素和神经学因素。

1. 遗传因素 研究证明，遗传因素对本症的发生也许起重要作用。一些研究证明，孤独症患儿的兄弟姐妹也具有较高的发病率，患病率是3%，患病几率比正常人群高出50倍。而同卵双胞胎的发病率（60%～90%）更远远高于异卵双胞胎的发病率（0～20%）。对患儿基因的研究发现，孤独症患儿具有一些不同于正常儿童的基因，并且基因不同，疾病的严重程度和表现形式也不同。

2. 神经因素 尚很难证明何种神经因素与孤独症的发生有关，但一些研究发现某些神经因素，如产后脑部感染、先天性风疹、苯丙酮尿症、脆性X染色体综合征可能与孤独症的发病有关。一些研究还揭示了本症存在脑器质性或功能性的异常，如脑室扩大、左侧颞叶异常、糖代谢增强以及血5-羟色胺水平提高。

（三）环境因素

已经初步证明胚胎发育期间，孕妇服用某些镇静剂或抗惊厥类药物可影响胚胎发育而导致本症。

三、常见类型与临床表现

一般于3岁前发病，常为慢性病程，症状可一直持续到成人期。孤独症的基本特征为人际交往障碍，兴趣狭窄和行为方式刻板。其他症状虽也较常见，如各种程度的精神发育迟滞，但缺乏特异性。其症状的严重程度和表现的特殊性受患儿年龄和发展水平的影响。

（一）社会交往障碍

社会交往障碍是孤独症的核心，通常在与父母交往过程中被首次发现，如不与父母

Social difficulties are usually first apparent in the child's interaction with parents and may include failure to cuddle; an indifference or aversion to affection or physical contact; a lack of eye contact, facial responsiveness, or socially directed smiles; and a failure to respond to their parents' voices. Parents may initially be concerned that the child is deaf. Younger children may treat adults as interchangeable. Peer problems (e.g., lack of interest, inability to play cooperatively, failure to make friends) become evident in the preschool years.

拥抱；漠视或讨厌父母的关心和身体接触；缺乏眼神接触、面部表情和微笑；对父母的声音无反应等。父母最初会担心自己的孩子是否失聪，而孩子则认为与大人们无法沟通。同伴问题，如缺乏兴趣、不能合作、不善交朋友等，常在入学前出现，并且表现明显。

1. One of the earliest social deficits is in motor imitation. Young children with autistic disorder have been consistently found to have more difficulty imitating body movements and using objects than do developmentally matched control subjects. Although these skills tend to improve with age, subtle deficits in the imitation of body movements have been found even in high-functioning autistic adolescents. Deficits in eye-to-eye gaze represent another early-developing social behavior associated with autistic disorder. Recent research suggests that children with autistic disorder differ from control subjects not in the absolute amount of eye contact, but rather in the ways it is used, particularly for social or communicative purposes, such as sharing enjoyment or directing another person's attention.

1. 最早出现的社会缺陷为动作模仿方面。与正常儿童相比，孤独症儿童常被发现很难模仿身体运动和使用物体。另外，孤独症儿童缺乏眼与眼的对视，这代表着一种早期发展的社会行为损害。与正常儿童相比，二者的差别主要体现在目光接触的方式而不是数量上。

2. A variety of deficits in the recognition and use of affect are associated with autistic disorder. Young autistic children, compared to control subjects, display less positive affect, more neutral affect, and more incongruent combinations of affect. Positive affect occurs more often during solitary activities than during social interaction. Children with autistic disorder smile less often in response to their mothers' smiles and pay less attention to an adult simulating distress. Unusual affective expressions and difficulty with affective understanding and empathy have also been noted in older, high-functioning individuals with autistic disorder.

2. 孤独症儿童的另一表现是在情感的再认和利用方面。与正常儿童相比，他们很少表现出积极的情感，大多为中性，或与现实不协调。他们多于独处时表现得更为高兴，对父母的微笑或成人假装的悲伤情绪无动于衷。而年长儿童，以及功能水平较高儿童常见情绪表达异常，对情绪理解困难，以及缺乏同情心。

3. About 50% of autistic individuals fail to develop functional spoken language. Those who do acquire spoken language often exhibit delayed milestones and a deviant pattern of development. A number of unusual language features may be present, including immediate and delayed echolalia, pronoun reversal, repetitive language, idiosyncratic use of words and phrases, and abnormal prosody (i.e., eccentric pitch, stress, rate, and rhythm). Deficits in the pragmatic aspects of language (i.e., the ability to use speech and gesture in a communicative and socially appropriate manner) are also common (e.g., pedantic speech, one-sided rather than reciprocal conversation, difficulty in using and understanding facial

3. 语音和语言障碍是孤独症的另一个主要特点。50% 孤独症儿童也多表现为言语发育障碍。即使获得语言能力的儿童，也通常表现为说话延迟和异常的发展模式。言语发育障碍主要表现为以下几种形式：立即或延迟模仿语言、代词颠倒、重复语言、词和词组的特异应用以及异常韵律等。另外，在语言运用中的障碍也很常见，如在应用符合常规的语言和非语言交流方式进行沟通方面常有障碍。相反，在语义学方面，如语法和句法

expressions or gestures, and a tendency to perseverant on particular topics). In contrast, the semantic aspects of language, such as syntax and grammar, are relatively unimpaired.

相对受损较少。

ii. Stereotyped Behaviours

Stereotyped movements, sensory abnormalities, and an insistence on complex routines impose some degree of regularity or invariance on a perceptually confusing or unstable environment (figure 13-1). The most common motor stereotypes are arm, hand, or finger flapping; head or body rocking; and spinning. Sensory abnormalities include hypereactivity, heightened awareness, and heightened sensitivity in one or more modalities.

（二）刻板、僵硬的行为方式

孤独症儿童倾向于刻板、重复的行为和特殊古怪的动作姿势（图 13-1）。表现为来回踱步、反复旋转自己的身体、搓弄手指、拍手或摇晃身体，有时摩擦、拍打、撞头、咬硬东西、转圈走、重复地蹦跳、注意力涣散、东张西望、活动过度。

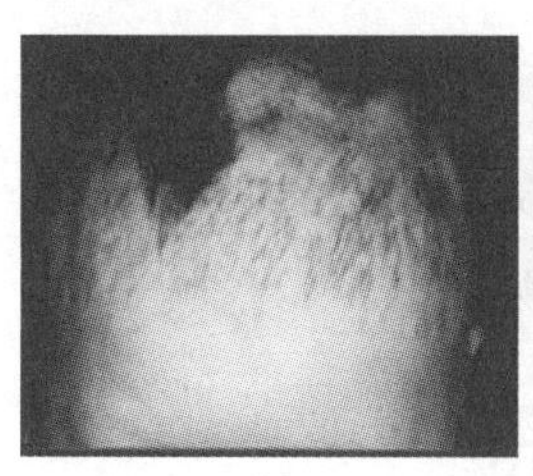
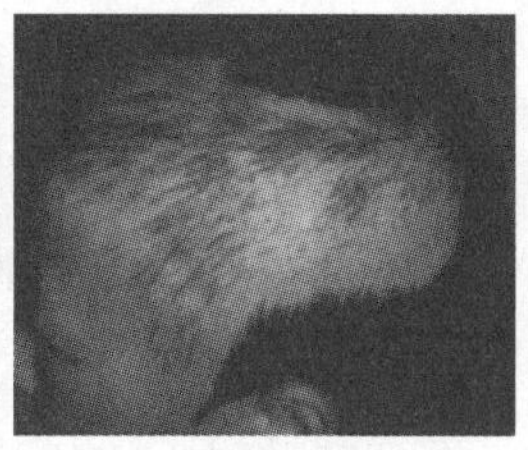
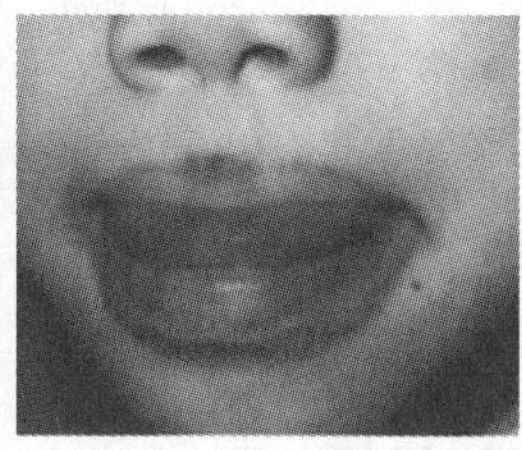
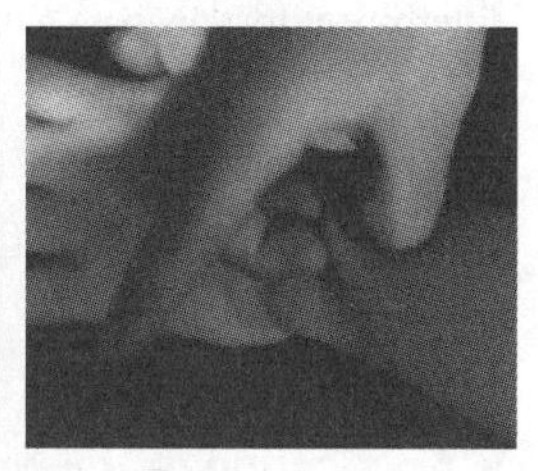

Figure 13-1 Stereotyped movements Trichotillomania, licking lip and pinching skin

iii. Restricted Interests

Restricted and repetitive forms of play are common in younger children with autistic disorder. Young autistic children demonstrate less diverse, less functional, and more sensory-based play (e.g., spinning, shaking, or twirling toys) than do control children. They also exhibit less play with dolls and less pretend play.

（三）兴趣范围狭窄

兴趣狭窄和重复性的游戏在孤独症患儿中是常见的。患儿对一般儿童所喜欢的玩具、游戏常缺乏兴趣，相反，对某些不是玩具的物品及游戏活动具有特别兴趣和迷恋，尤其是可以旋转的物品，如锅盖、瓶盖、车轮，观察旋转的电扇、奔驰的车轮达到着迷的程度。

IV. Treatment

There is no cure for autistic disorder. The primary goals of treatment are to promote social, communicative, and adaptive living skills; to reduce the frequency and intensity of maladaptive behavior such as rigidity and stereotypies; and to alleviate family stress. The best-established treatments for children with autistic disorder use educational and behavioral interventions. Early intervention programs appear to be beneficial. The following are effective in promoting learning and development, especially if begun early: a structured learning environment; specialized individually and developmentally based programming; the use of non-disabled peers as intervention agents; the use of behavioral techniques for the acquisition and generalization of new

四、治　疗

孤独症尚无特效治疗。治疗的主要目的为提高孤独症儿童的社会、交流和适应性生活技能，减少刻板行为等适应不良行为的发生频率和强度，缓解家庭压力。目前较好的治疗为教育和行为疗法。早期干预效果较好。以下为促进学习和发展中较为有效的策略：结构化的学习环境，有针对性的个别指导，以发展为基础的项目，以正常发育的同伴作为干预者，利用行为技巧，如游戏获得新技能的学习和推广以及父母参与等。

skills; and the involvement of parents in their child's treatment.

Pharmacotherapy is not a routine component of treatment, although in some cases it can be a useful adjunct. Haloperidol is an antipsychotic medication frequently used in the treatment of schizophrenia and has been shown in some controlled studies to reduce social withdrawal, stereotyped motor behavior, and some maladaptive behaviors such as self-mutilation and aggression. However, the drug has not proven effective in the treatment of abnormal interpersonal relationships and language impairments. Most importantly, long-term studies have show that over 30% of autistic children treated with haloperidol developed drug-related jerky muscle disturbances (dyskinesias), although most went away after the drug was discontinued.

目前药物治疗尚无法改变孤独症病程，但可能在某种程度上控制某些症状。例如研究证明用于治疗精神分裂症的抗精神病药物氟哌啶醇，能减少患者的社会缺陷、刻板行为及某些自残或伤害性的不良行为。但尚未证明该药物对治疗患者异常的人际交往关系和语言障碍有效，且一些长期的研究表明有30%的患儿应用氟哌啶醇后可伴发运动障碍，但大部分患儿停止用药后其运动障碍会消失。

At this point, however, research indicates that pharmacological treatment of autism is less effective than behavioural treatments.

然而，研究证明对孤独症的治疗，行为治疗的效果要好于药物治疗。

V. Application of the Nursing Process

五、护理程序的应用

i. Nursing Assessment

（一）护理评估

Assessment of children with autistic disorder is a complex endeavor. Critical elements include intellectual ability, linguistic competence, and adaptive functioning. The psychiatric nursing assessment begins with observing the child's behavior and the child's interactions with the family members.

评估内容主要包括智力、语言能力和社会适应能力。此外，患儿的身体状况和神经系统状况，尤其是协调能力、儿童期患病情况、损伤和住院情况等都要加以评估。睡眠、食欲、活动形式等也应包括在对这类儿童评估的范围内。

Keen observation is critical to evaluate the child's ability and relationship to others, to select age-appropriate activities, and to watch for the presence of stereotypic behavior. Assessment should also include a review of physical health and neurological status with particular attention to coordination, childhood illnesses, injuries, and hospitalizations. Sleep, appetite, and activity patterns should be assessed because they may be disturbed in these children.

评估过程中护理人员应注意观察患儿的行为，及其与家庭成员的交往方式。尤其应注意观察患儿与其年龄相符的活动，观察其刻板、僵化行为的表现。

These children exhibit a variety of behavioral problems and have varying degrees of adaptive deficits. Therefore, the assessment should include a review or the child's capacity for self-care and both adaptive and maladaptive behaviors.

这类儿童往往表现为较多的行为问题和各种程度的适应缺陷，所以对儿童自理能力和适应不良行为的评估也不容忽视。

Another important domain to be considered in the nursing assessment is the impact of the child's developmental delays on the family. After making the decision to place a child into a residential facility, family members may experience guilt, loss, and a sense of failure

当患儿家长由于无力在家庭中对儿童进行治疗和护理，不得不把患儿送到一些专门机构时，家庭成员大多会有犯罪感、失落感，或者失败感。所以，另一评估的重点是患儿

concerning their inability to manage the child at home.

ii. Nursing Diagnosis

Appropriate nursing diagnoses for the autistic disorder client include:

1. Impaired social interaction with peers and parents related to withdrawal.

2. Impaired verbal communication related to inadequate verbal skills.

3. Risk for self-mutilation related to neurological alterations.

iii. Nursing Care Planning and Implementation

Planning for nursing and other interventions should be a collaborative effort that includes the parents and, whenever possible, the child and may require the involvement of professionals from other disciples and representatives of community support agencies. To ensure that fragmentation of care does not occur, the psychiatric nurse assumes the role of case manager.

1. Outcome Identification The following criteria may be used for measurement of outcomes in the autistic disorder client.

The client:

(1) Demonstrates trust in at least one staff member;

(2) Is able to communicate so that he or she can be understood by at least one staff member;

(3) Exhibits no evidence of self-harm.

2. Nursing Intervention

(1) Common nursing interventions: Many factors such as establishing of a therapeutic relationship and being a good role model affect the outcome of nursing intervention (the detailed nursing activates presented in Unit 1 "Mental Retardation").

(2) Special nursing interventions: A successful health care visit for a child with autistic disorder (AD) can be accomplished by employing specific behavioral interventions. The goal is to help the child comply with the assessment or treatment using behavioral strategies. The following behavioral interventions were successfully implemented during our study by the nursing staff to obtain physical exams, vital signs, phlebotomy, and IV insertion.

1) Imitation/role-modeling paired with reinforcement: Modeling is a procedure that presents a sample of a given behavior to an individual to induce that individual to engage in a behavior. The nurse or parent demonstrates the desired action to the child. When the child imitates the action, the parent and/or nurse gives a "reinforcer" such as verbal praise.

发展上的延迟对其家庭的影响。

（二）护理诊断

针对儿童孤独症可能的护理诊断包括：

1. **与同伴和父母社会交往障碍** 与退缩性有关。

2. **语言交流障碍** 与缺乏语言技巧有关。

3. **潜在自残** 与神经性改变有关。

（三）护理计划与措施

护理计划的实施需要与服务对象及其父母的合作努力来完成，如果可能，还需要包括其他专业人员和社区支持机构的人员。在这一过程中护理工作者应担当起个案管理者的角色，以避免护理的中断。

1. **护理目标** 针对孤独症儿童的主要护理目标如下：

儿童能够：

（1）至少对一名医护人员表现出信任；

（2）能够通过交流得到至少一名医护人员的理解；

（3）没有发生自伤的行为。

2. **护理措施**

（1）一般护理措施：许多因素，如建立治疗性关系、成为良好的角色榜样等，都会影响护理措施的效果（具体护理措施见本章第一节“精神发育迟滞”的护理）。

（2）特殊护理措施：为保证孤独症患儿的医疗保健访视顺利进行，我们可以使用一些行为干预技巧。使用行为干预的目的是帮助孩子配合身体评估或治疗，提高治疗依从性。

1）模仿/榜样与强化：榜样是给个体展示一种行为过程，诱导个人参与这个行为。护士或家长对孩子演示所需的行动，当孩子模仿动作，父母和/或护士给口头表扬等“激励”。

2) Rewards: A reward is synonymous with a positive reinforcer. A reward is something that a child is motivated to obtain, which could be parental attention, praise, food, a break, a favorite activity, or a toy. The key is choosing a reward that is motivating. The parent usually knows these items and is typically the most appropriate person to deliver the rewards to the child.

3) High-probability requests/low-probability requests: High probability requests (high-p) are requests that have a high likelihood of compliance; low probability requests (low-p) are those with less expectation of compliance. "Touch your head" "Say Mom" or "Blow Mom a kiss" is examples of high-p requests. Once the momentum of compliance is established, a low-probability request is made, such as "Hold still". When completed, praise and delivery of the next request in the sequence immediately follows. After the child holds still (low-p request), allowing the procedure step to be completed, the child's mother holds or plays with the child for 5 seconds. This gives the child the best reward for the toughest task (to hold still). If the child is not compliant with a low-p request, no praise or reward should be given. The child's undesirable behaviors (e.g., kicking, hitting, screaming, crying) should be ignored or put on extinction. Extinction is a technical term of showing no observable or subjective response to the behavior.

4) Choices: It is important for children with AD to express preferences and make choices to increase personal autonomy and quality of life. Research has found that choice making can help decrease avoidance behavior and improve task performance. Research has indicated that individuals with severe developmental disabilities have not been offered many opportunities of choice by their educators or caregivers.

5) Visuals: Children who have AD are usually visual learners. When information is presented with a visual as opposed to verbal cues, children with AD are more successful at accomplishing the presented task.

6) Distraction techniques: Some researches described successful pre- and post-operative techniques of role-playing and distraction techniques to manage the operative course for tonsillectomies and adenoidectomies with children with autism. Distraction techniques can be used to decrease the amount of anxiety related to the procedure. Examples of distraction techniques include the following: Conversation, Singing, Counting and reciting the alphabet, Toys.

iv. Nursing Evaluation

Reassessment data may include information gathered by asking the following questions:

2）奖励：奖励是一种积极强化物的同义词。奖励是一个孩子希望获得的某些东西，这可能是父母的关注，赞美，食物，休息，最喜欢的活动或者一个玩具。关键是选择一个激励的奖励。父母通常知道这些东西，是最合适提供孩子奖励的人。

3）高概率/低概率的请求：高概率的请求是有很高的依从可能性；低概率的请求是有很低的依从可能性。例如“摸你的头”“叫妈妈”或“给妈妈一个吻”是高概率的请求。一旦建立了顺从的势头，一个低概率的请求，如“静静不动”完成时，立即赞扬和给与下一个要求。当后续的动作进一步完成，母亲拥抱孩子或和孩子玩5秒。这是孩子完成最艰难的任务后最好的奖励。如果孩子不顺从低概率要求，不应给予表扬或奖励。孩子的不良行为（如踢、打、尖叫、哭泣）应该被忽略或灭绝。灭绝是一个技术术语表示没有可观察到的或主观的反应行为。

4）选择：表达喜好和做出选择对孤独症患儿是很重要，能增加个人自立和生活质量。研究发现，选择能帮助孤独症患儿减少回避行为，提高任务绩效。研究表明，患有严重发育障碍的患者没有被教育工作者或看护者提供很多选择的机会。

5）视觉效果：有孤独症的孩子通常是视觉型学习者。当信息是视觉提示而不是口头提示，孤独症患儿能更成功地完成任务。

6）分散注意力技巧：有研究描述了成功的术前和术后角色扮演技巧和分散注意力技巧来管理孤独症儿童扁桃腺切除术和腺样体切除术的手术过程。分散注意力技巧可用于减少焦虑。分散注意力技巧的例子包括以下几点：对话、唱歌、计数和背诵字母表、玩具等。

（四）护理评价

评价过程是一个持续进展的过程。在评价阶段护理人员应提出以下问题：

1. Has the child been able to establish trust in at least one caregiver?

2. Have nursing actions directed toward preventing mutilating behaviors been effective in protecting the client from self-harm?

3. Has the child attempted to interact with others? Has he or she received positive reinforcement for these efforts?

4. Has eye contact improved?

5. Has the child established a means of communicating his or her needs and desires to others?

6. Have all self-care needs been met?

7. Does the child demonstrate an awareness of self as separate from others? Can he or she name his/her own body parts and body parts of caregiver?

8. Can he or she accept touch from others? Does he or she willingly and appropriately touch others?

1. 患者是否能够与至少一名照护者建立起信任的关系？

2. 是否建立了有效保护患者免于自伤的预防行为？

3. 患者是否试图与他人进行交往？当他朝这方面努力时是否得到了护理人员的积极强化？

4. 患者在应用目光接触方面是否有所进步？

5. 患者是否建立了一种表达其需要的交流方式？

6. 患者全部的自护需要是否得到了满足？

7. 患者是否意识到了自己与他人的隔离？能否说出自体及看护者的身体部分的名称？

8. 患者能否接受来自他人的触摸？他是否愿意并恰当地触摸他人？

Section 3 Nursing Management for Children and Adolescents with Attention Deficit and Hyperactivity Disorder

第三节　注意缺陷与多动障碍患者的护理

I. Introduction

一、概　述

i. Definition

Attention deficit and hyperactivity disorder (ADHD) is characterized by a combination of pervasive manifestation of over activity, marked inattention and lack of perseverance in task performance since early childhood. However, because the characteristic behavior of children younger than ages 4 or 5 years is so variable, it is difficult to establish this diagnosis in especially young children and the possibility of this disorder is often not considered until the child has entered kindergarten or the early grade school years. Nonetheless, it should be noted that in ordinary circumstances, even the attention of toddlers can be held in a variety of situations (for example, the average 2- to 3-year old child can typically sit with an adult looking through picture books). The clinical features should be evident in more than one situation (e.g., home, classroom, clinic, etc.)

（一）概念

注意缺陷与多动障碍是指发生于儿童早期明显的注意力不集中、与年龄不相称、与处境不相宜的活动过度和缺乏完成一件任务的毅力为主要特点的一组综合征。由于4～5岁之前儿童的行为非常多变，因此，在进入幼儿园和上学前，很难诊断此症。但在正常情况下，即使初学走路的孩子都会在不同情况下控制其注意力，例如平均2～3岁的儿童能坐在大人的身边看有图片的书。此症可发生于多种场所，如家庭、学校以及门诊等。

ii. Epidemiology

Because of the wide range of factors involved in establishing a diagnosis, estimates of prevalence rates for

（二）流行病学

由于诊断儿童多动症受多种因素广泛影响，患病率报告有很大差异。根据DSM- Ⅳ -

AD/HD have varied widely. The DSM-Ⅳ-TR put rates at 3% to 5%. However, other estimates vary from 2% to 7% in the United States with somewhat higher rates found in India and China. It should be noted, however, that using the same criteria may not adequately capture cultural differences. The general consensus is that about 3% to 7% of school-age children worldwide currently have ADHD. In China, the reported prevalence rate is variously reported at 1.3%-13.4% in school-aged children.

TR，该症患病率报告为3%～5%，也有报告该症在美国的患病率为2%～7%，高于印度和中国。但需要指出使用相同的诊断标准不足以反映文化的差异。总之，该症在世界范围内在学龄期儿童的患病率为3%～7%。我国报告的学龄期儿童患病率为1.3%～13.4%。

Evidence indicates that ADHD is more common in boys than in girls, but, again, exact figures depend on whether the sample is taken from clinical referrals or from the general population and, boys are more likely to be referred to clinics because of a higher likelihood of aggressive and antisocial behaviors.

调查证明该症男孩多于女孩，但需要考虑报告是来源于临床还是普通人群，因为，男孩常常会由于其侵略性和反社会行为而就诊，因此临床资料中男孩多于女孩。

II. Etiology and Mechanism

二、病因及发病机制

The determination of the causes of ADHD is complicated by the heterogeneity of children given this diagnosis; any factor found to be associated with the syndrome is probably linked with only some of those judged to have ADHD. It is clear that the etiology of ADHD may be multifactorial.

儿童多动症的病因和发病机理非常复杂，通常认为本症的发生是多因素的。

i. Genetics

（一）遗传因素

A number of studies have revealed supportive evidence of genetic influences in the etiology of ADHD. When parents have ADHD half of their children are likely to have the disorder. Moreover, numerous large-scale twin studies indicate a genetic component to ADHD, with heredity estimates as high as 70% to 80%.

一些研究证明遗传因素与本症的发生有关。当父母有多动症时，其子女有一半也会发病。此外，许多对双胞胎的研究亦证明遗传因素与本症有关，其遗传性可高达70%～80%。

ii. Biochemical Influences

（二）生化因素

Studies have implicated a deficit of the catecholamines, dopamine and norepinephrine in the overactivity attributed to ADHD.

研究表明多动症患者体内儿茶酚胺、多巴胺、去甲肾上腺素明显低于正常儿童。

iii. Prenatal, Perinatal and Postnatal Factors

（三）母亲产前、围产期及产后因素

While low birth weight is a specific predictor of the development of ADHD, the impact of low birth weight on later symptoms can be mitigated by greater maternal warmth. Maternal smoking during pregnancy has been consistently associated with ADHD. Some researchers hypothesize that maternal smoking can affect the dopaminergic system of the developing fetus, resulting in behavioral disinhibition and ADHD. Intrauterine exposure to toxic substances, including alcohol, can produce effects on behavior.

出生时低体重是多动症的致病因素，但母亲的温暖可以减少本症的发生。研究证明孕母吸烟与本症密切相关，研究者认为孕母吸烟可影响发育中胎儿的多巴胺能系统，最终导致多动症。此外，孕母接触有毒物质，包括饮酒，亦与多动症的发生有关。

iv. Environmental Influences

（四）环境因素

Studies continue to provide evidence of the adverse effects on cognitive and behavioral development in children with elevated body levels of lead. However,

研究表明体内过高的铅水平可对儿童认知、行为造成不良影响。但一些研究也表明，

although some evidence suggests that lead poisoning may be associated to a small degree with hyperactivity and attention problems, most children with lead poisoning do not develop ADHD, and most children with ADHD do not show elevated levels of lead in the blood. The possible link between food dyes and additives, such as artificial flavorings and preservatives, was introduced in the mid-1970. However, studies examining theories once popular in the 1970s-the 1990s associating food additives with upsets in the central nervous system of children have found that very few children with ADHD responded positively to diets free of the specific additives.

虽然铅中毒可导致儿童轻度多动和注意障碍，许多铅中毒的儿童并未发展为多动症，且许多多动症儿童亦未显示血中铅水平增高。在70年代中期，有人提出食物中的染料和添加剂（例如调味品和防腐剂）会引起儿童过度活动、冲动和学习问题。但在70年代到90年代，一些检测食物添加剂与儿童中枢神经系统障碍的研究显示，多动症儿童中很少存在对某些食物添加剂的阳性反应。

III. Types and Clinical Manifestation

三、常见类型与临床表现

Because ADHD is a developmental disorder, symptom manifestations are highly individualistic and core symptoms may shift with age. Hyperactivity and impulsivity tend to become less apparent as children get older and attention and cognitive problems move into the foreground. Secondary symptoms such as perceptual and emotional immaturity, poor social skill, and motor coordination problems may be observed. Academic underachievement is often further enhanced by commonly comorbid language and learning disorders. Disruptive and impulsive behaviors often lead to peer rejection and low self-esteem, and emotional and social complications frequently are the dominant features manifested by adolescents, whether or not the core symptoms persist.

由于儿童多动症是儿童发展性障碍，临床表现因人而异，主要症状常随年龄改变而改变。多动和冲动行为常随儿童年龄增长而减轻，而注意和认知问题却表现正相反。其他症状，如感知和情绪的不成熟、社会技能欠缺以及动作协调性差等问题也会出现。语言和学习障碍严重制约学业成就。捣乱和冲动的行为常引起同伴的拒绝和低自尊的发生。到了青春期，不管核心症状是否存在，本症的显著特征是情绪和社会问题。

IV. Treatment

四、治　疗

i. Principle of Treatment

Documented efficacious interventions for children with ADHD fall into three broad categories that should be used together: stimulant medication, behavior modification, and educational modifications. Undocumented treatments have also been proposed.

（一）治疗原则

儿童注意缺陷和多动障碍应给予综合治疗，主要包括以下三大方面，即药物治疗、行为矫正和教育调整。另外，还有其他非正式的方法。

ii. Treatment Measures

1. Stimulant Medication The most extensively prescribed and studied medications used to treat ADHD are CNS stimulants (in particular, methylphenidate, or Ritalin), which have been prescribed since the early 1960s, and, to a much lesser degree, tricyclic antidepressants and α-adrenergic agonists (primarily clonidine). Antipsychotic drugs were used in the past but have fallen into disuse because of their significant potential for serious side effects. Stimulants are the most popular form of psychotropic medication prescribed for children

（二）治疗措施

1. **药物治疗** 最常用于治疗多动症的药物是中枢神经兴奋剂（如哌醋甲酯，利他林），最早于60年代初便开始用于治疗该症，此外，三环类抗抑郁药和α肾上腺素能激动剂亦用于治疗多动症。过去某些抗精神病药物也用于治疗本症，但因其潜在的严重并发症现已较少使用。在美国，中枢神经兴奋剂是目前用于治疗儿童多动症的最常用精神药物，

in the United States and are by far the drugs of choice for ADHD. Methylphenidate (Ritalin) is the most popular and extensively researched stimulant; dextroamphetamine and pemoline are used much less frequently.

哌醋甲酯（利他林）最为常用，而右旋安非他命和匹莫林则较少使用。

2. Behavioral Modification Like pharmacological interventions, behavioral interventions are essentially designed to reduce symptoms and are effective only as long as they are being applied. The programs generally consist of targeting appropriate behaviors for increase and inappropriate behaviors for decrease or extinction. The appropriate behaviors are rewarded with praise as well as points or tokens as part of a reward system. Inappropriate behaviors cause loss of points or tokens or result in a punishment such as "time out". Social skills training, preferably in peer groups and within the school setting, is important because most children with ADHD have weak social skills.

2. 行为矫正 与药物治疗一样，行为治疗本质上是减少症状，是行之有效的。通过奖惩分明的正性强化或负性强化手段来完成。在行为矫正过程中，应注意社会技能的培养，在有条件情况下，让多动症儿童多与伙伴接触，参加适当的集体活动，使其适应社会化环境。

3. Educational Modification Modifications of the classroom environment and academic tasks and goals are significant aspects of the treatment plan. The effect of ADHD on academic and cognitive performance had been acknowledged and necessary classroom modifications must be specified in an Individualized Educational Plan for children certified as having ADHD and educational impairment.

3. 教育调整 调整教室环境、学习任务和学习目标是治疗计划的重要方面。多动症对于学校成绩和认知能力的影响是公认的。教育计划应注意结合多动症儿童的特点，保证个体化和有针对性的实施。

4. Undocumented Treatments In response to observations that some children show hyperactive behavior associated with certain foods, especially sugar, chocolate, food dyes, and other additives, various diet restrictions have been used with variable clinical success and, as rule, these studies have not received widespread acceptance in the professional field. More recently, biofeedback training has been promoted by a small group of therapists as improving ADHD symptoms. The psychotherapy has also been adapted to treat the children with ADHD symptoms.

4. 其他 由于发现多动症儿童的多动行为与某些食物有关，如糖、巧克力、食物染料或添加剂等，因此近来有通过限制儿童一些食物来进行治疗。此外，生物反馈以及心理治疗等手段也用于治疗儿童注意缺陷和多动障碍等。

V. Application of the Nursing Process

五、护理程序的应用

i. Nursing Assessment

Usually the nurse collects assessment data on the ADHD child through direct interview and observation of the child. Because children with ADHD may have difficulty in sitting through long sessions, interviews are typically brief. Parents and teachers are extremely important sources for assessment data.

（一）护理评估

一般通过观察和会谈进行评估。由于多动症儿童注意时间较短，常通过由父母及教师填写量表的方式进行评估。

Like other psychiatric disorders with onset in childhood, nursing assessment of children with ADHD begins with an identification and exploration of the presenting problem. The assessment includes contents

与其他儿童期发病的精神障碍患儿的护理评估相似，注意缺陷障碍及多动患儿应从对问题的确认和对现病史的评估开始。主要

below:

1. A review of the child's developmental course, the onset and pattern of the current symptoms, factors that have worsened or improved the child's problems, and prior treatment or self-initiated efforts to remedy the situation.

2. Language development and current linguistic functioning should be carefully considered.

3. Medical history is also essential and should include a complete account of pregnancy and perinatal factors, childhood illnesses, hospitalizations, injuries, seizures, tics, physical growth, general health status, and timing of the child's last physical examination.

4. Because ADHD often occurs in the context of disruptive, oppositional, and defiant behavior, it is important to review the family situation including parenting style, stability of membership, consistency of rules and routines, as well as life events. Identification of these factors can be useful in shaping a care plan that builds on potential strengths and mitigates the impact of environmental factors that may perpetuate the child's disruptive behavior.

ii. Nursing Diagnosis

Possible nursing diagnoses include:

1. Risk for injury related to impulsive and accident-prone behavior and the inability to perceive self-harm.

2. Impaired social interaction related to intrusive and immature behavior.

3. Self-esteem disturbances related to dysfunctional family systems and the absence of parent-infant bonding.

4. Non-compliance with task expectations as a result of low levels of tolerance for frustration and short attention spans.

iii. Nursing Care Planning and Implementation

1. Outcome Identification The following criteria may be used for measurement of outcomes in the ADHD client. The client:

(1) Has experienced no physical harm;

(2) Interacts with others appropriately;

(3) Verbalizes positive aspects about self;

(4) Cooperates with staff in an effort to complete assigned tasks.

内容包括：

1. 儿童发展史回顾，起病情况及症状的表现形式，缓解和加重症状的影响因素，以及治疗情况等。

2. 语言发育情况，以及目前的言语功能都应被仔细评估。

3. 医学史的评估很重要，包括产前、儿童期患病、住院、损伤以及一般健康情况等。

4. 由于注意缺陷障碍及多动患儿经常表现为破坏性、反社会性和对抗性行为，对其家庭情况，如父母养育方式、家庭成员稳定性、管教方式的一致性等的评估必不可少。这些因素的确立将有利于针对性制订护理计划，从而缓解环境因素对儿童行为的长期影响。

（二）护理诊断

针对儿童注意缺陷和多动障碍的护理诊断如下：

1. **潜在受伤的可能** 与冲动性行为和不能感知危险有关。

2. **社会交往受损** 与攻击性和不成熟行为有关。

3. **自尊受损** 与家庭系统功能不良及与父母亲密关系缺乏有关。

4. **不能完成所交给任务** 与对挫折承受力较低和注意力集中时间较短有关。

（三）护理计划与措施

1. **护理目标** 针对儿童注意缺陷和多动障碍的主要护理目标如下：

儿童能够：

（1）不发生身体受伤；

（2）与他人进行适当的交往；

（3）用语言表达对自身优点的认识；

（4）与医护人员合作努力完成所分配的任务。

2. Nursing Intervention

(1) Common nursing interventions: Many factors such as establishing of a therapeutic relationship and being a good role model affect the outcome of nursing intervention (the detailed nursing activates presented in unit 1 "Mental Retardation").

(2) Special nursing intervention: A multifaceted approach has been shown to be the most effective treatment for ADHD. The nurse's role is to develop a structured environment that enables the child or adolescent to alter or improve his or her reaction to environmental stimuli. The nurse may also work with the family or teachers to plan a firm, consistent environment in which limits and standards are set. Behavior modification and behavior contrasts are used to promote positive behavior. Social skills training are used with children who exhibit aggressive, impulsive, and socially damaging behaviors. The goal is to change the relationships between children who are socially isolated and their peer groups by showing children how their behavior affects others. The psychiatric nurse may provide psychotherapy, because some children or adolescents with ADHD exhibit anxiety, depression, self-esteem problems, and other emotional difficulties. Family therapy may be helpful in dealing with sibling concerns or other family problems such as divorce or the loss of a loved one. Medication remains one of the most successful treatments for the client with ADHD. The nurse educates the child or adolescent, family, and school personnel (when necessary) about the various types of medication that are used. The parents are then asked to complete a form to evaluate the client's response to medication. These observations enable the nurse to determine which medications and doses are most efficacious.

2. 护理措施

（1）一般护理措施：许多因素都会影响护理措施的效果。如建立治疗性关系、成为良好的角色榜样等（具体护理措施见本章第一节“精神发育迟滞”的护理）。

（2）特殊护理措施：多种方法联合治疗对多动症最有效。护理工作者需要帮助建立一个结构式环境，以改变和提高儿童对环境刺激的反应能力。可与家庭成员或教师合作计划一个固定的、前后一致的环境，确立标准和限制。应用行为矫正和行为对比来促进正性行为。另外，可利用社会技能训练帮助有攻击性、冲动性和社会损害行为的儿童，使其改变与他人关系，并了解他们的行为对别人的影响。此症儿童常伴有焦虑、抑郁、自尊心问题以及其他情绪障碍，心理治疗也是护理的一部分。对于有些离婚或丧偶的家庭，应用家庭治疗可能有益。药物治疗是对该症儿童最成功的治疗方法之一。药物治疗过程中，一般要求父母填写药物反应表，以协助护理人员确定哪种药物和剂量最有效。

BOX 13-1 Learning More

Tips for Helping Your Child Control His or Her Behavior

1. Make sure your child has a daily schedule. Try to keep the time that your child wakes up, eats, bathes, goes to school, and goes to bed the same every day.
2. Help your child adhere to the "task". Use charts and checklists to track progress with homework or chores. Keep instructions brief. Offer frequent, friendly reminders.

3. Reduce distractions. Loud music, computer games, and TV can be over stimulating to your child. Make it a rule to keep the TV or music turning off during mealtime and while your child is doing homework. Don't set a TV in your child's bedroom.

BOX 13-1 知识拓展

帮助孩子控制行为的技巧

1. 保证孩子每天的日程安排。尽量保持孩子每天在同一时间醒来，吃饭，沐浴，上学，睡觉。
2. 帮助孩子坚持“任务”。使用图表和清单跟踪作业和家务进展。保持简短的指令。提供频繁、友好的提醒。
3. 减少干扰，大声的音乐、电脑游戏和电视可能刺激孩子。规定孩子做作业、吃饭时关掉电视或音乐。不要把电视放在孩子的卧室里。

4. Set small, reachable goals. Focus on slow progress rather than instant results. Be sure that your child understands that he can learn to control himself step by step.

5. Reward positive behavior. Offer kind words, hugs, or small prizes for reaching goals in a timely manner or good behavior.

6. Find activities at which your child can succeed. All children need to experience success to feel good about themselves.

7. Develop a good communication system with your child's teacher so that you can coordinate your efforts and monitor your child's progress.

8. Use calm discipline. Physical punishment, such as spanking or slapping, is no help. Discuss your child's behavior with him when both of you are calm down.

4. 设定小的，可及的目标。注重于过程而不是结果。确保孩子知道他可以一步一步来学会控制自己。

5. 奖励积极的行为。对良好的行为或达到目标及时给予口头表扬，拥抱或小奖励。

6. 找到孩子能成功的活动。所有的孩子都需要经历成功和自我感觉良好。

7. 和老师建立一个良好的沟通系统，这样就可以调整你的努力和监督孩子的进步。

8. 使用平静的训导。体罚，如打屁股或抽耳光，是没有帮助的。当你和孩子两个都冷静下来时再讨论孩子的行为。

iv. Nursing Evaluation

The evaluation data may include information gathered by asking the following questions:

1. Have the nursing actions directed at client safety been effective in protecting the child from injury?

2. Has the child been able to establish a trusting relationship with the primary caregiver?

3. Is the client responding to limits set on unacceptable behaviors?

4. Is the client able to interact appropriately with others?

5. Is the client able to verbalize positive statements about self?

6. Is the client able to complete tasks independently or with a minimum of assistance? Can he or she follow after listening to simple instructions?

7. Is the client able to apply exercise self-control to decrease motor activity?

（四）护理评价

评价过程是一个持续进展的过程。在评价阶段护理人员应提出以下问题：

1. 护理行为是否有效地保护了患者的安全？

2. 患者是否与照护者建立了信任的关系？

3. 患者是否能够同意对不可接受行为制订的限制？

4. 患者是否能够与他人进行合适的交往？

5. 患者是否能够用语言表达对自身的积极看法？

6. 患者是否能独立或者借助最少的帮助完成任务，能否听从简单的指导？

7. 患者是否能应用自我控制技巧来减少动作行为？

Section 4 Nursing Management for Children and Adolescents with Conduct Disorder

第四节 品行障碍患者的护理

I. Introduction

一、概 述

i. Definition

Conduct disorders are characterized by a repetitive and persistent pattern of behavior in which the basic rights of others or major age-appropriate societal norms

（一）概念

品行障碍的特征是反复而持久的反社会性、攻击性或对立性品行。当发展到极端时，

or rules are violated. Such behavior is, by definition, more severe than ordinary childish mischief or adolescent rebelliousness. It may include, for example, excessive levels of fighting or bullying, cruelty to animals or other people; severe destructiveness to property; fire-settings; stealing; repeated lying, truancy from school and going away from home; unusually frequent and severe disobedience.

这种行为可严重违反相应年龄的社会规范，较之儿童普遍的调皮捣蛋或少年的逆反行为更严重。如过分好斗或霸道；残忍地对待动物或他人；严重破坏财物；纵火；偷窃；反复说谎；逃学或离家出走；长期的严重违拗等。

ii. Epidemiology

As with Attention deficit/hyperactivity disorder, cultural factors play a significant role in the determination/diagnosis of conduct disorder. For example, the rate of conduct disorders in Germany is estimated in some studies of Germany as 0.9% and much higher in the U.S. Nonetheless, conduct disorder is one of the most common problems diagnosed among children and adolescents. A review of epidemiological studies in the United States indicates that conduct disorder is fairly common with prevalence rates ranging from 4% to 16% for boys and 1.2% to 9% for girls. Serious lawbreaking appears to peak around age 17 and drop precipitously in young adulthood.

（二）流行病学

与儿童多动症一样，品行障碍的诊断受文化因素的影响。例如，在德国品行障碍的发病为 0.9%，但在美国，其发病率则很高。但总体来说，品行障碍是儿童和青少年中最常见的问题之一。据调查，在美国品行障碍非常常见，患病率在男孩为 4%～16%，女孩为 1.2%～9%，17 岁是违法的高峰年龄，以后在成人时期违法行为迅速减少。

II. Etiology and Mechanism

二、病因及发病机制

The factors found to be associated with conduct disorders is probably some of those following:

少年品行障碍是多种因素共同作用的结果。

i. Genetics

The DSM- Ⅳ notes that estimates from twin and adoption studies show that Conduct Disorder is influenced by both genetic and environmental factors. The risk for conduct disorder increases in children with a biological or adaptive parent with antisocial personality disorder or a sibling with conduct disorder. At the same time, the disorder appears to be more common in children of biological parents with alcohol dependence, mood disorders, or schizophrenia or biological parents who have a history of attention deficit/hyperactivity disorder or conduct disorder. Evidence from twin studies indicates that aggressive behavior (e.g., cruelty to animals, fighting, destroying property) is clearly heritable, whereas other delinquent behavior (e.g., stealing, running away, truancy) may not be. Other evidence suggests that the tie when antisocial and aggressive behaviors that begin in childhood are more heritable than similar behaviors that begin in adolescence.

（一）遗传因素

根据 DSM- Ⅳ，通过对双胞胎和收养儿童的一些研究表明品行障碍受遗传和环境因素的影响。如果儿童的亲生父母或养父母有反社会人格障碍或其兄妹中有品行障碍，则其患本症的危险性会明显增加。同时，本症在亲生父母有酒精依赖、情感障碍、精神分裂症或有多动症及品行障碍病史的儿童中更为多见。对双胞胎的研究表明，进攻性行为（如残害动物、好斗、破坏财物等）有明显遗传性，但其他一些违法行为（如偷窃、逃走、逃避等）则并非具有遗传性。一些研究指出如果在儿童时期就具有反社会和侵略性行为，则比那些在青少年时期才具有这些行为的人有明显的遗传性。

ii. Temperament

The term temperament refers to personality traits that become evident very early in life and may be present at birth. Evidence suggests a genetic component in temperament and an association between temperament and behavioral problems later in life.

（二）气质特点

气质特点是指人在出生时就可能有的并在早期生活中表现明显的个性特征。这些气质中的先天成分与儿童生活中的行为问题有关。

iii. Biochemical Factors

Various studies have reported a possible correlation between elevated plasma levels of testosterone and aggressive behavior. Testosterone may increase in response to aversive, stressful, or physically strenuous events.

iv. Family Influences

The following factors related to family dynamics have been implicated as contributors in the predisposition to this disorder: parental rejection, inconsistent management with harsh discipline, early institutional living, frequent shifting of parental figures, large family size, absent father, parents with antisocial personality disorder and/or alcohol/substance dependence, and association with a delinquent subgroup. In addition to these aspects, family dynamics studies have reported additional family influences in the predisposition to conduct disorder. They include marital conflict and divorce, inadequate communication patterns, and parental permissiveness.

（三）生化因素

许多研究均说明雄性激素在攻击性行为中起重要作用，不论儿童还是成人，雄性激素会增加人压力环境下的攻击性。

（四）家庭因素

大量研究表明先天的性格可在一定程度上受到环境的影响，尤其是家庭养育环境的影响。儿童的行为模式及规范受家庭的影响最大，有学者发现，品行障碍的儿童通常来自于不稳定的、不安全的、丧失教育权利和社会经济地位差的家庭。以下因素与儿童品行障碍有关：① 父母排斥；② 父母教养方式粗暴，常被体罚；③ 早期寄养；④ 儿童期受虐待；⑤ 儿童在某种程度上被忽略；⑥ 家庭对儿童过分溺爱，对患儿行为放任不管；⑦ 父母离婚；⑧ 家庭成员缺乏有效的沟通；⑨父母具有不良的品行或酒精依赖。

III. Types and Clinical Manifestation

Children with conduct disorder are usually referred for evaluation during childhood or adolescence by parents; care givers; pediatricians; or educational, childcare, or juvenile justice authorities because their behavior has become intolerably disruptive or dangerous at home, in school, or in the community. Often the referral occurs in response to threatened or actual suspension from school. According to *CCMD-3*, conduct disorder is classified into dissocial conduct disorder, oppositional defiant disorder, and other or unspecified conduct disorders.

i. Dissocial Conduct Disorder

The classic characteristic of conduct disorder is the use of aggression in the violation of the rights of others. The behavior pattern manifests itself in virtually all areas of the child's life. Stealing, lying, and truancy are common problems. The child lacks feelings of guilt or remorse. The use of tobacco, liquor, or non-prescribed drugs, as well as the participation in sexual activities, occurs earlier than the peer group's expected age. Projection is a common defense mechanism. Low self-esteem is manifested by a "tough guy" image. Characteristics include poor tolerance of frustration, irritability, and frequent temper outbursts. Symptoms of anxiety and depression are not uncommon. Levels of academic achievement may be low in relation to age and IQ. Features associated with ADHD (e.g.,

三、常见类型与临床表现

由于其捣乱和危险行为在家庭、学校和社区等场所达到令人难以忍受的程度，品行障碍儿童通常是因父母、照护者、儿科医生、教育者的建议来诊。*CCMD-3* 主要将其分为反社会性品行障碍、对立违抗性障碍和其他待分类的品行障碍。

（一）反社会性品行障碍的表现

它指那些不符合道德规范和社会准则，造成对他人权利侵犯的违法行为。常见的表现包括偷盗、说谎、流浪不归和逃学。这类儿童经常采取进攻性行为，对家庭、学校和社区造成很大威胁，而他们自己却没有犯罪感，不思悔改。常早于同龄人出现吸烟、酗酒、吸毒及性行为等。常表现为较低自尊心、易激惹、经常发脾气等。焦虑和抑郁较常见，学习成绩和智商水平低于同龄人。常伴有注意缺陷和多动障碍，如注意力难以集中、易冲动、活动过度等。

attention difficulties, impulsiveness, and hyperactivity) are very common in children with conduct disorder.

ii. Oppositional Defiant Disorder

This condition usually first presents before 10 years old and is characterized by a persistent pattern of defiant and provocative behavior in the absence of severe dissocial or aggressive activities that violate the law or the rights of others. The focal issue of oppositional defiant disorder is passive aggression and is exhibited by obstinacy, procrastination, disobedience, carelessness, negativism, resistance to change, violation of minor rules, blocking out communications from others, and resistance to authority. Other symptoms that may be evident are enuresis, encopresis, elective mutism, running away, school avoidance, school underachievement, eating and sleeping problems, temper tantrums, fighting, and argumentativeness.

Usually these children do not see themselves as being oppositional but view the problems as arising from others whom they believe are making unreasonable demands on them. Interpersonal relationships are fraught with difficulty, including those with peers. These children are often friendless, perceiving human relationships as negative and unsatisfactory. School performance is usually poor because of their refusal to participate and resistance to external demands.

（二）对立违抗性障碍的表现

常在10岁之前首次发病，主要表现为明显不服从、违抗或挑衅行为，但没有更严重的违法或冒犯他人权利的社会性攻击行为。主要问题为被动进攻，常表现为顽固、拖延、不服从、粗心、消极、违反规章制度、打断他人谈话、反抗权威等。其他症状明显的是遗尿、大便失禁，选择性缄默症，逃跑、逃避学校、学校学习成绩不良，饮食和睡眠问题，发脾气等。

通常这些孩子不认为自己是对抗的反而认为是别人找茬，是对他不合理的要求。人际关系困难重重，包括同伴关系。这些孩子往往是没有朋友的，感知人际关系是负面和不满意。因为他们拒绝参与和抵抗外部的要求，在学校的表现通常很差。

IV. Treatment

Conduct disorder is too complex a group of problems to be treated by a single method. Individually tailored combinations of biological, psychosocial, and ecological interventions generally prove to be most effective. The task is to find the most effective treatment combinations for different groups of children and adolescents with conduct problems. The following sections discuss the most common approaches to prevention and treatment.

i. Early Intervention Programs

Early intervention programs such as Head Start may have a preventative function. Head Start programs attend to the child's physical health and provide an early education program that prepares the child for elementary school. They also educate parents about child development and offer support in times of crisis. Early mental health intervention programs identify aggressive children and provide intensive parent education to counteract the poor communication, inconsistency, lack of follow through, coercive discipline, and failure to model or reward prosocial behavior that so frequently accompany

四、治　疗

儿童品行障碍尚无特殊的治疗方法，针对其问题的复杂性，治疗上也多为集生物、社会及环境为一体的综合治疗，最重要的是为儿童找出恰当的治疗方案。目前最常用的针对儿童和青少年的治疗手段为以下几种：

（一）早期干预项目

一些早期的干预项目，如起步教育项目，在儿童进入小学前进行，以达到预防性作用。该项目主要针对儿童的身体健康，通过早期教育做好儿童入小学前的准备。对有攻击性的儿童及其父母进行教育，使其了解儿童的发展状况和要求，在出现问题时提供帮助。一些具体的精神健康干预项目，通过对儿童及其父母的具体指导，帮助解决家庭中不良的交流方式、教养的不一致性、缺乏恒心和

nascent conduct disorder.

毅力、强制、缺乏榜样作用等问题，以期纠正儿童不良行为，促进良好的社会行为，最后能够顺利进入小学。

ii. Treatment Programs for School-Aged Children

Behavioral programs targeting parental effectiveness and the child's social problem-solving capacity, social skills, prosocial behavior, and academic functioning are more effective in the short term which is nonspecific treatment methods.

（二）对学龄儿童的治疗项目

这些项目对于短期内改善父母教养的有效性和儿童社会问题解决能力、社会技巧、学业表现等方面有效。

iii. Treatment Programs for Adolescents

A family therapy approach has been shown to have the greatest success in the treatment of adolescent oppositional disorder. In the problem solving communication training (PSCT) program, the family is first assessed with regard to the nature of the presenting problems: molecular (i.e., family communication problems and poor problem solving) or molar (i.e., family structural and functional problems). Molecular issues require the specific goals and objectives of therapy, while molar issues determine strategy and tactics.

（三）对青春期少年的治疗项目

对于品行障碍的青春期少年，家庭治疗是最有效的。在解决问题的沟通培训（PSCT）计划中，首先对家庭中的问题进行评估：分子（例如：家庭沟通问题和解决问题无效）或摩尔（例如：家庭结构和功能问题）。分子问题需要确立治疗的具体目标，而摩尔确立策略和手段。

Family communication and problem solving are addressed by eliciting the common causes of family disagreement and then ranking them in order of seriousness or difficulty. The family is directed to address one cause of dispute per session, starting with the least acrimonious, using an established formula for problem solving. As the family addresses these problems, family communication difficulties can be remediated with the use of feedback, instruction, modeling, and behavioral rehearsal. Sometimes the family's communication patterns are so destructive that they must be addressed before PSCT can begin.

在评估家庭沟通和解决问题过程中寻找导致家庭分歧的常见原因，并按问题的严重程度和解决难易排序。每次会话指导家庭解决争端的一个原因，从最容易解决的问题开始，使用已经建立的准则解决问题。当家庭解决了这些问题时，通过反馈、指导、示范、行为训练等方式，家庭沟通困难可望得到缓解。有时家庭沟通模式有如此大的破坏性，他们必须在 PSCT 开始之前就解决。

Problem-solving communication includes both assessment and treatment.

解决问题的沟通包括评估和治疗。

1. Assessment

(1) What are the specific issues that provoke discord in the family?

(2) How effective are the family's communication patterns?

(3) Is the family involved in coercive interactions?

(4) Do the parents model and convey effective problem-solving techniques?

(5) Does the family endorse negatively biased, inflexible beliefs about each other (e.g., "catastrophizing", perfectionism).

(6) Are structural problems evident in the family (e.g., misalignments, coalitions, triangulation,

1. 评估

（1）致家庭不和谐的特殊因素；

（2）目前家庭沟通形式的有效性；

（3）家庭成员的交往中是否有强制性表现；

（4）父母是否在有效解决问题的技巧方面起到了表率作用；

（5）家庭成员之间是否存在否定的偏见，对彼此看法僵化不变；

（6）家庭中是否存在结构性问题，如不配合、分帮结派、冲突等；

disengagement, enmeshment, conflict)?

(7) What functional purpose does the adolescent's behavior serve (e.g., to distract parents who would otherwise quarrel, or to drive parents apart, or to attract attention away from a sibling regarded as more favored)?

（7）少年的行为目标，是为了避免父母吵架，还是促使父母分开，还是为了引起注意等。

2. Treatment Objectives

2. 治疗目标

(1) Promote better family communication and more effective problem solving.

（1）进行更有效的家庭交流和问题解决；

(2) Help the family generalize their skills to the home.

（2）帮助家庭总结他们对于家庭所应用的技巧；

(3) Reverse or neutralize structural and functional problems.

（3）减少或使家庭的结构功能问题趋于缓和。

3. The Steps of Problem Solving for Families

3. 家庭中问题解决的步骤主要包括：

(1) Define the problem. Each family member tells the others what the problem is and why it is a problem. The other family members paraphrase the statement to check their understanding of it.

（1）每一名家庭成员告诉其他的家庭成员他所认为的目前家庭中所存在的问题及原因，其他家庭成员确认是否理解他的说法，最终确定家庭的问题到底是什么。

(2) Generate alternative solutions, taking turns.

（2）由每名家庭成员轮流说出解决问题的方法。

(3) Take turns evaluating each proposed solution either positively or negatively. The solution with the greatest number of positive ratings wins.

（3）由每名家庭成员轮流说出对所设想的措施的评价，确定同意率最高的方法。

(4) Implement the solution and check its effectiveness.

（4）实施并评价其有效性。

4. In the course of treatment, the family's rigid, biased beliefs will be revealed and targeted for cognitive restructuring. In cognitive restructuring, the therapist challenges each dysfunctional belief, suggests a more reasonable alternative, and helps the family to conduct an "experiment" that will disconfirm the belief. Dysfunctional beliefs of parents and children include the followings:

4. 在治疗过程中，家庭的僵化、偏见问题将暴露，通过认知重建，可改变以往的状态，代之以更加合理有效的方法。

(1) Parents:

（1）家庭中需要纠正的来自父母的传统观念为：

1) If my adolescent is given freedom, he or she will be ruined.

1）孩子若给予太多的自由，他就会被荒废了；

2) My adolescent should obey me.

2）孩子就应该绝对服从家长；

3) My adolescent should always make the right decision.

3）孩子不允许做错误的决定；

4) My adolescent is out to upset and hurt his or her parents.

4）孩子不应有不良情绪，不应伤害其父母；

5) If my adolescent does wrong, I must be to blame.

5）孩子一旦做了错事，做父母的应该加以谴责。

(2) Adolescents:

（2）家庭中需要纠正的来自孩子的常见观念为：

1) Rules are unfair.

1）规则对我不公平；

2) Rules will ruin my life.

2）太多的规则毁了我的生活；

3) I should be allowed complete freedom.

3）我应该有完全的自由；

4) People should always be fair to each other.

4）人们之间应该永远是公平的；

5) If my parents loved me, they would always trust me.

6) I should never upset my parents.

5. The following is a detailed introduction to effective parenting techniques both for children and adolescents.

With children under 12 years of age, treatment is provided primarily through the parents. Parents are educated concerning the origin and meaning of oppositional defiant behavior and are trained to replace coercive discipline with more effective child-rearing techniques. The essentials of effective parenting with oppositional defiant children are as following.

(1) Provide positive attention with praise and reinforcement of desirable behavior.

(2) Ignore inappropriate behavior unless it is serious.

(3) Give clear, brief commands, reduce task complexity, and eliminate competing influence (e.g., television).

(4) Establish a token economy at home with tokens or points awarded for compliance; tokens are "cashed in" on a weekly bases. Initially, tokens are not removed/taken away for noncompliance; and, the token economy is maintained for at least 6-8 weeks.

(5) When the token economy has been well established, use response cost (removal of tokens) or time out, contingent on noncompliance and applied soon after the noncompliance (1-2 minutes time out per year of age). Do not release the child from time out until he or she is quiet and agrees to obey.

(6) Extend time out to noncompliance in public places.

5）如果我的父母爱我，就应该永远尊重我；

6）我永远都不应该让父母伤心。

5. 下面具体介绍针对品行障碍儿童和青少年教育有效的父母参与技巧。

对于12岁以下的儿童，治疗基本上是通过父母完成的。通过教育使父母了解孩子反抗对立的根本原因，学会有效的教养技巧，改变以往强制惩罚。对于品行障碍的儿童有效的父母干预应注意以下几点：

（1）积极的眼光注意儿童，并对其良好表现给予表扬和正性强化。

（2）如果不是很严重，不要过分关注那些不合适行为。

（3）对儿童分配的任务要努力做到清楚、简单，避免复杂性和竞争性。

（4）在家庭建立一种奖励经济制度，对于好的行为给予奖励，如给予代用币或加分，反之则不给。

（5）当奖励机制建立后，对于儿童的不良行为可给予减分或取回代用币的方法，或者在一段时间内禁止儿童做此事。一般按年龄，每增加1岁，时间延长1～2分钟，直到儿童同意遵守要求为止。

（6）在公共场合，时间延长得还要多些。

V. Application of the Nursing Process

i. Nursing Assessment

Adolescents with conduct problems may be hostile, sarcastic, defensive, and provocative and calm, outgoing, and engaging at other times. Inconsistencies, distortions and lies are not unusual when interviewing these children, making it difficult to obtain a clear history. Therefore, instead of asking if an event or behavior occurred, it may be better to ask when it occurred. These adolescents are masters at changing the subject and diverting discussions away from sensitive issues. They often use denial, projection, and externalization of anger as defenses when asked to self-disclose. The assessment may take several sessions and should be conducted in a nonjudgmental fashion.

五、护理程序的应用

（一）护理评估

品行障碍儿童对人通常充满敌意、讽刺、挖苦、挑衅性，有时又表现得很安静、开朗和可爱。当与其会谈时，歪曲事实或撒谎时有发生，所以，在评估时很难得到一个清晰的历史。最好的提问方式是"这件事是何时发生的？"而不是问"如果这件事发生你将如何？"当对一些敏感性问题进行提问时，这类儿童经常会使用否认、影射、把气愤归咎于外因等防御性机制，护理评估也许会进行多次，评估者应认识到儿童这一特点而采

The assessment should include data from multiple sources and multiple domains including biological, psychological (mood, behavioral, cognitions) and social. Another important goal of assessment is to rule out comorbid conditions that may partially explain or complicate their lack of behavioral control.

用非评判性的态度进行评估。

护理评估内容包括生理、心理（包括情绪、行为、认知等）、社会各个领域，信息可从父母、教师、本人等多个渠道获得。同时，应评估患儿有无其他问题，如多动障碍伴注意缺陷、学习障碍、抑郁、焦虑等，这些都将影响患儿的表现。

ii. Nursing Diagnosis

Possible nursing diagnoses include:

1. Impaired social interaction related to negative parental role models, impaired social cognition, underlying hostility, manipulation of others.

2. Defensive coping related to low self-esteem and a dysfunctional family system.

3. Self-esteem disturbance resulting from a lack of positive feedback and unsatisfactory parent-child relationship.

4. Noncompliance with therapy related to negative temperament, denial of problems, underlying hostility.

5. Risk for violence directed toward others related to characteristics of temperament, peer rejection, and negative parental role models.

（二）护理诊断

品行障碍儿童可能的护理诊断包括：

1. **社会交往受损**　与负向父母角色功能、社会认知缺陷、敌意和控制他人倾向有关。

2. **防御性应对**　与低自尊和家庭系统功能受损有关。

3. **自尊障碍**　与缺乏积极反馈及对与父母关系不满有关。

4. **对治疗不依从**　与负性气质特征、拒绝承认问题、对他人存敌意有关。

5. **对他人施以暴力的潜在危险**　与性情特点、遭同伴拒绝、负向父母角色功能有关。

iii. Nursing Care Planning and Implementation

1. Outcome Identification　The following criteria may be used to measure outcomes in the client with conduct disorder.

(1) Interacts with others in a socially appropriate manner.

(2) Accepts directions without becoming defensive.

(3) Demonstrates evidence of increased self-esteem by discontinuing exploitative and demanding behaviors toward others; verbalizes positive aspects about self.

(4) Complies with treatment by participating in therapies without negativism.

(5) Has not harmed self or others.

2. Nursing Intervention　Planned interventions focus on maintaining safety and helping the child or adolescent develop internal limits, problem-solving skills, and self-responsibility for acts of antisocial behavior, which may include physical violence, theft, fire setting, assault, or manipulative behavior. Young clients with conduct disorder often have underlying medical problems; therefore, nursing interventions may include the treatment of a medical condition such as epilepsy or a closed head injury. Because conduct disorders do not be resolved without intervention, and appropriate planning and

（三）护理计划与措施

1. **护理目标**　针对品行障碍儿童的主要护理目标如下：

儿童能够：

（1）与他人用适宜的方法进行社会交往。

（2）接受他人的指导而不怀有敌意。

（3）通过终止对他人的侵犯性行为表现出自尊心的改善；用语言表述自己好的一面。

（4）服从治疗。

（5）不伤害自己和他人。

2. **护理措施**　对品行障碍儿童护理计划重点在于如何保护儿童的安全，以及帮助他们发展内在的自我限制、问题解决技巧，并能够对自己行为负责。该症儿童经常有原发病，如癫痫或闭合性颅脑损伤，因此，护理干预中常包括疾病治疗的护理内容。护理实施中应注意以下几点：通过建立相互信任的关系；通过设立限制保持对操纵性等行为的控制；各种要求和限制应保持前后一致；尊

treatment is essential. The following suggested approaches have been incorporated into nursing intervention: establish trust by being honest; maintain control by setting limits for manipulative, acting-out behavior; be consistent with limit setting; respect the client's age and maintain an adult-child or adult-adult relationship, whichever is appropriate; establish realistic expectations, discuss such expectations with the client and encourage verbalization of feelings. Additional nursing interventions aimed at helping young people realize and understand the effect their behavior has on others may include behavior therapy or psychotherapy in either individual or group sessions. Medications may also be used to alleviate clinical symptoms of depression or other comorbid disorders such ADHD and posttraumatic stress disorder.

重儿童的年龄，与其保持合适的成人－儿童，或成人－成人的关系；建立现实的期望，并与儿童讨论其感觉，鼓励其表达感受。此外，可通过个人或小组的行为治疗和心理治疗帮助儿童或青少年认识和理解其行为对他人所造成的影响。对于存在临床症状者，如抑郁或其他伴发儿童多动症症状或创伤后压力的还可应用药物治疗。

Most children or adolescents with the diagnosis of conduct disorder come from households in which discipline was inconsistent and sometime brutal. Rarely are such children held accountable for their action; parents often surrender to the demands of the child or adolescent. Children said to have conduct disorder may just need help fitting into society through appropriate discipline, mentoring, job training, and coaching in independent living skills.

许多品行障碍的儿童或青少年都来自于有矛盾甚至暴力家庭，对儿童的教育及要求前后不一致，甚至有暴力教育，因此，儿童很少为自己的行为负责，而父母则往往屈服于他们的无理要求。护理工作者应帮助这些孩子，通过恰当的训练、指导和工作技能培训以提高其独立生活的能力。

iv. Nursing Evaluation

（四）护理评价

Nursing evaluation is performed by asking the following questions:

在评价阶段护理人员应提出以下问题：

1. Is the client cooperating with the schedule of therapeutic activities? Is the level of participation adequate?
2. Is the client's attitude toward therapy less negative?
3. Is the client accepting responsibility for problem behavior?
4. Is the client verbalizing the unacceptable nature of his or her passive-aggressive behavior?
5. Is he or she able to identify which behaviors are unacceptable and substitute more adaptive behaviors?
6. Is the client able to interact with staff and peers without defending behavior in an angry manner?
7. Is the client able to verbalize positive statements about self?
8. Is increased self-worth evident with fewer manifestations of manipulation?
9. Is the client able to make compromises with others when issues of control emerge?
10. Are anger and hostility expressed in an appropriate manner? Can the client verbalize ways of releasing anger adaptively?

1. 患者对治疗计划是否合作，其参与程度是否足够?
2. 患者对治疗的消极态度是否有所减轻?
3. 患者是否能够对自己的行为负责?
4. 患者是否用语言表达出那些消极进攻性行为是不能令人接受的?
5. 患者是否能确认哪些行为是不可接受的，而代之以更加适应性行为?
6. 患者是否能与医护人员或伙伴用适当的方式交往?
7. 患者是否能够对自己进行积极评述?
8. 患者自我价值感是否有所增强，操纵性行为是否有所减少?
9. 当争端发生时患者能否与他人协议解决?
10. 患者是否能够用适当的方式表达愤怒和敌意，患者是否能说出适当的释放愤怒的方式?

11. Is he or she able to verbalize true feelings instead of allowing them to emerge through use of passive-aggressive behaviors?

11. 患者是否能用语言表达真正的感觉而不是轻易采取消极进攻性行为？

Section 5 Nursing Management for Children and Adolescents with Tic Disorders

第五节 儿童抽动症患者的护理

I. Introduction

i. Definition

Tic disorders are sudden, rapid, repetitive, stereotyped motor movements or vocalizations. A tic is an involuntary, rapid, recurrent, non-rhythmic motor movement usually involving groups of muscles. It can take the form of abrupt purposeless vocalization.

ii. Epidemiology

The age at onset of tics can be as early as age 2 years but occurs most commonly during childhood or early adolescence, with the median age being 7 years. Most cases occur before the age of 14 years. The prevalence of tics is estimated to be between 0.5/1 000 and 1/1 000, with boys being affected three to six times more often than girls.

一、概 述

（一）概念

儿童抽动症是指发生在儿童时期的不自主运动和运动障碍，是一种突发、快速、重复、非节律性、刻板的单一或多部位肌肉运动或发声，一般为不可自控性及无目的性。

（二）流行病学

本病发病年龄最小为 2 岁，但多发生在儿童期或青春早期，大多在 14 岁以前，平均年龄为 7 岁。估计一般人群中患病率为 0.5‰ ~ 1‰，且男孩是女孩的 3 ~ 6 倍。

II. Etiology and Mechanism

i. Genetics

Tics are noted in two thirds of relatives of Tic clients. Twin studies with both monozygotic and dizygotic twins suggest an inheritable component.

ii. Biochemical Factors

Abnormalities in levels of dopamine, serotonin, gamma-aminobutyric acid (GABA), and acetylcholine have been associated with Tic.

iii. Structural Factors

Neuro-imaging/brain studies have been consistent in finding dysfunction in the area of the basal ganglia. Enlargement has been found in the caudate nucleus and decreased cerebral blood flow in the left ventricular nucleus.

iv. Environmental Factors

Retrospective studies have implicated a number of factors in the etiology of tic disorders including increased prenatal complications and low birth weight. Greater emotional stress during pregnancy and more nausea and vomiting during the first trimester of pregnancy have been

二、病因及发病机制

（一）遗传因素

本症的 2/3 发生于患者的亲属当中，通过对单卵双生和异卵双生的双胞胎研究表明本病具有家族遗传的特点。

（二）神经生化改变

抽动障碍患儿中发现有多巴胺、5- 羟色胺、γ- 氨基丁酸、乙酰胆碱的水平异常。

（三）神经系统结构异常

通过对神经系统的检查发现基底神经节功能异常，尾状核扩大和左豆状核血液供应减少等改变。

（四）环境因素

回顾性研究发现，抽动症患儿母亲产前并发症以及新生儿低体重的发生比率较高。另外，抽动障碍患儿母亲在怀孕期间经受较高压力以及怀孕早期出现恶心、呕吐等症状

noted in the mothers of these children. It is speculated that these environmental factors may temper the genetic predisposition to tic.

的较多。

III. Types and Clinical Manifestation

三、常见类型与临床表现

A tic disorder is a general term encompassing several syndromes that are chiefly characterized by motor and/or phonic tics.

Motor tics are usually quick, jerky movements of the eyes, face, neck, and shoulders, and may include eye blinking, neck jerking, shoulder shrugging, facial grimacing, and coughing. Common complex motor tics include touching, squatting, hopping, skipping, deep knee bends, retracing steps, and twirling when walking.

Phonic tics typically include repetitive throat clearing, grunting, or other noises but may also include more complex sounds such as words, parts of words, and obscenities in a minority of patients.

抽动障碍的表现主要包括运动和 / 或发声抽动。

运动和发声抽动都可分为简单和复杂两类，但界限不清。如眨眼、斜颈、耸肩、扮鬼脸、咳嗽等属于简单的运动抽动；触摸、蹲坐、蹦、跳、膝部过分弯曲、行进中折回或转圈等属于复杂的运动抽动。

典型的发声抽动包括清喉声、咕哝声、吼叫、吸鼻动作等，这些属于简单的发声抽动；少部分患者也有重复言语、模仿言语、秽语等复杂的发声抽动。

The movements and vocalizations are experienced as compulsive and irresistible but can be suppressed for varying lengths of time. They are exacerbated by stress and attenuated during periods in which the individual becomes totally absorbed by an activity. Tics are usually markedly diminished during sleep.

各种形式的抽动是强制的、不可压制的，但可在短时间受意志控制，在应激下加重，在注意力集中或睡眠时减轻或消失。

Tics can be further divided into transient tic disorder, chronic motor or vocal tic disorder, and combined vocal and multiple motor tic disorder (Tourette's syndrome) depending on the clinical manifestation and age of onset.

根据发病年龄、临床表现、病程长短和是否伴有发声抽动而分为短暂性抽动障碍、慢性运动或发声抽动障碍及发声与多种运动联合抽动障碍（图雷特综合征）。

i. Transient Tic Disorder

Transient tic disorder is the most common form of tics; it is characterized by acute and simple tics, which are usually limited to one or two muscle groups with onset in early school years.

（一）短暂性抽动障碍（抽动症）

这是儿童期最常见的抽动障碍。临床上表现为急性的单纯的运动抽动，极少数患儿可以为单纯发声抽动。常限于某一部位一组肌肉或两组肌肉群发生运动或发声抽动。

ii. Chronic Motor or Vocal Tic Disorder

Chronic motor or vocal tic disorder is a tic disorder characterized by motor or vocal tics (but not both), which may be either single or multiple (but usually multiple).

（二）慢性抽动障碍

这是以限于一组肌肉或两组肌肉群发生运动或发声抽动，但两者不并存为特征的一种抽动障碍，抽动可以是单一的，通常是多种的。

iii. Tourette's Syndrome

Tourette's syndrome is a progressive childhood and adolescent onset disorder with both motor and vocal symptoms. The most commonly recognized associated features are echopraxia, echolalia, compulsion, attention deficit, emotional disturbance and aggression. Onset is in childhood.

（三）发声与多种运动联合抽动障碍

它又称抽动秽语综合征（图雷特综合征），是以进行性发展的多部位运动和发声抽动为特征的抽动障碍，部分患儿伴有模仿言语、模仿动作，或强迫、攻击、情绪障碍及注意缺陷等行为障碍，起病于童年。

IV. Treatment

Medications are used to reduce the severity of tic disorders. Pharmacotherapy is most effective when it is combined with other forms of therapy, such as education and supportive intervention, individual counseling or psychotherapy, and family therapy. A number of medications have been used to treat tics. The most common ones are Haloperidol (Haldol), Pimozide (Orap) and Clonidine (Catapres).

四、治 疗

对抽动障碍的患者多采用药物治疗，常用的药物有氟派啶醇、匹莫齐特、可乐定。但药物治疗综合其他治疗效果更好，如教育、支持性干预、个别咨询或心理治疗，以及家庭治疗等。

V. Application of the Nursing Process

i. Nursing Assessment

Nursing assessment of a child with tics includes a review of the onset, course, and current level of the symptoms. The goal of the assessment is to identify the frequency, intensity, complexity, and the impact on the child's functioning; identify the child's strength and weaknesses; identify the social supports for the child and family. Another important aspect of assessment is to determine the impact of the tic symptoms on the child and family. Therefore, in addition to inquiring about tics, the child's overall development, activity levels, capacity to concentrate and persist with a single task, as well as the presence of repetitive habits and recurring worries should be assessed.

ii. Nursing Diagnosis

1. Risk for violence directed at self or others related to low tolerance for frustration.

2. Impaired social interaction related to impulsiveness, oppositional and aggressive behavior

3. Disturbances in self-esteem associated with tic behaviors.

iii. Nursing Care Plan and Implementation.

1. Outcome Identification

(1) Has not harmed self or others during times of increased tension;

(2) Interacts with with staff and peers in a socially appropriate manner;

(3) Verbalizes positive aspects about self, particularly as they relate to his or her ability to manage the illness.

2. Nursing Intervention

(1) Observe client's behavior frequently through routine activities and interactions. Become aware of behaviors that indicate a rise in agitation (Stress commonly increases tic behaviors. Recognition of behaviors

五、护理程序的应用

（一）护理评估

儿童抽动症患者的评估包括起病情况，病情的发展状况及现在的症状。其目的在于了解发病的频率、强度、复杂性，儿童的适应情况和各方面表现，以及儿童及家庭的社会支持情况。另外还应评估抽动对儿童及家庭的影响、儿童的整体发展水平、运动水平及行为习惯。

（二）护理诊断

1. **对自己或他人施以暴力的潜在危险** 与患儿对挫折忍耐力较低有关。

2. **社会交往受损** 与患儿易冲动、违抗性及进攻性行为有关。

3. **自尊受损** 与抽动行为导致的羞耻感有关。

（三）护理计划与措施

1. 护理目标

（1）在面对增加的压力时，患者能够克制自己而未导致对自己或他人造成伤害；

（2）患者能够与医护人员或同伴以合适的方式进行交往；

（3）患者能够用语言表达出自己的优点，尤其是有关应对疾病能力方面的优点。

2. 护理措施

（1）密切观察患者的行为和交往，以便及时发现患者兴奋性增高的先兆，因为压力通常会增加冲动行为发生的可能，早期发现早

that precede the onset of aggression may provide the opportunity to intervene before violence occurs).

期预防可避免暴力行为的发生。

(2) Monitor for self-destructive behavior and impulses. A staff member may need to stay with the client to prevent self-mutilation. Provide hand coverings and other restraints that prevent the client from self-mutilating behaviors.

（2）密切观察患者是否有自残或冲动行为发生。应有一名护理人员陪伴患者身边，以避免上述行为的发生。必要时可通过一些限制手段预防自残行为的发生。

(3) Redirect violent behavior with physical outlets for frustration. (Excess energy is released through physical activities and a feeling of relaxation is induced.)

（3）指导患者进行一些体育活动代替那些暴力行为。通过体育活动释放患者能量能够使患者达到放松。

(4) Develop a trusting relationship with the client. Convey acceptance of the person separate from the unacceptable behavior. (Unconditional acceptance increases feeling of self-worth.)

（4）与患者建立一种相互信任的关系。让患者知道他是被接受的，不被接受的仅仅是那些不良行为。因为无条件接受会增加患者自我价值。

(5) Discuss with client which behaviors are and are not acceptable. Describe in matter-of-fact manner the consequences of unacceptable behavior. Follow through. (Negative reinforcement can alter undesirable behaviors.)

（5）与患者讨论哪些行为是可接受的，哪些是不被接受的。以事实为依据描述那些不被接受的行为所导致的结果。

(6) Provide group situations for client. (Appropriate social behavior is often learned from the positive and negative feedback of peers.)

（6）为患者提供与同伴相处的机会。因为适当的社会行为通常是从来自同伴的正性或负性反馈中学习到的。

(7) Set limits on manipulative behavior. Take caution not to reinforce manipulative behaviors by providing desired attention. Identify the consequences of manipulation. Administer consequences matter-of-factly when manipulation occurs. (Aversive consequences may work to decrease unacceptable behaviors.)

（7）对操纵性行为制订规定。注意不要通过关注来加强操纵性行为。确定操纵性行为的结果。当其发生时应根据事实处理。

(8) Help client understand that he or she uses manipulation to try to increase his or her own self-esteem. Interventions should reflect other actions to accomplish this goal. (When client feels better about his or her self, the need to manipulate others will diminish.)

（8）帮助患者弄清他或她实施操纵性行为只是为了增加自尊。帮助患者采取其他有利于自尊提高的措施。当患者自我感觉好转时，对他人操纵的需要将减轻。

(9) If the client chooses to suppress tics in the presence of others, provide a specified "tic time" during which he or she "vents" tics, feelings, and behaviors (alone or with staff). (Allow for release of tics and assists in sense of control and management of symptoms.)

（9）对于当他人在场时压抑抽动发生的患者，可为其提供一个特殊的时间使抽动、感觉或行为得以释放。这样可允许抽动释放，帮助增加控制感和对症状的管理。

(10) Ensure that client has regular one-to-one time with RN staff. (Provides opportunities for educating about illness and teaching management tactics. Assists in exploring feelings around illness and incorporating illness into a healthy sense of self.)

（10）保证患者有规律的时间与护理人员独处。这样可了解患者对疾病的认识和感觉，同时提供机会对患者进行疾病知识和管理技巧的教育。

iv. Nursing Evaluation

（四）护理评价

Reassessment data may include information gathered by asking the following questions:

在评价阶段护理人员应提出以下问题：

1. Has the client refrained from causing harm to self or others during times of increased tension?

1. 在面对增加的压力时，患者是否能够抑制自己而未导致对自己或他人的伤害？

2. Has the client developed adaptive coping strategies for dealing with frustration in order to prevent resorting to self-destruction or aggression to others?

2. 在面对挫折时患者是否发展了适应性应对策略而不是用对自己或他人造成损害的方法去处理？

3. Is the client able to interact appropriately with staff and peers?

3. 患者是否能够与医护人员或同伴以合适的方式进行交往？

4. Is the client able to suppress tic behaviors when he or she chooses to do so?

4. 患者是否能够压抑抽动行为？

5. Does the client set a time for "release" of the suppressed tic behaviors?

5. 患者是否为压抑的抽动行为设立了一个"释放"的时间？

6. Does the client verbalize positive aspects about self, particularly as they relate to his or her ability to manage the illness?

6. 患者是否用语言表达出自己的优点，尤其是有关应对疾病的能力方面的优点？

7. Does the client comply with treatment in a non-defensive manner?

7. 患者是否能够以非防卫的方式配合医护人员的治疗护理？

Section 6 Nursing Management for Children and Adolescents with Emotional Disorder

第六节　儿童情绪障碍患者的护理

I. Introduction

一、概　述

i. Definition

（一）定义

According to *CCMD-3*, emotional disorder requires a persistence of the predominant emotional symptoms such as anxiety, phobia, obsession, compulsion and social withdrawal with their manifestations closely related to the developmental stage and social situation of the patient, and, in general, there is no definite continuity between this disorder and the adult neurotic disorder.

CCMD-3 对儿童情绪障碍的定义为："起病于儿童时期的焦虑、恐惧、强迫或羞怯等情绪异常，与儿童的发育和境遇有一定的关系，与成人期神经症无连续性。"

ii. Epidemiology

（二）流行病学

The emotional disorder is one of most popular mental disorders in children and its prevalence is just inferior to conduct disorder with 2.5% of such disorder occurred in children of 10-11 years. Separation anxiety disorder occurs in 2%-4% of children and adolescents. Separation anxiety disorder may be slightly more prevalent in girls and in families of lower socioeconomic status. The prevalence of social anxiety disorder among children and adolescents is 0.9%-1.1%. Girls predominate over boys in a ratio of about 7:3.

儿童情绪障碍是非常常见的儿童精神障碍，其发生率仅次于儿童行为障碍。在 10～11 岁儿童中的患病率为 2.5%。分离性焦虑在一般儿童和青少年人口中发生率约为 2%～4%，女孩和社会经济地位较低下家庭的儿童发生率较高。儿童社交恐惧症的患病率约为 0.9%～1.1%，男女之比为 3∶7。

II. Etiology and Mechanism

i. Genetics

Studies have shown that a greater number of children with relatives who manifest anxiety problems develop anxiety disorders themselves than do children with no such family patterns. Studies indicated that, from a hereditary perspective, individual differences in temperaments may be related to the development of fear and anxiety disorder in childhood.

ii. Environmental Influences

Studies have shown a relationship between life events and the development of anxiety disorders.

iii. Family Influences

Various theories account for the development of anxiety disorders in children and many of these contend that anxiety disorders in children are related to an over-attachment of the child to his/her mother. Children with separation anxiety disorder are believed to come from close-knit families. It is believed that some parents instill anxiety in their children by overprotecting them from expectable dangers or by exaggerating present and future dangers in the environment. Some theorists also contend that parents may transfer their fears and anxieties to their children through role modeling.

III. Types and Clinical Manifestation

According to *CCMD-3*, childhood emotional disorder is mainly divided into separation anxiety disorder, phobic anxiety disorder, social anxiety disorder.

i. Separation Anxiety Disorder of Children

This disorder describes a condition in which separation from attachment figures induces excessive anxiety during the early years of childhood.

The average age at onset is 8-9 years. Children with separation anxiety disorder exhibit severe distress when separated or threatened with separation from their parents, usually the mother. Fearing that harm will befall the attachment figure or themselves, they typically want to sleep in the parental bed, refuse to be alone, plead not to go to school, have nightmares about separation, and exhibit numerous somatic symptoms when threatened with separation. For example, when it is time to go to school these children complain of abdominal pain, nausea, vomiting, diarrhea, urinary frequency, and heart palpitations. Sometimes they have to be forced to leave the house. In order to avoid greater separation, they may also

二、病因及发病机制

（一）遗传因素

很多研究表明，家庭中有焦虑问题的亲属其儿童焦虑的发生率要高于家庭中没有此类问题的儿童。另外，从遗传的角度来说，焦虑、恐惧等障碍发生也与个人的气质有关。

（二）环境因素

研究表明焦虑障碍的发生也与压力性生活事件的发生有关。

（三）家庭影响

有许多研究儿童焦虑的理论认为儿童焦虑障碍的主要原因是患儿存在对其母亲的过度依赖。那些具有分离焦虑的儿童多来自于组织严密的家庭，其父母多表现为对儿童的过度担心和保护，对危险的过度夸张。一些理论家认为，父母可通过其角色榜样作用，将恐惧和焦虑传递给儿童。

三、常见类型与临床表现

CCMD-3 将儿童情绪障碍主要分为以下几个类型：儿童分离性焦虑障碍、儿童恐惧症和儿童社交恐惧症等。

（一）分离性焦虑障碍

此症儿童主要表现为与主要的依恋对象（常为父母，尤其以母亲为主）、家庭或其他熟悉的环境分离时出现过分焦虑。一般情况下，婴幼儿期与父母分离产生焦虑是正常的。但到了 3 岁以后，随着儿童与外界交往的日益扩大，对父母的依恋逐渐减少，如果再出现焦虑，且持续 2 周以上，则属病态。分离性焦虑的平均发病年龄为 8～9 岁，主要表现为担心什么事伤害父母，担心与父母分离后将不再回来，故拒绝上学或上床睡觉，不敢离开家；如果与主要依恋对象将要分离时，则出现头痛、胃痛、恶心及呕吐等躯体症状，渴求父母对其关注。

run away and hide near the home.

ii. Phobic Anxiety Disorder of Children

This diagnostic entity describes specific phobias in childhood in different developmental phases. Typically symptoms are episodes of hyperventilation, trembling, palpitations, shortness of breath, sweating, numbness, depersonalization, chest pain, choking, fear of dying, dizziness, and fainting.

（二）儿童恐惧症

此症儿童对某些物体或某些特殊情景产生异常的恐惧，而正常儿童对此无异常情绪反应。主要表现为对新环境或陌生人产生恐惧、焦虑情绪和回避行为，如害怕动物、死亡、昆虫、黑暗、噪声。常见症状为过度通气、颤抖、心悸、呼吸短促、出汗、麻木、人格解体、胸痛、窒息、害怕死亡、头晕眼花，甚至晕厥。

iii. Social Anxiety Disorder of Children

Children with social anxiety disorder experience anxiety in the company of other people or when expected to perform in some way. For example, when unfamiliar visitors arrive, they hide; they prefer single playmates; they avoid sports events and parties; and they detest taking examinations, reading aloud in class, eating in front of others, using public toilets, answering telephones, or speaking up to people in authority. Most of these children are afraid of two or more situations. When threatened, they experience the somatic features of anxiety (e.g., rapid breathing, palpitations, shakiness, chills, sweating, nausea).

（三）儿童社交恐惧症

此症儿童对新环境或陌生人产生恐惧、焦虑情绪和回避行为。与陌生人接触时持续和过分地退缩，达到妨碍同伴关系、社会功能的严重程度。主要表现为躲避、愿意单独玩耍，避免运动项目，避免参加聚会，厌恶参加考试、在班级同学面前大声朗读，不愿意使用公共盥洗室、打电话或与权威者大声说话；患儿在与陌生人接触时，表现为困窘、脸红或保持沉默。大多数儿童通常对两种或两种以上情境有恐惧心理，当被强迫做上述事情时，他们会表现出躯体症状，如呼吸加快、心悸、颤抖、寒战、出汗、恶心等。

IV. Treatment

It is reasonable to start with behavioral treatments and to try medication only if such treatments are unsuccessful. Family treatment, individual psychotherapy for unresolved conflicts, and liaison with the patient's school are also commonly required. The behavioral techniques most often used are systematic desensitization and exposure, operant conditioning, modeling, and cognitive-behavioral therapy.

四、治　疗

儿童情绪障碍往往以一种或多种形式出现，因而治疗形式多样。首选行为治疗，当效果不佳时可考虑药物治疗。家庭治疗、个别心理治疗及联合学校治疗也是常用的。行为疗法最常用的是系统脱敏疗法、暴露疗法、生物反馈治疗、模拟训练和认知行为治疗。

V. Application of the Nursing Process

i. Nursing Assessment

Nurses should assess the onset, duration, symptoms, sign, and its impact on social and academic functioning.

五、护理程序的应用

（一）护理评估

评估阶段应注意了解患儿的起病情况、病情进展，以及病情对社会适应和学习的影响。另外，也应评估家庭，如父母的养育方式等。

ii. Nursing Diagnosis

Symptoms that should be considered by nurses in forming a diagnosis include:

1. Anxiety (severe) related to family history, temperament, over attachment to parents, and negative role modelling.

2. Ineffective individual coping related to unresolved separation conflicts and inadequate coping skills evidenced by numerous somatic complaints.

3. Impaired social interaction related to reluctance to be away from the attachment figure.

iii. Nursing Care Planning and Implementation

Planning for nursing and other interventions should be a collaborative effort that includes the parents and the child. To ensure that fragmentation of care does not occur, the psychiatric nurse assumes the role of case manager.

1. Outcome Identification The following criteria may be used for the measurement of outcomes in the treatment of the emotional disorder client.

The client:

(1) Is able to maintain anxiety at manageable level.

(2) Demonstrates adaptive coping strategies for dealing with anxiety when separation from attachment figure is anticipated.

(3) Interacts appropriately with others and spends time away from attachment figure to do so.

2. Nursing Intervention The following provides a treatment plan for the care of the child or adolescent with separation anxiety disorder, using nursing evaluations of symptoms common to this disorder, appropriate nursing interventions and rationales.

(1) Anxiety (severe)

1) Establish an atmosphere of calmness, trust, and genuine positive regard. (Trust and unconditional acceptance are necessary for satisfactory nurse-client relationship. Calmness is important because anxiety is easily transmitted from one person to another.)

2) Assure client of his or her safety and security. (Symptoms of panic and anxiety are very frightening.)

3) Explore the child's or adolescent's fears of separating from the parents. Explore with the parents possible fears they may have of separation from the child. (Some parents may have an underlying fear of separation from the child, of which they are unaware and which they are unconsciously transferring to the child.)

（二）护理诊断

针对儿童分离性焦虑障碍可能的护理诊断包括：

1. **焦虑** 与家庭历史、性情特点、对父母过度依恋、负向角色榜样有关。

2. **个人应对无效** 与分离冲突不能解决和应对技巧不足等有关。

3. **社会交往受损** 与不愿与依恋的人分离有关。

（三）护理计划与措施

护理计划的实施需要与服务对象及其父母的合作共同完成，在此过程中护理工作者应充当个案管理者的角色，以避免护理的中断。

1. **护理目标** 针对儿童分离性焦虑障碍的主要护理目标如下：

儿童能够：

（1）将焦虑水平控制在可管理范围内；

（2）与所依恋人分离时用适应性策略来处理；

（3）用适当的方式与他人交往，即使当所依恋人不在场时。

2. **护理措施** 以下以儿童分离焦虑症为例，针对其主要护理诊断，提出护理措施，同时指出措施的合理性。

（1）焦虑（严重）

1）建立一种平静的、信任的、诚恳的、积极认可的气氛。（信任和无条件接受对于建立满意的护患关系非常必要。因为焦虑情绪很容易从一个人影响到他人，因此，平静的气氛很重要。）

2）向患者保证能保护其安全。（焦虑的症状会令患者非常害怕。）

3）与儿童或青少年探讨其与父母分离时的恐惧，与父母探讨他们与孩子分离时内心的感受。（一些父母可能并未意识到与孩子分离时自己的不良感觉，同时他们又把这种感觉在无意识状态下传染给了孩子。）

4) Help parents and child initiate realistic goals (e.g., child to stay with sitter for 2 hours with minimal anxiety stay at friend's house without parents until 9 PM without experiencing panic anxiety). (Parents may be so frustrated with child's clinging and demanding behaviours that assistance with problem-solving may be required.)

4）帮助父母或孩子确立现实的目标，如儿童能够与临时看管人在一起2个小时，而保持最低程度的焦虑；或者儿童能够在朋友家到晚上9点而没有恐惧发生。（当孩子过分依恋父母时，父母会有受挫感，因而帮助其解决问题是必要的。）

5) Give, and encourage parents to give, positive reinforcement for desired behaviours. (Positive reinforcement encourages repetition of desirable behaviours.)

5）鼓励父母对儿童表现出的好的行为给予积极的强化。（积极的强化可鼓励良好行为的重复性。）

(2) Ineffective individual coping

（2）个人应对无效

1) Encourage child or adolescent to discuss specific situations in life that produce the most distress and describe his or her response to these situations. Include parents in the discussion. (Client and family may be unaware of the correlation between stressful situations and the exacerbation of physical symptoms.)

1）鼓励儿童或青少年讨论生活中导致不良情绪反应的情境及描述他们对这些情境的反应。讨论邀请父母参加。（患者及其家庭可能并未意识到应激情境和身体症状之间的相关性。）

2) Help the child or adolescent who is a perfectionist to recognize that self-expectations may be unrealistic. Connect times of unmet self-expectations to the exacerbation of physical symptoms. (Recognition of maladaptive patterns is the first step in the change process.)

2）帮助具有完美主义倾向的儿童或青少年认识到自我期望可能是不现实的。帮助其将自我期望没有满足与身体症状的加重联系到一起。（对适应不良行为的认识是疾病变化过程的第一步。）

3) Encourage parents and child to identify more adaptive coping strategies that the child could use in the face of anxiety that feels overwhelming. Practice through role-playing. (Practice facilitates the use of the desired behaviour when the individual is actually faced with the stressful situation.)

3）鼓励父母和儿童寻找面对焦虑事件时更适应的策略。通过角色扮演加以训练。（实践将有助于面对应激情境时采取积极行为。）

(3) Impaired social interaction

（3）社会交往受损

1) Develop a trusting relationship with client. (This is the first step in helping the client learn to interact with others.)

1）与患者建立相互信任的关系。（这是帮助患者学会与他人交往的第一步。）

2) Attend groups with the child and support efforts to interact with others. Give positive feedback. (Presence of a trusted individual provides security during times of distress. Positive feedback encourages repetition.)

2）鼓励儿童参加集体活动，对交往给予支持，提供积极反馈。（信任人员的存在有助于提高安全感。积极反馈可鼓励良好行为的重复。）

3) Convey to the child that it is acceptable (but not desirable) for him/her not to participate in groups initially. Gradually encourage small contributions until client is able to participate more fully. (Small successes will gradually increase self-confidence and decrease self-consciousness, so that client will feel less anxious in the group situation.)

3）采取循序渐进的原则，对儿童开始的不参与表示接受，逐渐鼓励其增加参与的程度。（小的成功将逐渐增加自信，使儿童在集体环境中焦虑水平下降。）

4) Help client set small personal goals (e.g., "Today I will speak to one person I don't know.") (Simple, realistic goals provide opportunities for success that increase self-

4）帮助儿童设立小的个人目标，如今天我将与一位不认识的人说话。（简单的、现实

confidence and may encourage the client to attempt more difficult objectives in the future.)

的目标提供成功的机会，有助于提高自信，鼓励更高目标的完成。）

iv. Nursing Evaluation

Reassessment data may include information gathered by asking the following questions:

（四）护理评价

评价过程是一个持续进展的过程。评价过程中应考虑儿童的发展阶段，判断情绪和行为是否发生了变化，药物治疗是否有效，家庭动力情况有否改善，社会化情况和学校技能方面有否进步等。在评价阶段护理人员应提出以下问题：

1. Is the client able to maintain anxiety at a manageable level?

2. Have complaints of physical symptoms diminished?

3. Has the client demonstrated the ability to cope in more adaptive ways in the face of escalating anxiety?

4. Have the parents identified their role in the separation conflict? Are they able to discuss more adaptive coping strategies?

5. Does the client verbalize an intention to return to school?

6. Have nightmares and fears of the dark subsided?

7. Is the client able to interact with others away from the attachment figure?

8. Have the precipitating stressors been identified? Have strategies for coping more adaptively to similar stressors in the future been established?

1. 患儿是否能够控制焦虑在可管理水平？

2. 患儿是否自诉躯体症状减少了？

3. 随着焦虑程度的加深患儿是否能够用更适应的方式来应对？

4. 患儿的父母是否认识到他们在分离冲突中的角色？他们是否能够讨论出更具适应性的应对策略？

5. 患儿是否用语言表达回到学校的愿望？

6. 患儿是否做噩梦和害怕黑暗的次数和水平有所减少或降低？

7. 当所依恋的人不在时，患儿是否能够与他人较好相处？

8. 是否找出了压力源，是否建立了应对未来同样压力的策略？

Child psychiatry is an area in which nursing can make a valuable contribution. Nurses who choose this field have an excellent opportunity to serve in the promotion of emotional wellness for children and adolescents.

在儿童青少年精神科护理领域，护理人员担负着重大使命，所有护理工作者都应为促进儿童青少年的健康情绪做出自己最大的贡献。

(Fang Hua)

（方 华）

Key Points

1. Although studies regarding the development of psychiatric disorders in children and adolescents have been limited due to the overlap of one or more syndromes, theories have identified some generic and biologic factors contributing to the development of disorders such as autistic disorder, ADHD, conduct disorder.

2. Environmental factors such as schools and neighbourhoods can influence the development of behavior disorders.

内容摘要

1. 虽然儿童、青少年精神障碍的症状重叠性限制了相关研究的进行，但是现有研究已经表明一些障碍，如孤独症、注意缺陷和多动障碍、行为障碍等症与生物和遗传因素有关。

2. 环境因素，如学校和邻里环境等可影响行为障碍的发展。

3. Mental retardation is a developmental disorder in which the client exhibits impairment in areas such as communication, activities of daily living, socialization, and functional academic or occupational skills.

3. 精神发育迟滞是以在沟通、日常生活能力、社会化、学业和职业技能方面受损为主要表现的发育障碍。

4. Two commonly diagnosed disorders in childhood and adolescence are ADHD and conduct disorder.

4. 儿童和青少年期最常见的两大障碍为注意缺陷和多动障碍以及行为障碍。

5. The incidence of autistic disorder, an incurable and lifelong pervasive developmental disorder, has increased over the past years.

5. 孤独症是不可治愈、持续终生的广泛性发育障碍，其发病率在近年有增高趋势。

6. The assessment of a young client is often complicated by the interaction of psychopathology with the child's environment and developmental processes.

6. 精神病理情况与儿童环境和发展阶段的相互作用导致护理评估的复杂性。

7. Stating a nursing diagnosis for children or adolescents who exhibit a mental disorder can be difficult because of changing or inconsistent behavior, discomfort in the presence of the examiner, developmental changes, and the influence of parents.

7. 由于儿童和青少年行为的不断变化和不一致性，检查者在场时引起的不适，自身发展的变化以及父母的影响，加大了护理诊断的难度。

8. Planning interventions is a collaborative effort with the client and parents and may include efforts and cooperation in multidisciplinary teams and community. Nursing plans and interventions should individually meet the need of client.

8. 护理计划和实施是需要服务对象、父母、其他团队、社区共同努力合作完成的。护理计划和实施需满足每位服务对象的个体化需要。

9. Psychopharmacology has been approved as adjunctive therapy in the treatment of some certain disorders and remains one of the most successful treatments for ADHD.

9. 精神药物已被证明是某些特定障碍的辅助治疗手段，是注意缺陷和多动障碍的最为有效的治疗方法。

Exercises

思考题

(Questions 1 to 2 share the same question stem)

A 2- year-old child is brought into the physician's office by her parents who are concerned by her behavior. They state that she resists their affection, twirls around frequently, and refuses to respond to other children and adults.

1. What medical diagnosis would the nurse suspect?
2. What would be the possible nursing diagnoses?

（1～2题共用题干）

一个2岁孩子被父母带进医生办公室，他们对她的行为表示担忧。他们说孩子抗拒他们的爱，经常旋转并拒绝回应其他儿童和成人。

1. 护士认为最可能的医疗诊断是什么？
2. 考虑什么护理诊断？

(Questions 3 to 4 share the same question stem)

The parents of a 15-year-old girl bring their daughter for admission to the mental health center. She was recently expelled from school for repeated behavior problems and truancy. She was also arrested for vandalism and prostitution in the past week.

3. What medical diagnosis would the nurse suspect?
4. What would be the possible nursing diagnoses?

（3～4题共用题干）

一名15岁女孩被父母带到精神卫生中心，她最近因为反复出现行为问题和逃学被学校开除，上周又因破坏和卖淫被拘捕。

3. 护士认为最可能的医疗诊断是什么？
4. 考虑什么护理诊断？

(Questions 5 to 6 share the same question stem)

A 6-year-old female student is brought to the school nurse for refusal to sit in class. She denies feeling sick but insists that her mother be called so she can go home. She

（5～6题共用题干）

一名6岁女学生因拒绝坐在教室被送去见学校护士。她说自己没有生病但她坚持要给母

is pacing and chewing on a fingernail. This has occurred daily since school began 4 weeks ago. She tells the nurse that she is afraid something bad is going to happen to her mother.

5. What medical diagnosis would the nurse suspect?

6. What would be the possible nursing diagnoses and nursing intervention?

亲打电话接她回家。她咬着手指甲在教室里走来走去，从开学4周到现在每天都如此。她告诉护士她担心母亲发生不幸的事情。

5. 护士认为最可能的医疗诊断是什么？

6. 考虑什么护理诊断和护理措施？

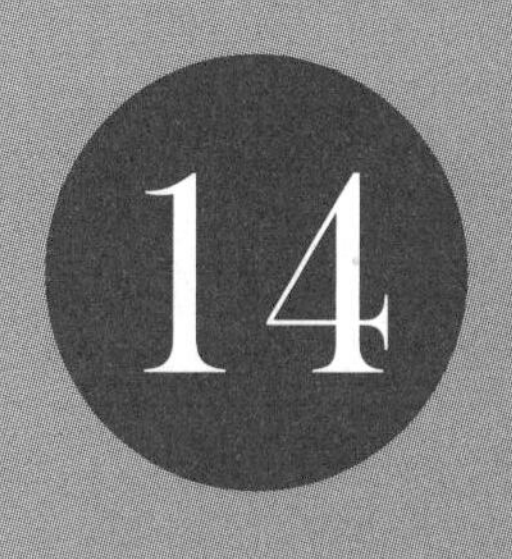

Chapter 14 Nursing Management of Clients with Physiological Disorders Related to Psychological Factors

第十四章　心理因素所致生理障碍患者的护理

Learning Objectives

Memorization

1. Describe concepts of anorexia nervosa and insomnia.
2. Summarize the causes of eating disorders and sleep disorders.

Comprehension

1. Identify the mental symptoms of anorexia nervosa and neurological bulimia.
2. Explain the mental factors of the insomnia and circadian rhythm sleep disorder.

Application

1. Make a meal plan for the client with anorexia nervosa through negotiation based on information acquired from nursing assessment.
2. Make non-drug treatment plan for the client with insomnia based on nursing program and assess the rehabilitation program.

学习目标

识记

1. 能准确描述神经性厌食症和失眠症的概念。
2. 能正确概述进食障碍和睡眠障碍的病因。

理解

1. 能识别神经性厌食症与神经性贪食症的精神症状。
2. 能用实例说明失眠症与昼夜节律障碍发生的精神因素。

运用

1. 能运用护理评估获得的信息与神经性厌食症患者商议制订一份饮食计划。
2. 能运用护理程序为失眠症患者制订非药物治疗的康复计划并进行评价。

14章

Kelly, a 17-year-old girl, a high school student, was brought into hospital because she ate little, looked skinny and suffered amenorrhea for one year. One year ago, Kelly was teased as a "fat girl" by classmates, so she began to lose weight and refused to eat staple food. Afterwards, she even didn't eat fruits. She was 167cm in height and 42 kg in weight when she was hospitalized. Morgan, the nurse who took care of Kelly always tries to convince Kelly to eat food, but Kelly was very indifference to her and won't cooperate with her treatment. Kelly cried in the ward at dinner time, but when Morgan entered the room to console her, she pushed away the dishes to the ground, and cried, "I won't eat, can't you see how fat I am. I could become a balloon if I eat more foods!"

Please think about the following questions based on the case:

1. What might be the potential nursing diagnoses for Kelly?
2. How does Morgan provide effective care for helping Kelly to eat food?

患者凯莉，女，17岁，是一名高中学生，因进食少、消瘦闭经1年而入院。1年前，凯莉在学校被同学取笑是“胖女孩”，从此，凯莉开始减肥，不吃主食，后来连水果也吃不下去了，入院时凯莉身高167 cm，体重42 kg。摩根是照顾凯莉的护士，总是劝说凯莉多吃点饭，可凯莉一直对她很冷淡，不太配合。到了晚餐时间，凯莉在病房里哭泣，摩根过来劝慰她时，她把饭菜推到了地上，哭着说：“我不要吃，你看我都多胖了，再吃就要吃成气球了！”

请思考：

1. 患者目前及潜在的护理诊断是什么？
2. 护士可以采取什么方法帮助患者进食？

In modern society, more and more people start to pay attention to figure, especially some females, they even think "the slimmer, the better". However, if we pursue for "bony beauty" and neglect whether the figure conforms to heath standard, it is likely that we will be trapped in the situation of "anorexia nervosa". In 2010, French "bony" model Isabelle Caro who once took naked photo to fight with anorexia nervosa dead at the age of 28. She was 1.65 meters in height, but only weighted 32 kg.

现代社会越来越多的人开始关注自己的身材，尤其是某些青年女性，甚至认为“越瘦越好”。然而，盲目沉迷于“骨感美”而不注重身体是否符合健康标准会使人们不知不觉地陷入“神经性厌食症”的深渊。2010年，被称为“皮包骨”的法国模特伊莎贝尔·卡罗（Isabelle Caro）去世，她生前曾拍摄裸照对抗神经性厌食症。年仅28岁，身高1.65 m的她死时体重仅32 kg。

With the rapid development of the society, people are facing with increasing pressure, and many people couldn't fall asleep in the night although they have worked for a whole day. As time goes by, the living and working levels of the public decline, and their physical and mental health are affected seriously, which makes "Have a good sleep." a hope for many people.

社会的快速发展使得人们的压力越来越大，人们在经过一天的辛苦工作后晚上反而睡不着，久而久之，生活和工作水平都会下降，严重影响身心健康，“好好地睡上一觉”成了不少人的奢望。

Sleep and eating are basic human functions closely related to physical and mental health. Both psychological disorders and physical illnesses often manifest as disturbances in these functions. But, even in the absence of general psychiatric or physiological diagnoses, independent disorders of eating and sleep can occur.These disorders may present in psychiatric nursing practice or in other care settings.This chapter provides an introduction to some of the most common of such disorders of regulation and how to provide care to the people with these disorders.

饮食和睡眠是人类的基本功能，与身心健康密切相关，许多生理和心理疾病都会表现出上述功能障碍。这些障碍可单独出现，也可伴随其他疾病同时出现；既可发生在精神疾病，也可发生于躯体疾病。本章将重点介绍进食障碍及睡眠障碍患者的护理。

Section 1 Eating Disorders

第一节　进食障碍

Food is essential to life because it supplies needed nutrients and energy. As an activity of self-regulation, eating can also assume importance and meaning beyond that of nutrition and become associated with biopsychosocial processes that promote or inhibit adaptive functioning. Properly controlled eating contributes to psychological, biological, and sociocultural health and well-being. Adaptive eating responses are characterized by balanced eating patterns,appropriate caloric intake,and body weight that are appropriate for height.

食物是生命的必需品，机体需要不断摄取食物来获得营养以维持生命，作为一种可自我控制的行为，进食不单是一种摄取营养的行为，而成为与生理、心理、社会有关的过程。适宜的摄食行为有助于身心健康和维持良好的社会文化功能，其特征表现为所摄取的食物种类均衡、热量适当、体重与身高比例协调。

Although eating is common occurrence,society appears to have difficulty in understanding the idea of unregulated eating. Sociocultural ideals concerning body size can cause eating disorders by influencing a person to perceive his or her body size as being larger or smaller than it actually is. This distorted body image may lead to an attempt to attain an unrealistic body size. Abnormal eating behavior may arises as an attempt to calm and soothe unpleasant emotions, as an effort to resolve intrapsychic conflicts around aggression, sexuality, and interpersonal relationships, or as an attempt to act out issues on behalf of a dysfunctional family. The inability to regulate eating habits and the frequent tendency to overuse or underuse food interferes with biological, psychological, and sociocultural integrity. Illnesses associated with maladaptive eating regulation responses include anorexia nervosa and bulimia nervosa.

尽管进食是一项普通的事情，但人们似乎很难理解无节制进食行为的发生。社会文化对理想体重的标准和关注，使人们对自己的身材有不恰当的认识和不切实际的要求，并试图通过过度地限制或增加进食来达到目的；此类人群采用过度进食来缓解压力或减轻内心冲突，这些不恰当的摄食习惯，会使个体的生理、心理、社会功能的完整性和协调性遭到破坏，这就是所谓的进食障碍，包括神经性厌食症和神经性贪食症。

These disorders can cause biological changes that include altered metabolic rates, profound malnutrition, and possibly death. Obsessions about eating can cause psychological problems that include depression, isolation, and emotional lability.

其结果常导致生理变化，如代谢率改变、营养失调，甚至死亡；心理学方面则出现抑郁、孤立和情绪不稳。

Eating disorders are more commonly seen among females, with a male-female ratio ranging from 1∶6 to 1∶10. Eating disorders appear to be about as common in young Hispanic women as in whites, more common among Native Americans, and less common among blacks and Asians.

进食障碍较易发生在女性群体中，男女比例大约为1∶6～1∶10。进食障碍在美洲土著人中的发生率最多，其次是白人和西班牙女性，在黑色人种和黄色人种中的发生率较少。

I. Anorexia Nervosa

一、神经性厌食症

Anorexia nervosa is a complex eating disorder characterized by the client's refusal to maintain body weight appropriate for height, morbid fear of gaining weight or becoming fat, a severely distorted concept of body image, and unrelenting pursuit of thinness. Anorexia nervosa occurs in approximately 0.4% of the female population.Its onset is usually between 13 and 20 years of age, but the illness can occur in any age-group, including

神经性厌食症的特征为个体对自身体像的感知有歪曲，因担心发胖而故意节食，以致体重显著下降。在年轻女性中神经性厌食症的12个月患病率约为0.4%，女性与男性比率约为10∶1。初发年龄一般为13～20岁，但其他年龄段的人群也可发生，包括老年人和

the elderly and prepubertal children. Males with anorexia nervosa are thought to make up on 5% to 10% of the anorectic population. The mortality from anorexia nervosa is estimated to be approximately 5%.

青春前期儿童。神经性厌食症的病死率大约为 5%。

Specific diagnostic criteria include body weight less than 85% of expected body weight for age and height, amenorrhea, preoccupation with food and food-related activities, and obsessive behaviors to prevent weight gain such as restricting food intake, excessive exercise,or purging methods such as self-induced vomiting,use of laxatives,emetics,enemas, or diuretics.

诊断标准包括体重低于标准体重的 85%；有意控制进食量，或采取过度运动、引吐、导泻等方式以减轻体重；无月经。

i. Etiology

Numerous biologic, psychological, and sociocultural factors contribute to the development of anorexia nervosa. A possible genetic vulnerability may predispose the individual to a number of neurochemical changes, but these changes are difficult to separate from psychological and environmental stressors. Rigid, perfectionistic family systems with enmeshed boundaries may further exacerbate the symptoms, resulting in a sense of helplessness, fear of isolation, fear of losing control, and low self-esteem. These stressors occur in the context of a society that idealizes thinness and often views "fat" as a personal or moral failing, an underlying psychological trauma that can greatly contribute to a young woman's emotional conflict and distress over body image,which seem to be at the root of eating disorders.

（一）病因

多种生物、心理、社会文化因素都与神经性厌食症的发生有关系。遗传因素可能导致相关的神经化学变化，心理紧张、环境压力也可能会引起这些变化。家庭教育方式不当，如过分严格或追求过度完美所导致的无助感、孤独感、失控感和低自尊则会进一步加重症状。社会习俗对苗条美的崇尚，并且把肥胖视为一种个人或者道德上的失败，潜在精神创伤给年轻女性造成情感冲突和对体形的担忧被认为是进食障碍的根本原因。

ii. Signs and Symptoms

Individuals with anorexia nervosa go to incredible extremes to lose weight. They begin by drastically reducing caloric intake, with virtually complete avoidance of high-carbohydrate and fat-containing foods. They exercise incessantly walking, running, swimming, cycling, dancing, and performing calisthenics. Even when weight loss has resulted in cachexia, hyperactivity is dramatic and persists. Some clients alternate fasting with bulimia-episodes of uncontrolled gorging without awareness of hunger or satiation. Self-induced vomiting often follows such eating binges. Huge quantities of laxatives are commonly consumed. Diet pills and diuretics may also be abused in the effort to lose weight. Two-thirds of clients with anorexia nervosa are also diagnosed with at least one mood disorder. Up to 60% of clients with anorexia nervosa are diagnosed with major depression and about 33% with anxiety disorders. Obsessive-compulsive,phobias,and panic disorder are also common. Personality disorders are diagnosed in at least 20% and as many as 80% of clients with anorexia nervosa.The patient's distorted cognition of eating and weight promotes excessive attention to body shape and intense fear of obesity. Table 14-1 lists the cognitive distortions related to eating disorders.

（二）症状和体征

神经性厌食症患者采用不可思议的极端方式来减轻体重，起初是大大减少热量的摄入，基本不吃高热量的和含脂肪的食物。为了减轻体重而不停地走动、跑步、游泳、骑脚踏车、做健美操，即使身体十分虚弱仍坚持进行过度运动。有的患者由于过度节食，可出现无法控制的强烈进食欲望而间歇贪食，但进食后立即自行引吐或使用大量泻药、利尿剂，以减轻体重。大约三分之二的患者合并一种或多种情绪障碍，其中约 60% 患有抑郁症，33% 有焦虑症状。强迫症、惊恐发作、恐惧也较常见。大约 20%～80% 的患者伴有人格障碍。患者对进食、体重等歪曲的认知，促使其对体型的过分关注和对肥胖的强烈恐惧。表 14-1 列举了与进食障碍有关的认知扭曲。

Table 14-1 Cognitive distortions related to eating disorders

Cognition	Example
Overgeneralization: A single event affects unrelated situations	"He didn't ask me out. It must be because I'm fat." "I was happy when I wore a size 6.I must get back to that weight."
All-or-nothing thinking: Reasoning is absolute and extreme, in mutually exclusive terms of black or white, good or bad	"If I have one Popsicle, I must eat five." "If I allow myself to gain weight, I'll blow up like a balloon."
Catastrophizing: The consequences of an event are magnified	"If I gain weight, my weekend will be ruined." "When people say I look better, I know they think I'm fat."
Personalization: Events are overinterpreted as having personal significance	"I know everybody is watching me eat." "People won't like me unless I'm thin."
Emotional reasoning: Subjective emotions determine reality	"I know I'm fat because I feel fat." "When I'm thin,I feel powerful."

表 14-1 与进食障碍有关的认知扭曲

认知	例子
以偏概全：把某单一事件认为和其他不相关的事件有关	"他没有约我出去，一定是因为我胖。" "当我穿 6 号衣服时我很高兴，我必须回到那时候的体重。"
极端认知：推理是绝对的和极端的，非黑即白，非好即坏	"如果我有一根冰棒，我一定要吃五个。" "如果我允许自己发胖，我会像气球一样爆炸。"
大祸临头感：放大事件的后果	"如果我的体重增加，我的周末就毁了。" "当人们说我很好时，我知道他们觉得我胖了。"
过度自我化：把事件过度诠释与自己有关	"我知道每个人都在看着我吃。" "人们不会喜欢我，除非我很瘦。"
推理情绪化：主观情绪决定现实	"我知道我胖是因为我觉得我胖了。" "当我瘦的时候，我觉得自己很强大。"

In addition to weight loss, a number of physical signs of anorexia nervosa can be result from malnutrition. Amenorrhea or oligomenorrhea, independent of weight loss and often preceding initial weight loss, is always present in women. Anorexia nervosa with premenarcheal onset often results in short stature and delayed breast development. Prolonged amenorrhea in women with anorexia nervosa may lead to the development of osteoporosis. Vomiting, constipation, cold intolerance, headache, polyuria, and sleep disturbances are also commonly reported. In addition to emaciation, physical findings may include edema, lanugo, dehydration, low blood pressure, bradycardia, arrhythmias, diminished cardiac mass, and infantile uterus. Males with anorexia frequently have hemorrhoids and experience loss of sexual desire.

除了体重减轻，严重的营养不良还会导致一系列的体征。女性月经不调或月经稀少可出现在体重减轻之前、同时或之后。如果厌食症发生在月经初潮前，则会导致患者身材矮小、乳房发育不良，长期闭经还会引起骨质疏松。呕吐、便秘、畏寒、头痛、多尿和睡眠障碍等症状也很常见。体格检查可发现水肿、低血压、脱水、阴毛稀疏、脉搏迟缓、心律失常和幼稚子宫。男性常出现痔疮和性欲丧失。

Laboratory findings include abnormalities of vasopressin secretion, prepubertal plasma levels of follicle-stimulating hormone and luteinizing hormone,

实验室结果显示抗利尿激素分泌异常，促性腺激素分泌减少，皮质醇无昼夜节律变

and a diminished response to gonadotropin-releasing hormone,estrogen is at postmenopausal levels, males have low testosterone. There is abolition or reversal of the normal circadian rhythm of plasma cortisol. Plasma levels of triiodothyronine (T_3) are reduced. Hypercholesterolemia and hypomagnesemia are common findings. Electroencephalographic patterns may be abnormal, and the electrocardiogram may show flat or inverted T waves, ST depression, and increased Q-T intervals.

化，血清 T_3 下降，血脂高，血镁低。脑电图检查可能有异常，心电图显示 T 波低平或倒置，ST 下移，Q–T 间期延长。

The number of people with anorexia nervosa who fully recover is small. Although some clients improve symptomatically over time, most continue to have disturbances with body image, disordered eating, and other psychiatric problems. Death, which occurs in 10%-22% of clients, is caused by starvation and its complications (including pneumonia and other infections, cardiac arrhythmia, congestive heart failure, and renal failure) or by suicide. Clients who purge by vomiting or by abusing laxatives or diuretics are at risk for sudden death due to fluid and electrolyte imbalance.

完全治愈的病例不多，部分患者症状虽有好转，但大部分患者仍会持续存在体像障碍、进食障碍和心理问题。本病的病死率为 10%～22%，死因主要是营养不良及其并发症，包括肺炎、心律失常、充血性心衰和肾衰竭或自杀。长期使用泻药、利尿剂和自行引吐的患者还会由于水、电解质失衡而发生猝死。

iii. Treatment

（三）治疗

A multidisciplinary approach is essential in treating anorexia nervosa, which includes medication, behavioral therapy, cognitive therapy and family treatment. Clients may require acute intensive medical intervention to correct fluid and electrolyte imbalances, cardiac problems,and organ failure.

本病的治疗主要是综合治疗，包括行为治疗、药物治疗、认知治疗和家庭治疗。急性期患者需尽快住院治疗，以纠正水、电解质失衡和心肾衰竭。

1. Behavioral Therapy There is general agreement that weight restoration should be a central goal for the seriously underweight client,and most of these clients will require inclient management, during which controlled conditions can be achieved. The dietary regiment for the anorexic client generally involves a slow,s teady weight gain of no more than 2 pounds per week. Too-rapid weight gain can put undue stress on the heart and precipitate complications.

1. **行为治疗** 恢复理想体重是最主要的目标。体重增加的速度不能过快，以每周不超过 2 磅（0.907 2 kg）为宜，太快会增加心脏负担，加重并发症。行为治疗对短期内增加体重有一定的治疗效果，这种方法应该与大多数厌食症的组织治疗方法结合使用。

2. Pharmacotherapy Although there have been many drugs used to treat anorexia nervosa,no medication has been shown to be effective in maintaining weight gain, change anorectic attitudes, or preventing relapse either by itself or as an adjunct for treating anorexia nervosa. Antidepressants, neuroleptics, cyproheptadine, and lithium, may be helpful adjuncts, especially for clients who have coexisting depressive or psychotic features. Behavioral therapy is effective in inducing short-term weight again in anorectic clients, and this approach is incorporated into most structured treatment programs for anorexia.

2. **药物治疗** 目前很多药物可以用来治疗神经性厌食症，但尚无确切有效的药物来维持体重的增加、改变进食态度和防止复发。抗抑郁药、安定类药、赛庚定和锂盐可用于合并精神障碍的患者。

3. Cognitive Therapy Cognitive therapy helps clients challenge the validity of distorted beliefs and perceptions that are perpetuating their illness. The

3. **认知治疗** 帮助患者正确认识自己的体像和疾病，方法是先探讨和了解患者的错

modification of cognitive techniques for the treatment of anorexia nervosa includes examining underlying assumptions,modifying basic assumptions, reinterpreting body image misperceptions. Family therapy is advocated not as a single mode of treatment, but as an adjunct therapy, especially for anorectic clients with an early age of onset (younger than 18 year).

误感知，然后向患者解释，纠正他们对体形的错误观念。家庭治疗作为一种辅助治疗手段而不是单独的治疗方法，对于发病年龄早（18 岁前）的病例有一定效果。

II. Bulimia Nervosa

二、神经性贪食症

Bulimia nervosa is an eating disorder that involves the individual engaging in recurrent, uncontrolled episodes of binge eating and compensatory behavior to avoid weight gain through purging methods such as self-induced vomiting or use of laxatives, diuretics, enemas, emetics, or through purging methods such as fasting or excessive exercise.

神经性贪食症是指反复发作的强烈的、无法控制的摄食欲望和行为，患者每次可进食大量食物，但事后又担心发胖，进而采取自我诱吐、导泄、过度运动的方法防止体重增加。

i. Etiology

（一）病因

As with anorexia and many other psychiatric and medical disorders, bulimia nervosa has no single etiologic cause. Genetic factors and environmental factors such as conflicting family relationship may make an individual more susceptible. Multiple neurochemical alterations precede or are a result of the manifestations of the disorder.

和厌食症以及其他精神或功能失调一样，神经性贪食症的病因和发病机制尚未清楚。遗传因素、环境因素如家庭关系紧张都会增加个体的易感性。多种影响神经系统的化学物质改变都会导致疾病的发展。

ii. Symptoms and Signs

（二）症状和体征

1. Uncontrolled Gorging of Large Quantities of Food in Short Periods of Time The essential feature of bulimia nervosa is the episodic, uncontrolled gorging of large quantities of food in short periods of time. Clients are aware of their disordered eating habits and distinguish eating binges from simple overeating. The food consumed during a binge often has a high caloric content,a sweet taste, and a soft or smooth texture that can be eaten rapidly, sometimes even without being chewed. The binging episodes often occur in secret and are usually only terminated by abdominal discomfort, sleep, social interruption, or self-induced vomiting. Binges are usually preceded by depressive moods in which the client feels sad, lonely, empty,and isolated; or by anxiety states with overwhelming tension. These feelings are usually relieved during the binges, but afterward clients typically report a return of depressive mood with disparaging self-criticism and feelings of guilt.

1. 不可控制的暴食发作 是本病的主要特征。暴食发作时，患者食欲大增，吃得又多又快，甚至来不及咀嚼，较喜欢高热量的松软甜食，每次均吃到腹部胀痛或恶心为止。患者进食时常常避开他人，在公共场所尽量克制。暴食前患者通常会有抑郁心境或因进食冲动所致的内心紧张，暴食可以帮助患者缓解这种紧张感，但过后患者会感到更抑郁，甚至悔恨、内疚。

2. Purging Behaviors In order to rid the body of the excessive calories, the individual may engage in purging behaviors (self-induced vomiting, or the misuse of laxatives, diuretics, or enemas) or other inappropriate compensatory behaviors, such as fasting or excessive exercise. Those who do vomit may use emetics such as ipecac syrup or induce vomiting by activating the gag

2. 清除行为 为了抵消暴食引起的体重增加，患者常采用自我诱吐、导泄、禁食、过度运动的方法减少热量的摄入。自我诱吐是借助催吐剂或用手指刺激咽后壁后发生，因此，患者手背上常带有特征性的损伤。随着病程的发展，部分患者甚至可以不借助任

reflex. Lesions on the back of the hand may be evidence of this. Many report that they no longer need chemical or mechanical stimulants to induce emesis, as they can simply vomit at will. There is a persistent overconcern with physical appearance, particularly regarding how they believe others perceive them. Weight fluctuations are common. Most clients experience weight fluctuations because of the alternating binges and fasts. However, most bulimics are within a normal weight range, some slightly underweight, some slightly overweight.

3. Complication Frequent vomiting and laxative/diuretic abuse may lead to problems with dehydration and electrolyte imbalance. Gastric acid in the vomitus also contributes to the erosion of tooth enamel. In rare instances, the individual may experience tears in the gastric or esophageal mucosa. Some people with this disorder are subject to mood disorders, anxiety disorders. Other symptoms associated with bulimia include headache, sore throat, painless or painful swelling of parotid and salivary glands, feelings of fullness, abdominal pain, and lethargy and fatigue. Menstrual irregularities are common, but amenorrhea is usually not sustained. Deaths from gastric dilatation and rupture have been reported.

Bulimia and anorexia may be present in the same client.As many as 50% of individuals with anorexia develop bulimic symptoms, and some people with bulimia develop anorexia. Bulimia nervosa is more common than anorexia, with an estimated occurrence of 1% to 4% of the population and 4% to 15% of female high school and college students.The age of onset is typically 15 to 18 years of age.It is estimated that men make up only 10% of the bulimic population. The long-tern outcome of bulimia nervosa is not known. Research suggests that 30% of clients with bulimia nervosa rapidly relapse, with up to 40% remaining chronically symptomatic.

iii. Treatment of Bulimia Nervosa

Treatment of bulimia nervosa is currently accomplished by a variety of approaches. Clients who demonstrate major electrolyte disturbance, who have depression with suicidal ideation, or who have not responded to general client management need inclient treatment. Hospitalization is rarely required for uncomplicated bulimia nervosa. Many psychosocial approaches have value in the treatment of this disorder. Cognitive-behavioral therapy has been found to be the single most effective treatment for clients with eating disorders. Other therapeutic approaches include group psychotherapy and family therapy. Several types of agents have been studied in clients with bulimia nervosa. Lithium and anticonvulsants yielded unimpressive changed in

何方法，随心所欲地吐出食物。患者对自己的体像非常关注，很在意他人对自己身材的评价，其体重常由于反复暴食和禁食而发生波动，但大多限于正常范围内。

3. 并发症 频繁的呕吐和泻药、利尿剂的滥用，可引起一系列躯体并发症，导致患者脱水和电解质失衡，胃酸和呕吐物致牙釉质腐蚀，少数病例可发生胃、食道黏膜损伤。部分患者可合并精神障碍，如焦虑、心境障碍等。其他的症状还包括头痛、咽喉肿痛、唾液腺肿、腹痛腹胀、软弱无力。月经紊乱、闭经也较为常见。因胃扩张和胃破裂而致死也可发生。

贪食症和厌食症可同时发生于同一个体，约 50% 的厌食症患者合并贪食症状。贪食症较厌食症为多见，在年轻女性中 12 个月患病率为 1%～1.5%，女性与男性患病率比率约为 10∶1。其中 4%～15% 为女性中学生和大学生，初发年龄一般为 15～18 岁。该病的长期预后还不太清楚，有研究显示 30% 的患者较易复发，40% 的患者会残留症状。

（三）治疗

贪食症的治疗常需多种方法联合使用。有电解质紊乱、抑郁伴自杀倾向，对一般治疗无效的患者需要住院治疗。其他患者可以进行院外治疗。许多社会心理治疗方法对贪食症的治疗有一定的疗效。认知行为治疗是其中最为有效的方法。其他的方法还包括小组治疗和家庭治疗。药物治疗中，抗抑郁药被证实对治疗贪食症有效，包括三环类、单胺氧化酶抑制剂、曲唑酮及 SSRIs 等都能有效减少贪食症的症状。

symptomatology. Only the antidepressants have proven efficacious with bulimic symptoms.Antidepressants of every class, including tricyclics, monoamine oxidase inhibitors, trazodone, and selective serotonin reuptake inhibitors, have demonstrated efficacy in reducing bulimic symptoms.

Section 2 Sleep Disorders

Sleep, an experience that occupies nearly one-third of our lives, is a recurrent, altered state of consciousness that occurs for sustained periods, restoring a person's energy and well-being. Sleep is not a quiescent state,but a complicated process integrating behavioral, mental and physical factors. The need for sleep decreases with age: newborns should sleep for 18 or more hours a day; school-age children and teens sleep for about 10 to 12 hours; adults sleep for 7 to 9 hours; and elderly people sleep for about 6 hours per night with additional napping during the day.

Sleep is needed for body restoration and repair,and the subjective sense of being well rested is ventral to a person's perception of well-being. Sleep disorders put an individual at risk for experiencing a change in the quantity or quality of rest and sleep as related to biologic and emotional needs. Adverse physical, mental, and emotional changes may occur if normal rest and sleep patterns are interrupted. Most people have suffered from at least transient sleep disturbances. Many factors lead to poor sleep, such as the environment of the sleeping area (levels of sound, light, and temperature), the age and general physical and psychological condition of the client, and recent stressful events.

BOX 14-1 Learning More

The Major States of Normal Sleep

Normal sleep consists of two major states: REM sleep and NREM sleep. REM sleep is also sometimes called dreaming sleep (because it is associated with dreaming). NREM sleep conforms to traditional concepts of sleep as a time of decreased physiologic and psychological activity and is further divided into four sleep stages on the basis of scored EEG patterns.

Stage I NREM: It is a transition from wakefulness to sleep. About 5 percent of sleep time is spent in adults in the phase. Person feels every drowsy and musculature relaxe.

第二节　睡眠障碍

人的一生约有三分之一的时间在睡眠中度过。睡眠是一种周期性的现象，对维持人们的身体健康和维持精神活动的进行有重要作用。睡眠并不是人体的静止状态，而是一个贯穿着行为、心理及生理活动的复杂变化过程。随着年龄的增长，人的睡眠需要逐渐减少。新生儿每天需睡 18 小时或更多，学龄儿童和青少年一般需 10～12 小时，成人为 7～9 小时，老年人如在白天小睡只需 6 小时。

良好充分的睡眠，可以使人精力充沛并产生心理上的满足感。如果存在睡眠障碍就会导致睡眠的质和量的不足，从而使个体感到倦怠、不适，出现一系列的躯体、心理症状。造成睡眠障碍的因素很多，一般包括生理、心理、社会、环境等多种因素。

BOX 14-1　知识拓展

正常睡眠的时相

正常睡眠分为快速眼球运动睡眠（REM）和非快速眼球运动睡眠（NREM）两种时相。REM 也称为造梦睡眠。NREM 是指传统概念中的睡眠，即生理和心理活动减少的状态，根据脑电图的变化又将其细分为 4 个期：

第Ⅰ期　是从清醒到入睡的过渡阶段，约占成人睡眠时间的 5%，机体反应为感觉昏沉、肌肉松弛，对外界仍有反应。

Stage II NREM: These stages occupies about 50 percent of sleep time;muscles relax further; cerebral activity decreases.

Stage III NREM: This stage occupies about 10% to 23% of sleep. Physiologic changes are evident; vital signs decrease.

Stage IV NREM: Deepest level of sleep with lowest level of body function.

During an eight-hour sleep period, the cycle of NREM and REM sleep repeats itself five or six times. REM sleep occurs cyclically throughout the night, alternating with NREM sleep about every 80 to 100 minutes, lasts about 5 to 30 minutes, and is associated with dreaming that is remembered. REM sleep increases in duration toward the morning. This cycle changes as the sleeping progresses. In the first cycle, the amount of REM sleep is brief. With each succeeding cycle, the amount of time spent in REM sleep lengthens until it seems to dominate at the end of the sleep period.

第Ⅱ期　约占睡眠时间的50%；肌肉进一步松弛，大脑活动减少。

第Ⅲ期　约占睡眠时间的10%～23%。生理变化比较明显，生命体征下降。

第Ⅳ期　此期睡眠最深；机体功能也降到最低。在整个睡眠过程中，REM和NREM相互交替出现5～6次，REM每次持续5～30分钟，NREM每次持续80～100分钟。随着睡眠时间的发展，NREM越来越短，REM越来越长，在快醒时成为主要时相。

Sleep disorders are classified by the Association of Sleep Disorders Centers (ASDC) into four major groups with considerable overlap:

1. Disorders of initiating or maintaining sleep, also known as insomnia. Anxiety and depression are major causes of insomnia.

2. Disorders that manifests as excessive amounts of sleep and excessive daytime sleepiness, also known as hypersomnia. This category includes narcolepsy, sleep apnea, and nocturnal movement disorders.

3. Disorders of the sleep-wake schedule, characterized by normal sleep but at the wrong time. Sleep-wake schedule disturbances occur when there is a disruption in an individual's regular pattern of fluctuation in physiology that is linked to the 24-hour light-dark cycle. This commonly occurs in individuals whose jobs require rotating shifts and in those who frequently travel long distances over a short period of time.

4. Disorders associated with sleep stages, also known as parasomnia. This category includes conditions such as sleepwalking, night terrors, nightmares, restless legs syndrome, and enuresis. These sleep problems are often experienced by children and can have a significant effect on functioning and well-being. These disorders primarily begin in childhood but can also affect adults.

按照美国睡眠障碍协会的标准，睡眠障碍可分为以下四大类：

1. 入睡和维持睡眠障碍，即失眠症，主要由焦虑和抑郁引起。

2. 睡眠过多，或日间睡眠过多，即嗜睡症，包括睡眠发作、睡眠呼吸暂停等。

3. 睡眠的昼夜节律障碍，通常发生于长期值夜班和长途旅行造成的时差等情况。

4. 异常睡眠，包括梦游、梦魇、不宁腿综合征、遗尿等。它主要见于儿童，也可见于成人，对身体健康有重要影响。

I. Primary Insomnia

Insomnia refers to difficulty in falling asleep, trouble with maintaining sleep. It is the most prevalent sleep

一、失眠症

失眠症是指入睡困难和睡眠维持困难，是最常见的睡眠障碍。它既是单独的疾病，

disorder.The word insomnia is used in two different circumstances:as a symptom and a disorder.Insomnia as a symptom can lead to the diagnosis of another disorder (depression, breathing-related sleep disorders). The term primary insomnia is given to the condition in which there is no known external cause of the inability to sleep. Insomnia is the most commonly disease among all sleep disorders.

也是其他疾病的临床表现之一。原发性失眠症是指没有明显的外在因素所导致的失眠。在所有睡眠障碍中，失眠症最为常见。

i. Etiology

There are many causes resulting insomnia. Insomnia may be related to heredity, circumstance, physical factor and personality.But the most common cause is mental disorder such as anxiety, tension and fear. Insomnia could be situational, continuous or recurrent, and it can also be intermittent. Situational insomnia is usually related to life events or the rapid change of sleep time or environment. Generally, situational insomnia lasts for several days or several weeks. Insomnia disappears when the emergency does not exist anymore. Recurrent insomnia usually is related to stressful events. One third of the adults in DSM-V report have suffered insomnia, and 10%-25% individuals have reflected relevant functional lesion in daytime, while 6%-10% individuals conform to the diagnosis standard of insomnia.

（一）病因

引起失眠的原因很多，可能与躯体因素、环境因素、人格特征、遗传因素等有关。但最常见的原因是精神紧张、焦虑恐惧等所致。失眠可以是情境性的、持续的或反复发作的，也可能是间歇性的。情境性失眠通常与生活事件或快速改变的睡眠时间或环境有关，一般只持续数天或数周。当初始的突发事件消失后，失眠也会消失。间歇性的反复发作通常与应激性事件的出现有关。DSM-V 报告约三分之一的成年人有失眠的症状，其中 10%～25% 的个体表现出相关的日间功能损害，而 6%～10% 的个体符合失眠症的诊断标准。

ii. Symptoms and Signs

On occasion, almost everyone experiences difficulties getting to sleep or staying asleep. Even a few days of insomnia while acutely unpleasant, are far from abnormal. Insomnia is considered a psychological problem if it lasts sufficiently long to impair functioning. In many individuals, insomnia does lead to anxiety, arousal, and preoccupation with the process of falling to sleep. The disorder might have taken a long time to conquer, if it had been faintly experimented on in bed. Worrying about sleeplessness while in bed can prolong an episode of insomnia. Some individuals fall asleep easily and remain asleep through the night but do not feel in the morning as if they have had a restful or restorative night of sleep. Clients with primary insomnia report daytime fatigue, difficulty with concentration,and poor mood but do not demonstrate signs of sleepiness. The type of insomnia changes with age, while many young people found it is very difficult to fall asleep, while middle aged people and the old-aged often are difficult to keep sleeping.

（二）临床表现

几乎所有的人都有过难以入睡或睡眠不深的经历，但这只是一过性的，属于正常现象，如果这种情况持续时间较长，并影响了躯体功能，就应考虑为失眠症。失眠症患者最常见的主述是难以入睡，其次是维持睡眠困难和早醒。患者在就寝时感到紧张、焦虑而无法入睡。原发性失眠的患者醒后常感到心身憔悴，白天感到疲乏、注意力不集中、情绪不佳，但又没有睡意。失眠的类型随着年龄而改变，在青年人中入睡困难较常见，而在中老年个体更经常出现维持睡眠的问题。

Requirements for sleep vary widely. Most adults' need the traditional 7 to 9 hours of sleep a night, but some adults are "short sleepers" and function well on only 3 or 4 hours. Persons who function well despite little sleep are not diagnosed with primary insomnia. Primary insomnia is usually diagnosed on the basis of an individual's

睡眠时间和深度有很大的个体差异，大部分成人需 7～9 小时，有的人长期睡眠时间为 3～4 小时，但自感精力充沛无任何痛苦感。部分人虽然睡眠时间没有变化，但睡眠质量差。人对自身睡眠的主观评定很不可靠，因

subjective complaint, but quality and quantity of sleep are difficult to judge objectively outside the sleep laboratory. Many people overestimate the amount they actually get during a restless night. So correct diagnosis should be based on subjective and objective assessment.

此，要得出较为准确的诊断，最好结合失眠的主观标准与客观标准。

iii. Treatment

Interventions usually involve a combination of approaches. Short-term use of hypnotics may provide immediate relief, but long-term use is detrimental. Interventions focus on teaching clients to develop and maintain good sleep habits. Behavioral interventions described below include stimulus control; sleep restriction,and relaxation therapy.

（三）治疗

失眠的治疗主要采用综合疗法。短期使用安眠药物，可迅速缓解失眠症状，但是长期使用会对身体造成损害。治疗的重点是帮助患者形成和保持良好的睡眠习惯。行为治疗包括刺激控制训练，睡眠限制疗法和放松疗法。

1. Pharmacotherapy Pharmacotherapy of insomnia generally includes hypnotics and sedatives used for short periods of time. The most widely used sedative-hypnotics are benzodiazepines. They usually have characteristic effects on sleep that include shortening of sleep latency, improvement of sleep continuity, elevation of stage Ⅱ sleep (with increase spindles), decreased slow-wave sleep, and decreased REM sleep. Long-term administration can lead to tolerance and need larger doses. Recreational use of benzodiazepines is rare. Abuse is more often associated with simultaneous use, for example, with alcohol and stimulants. Short-term use of benzodiazepines to treat insomnia and long-term use to treat anxiety disorders are usually not associated with serious clinical problems.

1. 药物治疗 失眠的药物治疗包括短期使用催眠药和镇静剂。药物作为辅助治疗可短期使用，应避免长期用药，尤其慢性失眠患者，长期用药往往无效，并可导致药物依赖。常用催眠药物主要为苯二氮䓬类，该类药物可缩短入睡潜伏期，减少夜间醒转次数，使 REM 时间缩短但次数增加。其缺点是易形成药物依赖。

2. Cognitive and Behavioral Therapy

(1)Stimulus control: Stimulus control is a technique that is used when the bedroom environment no longer provides cues for sleep but has become the cue for wakefulness. Clients are instructed to avoid behaviors incompatible with sleep-watching television, performing homework, or eating in the bedroom, which allows the bedroom to be reestablished as a stimulus for sleep.

(2)Sleep restriction: Insomniac clients often increase their time in bed to prove more opportunity for sleep. This results in fragmented sleep. Irregular sleep schedules result in poor sleep efficiency. Clients are proposed to spend less time in bed and avoid napping. Clients are asked to estimate how many minutes of sleep they actually obtain and then are instructed to spend only that amount of time in bed. A client who reports spending 10 hours in bed but estimates getting only 5 hours of sleep is then prescribed 5 hours in bed. The minimal amount of time restricted is 4.5 hours. Rising time is kept constant; bedtime is manipulated to meet the restriction. When sleep efficiency reaches 85% to 90% over the past 5 to 7 days, the bedtime

2. 认知行为治疗

（1）刺激控制训练：属于行为疗法的一种，主要是帮助失眠者减少与睡眠无关的行为和建立规律性睡眠－觉醒模式的手段。把卧室当作睡眠的专用场所，不在卧室从事与睡眠无关的活动，如看电视、做作业和吃饭等。

（2）睡眠限制疗法：主要目的是指导失眠者减少在床上的非睡眠时间。失眠症患者为了增加睡眠机会和时间，会在睡不着的时候也躺在床上，结果睡眠断续不完整，而不规律的睡眠节律会导致睡眠效率差。指导患者首先估计他每天的实际有效睡眠时间，然后按照估计的时间进行睡眠指导。例如患者每晚卧床 10 个小时里只睡着 5 小时，则睡眠效率为 50%，那么规定患者每天只能卧床 5 小时（最少 4.5 小时）。当本周睡眠效率达到 85%～90% 时，下周可提早 15 分钟卧床。根据患者

is advanced 15 minutes earlier. As sleep becomes more consolidated, the client is allowed to gradually increase time in bed.

(3)Relaxation training: Relaxation training is used when clients complain of difficulty in relaxing, especially if they are physically tense or emotionally distressed. A variety of procedures to reduce somatic arousal can be used (e.g., progressive muscle relaxation, autogenic training, and biofeedback). The application of these techniques can play an important role in the management of difficulties in falling asleep.

睡眠改善的情况，逐渐延长睡眠时间。

（3）放松疗法：当患者在躯体紧张或精神上有压力难以放松下来时可以采用放松训练，如渐进式肌肉放松法、自控放松、生物反馈法等。通过训练使患者学会有意识地控制自身的心理生理活动，降低唤醒水平，以改善机体功能紊乱。

II. Primary Hypersomnia

The essential characteristic of primary hypersomnia is excessive sleepiness for at least 1 month demonstrated by either daytime sleep episodes or sleeping extended periods at night. Sleepiness occurs almost on a daily basis. This diagnosis is reserved for individuals who have had no other causes of daytime sleepiness. The exact cause of the primary hypersomnia isn't known. DSM-V report is used on the out-patient department of sleep disorders in America, and about 5%-10% people are diagnosed with lethargy and the prevalence rate of man and woman are nearly the same.

i. Symptoms and Signs

People with primary hypersomnia typically sleep 8 to 12 hours one night. They fall asleep easily and sleep through the night, but often have problems awakening in the morning. Sometimes they are confused or even combative on awakening. This difficulty in making the transition from sleep to wakefulness is sometimes referred to as "sleep drunkenness". They often have difficulty in meeting morning students have trouble with attending morning classes or working people are continually late for work. They also exhibit excessive daytime sleepiness usually demonstrated by taking unintentional or intentional naps, which may last an hour or more, but usually they do not feel refreshed after awakening. People typically report feeling embarrassed by nodding off at work and may even describe dangerous situations that resulted from their falling asleep, such as being sleepy while driving or operating heavy machinery. Poor concentration and memory are reported as well.

ii. Treatment

Stimulant medications often do not provide relief. In some cases, however, methysergide has been clinically useful.The difficulty in prescribing appropriate treatment comes from the lack of clear etiology for this disorder.

二、嗜睡症

嗜睡症是指在不存在睡眠量不足的情况下至少 1 个月几乎每天发生白天睡眠发作或夜间睡眠时间过多，目前病因不明。DSM-V 报告美国就诊于睡眠障碍门诊并有日间困倦主诉的个体中，约 5%～10% 被诊断为嗜睡症，男女患病率相当。

（一）临床表现

本病表现为白昼睡眠时间延长，夜间通常每晚要睡 8～12 小时，容易入睡，睡一整晚后醒转时要想达到完全的觉醒状态却非常困难，常常导致上课或工作迟到，醒转后常有短暂意识模糊，呼吸及心率增快，常可伴有抑郁情绪。部分患者可有白天睡眠发作，发作前多有难以控制的困倦感，如患者可在工作时打盹，甚至在操作重型机械等危险状况下睡着，常影响工作、学习和生活，患者常为此感到苦恼。

（二）治疗

嗜睡症主要是对症治疗，首先消除发病的诱导因素，可适当给予中枢神经兴奋剂。辅以支持疗法和疏导疗法，以达到治疗和预防疾病的目的。

III. Circadian Rhythm Sleep Disorder

The prime feature of a circadian rhythm sleep disorder is the mismatch between the individual's internal sleep-wake circadian rhythm and the desired sleep-wake rhythm for the environment. People with these disorders complain of insomnia at night and excessive sleepiness during day. This diagnosis is reserved for those individuals who present with marked sleep disturbance or significant social or occupational impairment. Circadian rhythm disorders are caused by the dissociation of the internal circadian pacemaker and conventional time. The cause might be intrinsic such as delayed sleep phase or extrinsic as in jet lag and shift work. Each results in overflowing wakefulness at night. There are no data about the prevalence of circadian rhythm disorders in the general population.

i. Symptoms and Signs

The *DSM- V* identifies a broad group of subtypes including delayed sleep phase type, jet lag type, shift work type, and unspecified type.

1. Delayed Sleep Phase Type Individuals with delayed sleep phase type tend to be unable to fall asleep before 2 to 6 a. m; hence, their whole sleep pattern shifts and they have difficulty in awakening in the morning. They are often referred to as "night owls". These people are "locked in"to late sleep hours and cannot adjust their sleep time to an earlier time. When left to their own schedule on the weekends or vacation, they usually go to bed late, and if they are not sleep deprived, will sleep about 8 hours and awaken spontaneously and feel refreshed. They often devise elaborate strategies to get up in the morning for work-setting multiple alarm clocks around the bedroom, enlisting others to awaken them by person or telephone.

2. Jet Lag Type Most people have experienced jet lag when they must travel across time zones, particularly in coast-to-coast and international travel. This type of circadian disorder occurs when the person's normal endogenous circadian sleep-wake cycle does not match the desired hours of sleep and wakefulness in a new time zone. Chief symptoms include headache, fatigue, and indigestion; severity is proportional to the number of time zones traveled. Individuals traveling eastward are more prone toward jet lag because this involves resetting one's circadian clock to an earlier time. It is easier to delay the endogenous clock to a later time period than an earlier one.

3. Shift Work Type In this type of disorder,the endogenous sleep-wake cycle is normal, but mismatched to the imposed hours of sleep and wakefulness required by

三、睡眠的昼夜节律障碍

昼夜节律障碍是指个体的昼夜节律与通常的昼夜节律之间不同步，导致患者失眠或嗜睡而影响了生活或工作的一种睡眠障碍。引起这一障碍的原因很多，如心理社会、外界环境、某些药物等都可能造成个体的昼夜节律与特定社会中的正常情况及同一文化环境中为大多数人所认可的昼夜节律不同步。目前还缺乏对该病的流行病学资料。

（一）临床表现

DSM-V 将该病分为睡眠时相延迟型、时差紊乱型、轮班紊乱型和其他型。

1. **睡眠时相延迟型** 睡眠时相延迟的人在凌晨 2～6 点以前很难入睡，在早晨该醒时又很难清醒，其整个睡眠时相均比常人晚，即俗话所说的“夜猫子”。他们很难将自己的睡眠时相调整到正常，只能依靠闹铃或他人将自己唤醒，因此长期处于睡眠不足状态，而影响了社会职业功能。

2. **时差紊乱型** 由于长途旅行（尤其是国际旅行必须跨越时区）所导致的时差与个体固有的生物钟不协调，个体会产生不适感，包括疲倦、头痛、消化不良等，症状的严重程度与时差的长短成正比，对相同的时间差来说，时差提前（向东旅行）比延后严重。

3. **轮班紊乱型** 轮班紊乱型的睡眠－觉醒周期正常，只是因为长期倒班，使睡醒时间变化不定而导致的睡眠不足或睡眠质量差，

shift work. Rotating shift schedules are disruptive because any consistent adjustment is prevented. Compared with day-and evening-shift workers, night and rotating-shift workers have a shorter sleep duration and poorer quality of sleep. They may also be sleepier while performing their jobs.This disorder is further exacerbated by insufficient daytime sleep attribute to social and family demands and environmental disturbances (traffic noise, telephone).

并引起头晕、乏力等不适，使工作、生活能力受到影响。

ii. Treatment

First, an attempt should be made to synchronize sleep and wakefulness to the underlying phase position of the circadian clock. Light therapy is used to treat delayed sleep phase and shift work. Bright light, a powerful zeitgeber, manipulates the circadian system. Light is measured in lux units of illumination. Indoor light is about 150 lux. Therapeutic light has a potency of 2 500 to 10 000 lux and is produced by commercially prepared light boxed (Gulebas, 1996). The client sits at a distance of 3 feet from the box for a prescribed amount of time at specific times. Headache, dizziness, and hyperactivity are evidence of treatment overdose. Light therapy may be useful in the management of shift work schedules and jet lag syndrome.

（二）治疗

睡眠昼夜节律障碍的治疗首先应针对病因，消除或减轻各种致病因素，使睡眠和觉醒时间与个体的生物钟同步。光照疗法对该病尤其是时差紊乱型和轮班紊乱型有一定疗效，其照明强度是普通灯光的17～67倍，方法为患者在特定时段内，坐在0.9 m远的地方接受一定时间的照射。如果光照时间过长或强度过大，会引起头痛、眩晕、兴奋等副作用。

Recently, melatonin has been promoted as a natural product that resets the circadian clock. When correctly timed, melatonin induces both phase advances and delays in the circadian rhythm system. If incorrectly timed, melatonin has the potential to induce adverse effects. There are no long-term safety data. The optimal dosage and formulation have not been established. To date, little research validates the use of this hormone in manipulating biologic rhythms. Further, production of melatonin supplied to health food stores undergoes no quality controls (Culebas, 1996). Treatment with both bright light and melatonin would need to be carefully timed, because the sensitivity of the biological clock undergoes a circadian variation.

近年来，褪黑素也常用来治疗该病，它既可以将人体生物钟提前亦可以将其推迟，但应用不当也会发生副作用。目前，其最佳剂量和最佳用法还没有定论。不管是光疗还是褪黑素，都需谨慎应用，以免加重机体生物钟的紊乱。

IV. Sleepwalking Disorder

四、睡行症

Sleepwalking, also called somnambulism. Sleepwalking is common in children and peaks around age 11 to 12 years. There appears to be some genetic predisposition as those with relatives who sleepwalk are more likely to sleepwalk. Studies have shown that incidence of sleepwalking and related parasomnias (sleep terrors) increases when parents are affected.Internal stimuli (a full bladder) or external stimuli (noise) can precipitate an episode. Sleep deprivation, fever,and stress may increase the likelihood of an episode.

睡行症过去习惯称为梦游症，多发生于生长发育期的儿童，以11～12岁年龄段为最多。家系调查表明睡行症的患者中，其家族有阳性史的较多，说明该症与遗传因素有一定的关系。内部刺激如膀胱充盈和外部刺激如噪音等可以诱发睡行的发生，另外睡眠不足、发烧、精神压力等也与睡行症的发作有一定的关系。

i. Symptoms and Signs

Sleepwalking involves a pattern of behavior usually including getting out to bed, walking around in the bedroom or on occasion outside of the bedroom, and then returning to bed. While sleepwalking, people typically have a blank stare, are difficult to awaken. Some persons may be able to carry on rudimentary conversations during a sleepwalking episode. Sometimes sleepwalking behaviors are bizarre and stereotyped, occasionally including behavior such as urinating in unusual places. Like persons with sleep terrors, sleepwalkers are difficult to arouse during an episode and if awakened are often confused and without any specific recall of the events that led to their behaviors. In the morning, they have little or no recall of what has happened to them.If awakened during the episode, there is a brief period of confusion, followed by a full recovery. Frequently, a sleepwalker awakens in the morning to find himself sleeping in an entirely different bed or room than where he fell asleep the previous night. Episodes usually happen during the first third of the night.

（一）临床表现

主要表现为患者在睡眠中突然起身下床徘徊数分钟至半小时，或走出家门、进食、穿衣等，有的口中还念念有词，但口齿不清，常答非所问，无法交谈。有时睡行行为是怪异或刻板的，如在很奇怪的地方小便等。睡行时患者表情茫然、双目凝视，难以唤醒，一般历时数分钟或数十分钟，然后自行上床或随地躺下入睡，次日醒后对所有经过不能回忆，若在睡行期内强行加以唤醒，患者可有短暂的意识模糊。睡行症常发生在睡眠的前1/3期，次日醒来对发生经过不能回忆。

ii. Treatment

Treatment of Sleepwalking may include reducing the problem behavior itself or treating the cause (e.g., modification of psychosocial stressors or psychotherapy for nightmare disorders). Safety (to the client and others) is crucial in the treatment of sleepwalking. For example, clients and families should be counseled to remove or modify environmental dangers by padding sharp pieces of furniture, putting safety gates at the top of stairs,and so on. Sleepwalking have been treated, with variable success, with benzodiazepines or low-dose tricyclic antidepressants (which suppress slow-wave sleep to some extent).

（二）治疗

对睡行症的治疗包括减少发作次数，防止发作时意外事故的发生两方面。消除或减轻发病的诱发因素如减少心理压力，日常生活规律，避免过度疲劳和高度紧张，养成良好的睡眠习惯，以及某些药物如苯二氮䓬类、小剂量的三环抗抑郁剂等对减少睡行症的发作有一定疗效。另外，还要保证其睡眠环境的安全性，如睡前关好门窗、收好各种危险物品、清除障碍物等，以防睡行发作时外出走失或引起伤害自己及他人的事件。

Section 3 Application of the Nursing Process

第三节 护理程序的应用

I. Eating Disorders

一、进食障碍

i. Assessment

1. Biologic Assessment Physical examination shall be carried out carefully; more attention shall be paid to vital signs, weight, and the its proportion with height and age, skin and condition of cardiovascular system, especially the change of client's weight and idea weight in

（一）护理评估

1. **生理功能评估** 体格检查需详细进行，注意生命体征、体重与身高年龄比例、皮肤、心血管系统情况，尤其要重点评估患者的体重变化情况及患者认为的理想体重是多少。

the eyes of the client.

2. Psychological Assessment Clients with eating disorder usually have wrong recognition and behaviors about eating. Therefore, attention should be paid to its assessment:

(1) The client's eating habit and structure, including variety, quantity, preference and recognition about food;

(2) Diet, including the beginning date of the diet;

(3) The usage of emetic, cathartic drug, and other emetic methods;

(4) The client's opinion about his or her own figure, and image;

(5) The exercise and intensity of the exercise that the client is involved in order to lose weight;

(6) Mental situation and is there any intention to commit suicide or autolesion.

3. Social Assessment Usually, the clients with eating disorders are over-controlled or over-protected in the family, so their behaviors of eating disorders are used as a resistance against control. Therefore, it is necessary to evaluate the relation between the clients and their families, as well as their families' knowledge and attitude about the disease.

ii. Nursing Diagnosis

Nursing diagnoses related to eating disorders encompass biological, psychological, and sociocultural concerns; because of the complexity of these disorders, many NANDA nursing diagnoses may be appropriate. Among them there are four chief diagnoses:

1. Altered Nutrition: Less than body requirements Related to refusal to eat/drink; self-induced vomiting;abuse of laxatives/diuretics.

2. Altered Nutrition: More than body requirements Related to compulsive overeating.

3. Body Image Disturbance Related to dissatisfaction with appearance, distorted thoughts and inability to perceive body size and physical needs realistically, psychosocial factors, morbid fear of obesity, low self-esteem, feelings of helplessness and dysfunctional family system.

4. Ineffective Individual Coping Related to disturbance in impulse control.

iii. Nursing Objectives

The client(s):

1. Increase caloric and nutritional intake, and show gradual increases on a weekly basis. Gain no more than 1 to 2 pounds in the first week of refeeding, and no more than 3 to 5 pounds per week afterward. Will achieve and maintain at least 80%-85% of expected body weight. Vital signs, blood pressure, and laboratory serum studies are

2. 心理行为评估 进食障碍的患者往往在进食方面有不良的认知与行为方式，因此要重点评估：① 患者的饮食习惯和结构，包括种类、量、偏好及对食物的认识；② 节食情况，包括开始的时间等；③ 催吐剂、导泻剂及其他催吐方式的使用情况；④ 患者对自身身材和自我概念的看法；⑤ 患者为减轻体重所进行的活动种类和量；⑥ 情绪状况和有无自杀、自伤倾向。

3. 社会关系评估 进食障碍患者的家庭大多存在过度控制或过度保护，异常的进食行为是对控制的反抗。因此，要评估患者与家属的关系以及家属对疾病的知识和态度。

（二）护理诊断

1. 营养失调：低于机体需要量 与拒绝进食，自行诱吐，滥用泄剂、利尿剂有关。

2. 营养失调：高于机体需要量 与进食过多有关。

3. 自我形象紊乱 对自己的外表不满意；对自己的身材和实际的机体需要有错误的认识；心理因素；害怕长胖；低自尊；无助感和家庭功能障碍。

4. 个人应对无效 与冲动控制障碍有关。

（三）护理目标

患者能：

1. 在增加每周进食的基础上摄入热量和营养物质逐渐增加；体重在第一周增加 1～2 磅（0.453 6～0.907 2 kg），以后每周不超过 3～5 磅（1.360 8～2.268 0 kg）；能达到标准体重 80%～85%；生命体征、实验室检查结果在正

within normal limits.

2. Clients could express their anxiety and depression with language before they begin to eat too much food; other normal behaviors could be used to replace the behavior of eating too much food.

3. Describe a more realistic perception of body size and shape in line with height and body type.

4. Client will establish regular, nutritional eating habits. Demonstrate reduced number of behaviors that would sabotage treatment plan. Demonstrate more adaptive coping mechanisms. Verbalize ways in which he or she may gain more control of the environment and thereby reduce feelings of helplessness.

常范围内。

2. 患者能用语言表达暴食发作前的焦虑、抑郁情绪；能采用其他正常的方式替代暴食发作。

3. 患者对自己的体重和体形有更为现实的认识。

4. 患者能够建立健康的饮食习惯；配合治疗计划；显示适宜的应对机制；述说对环境的控制感增强，无助感减少。

iv. Nursing Interventions

（四）护理措施

1. Diet Nursing Care Diet nursing is the focus of nursing for patients with eating disorders. The goal is to maintain nutrition, restore and maintain a normal weight.

(1) Closely monitor and record vital signs, intake and output, electrocardiogram (ECG) and laboratory tests (electrolytes, acid-base balance, albumin, and others) until stable. Report abnormal values to primary clinician.

(2) Determine number of calories required to provide adequate nutrition and realistic weight gain. Obtain specific information from a client who purges, including method of self-induced vomiting, laxative,or diuretic use. Provide a pleasant, calm atmosphere at mealtime. Encourage him or her to select some foods. Set limits, however, on length of mealtimes (usually 30 min). Stay with client during meals and for at least 1 hour following meals to be sure food is actually eaten. Weigh client daily with same scale at same time. Set limits on dysfunctional behaviors such as strenuous exercise and use of bathroom after eating. Privileges are based on weight gain (or loss) when setting limits. When weight loss occurs, decrease privileges.

(3) When being severely malnourished and refusing nourishment, client may require tube feedings, either alone or in conjunction with oral or parenteral nutrition.

1. 饮食护理 饮食护理是进食障碍患者的护理重点，目的是保证营养，恢复并维持正常体重。

（1）密切观察和记录患者的生命体征、摄入和排出量、心电图、实验室检查结果（电解质、酸碱平衡、白蛋白等），直至平稳。如有异常，及时向其主管大夫汇报。

（2）评估患者达到标准体重和摄取合适的营养所需的热量，患者为了限制体重采取了何种措施，如自我诱吐、滥用泻药、利尿剂的情况。与营养师、患者一起制订饮食计划和体重增长计划，确定目标体重和每日应摄入的最低限度、热量以及进食时间。提供安静、舒适的进食环境，鼓励患者自行选择食物种类，但对进食时间加以限制，一般为30分钟；从患者进餐到餐后至少一小时都和患者在一起，以保证患者确实摄入食物；每天用同一个体重称，定时测量患者体重；限制患者过度运动和饭后使用盥洗室；当患者体重增加时，给予一定的奖励；体重减轻时，应限制其活动。

（3）如果患者严重缺乏营养又拒绝进食，在劝其进食的基础上可辅以胃管鼻饲或胃肠外营养的方式。

2. Psychological Interventions Demonstrate acceptance by use of support and concern to help the client feel lovable and accepted. Recognize the importance of developing a trusting relationship with client.

(1) Perception: Assess client's feelings and attitudes about being obese. Encourage client to express feelings,

2. 心理护理 护士首先要向患者表达关心和支持，与患者建立相互信任的关系，使患者感觉到爱心和有被接纳感。

（1）认知方面：评估患者对肥胖的感受和态度，鼓励患者表达对自己和对他人的看

especially about the way he or she thinks about or views himself or herself. Listen for signs of perfectionist thinking and explore ways to challenge unrealistic expectations. It is very important to know the clients' idea about which parts they like about their body and which they dislike, as well as their opinions when they are not in good shape. Help client to develop a realistic perception of body image and relationship with food.

(2) Behavior: Give the client factual feedback about the client's low weight and resultant impaired health, however, do not argue or challenge the client's distorted perceptions. Encourage discussion of positive personal traits, especially regarding client's body image. Encourage client to dress attractively and to use makeup and jewelry, as appropriate. Help client focus on short-term goals that he or she can achieve. Identify one area over which the client has some control. Reinforce coping abilities. Encourage client to make small decisions. This tends to empower the client and assists in imparting a sense of control and accomplishment. Educate family regarding the client's illness and encourage attendance at family and group therapy sessions.

3. Safety Interventions Assess client for depression,suicidal risk,and substance abuse, and intervene as appropriate.

Table 14-2 lists nursing interventions for anorexia nervosa.

法，特别是他人对自己的看法；了解患者对自己的身材哪些地方喜欢，哪些地方不喜欢，当身材有变化的时候患者是怎么想的；帮助患者形成更为现实的体像感受以及认识身材与食物之间的关系；了解亲属或朋友对患者的看法和态度对患者产生了哪些影响。然后，将患者实际的身体尺寸与其主观感受做对比，帮助患者认识到自我认知的偏差，主观判断是错误的。

（2）行为鼓励：向患者讲明过低的体重对健康的危害性，不对患者的错误认识进行指责；鼓励患者讨论自己的优点，尤其是身体形象方面的优点并鼓励患者进行适当的修饰和打扮；鼓励患者制订易达到的短期目标，做一些小决策，以帮助患者获得成就感和控制感；对患者家庭进行宣教，帮助他们关注患者的病情，并鼓励其参与家庭治疗和集体治疗。

3. 安全护理 评估患者的情绪反应，如有无抑郁，有无自杀的危险和滥用药物的情况并采取适当的措施。

表 14-2 列举了神经性厌食症的护理干预。

Table 14-2 Interventions for anorexia nervosa

Intervention	Rationale
1. Acknowledge the emotional and physical difficulty the client is experiencing	A first priority is to establish a therapeutic alliance
2. Assess for suicidal thoughts/self-injurious behaviors	The potential for a psychiatric crisis is always present
3. Monitor physiological parameters(vital signs,electrolyte levels)as needed	The life-threatening effect of weight restriction and/or purging needs to be monitored
4. Weigh client wearing only bra and panties/underwear only on a routine basis(same time of day after voiding and before drinking/eating). Some protocol includes weighting with the client's back to the scale	Weights are a high-anxiety time. The underweight client might try to manipulate the weight by drinking fluids or placing heavy objects in clothing before being weighted
5. Monitor client during and after meals to prevent throwing away food and/or purging	The compelling force of the illness makes it difficult to stop certain behaviors
6. Recognize the client's distorted Image/overvalued ideas of body shape and size without minimizing or challenging patient's perceptions	A straightforward statement that the nurse's perceptions are different will help to avoid a power struggle. Arguments and power struggles intensify the client's need to control
7. Educate the patient about the ill effects of low weight and resultant impaired health	The treatment goal of gaining weight is what the client most resistsFocus on the benefits of improved health and increased energy at a more normalized weight
8. Work with client to identify strengths	When clients are feeling overwhelmedthey no longer view their lives objectively

表 14-2　神经性厌食症的护理干预

措施	依据
1. 认同患者在情绪和身体上的体验	首先要建立一个治疗联盟
2. 评估自杀意念 / 自我伤害行为	精神科危机时刻可能存在
3. 监控必需的生理参数（生命体征，电解质水平等）	过度限制饮食对生命的威胁和 / 或清除行为需要时刻监控
4. 每天常规同一时间（排尿后，进餐前）给患者称重，称重时只能穿内衣裤	患者在称重时过度焦虑，低体重患者可能会试图在称重前大量饮液体或在衣服里放置重物来增加体重
5. 进餐期间和进餐后都要监控患者，以免患者把食物偷偷扔掉或吐出	这种疾病的强制力使患者很难阻止某些行为
6. 在不挑战患者的看法的情况下纠正患者的体象障碍	明确表明护士的看法是不一样的，将有助于减少冲突
7. 指导患者认识到低体重与它的不良后果对健康的威胁	增加体重的治疗目标是患者最抗拒的，护士可让患者关注改善健康状况对个体的益处，以及恢复正常体重让个体更有活力
8. 与患者一起找出她的优点	当患者不堪重负时不能客观地看待自己

v. Evaluation

1. Have normal eating patterns been restored?

2. Have the biological and psychological sequelae of malnutrition been corrected?

3. Has the client been able to develop a more realistic perception of body image?

4. Has the client developed adaptive coping strategies to deal with stress without resorting to maladaptive eating behaviors?

（五）护理评价

1. 患者正常的饮食形态是否恢复？

2. 重度营养不良造成的生理、心理损害是否已恢复？

3. 患者是否能客观地评价自己的形象？对体形建立更为客观的概念？

4. 患者是否学会使用正确的应对策略来应对压力而不是采取不当的进食行为？

II. Sleep Disorders

i. Assessment

1. Biologic Assessment The assessment of clients with sleep problems is multifaceted, involving a detailed history and medical and psychiatric examinations, extensive questionnaires, the use of sleep diaries or logs, and often psychological testing such as Pittsburgh sleep quality index scale (PSQI). It is not enough to ask, “Did you sleep well last night?” A nurse must inquire if the client has/had difficulty in falling asleep,experiences early awakening without the ability to return to sleep, and feels well rested in the morning. Further,the nurse should ask if the client feels fatigued and sleepy during the day.

2. Psychological Assessment It is necessary to evaluate the factors that induce or worsen sleep disorders in clients, and whether the clients has bad habits such as drinking strong tea, coffee, etc. A nurse should assess the clients' perception of sleep, such as whether the clients have too high expectation on sleep time and quality. And

二、睡眠障碍

（一）护理评估

1. 生理功能评估　了解患者的睡眠异常表现，有无早醒、入睡困难、睡眠维持困难、睡眠深度及使用药物的情况。必要时可用匹兹堡睡眠质量指数量表（PSQI）评定患者最近1个月的睡眠质量。

2. 心理行为评估　了解患者诱发或加重睡眠障碍的原因，有无不良的生活习惯如经常饮酒、饮浓茶、饮咖啡等习惯。评估患者对睡眠的认知，对睡眠时间与质量是否有过高的期望等。评估患者有无焦虑、恐惧、抑

the clients were assessed for anxiety, fear, depression and other psychiatric symptoms.

3. Social Assessment It is necessary to evaluate the relation between the clients and their families, as well as their families' knowledge and attitude about the disease.

ii. Nursing Diagnosis

Because of the complexity of sleep disorders, many NANDA nursing diagnoses may be applied. Chief among them are as follows:

1. Sleep Pattern Disturbance Related to sleeping in unfamiliar environment.

2. Impaired Rest-activity Pattern Related to hyperactivity, hallucinations, and other psychotic symptoms.

Other nursing diagnoses include anxiety, fear, hopelessness and ineffective individual coping.

iii. Nursing Objectives

1. The client sleeps at least 4 hours every night. The client will experience restful sleep and feel rested on awakening by two weeks.

2. The client remains awake during the day.

3. The client will understand the disorder and establish means of coping with it within his family.

iii. Nursing Interventions

1. Biologic Interventions Provide good circulation of air with comfortable room temperature and decrease background noise. Provide a calming environment.Limit coffee and other caffeine-containing foods and drinks such as tea, cola, or chocolate, especially after 4:00 p.m. Encourage the client to use decaffeinated products. Discourage daytime naps. During the day, encourage client to remain active. Provide structured activities during the day if needed. Take physical exercise, such as client's daily walks, in the early evening. Avoid reinforcing behaviors that encourage being awake at night such as not allowing eating, television, or socializing. Position clients comfortably; assist in turning and using bathroom as needed. Use hypnotics or sedatives only as a last resort. Do not use more than few days because sleep patterns can be further disturbed by frequent or chronic use of sleep medication.

2. Psychological Interventions Help to establish a sense of security, familiarize client with environment; walk around unit, and describe building. Assess the client's sleep for quantify and quality.Ask about client's normal sleep habits. Determine what is promoting or inhibiting client's sleep in the new environment. Establish a sleep routine for the client using familiar sleep habits if possible, such as special activities in preparation

郁等精神症状。

3. 社会关系评估 评估患者与家属的关系以及家属对疾病的知识和态度。

（二）护理诊断

由于睡眠障碍的复杂性特点，可能应用很多 NANDA 护理诊断。其中主要的有：

1. 睡眠形态紊乱 与陌生的睡眠环境、精神刺激有关。

2. 活动休息形态受损 与过度劳累、幻觉及其他精神征兆有关。

其他相关护理诊断包括焦虑、恐惧、绝望、个人应对无效。

（三）护理目标

1. 患者每晚睡眠至少达 4 小时以上；患者两周后恢复正常睡眠，感觉精力充沛。

2. 患者日间能保持清醒状态。

3. 患者能够理解这种失调的含义并且建立家庭应对方式。

（四）护理措施

1. 生理方面 保持病房空气流通，温度适宜，噪音低；提供安静的睡眠环境；限制咖啡和其他含咖啡因的饮料和食物如茶、巧克力、可乐等的摄取，特别是在下午四点之后，鼓励患者摄取不含咖啡因的食物；限制患者午间小睡，鼓励患者多活动；鼓励患者日间参加身体锻炼，如晚饭后散步；避免睡前易兴奋的活动，如看刺激紧张的电视节目、长久谈话、进食等；帮助患者采取舒适的卧位，必要时帮助患者翻身和洗漱；遵医嘱短期使用镇静催眠药，但不要长时间的使用，因为睡眠模式会因为使用这些药物而受到影响。

2. 心理护理 带领患者参观病房，向其介绍环境、设施，以增加患者对环境的熟悉度和安全感；评估患者睡眠的质和量，询问既往睡眠习惯，确定新环境中影响睡眠的因素并试图减轻或消除这些因素；用熟悉的物品或习惯帮助患者入睡，如听音乐、用固定的褥子等；如果一段时间后，患者睡眠仍未

for sleep, fixing the bedding, or playing music. If sleep-rest pattern continues to be disturbed after a reasonable amount of time for adjustment, reassess for other possible problems,such as depression or anxiety.

改善，应考虑是否有其他可能问题存在，如焦虑、抑郁等。

3. Safety Interventions To help the clients and their families to know more knowledge about sleeping, and help them to recognize sleep disorders, enhance safety consciousness, and prevention the occurrence of accident. For clients with sleep walking, it is very important to ensure their safety in sleeping environment in the night, for instance, close the window and door, prevent the client from walking outside in sleeping or getting lost; clean the obstacles in the environment, and prevent the client from stumble or hurt; put all kinds of dangerous things away, and prevent the client to hurt themselves or others. The clients with sleep walking shall avoid attending activity or work that might cause accident for falling asleep suddenly, such as driving or working high above the ground etc.

3. 安全护理 对患者和家属进行睡眠知识宣教，帮助他们认识睡眠障碍，增强安全意识，防范意外发生。对于睡行症患者，要保证夜间睡眠环境的安全，如给门窗加锁，防止患者梦游时外出、走失；清除环境中的障碍物，防止患者被绊倒、摔伤；收好各种危险物品，防止患者伤害自己和他人。嗜睡症患者要避免从事可能因突然进入睡眠而导致意外发生的活动和工作，如开车、高空作业等。

v. Evaluation

1. Do client report a satisfactory amount of sleep time and awaken feeling rested?

2. Dose the client report that there has been improvement in sleep?

(Zhao Wei)

（五）评价

1. 患者是否陈述睡眠充足，醒后无疲倦感？

2. 患者是否反映其睡眠有所改善？

（赵　伟）

Key Points

1. Adaptive eating regulation responses include balanced eating patterns, caloric intake, and body weight that are appropriate for height. Maladaptive responses include anorexia nervosa and bulimia nervosa.
2. Anorexia nervosa is characterized by an aversion to food and may result in death owing to serious malnutrition or other medical complications. The individual believes he or she is fat even when emaciated. The disorder is commonly accompanied by depression and anxiety.
3. Bulimia nervosa is an eating disorder characterized by the rapid consumption of huge amounts of food, and often in secret. Tension is relieved and pleasure is felt during the time of the"binge", which is soon followed by feelings of guilt and depression. Individuals with this disorder "purge" themselves of the excessive intake with self-induced vomiting or the misuse of laxatives, diuretics, or enemas. Serious medical consequences may occur because of alternating bingeing and purging. They are also subject to mood and anxiety disorders.
4. The expected outcome of nursing care for the client with eating disorders is that the client will restore healthy eating patterns and normalize physiological parameters related to body weight and nutrition.

内容摘要

1. 适宜的饮食形态表现为所摄取的食物种类均衡，热量适当，体重与身高成协调比例。不良的饮食形态包括神经性厌食症、贪食症。
2. 神经性厌食症的特征是患者厌恶进食，并由此发生重度营养不良和其他并发症而导致死亡。即使患者非常消瘦，仍认为自己太胖，常伴发抑郁和焦虑症状。
3. 神经性贪食症的临床特征是患者在短时间内摄入大量食物以缓解心理紧张，进食时常常避开他人，食后感到悔恨、担忧，为了抵消暴食引起的体重增加，患者常采用多种手段增加排泄、减少吸收，如食后催吐、使用泄剂、利尿剂或是灌肠剂等方法，常因此导致严重的躯体并发症，同时也会伴发情感障碍。
4. 对进食障碍患者的护理目标主要是帮助患者恢复正常饮食形态和身体健康状况。

5. Interventions include nutrition stabilization, exercise, cognitive behavioral interventions, family involvement, group therapy, and medications.

5. 进食障碍的治疗措施主要是保持营养摄入的稳定性，体育锻炼，并辅以认知行为治疗、小组治疗和家庭治疗。

6. Insomnia is a sleep disorder characterized by either difficulty in falling asleep or in staying asleep. It is the most prevalent sleep disorder and is often precipitated by feelings of stress or tension. The term "primary insomnia" is given to the condition in which there is no known external cause of the inability to sleep.

6. 失眠症是指入睡困难和睡眠维持困难，是最常见的睡眠障碍，常由精神紧张、压力引起。如果没有明显的发病原因，即称为原发性失眠症。

7. Assessment includes a thorough sleep history-current sleeping patterns, previous sleep patterns prior to sleep difficulties, medical problems, current medications,current life events, and emotional and mental status as well as assessment of the details of the sleep complaint including description,duration, and stability and intensity of the problem.

7. 对睡眠障碍患者的评估应包括完整详尽的睡眠史，包括既往和现存的睡眠形态、近期生活事件、目前的用药史、身体状况和情绪状况等。评估还应包括睡眠障碍的详细情况、持续时间、稳定性和严重程度等。

Exercises

思考题

(Questions 1 to 2 share the same question stem)

The nurse Morgan shall invite students of the eighth grade in a middle school to attend the lecture about nutrition and anorexia nervosa.

（1～2 题共用题干）

护士摩根应邀去一所中学为八年级学生做一场关于营养与神经性厌食症的讲座。

1. Which group of people shall Morgan list as main affected group of anorexia nervosa while making her lecture plan?

1. 摩根在制作讲座计划时，应把哪些人列为神经性厌食症的主要影响人群？

2. Which key words shall Morgan mention to describe the characteristics of anorexia nervosa?

2. 摩根可以列举出哪些关键词来为学生描述神经性厌食症的特点？

(Questions 3 to 4 share the same question stem)

The client June, who is 1.65 m in height, 37 kg in weight with anorexia nervosa was sent to the mental health center, and Alice received her, and knew it was the second time that June was hospitalized based on their conversation.

（3～4 题共用题干）

琼，身高 1.65 m、体重 37 kg，因神经性厌食症被送到了精神卫生中心，护士艾莉丝接待了她，经交谈得知，琼已经是第二次入院了。

3. What nursing diagnosis shall June give priority to?

3. 对于患者琼来说，最优先考虑的护理诊断是什么？

4. At the second day since June was hospitalized, the nurse Alice made an agreement of behavior with June, and which aspects shall they reach consensus on?

4. 入院第二天，护士艾莉丝与患者琼谈论制订一份行为约定，她们需要在哪些方面达成一致意见？

(Questions 5 to 6 share the same question stem)

A client who was diagnosed with boulimia attended the team of nursing guidance in the center of mental health and she said the reason why she came here was, her husband will divorce with her if she doesn't turn to help. The client told the nurse shall usually eat a lot when she feel uncomfortable, and then vomit, so she didn't gain much weight. Several days later, the client trust on the nurse increasing, and she said, "I couldn't bear the way that I look."

（5～6 题共用题干）

一名刚被诊断为贪食症的患者参加精神卫生中心的护士指导小组，她说她来这里完全是因为她丈夫说如果她不来寻求帮助就离婚。患者告诉护士当她感到不舒适时会吃很多，然后呕吐，所以她体重没有增加多少。几天后，患者越来越信任护士，对护士说："我不能忍受我看起来的样子。"

5. What is the most important nursing problem for the client at present?
6. Which methods can be used to help the client to correct her wrong recognition?

5. 患者目前存在最主要的护理问题是什么?
6. 有哪些方法可以帮助患者改变不恰当的认知?

Chapter 15 Psychopharmacology and Nursing Care

第十五章　药物治疗及护理

Learning Objectives

Memorization

1. Accurately summarize the concept and classification of psychotropic drugs.
2. Correctly describe the representative drugs and indications of various kinds of psychotropic drugs.

Comprehension

Identify the side effects and adverse reactions of commonly used psychotropic drugs.

Application

In order to improve the compliance of drug treatment, work out a plan by means of nursing assessment, to take the drugs together with the client who is taking psychotropic drugs.

学习目标

识记

1. 能准确概括精神药物的概念与分类。
2. 能正确描述各类精神药物的代表药及适应证。

理解

能识别常用精神药物的副作用与不良反应。

运用

能运用护理程序与正在服用精神药物的患者商议，制订一份服药计划，以利于提高其药物治疗的依从性。

15章

Linda is a 38-year-old, married, female, middle school teacher. She was admitted into hospital due to "alternative onset of intermittent excitement, hypertalktiveness and sadness, hypotalktiveness for 8 years, additional onset for 3 months". She became gloomy with unsatisfactory title promotions 8 years ago, locking herself in home and forming an idea of suicide. It took 6 months for her to alleviate by herself and everything turned usual.

She got excited again after a year and voluntarily became a newspaper correspondent, staying up all night writing stories and poems. In May the following year she was sent into mental hospital for the first time and underwent special treatment. The mental health checks revealed she was in typical manic state, intellectually well, without illusions or delusion and lack of insight. After treatment with haloperidol for 1 month her symptoms disappeared, insight recovered and she was released from the hospital. 3 years ago she fell into mania again for no reason and was tied into hospital by family. She was cured by taking lithium carbonate for 2 months. The symptoms disappeared, her insight resumed, she was discharged form hospital and turned into an ordinary person. 6 months ago she began her alternative onset of joy and sorrow every 8 days. It took place by turn for 6 times within 3 months. In manic period she was irritable besides excitement and talkativeness. She often abused kids because of trivial things, slept less and became energetic. Her mania came up again as she stopped taking lithium carbonate for half a month. For the third time she was hospitalized for treatment. Admitting diagnosis: bipolar disorder.

Please think about the following questions based on the case:

1. What is the nursing diagnosis for the client at present and potentially?

2. How do nurses offer guidance on medicine according to different illness ?

患者琳达，女，38岁，已婚，中学教师。因"间歇性兴奋话多与愁闷少语交替发作8年，再次发作3个月"入院。8年前因职称晋升不顺而闷闷不乐，闭门不出，有轻生念头，半年后自行缓解，一切如常。

一年后又变得兴奋话多，毛遂自荐当了某报社义务通讯员，彻夜不眠地写报道、写诗歌，于次年5月第一次收入精神病院，接受专科治疗，当时精神状况检查为典型躁狂状态，智能良好，无幻觉妄想，自知力缺失。经氟哌啶醇治疗1个月上述症状消失，自知力恢复，痊愈出院。3年前无明显原因又出现躁狂发作，被家人捆绑入院。经碳酸锂治疗2月后症状消失，自知力恢复，痊愈出院，出院后如常人。6个月前开始欢乐与忧愁交替发作，各维持8天左右，3个月内交替6次。在躁狂期除话多、兴奋外，还易激惹，常因小事而打骂孩子，睡眠少而精力充沛，3月前因停用碳酸锂半个月再次出现躁狂发作，第3次进医院治疗。入院诊断：双相情感障碍。

请思考：

1. 患者目前及潜在的护理诊断是什么？

2. 护士如何针对患者病情不同进行服药知识指导？

In 1917, there was a high-fever therapy for mental disorders, followed by sleep therapy, insulin-coma therapy, electro-convulsive therapy (ECT) and psychiatric surgery therapy, but the efficacy of these treatments were not determined. Until the 1950s, the discovery of psychotropic drugs chlorpromazine, made the client get rid of the internees fate, and then there was a breakthrough on the prevention, treatment and rehabilitation for mental disorders. Because of taking convenience, reliable effect, reducing the recurrence rate, psychotropic drugs have become an important means of treatment of mental illness. Medication and nursing care become particularly

精神障碍继1917年开始的高热疗法后，陆续出现了睡眠疗法、胰岛素休克疗法、电抽搐治疗及精神外科治疗，但这些治疗方法疗效均不确定，直至20世纪50年代精神药物氯丙嗪的问世，精神障碍的预防、治疗、康复才有了突破性进展，使患者摆脱了被拘禁的命运。精神药物因服用方便，疗效可靠，降低了复发率，已成为当今治疗精神疾病的重要手段，药物的治疗及护理亦因此成为了精神科护士的重要护理内容之一。本章重点

important in the field of psychiatric nursing. This chapter focuses on the application of psychotropic drugs in the treatment of mental diseases and nursing care of clients with psychiatric medication.

介绍精神药物在治疗精神疾病中的应用以及运用精神药物过程中的护理。

Section 1 Introduction

第一节 概 述

I. History of Psychiatric Medication

一、精神药物发展概况

All the studies on the efficacy of psychotropic drugs almost began in the mid-20th century. In 1886, John Aulde and Carl Lange recognized that lithium could be used to control symptoms of what was later called Bipolar Disorder. However, these early observations were forgotten, to be rediscovered by Cade and Schou in the mid-20th century. The basic chemical structure underlying both tricyclic antidepressants and phenothiazine antipsychotics was initially synthesized in 1889. It was not until the early 1950s that pharmacological investigation led to modifications of this iminodibenzyl structure. These modifications produced both antidepressant and antipsychotic medications from remarkably similar underlying molecular structures. Benzodiazepine drugs for treatment of anxiety were first synthesized in the mid-1950s and released for clinical use in 1960.

Much more recent pharmacological research has resulted in important therapeutic advances such as atypical antipsychotics (clozapine) and selective serotonin reuptake inhibitors [fluoxetine (Prozac) and others]. Current pharmacological treatments have serious deficiencies, of which the most important is that (as with many chronic diseases) they serve to control symptoms rather than to cure psychiatric disorders. Also, psychiatric drugs are not effective for, or tolerated by, a significant portion of affected individuals, often those with the most disabling symptoms. Despite these important limitations of current practice, the use of psychiatric medications offers great benefits to many clients. These benefits will continue to increase as ever more effective treatments are developed and brought into practice.

几乎所有精神药物药效的研究均始于20世纪50年代之后。锂盐的应用早在1886年就被John Aulde和Carl Lange所认识，用来控制后来被称为“双相障碍”的精神症状，但当时被人们所忽视，直到20世纪中期才由Cade和Schou再次发现，并逐步用于精神疾病的治疗。三环类抗抑郁药物和酚噻嗪类抗精神病药物早在1889年便被合成，也是直到20世纪50年代，药理学研究才发现了亚胺二联苄结构的异构体，这些合成的异构体与抗抑郁和抗精神病药物在分子结构上极为相似。用于治疗焦虑的苯二氮䓬类药物亦于20世纪中期被发现并合成，1960年投入临床应用。

近年来，随着药理学研究的不断进展，精神疾病的治疗方法有了突飞猛进的发展，如非典型抗精神病药（氯氮平）以及选择性5-羟色胺再摄取抑制剂（氟西汀）等的临床应用，使得更多的精神疾病患者得到有效医治。尽管如此，精神药物在治疗许多慢性精神疾病中仍存在诸多不足，大部分药物只能用来控制疾病症状，而不能达到治愈的目的，部分有致残性症状的患者使用精神药物效果并不理想或难以耐受其副作用。

BOX 15-1 History Corridor

The Discovery of Chlorpromazine

The advent of the chlorpromazine was legendary, since it is not a psychiatrist but a surgeon found that chlorpromazine could be used as a antipsychotic. In April

BOX 15-1 历史长廊

氯丙嗪的问世

氯丙嗪的问世颇具传奇色彩，因为发现氯丙嗪能够抗精神病的不是精神病科医生，而是

1949, a French naval surgeon Laib Litt was researching drugs on prevention of surgical shock. He found promethazine is more powerful than other drugs, and in addition to anti-shock function, it could take effect on central nervous system. This discovery of Laib Litt interested the researchers in Greenspan West Lab who produced promethazine. They synthesized chloride derivative of Sparine on the basis of previous studies. The pharmacological experiments showed that the derivative has significant activity and low toxicity. So they sent the sample to Laib Litt, who thought it as a ideal drug. He went on with a complete animal experiment, and then tried it on surgical patients.

外科医生。1949年4月，法国的一位海军外科医生莱伯利特在研究防止外科休克药时发现异丙嗪比其他药物作用强，异丙嗪除了有抗休克作用外，还可对中枢神经系统起作用。莱伯利特的这一发现，使生产异丙嗪的斯潘西亚实验室的研究人员产生了兴趣，他们在前人研究的基础上合成了普马嗪的氯化衍生物，药理实验表明该类衍生物低毒而有显著活性。于是他们把这一样品送到了莱伯利特那里，莱伯利特认为该药很理想，就进一步全面进行动物实验，接着又在外科手术患者身上试用。不久发现，使用该药抗休克的同时，患者手术后食欲恢复得很好，并且在手术前那种紧张情绪也消失了。莱伯利特想，这种抗休克药是否也能抗精神病呢？于是莱伯利特请同事在精神病患者身上做试验，以求取得结论。

It was not long before the drug was found to be preventive to shock, and the patient's appetite recovered well after the operation, furthermore, the tension before the surgery disappeared. Laib Litt thought, is the anti-shock drug can also be antipsychotic? So he asked his colleagues to do experiments on clients with mental disorder in order to reach a conclusion. In January 1952, psychiatry department director Harmon and other doctors used the drug on a client with mania. The client's agitated symptoms disappeared soon and the effect lasted for several hours. Since then, thousands of clients also took the drugs sent by Lee Teuk leber. Later, French psychiatrist Delay further applied the drug on treatment of a variety of mental illness. Thus heralding of a new era of psychotropic on treatment of mental diseases. The autumn of 1952 witnessed the launch of the new medicine in Paris market by Lenny G company, named Largaotil, suggesting its' variety of effects.

1952年1月，精神科主任哈蒙与其他医生用该药对一名躁狂症患者进行治疗后，患者狂躁不安的症状很快消失，作用持续了几个小时。此后，数以千计的这类患者也服用了莱伯利特送来的药物。法国精神病专家Delay还进一步将此药应用于多种精神病的治疗，从此开始精神药物治疗精神病的新纪元。1952年秋季，这一新药由隆尼普莱尼克公司在巴黎投放市场，取名氯普马嗪即氯丙嗪（Largaotil），意思是有多种作用。

II. Mechanism of Psychiatric Medication

二、精神药物的作用机制

i. Usage and Absorption of Drugs

Many psychiatric medications are given orally (p.o.), and some drugs can be administered via parenteral routes, usually through the intramuscular injection (i.m.). Only rarely are psychiatric medications given intravenously (i.v.) or subcutaneously (s.c.). Most drugs are absorbed quite predictably when given by a parenteral route, but

（一）给药途径及吸收

大部分精神药物经口服给药，部分经非肠道途径给药，通常为肌肉注射，极少数通过静脉或皮下注射给药。经非肠道给药的药物，大部分可被吸收，而口服药物的吸收受患者饮食、胃酸及药物自身性质的影响较大。

oral administration may be significantly affected by foods, stomach acidity (often modified by antacids), and the nature of the drug itself. Once absorbed, drugs distribute throughout the body depending on their solubility in water and fat and on their tendency to bind to proteins. Fat-soluble drugs tend to distribute widely in the body; protein-bound drugs may be very slow to diffuse out of the bloodstream. These characteristics affect drug actions.

药物吸收与其水溶性和脂溶性以及药物与蛋白质的结合力有关。脂溶性药物易全身分布，而与蛋白结合的药物在血中扩散缓慢，这些特征均影响药物的作用效果。

ii. Metabolism and Clearance of Drugs

Once in the body, most drugs are eliminated by excretion (usually into the urine by the kidney or into the bile or feces by the liver). Prior to excretion, drugs are almost always metabolized, most often by the liver but occasionally by lungs or even skin. Some substances have pharmacological activity only after they have been metabolized into biologically active metabolites, even more active than the original drugs. The potential effects of any drug are a complex balance of each of these factors: absorption, distribution, elimination and metabolism. Another term for this balance is pharmacokinetics. In most cases, the goal of drug administration is the achievement of a "steady" pharmacokinetic state (often called steady state) in which the amount of drug absorbed is constantly balanced by the competing processes of distribution, elimination and metabolism. The half-life may help estimate pharmacokinetics, especially when combined with knowledge of absorption, distribution, and elimination/metabolism. The half-life is the time (typically in hours) it takes or plasma concentrations of a drug to decrease to half of an initial value. After seven half-lives, less than 1% of a drug remains in the plasma. For a short-acting drug, such as triazolam, which has a half-life as short as 1.5 hours, seven half-lives may be very short (about 10 hours) whereas a long half-life drug such as fluoxetine (half-life of 3 days) may not be fully eliminated for several weeks.

（二）药物的代谢及清除

精神药物进入体内后经肝脏或肺代谢，可成为具有非生物活性的物质，并直接经肾由尿液排出，或经肝脏由胆汁或粪便排出体外。而部分药物经过代谢后则比原始药物生物活性更强，并具有更强的药理活性。药物在机体的吸收、分布、代谢及清除过程称为药物动力学。通常情况下，给药的目的在于发挥最大效应、达到稳定的药物动力学状态，这种状态又可称为稳态（即药物的吸收量在机体的分布、清除和代谢过程中保持恒定）。半衰期是测定药物动力学状态的常用指标，它是指药物在血清中浓度减少到原来一半时所需的时间。大多数精神药物经过 7 个半衰期后，残留在血清中的药物不足 1%。然而，不同精神药物其半衰期有所不同，如短效药物（如三唑仑）半衰期仅 1.5 小时，7 个半衰期仅 10 小时左右，而长效药物（如氟西汀）半衰期则需 3 天，有时经过数周也不能完全被清除。

iii. Application of Drug Mechanism in Nursing

Some psychiatric drugs are intended to have a significant effect after the first dose. Antipsychotic drugs, hypnotics and anxiolytics most commonly have rapid single-dose effects. Other psychiatric drugs only work after a steady state being achieved, typically several weeks after administration begins. Of course, onset clearly varies with the mode of administration and is typically shorter for drugs given parenterally (especially intravenously) than for drugs given orally. Most psychiatric drugs act on the central nervous system and must therefore leave the bloodstream to enter the interstitial fluid, the cerebrospinal fluid (CSF), and/or the cells of the brain. Howerver, many drugs circulate in the blood bound to protein, and these protein-drug complexes are almost completely excluded

（三）药物作用机制在护理中的应用

部分精神药物常在首次给药时效果就很明显，如抗精神病药、催眠药、抗焦虑药等具有迅速的单剂量效果；而另外一些精神药物仅在首次给药后数周，达到稳态后才起作用。当然，药物起效时间取决于给药途径，非肠道给药，特别是静脉给药的起效时间明显快于口服给药方式。大多数精神药物作用于中枢神经系统，必须经血液进入脑脊液（CSF）和 / 或脑细胞中，而许多药物在血中与蛋白质结合形成“蛋白质 – 药物复合物”，它是一种大分子物质，几乎完全被血 – 脑脊液

by the capillary barrier between blood and CSF. Fat-soluble drugs can often pass through capillary membranes, and many molecules are actively transported across capillary cell walls into the brain. Some drugs cannot cross the blood-cerebrospinal fluid barrier in an active form but will cross in an inactive form that is later changed into the active metabolite within the brain: Levodopa (L-dopa), used to treat parkinsonism, is metabolized to dopamine once it is transported across capillary walls. Therefore, the psychiatric nurses should improve the knowledge of mechanism of psychotropic drugs during the treatment and nursing of mental illness, these are helpful for them observing drugs' treatment effect and providing health guidance on drugs' knowledge.

屏障滤过。脂溶性药物常能透过毛细血管膜，经主动运输穿过细胞膜进入大脑。一些药物虽不能以活性状态穿过血－脑脊液屏障，但可以非活性状态进入，并在大脑中代谢为有活性的物质，从而发挥其药理效应，如常用于治疗帕金森综合征的左旋多巴，一旦穿过血－脑脊液屏障，即被代谢为多巴胺。因此，在精神疾病的治疗过程中，护理人员提高对精神药物作用机制的认识，有助于更好地进行药物治疗后的效果观察和药物知识的健康指导。

Section 2 Common Medications

第二节　常用药物

Acorrding to different application purpose, the commonly used psychotropic drugs can be divided into six categories according to the purpose: antipsychotics, antidepressants, mood stabilizers (antimanics), anxiolytics, psychostimulants and nootropic drugs (figure 15-1). This section mainly introduces antipsychotic drugs and medications for mood disorders.

目前，在临床上常用的精神药物按其使用目的可分为六大类：抗精神病药、抗抑郁药、心境稳定剂（抗躁狂药）、抗焦虑药、精神振奋药和促脑代谢药（图 15-1）。本节重点介绍抗精神病药和治疗心境障碍的药物。

I. Antipsychotic Drugs

一、抗精神病药物

Antipsychotic drugs, also called "major tranquilizers", are administered to control the symptoms of psychosis such as hallucinations and bizarre or paranoid behavior. These drugs tend to produce a calming effect without significantly sedating the client or reducing

抗精神病药物也称“强安定剂”，用于控制精神病症状，如幻觉、怪异或偏执行为。这些药物可使患者平静，且不伴有明显的过度镇静或降低警觉的作用。大部分抗精神分

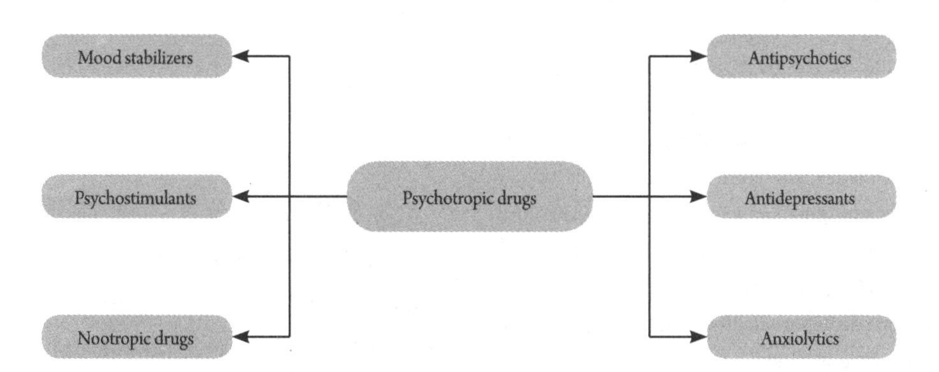

Figure 15-1　The classification of psychotropic drugs

alertness. A number of antipsychotic medications are considered in this section. There are nearly 20 antipsychotic drugs in clinical use.

裂症药属于此类。

i. Classification

（一）分类

1. Grouping by Chemical Class Antipsychotic drugs can be classed as phenothiazines, thioxanthenes, butyrophenones, dibenzoxazepines, dihydroindolones, dibenzodiazepines, and benzisoxazoles. The phenothiazines, together with the next four categories (thioxanthenes, butyrophenones, dibenzoxazepines and dihydroindolones),comprise the "typical" antipsychotic drugs. Dibenzoxazepines and benzisoxazoles comprise the "atypical" antipsychotic drugs (table 15-1). Due to the complexity of chemical names, which is difficult to memorize, mental health professionals find it practical to classify antipsychotic drugs into broad groups: phenothiazines and the other classical agents, the newest drugs(atypical agents)-clozapine (Clozaril), risperidone (Risperdal), olanzapine (Zyprexa) and quetiapine (Seroquel). Clozapine may effectively treat psychotic clients not helped by classical agents, but this benefit comes at the risk of occasional life-threatening bone marrow depression. Risperidone is a relatively new medication that at low doses has fewer serious side effects than phenothiazines and may be more effective under some circumstances.

1. 按化学结构分类 抗精神病药物按化学结构可分为酚噻嗪类、硫杂蒽类、丁酰苯类、二苯氧氮平类、苯甲酰类、二苯二氮䓬类、苯丙异噁唑类。其中酚噻嗪类、硫杂蒽类、丁酰苯类、二苯氧氮平类、苯甲酰类组成经典抗精神病药物。二苯二氮䓬类与苯丙异噁唑类组成非经典抗精神病药物（表 15-1）。由于化学名称复杂，难以识记，精神卫生专业人员又将抗精神病药物分为两大类：① 酚噻嗪类和其他经典类药物；② 新型药物（非经典类药物）：氯氮平、利培酮、奥氮平、喹硫平。氯氮平常用于治疗对经典类药物效果差的患者，且效果显著，但偶见骨髓抑制。利培酮是一种较新的药物，与酚噻嗪类相比，其服用剂量小，且副作用少，在某些情况下比酚噻嗪类更有效。

2. Grouping by Potency Class Antipsychotic medications are commonly grouped by the amount of drug required to achieve an effect. Two phenothiazines-fluphenazine(Prolixin)and trifluoperazine(Stelazine)-and a butyrophenone-haloperidol (Haldol)-are classified as "high potency" because only a few milligrams have significant antipsychotic effects. The "low-potency" drugs-chlorpromazine (Thorazine), thioridazine (Mellaril) and chlorprothixene (Taractan)-typically achieve effects comparable to a few milligrams of high-potency drugs with doses of approximately 100 mg. Beyond this 50-fold difference in absolute dose needed to achieve similar effects, there are some additional differences between potency classes. For example, the low-potency drugs are more sedating, whereas the high-potency drugs are more likely to produce certain troublesome complications. The majority of drugs falls into an intermediate potency range and also has intermediate sedative and adverse effects.

2. 按效能分类 抗精神病药物常按产生疗效所需的剂量分为高效能药物、中效能药物和低效能药物。高效能药物包括两种酚噻嗪类药物，即氟奋乃静和三氟拉嗪，以及一种丁酰苯类（氟哌啶醇），它们仅需几毫克便能产生明显抗精神病效果。低效能药物有氯丙嗪、硫利哒嗪、泰尔登，这些药物均需 100 mg 才能达到几毫克高效能药物所产生的效果。高效能与低效能药物除了所需剂量不同外，效能类别间还存在其他差别，例如，低效能药物镇静作用强，而高效能药物易产生并发症等。在临床，大多数药物都属于中效能药物，既具有中度镇静作用，又有中度的不良反应。

3. Grouping by Length of Action The third major classification divides drugs into short and long-acting preparations. Long-acting preparations: two drugs (fluphenazine decanoate and haloperidol decanoate) are given intramuscularly and have effects that last for several weeks. These drugs are compounded as decanoic acid

3. 按作用时间分类 抗精神病药物也可根据作用时间，将其分为短效和长效制剂。长效制剂如氟哌啶醇癸酸酯和氟奋乃静癸酸酯，其半衰期可达 10 天，肌肉注射后作用可持续数周。短效制剂如氯丙嗪、氟哌啶醇，

Table 15-1 Antipsychotic medications

GENERC NAME	MODE OF ADMIN-ISTRATION	SEDA-TION	EXTRA-PYRA-MIDAL	ANTI-CHOLIN-ERGIC	ORTHO-STATIC HYPO-TENSION	DOSE RANGE/($mg \cdot d^{-1}$)
Phenothiazines						
Chlorpromazine	p.o.,p.r., i.m.,i.v.	3+	2+	2+	2+	30-800
Thioridizine	p.o.	3+	1+	3+	3+	150-800
Fluphenazine	p.o., i.m./s.c.	1+	3+	1+	1+	5-40
Trifluoperazine	p.o.,i.m.	1+	3+	1+	1+	2-40
Thioxanthene						
Thiothixene	p.o.,i.m.	1+	3+	1+	1+	8-30
Butyrephenone						
Haloperidol	p.o.,i.m.	1+	3+	1+	1+	1-15
Dibenzoxazepine						
Loxapine	p.o.,i.m.	2+	3+	1+	2+	20-250
Dibenzodiazepines						
Clozapine	p.o.	3+	1+	3+	3+	300-900
Olanzapine	p.o.	3+	1+	3+	3+	5-10
Quetiapine	p.o.	3+	1+	3+	3+	300
Benzisoxazole						
Risperidone	p.o.	1+	3+	1+	1+	4-60

表 15-1 抗精神病药物

通用名	服药方法	镇静作用	锥体外系反应	抗胆碱能作用	体位性低血压	剂量范围 /（$mg \cdot d^{-1}$）
酚噻嗪类						
氯丙嗪	p.o.,p.r., i.m.,i.v.	3+	2+	2+	2+	30～800
硫利达嗪	p.o.	3+	1+	3+	3+	150～800
氟奋乃静	p.o., i.m./s.c.	1+	3+	1+	1+	5～40
三氟拉嗪	p.o.,i.m.	1+	3+	1+	1+	2～40
硫杂蒽类						
替沃噻吨	p.o.,i.m.	1+	3+	1+	1+	8～30
丁酰苯类						
氟哌啶醇	p.o.,i.m.	1+	3+	1+	1+	1～15
诺昔替林						
洛沙平	p.o.,i.m.	2+	3+	1+	2+	20～250
二苯并二氮䓬类						
氯氮平	p.o.	3+	1+	3+	3+	300～900
奥氮平	p.o.	3+	1+	3+	3+	5～10
喹硫平	p.o.	3+	1+	3+	3+	300
苯异噁唑						
利培酮	p.o.	1+	3+	1+	1+	4～60

esters so that their half-life may reach nearly 10 days. Short-acting preparations: chlorpromazine and haloperidol are also available in much shorter acting forms with half-lives of only a few hours. The remaining drugs have clinically significant effects for 24 hours or less.

半衰期仅为数小时，24 小时内起效。

ii. Drugs Actions

The pharmacological actions of antipsychotics are complex. In general, these medications have two major characteristics: They all bind to brain dopamine receptors; probably as a result of that binding, they produce a degree of indifference to both external and internal stressful stimuli. Other medications that induce a degree of indifference to stress (e.g., narcotics and sedatives) produce sedation or a direct blockade of pain perception. Antipsychotics, in contrast, exert a calming effect without reducing alertness or sensitivity to pain. Narcotics and sedatives typically produce dependence and/or addiction after frequent or prolonged use. Dependency does not occur with antipsychotic medications, but clients should typically be tapered off these medications rather than stopped abruptly.

（二）药理作用

抗精神病药物的药理学作用很复杂，总体上这些药物有两个主要特征：① 均与脑内多巴胺受体结合；② 造成对外源或内源性应激性刺激的反应淡漠。一些导致对应激性刺激反应淡漠的药物，如麻醉药和镇静药可产生过度镇静作用或直接阻断痛觉，而抗精神病药虽发挥镇静作用，但并不降低对疼痛的警觉和敏感性。频繁或长期使用麻醉镇静药可产生依赖和 / 或成瘾，虽然抗精神病药物不会引起药物依赖，但应避免突然停药，而应逐渐减量。

Much current evidence suggests that schizophrenia involves excessive activation of brain D_2 dopamine receptors. Antipsychotic drugs are all strong blockers of dopamine D_2 receptors in the brain. The “atypical” antipsychotic drugs block D_2 and serotonin (5-HT_2) receptors in the brain. For example, clozapine blocks D_2 and 5-HT_2 but also has effects on other dopamine receptors (D_1 and D_4)as several other neurotransmitter systems. This wider range of action may explain the enhanced effectiveness of clozapine, in comparison with other “classical” antipsychotics. The phenothiazines, thioxanthenes and dibenzoxazepines have a similar chemical structure, each with a central ring flanked on each side by two aromatic rings. Because their chemical structure typically lacks highly polar regions, the antipsychotic drugs are not very water soluble, and as a result they have a high affinity for fatty tissues such as lung, brain, and adipose stores. Because of this fat affinity, lower doses may be required in very thin persons.

近年来，许多研究证据表明精神分裂症与大脑多巴胺 D_2 受体功能亢进有关，而抗精神病药物都是强多巴胺 D_2 受体阻滞剂。新型的非典型抗精神病药物以 5-HT_2/D_2 受体的阻断作用为标志，如氯氮平不仅阻断 D_2 受体，而且还影响其他多巴胺受体（D_1 和 D_4）、5-HT_2 及其他神经递质系统。酚噻嗪类、硫杂蒽类和二苯氧氮平类具有相似的化学结构，均对脂肪组织具有高度亲合性，如肺、脑和贮脂组织，因其高亲脂性，低体重患者只需服较少剂量便可达到治疗效果。

iii. Clinical Use

1. Indications and Evidence for Effectiveness Antipsychotic drugs are mainly used in the treatment of schizophrenia and prevent the recurrence of schizophrenia, manic control. Since many medically induced psychotic states are transient, treatment may not be necessary for brief or mild psychosis. Symptoms for which antipsychotic treatment is often used include hallucinations, delusions, and disorganized thought processes, including paranoia. In the course of schizophrenic illness, such antipsychotic-

（三）临床应用

1. 适应证及疗效 抗精神病药物主要用于治疗精神分裂症和预防精神分裂症的复发、控制躁狂发作。许多躯体疾病导致的精神异常是一过性的，症状轻的可不必治疗，症状较重时可给予抗精神病药物治疗。在治疗精神分裂症状的过程中，阳性症状如幻觉、妄想、思维障碍等对经典抗精神病药物的反应

responsive symptoms are termed positive symptoms because they result in socially disruptive behaviors. The negative symptoms of schizophrenia (withdrawal, lack of initiative, failure to maintain hygiene) do not respond to classical antipsychotics, although they may briefly improve after treatment with the "atypical" antipsychotic clozapine (Clozaril).

良好，而阴性症状，如退缩、意志缺乏、生活懒散等则反应差，但经“非典型”抗精神病药氯氮平治疗后，症状可明显改善。

2. Dose and Administration The dosage of antipsychotics varies with the drug chosen and with the prescribing practice of the psychiatric clinician. In general, thioridazine (Mellaril), haloperidol (Haldol), chlorpromazine (Thorazine), risperidone (Risperdal) and olanzapine are commonly used preparations. Chlorpromazine and thioridazine dosages vary from 200 to 600 mg daily, whereas haloperidol doses range from 6 to 20 mg, risperidone 2-6 mg daily, olanzapine 5-20 mg daily (table 15-1). The guidelines suggest 1 to 3 years of treatment following a first psychotic episode and at least 5 years of treatment following recurrent episodes. Some clients with severe and recurrent disease need lifelong medication. Although oral onset time is generally 1-4 hours, than the muscle injection, which onset time is 15-30 minutes, the methods of administration are mainly oral, intramuscular injection or intravenous drip can also be used as appropriate.

2. 剂量与用法 抗精神病药物的种类不同，临床常规用法不同，其使用剂量也不同。例如，硫利达嗪、氟哌啶醇、氯丙嗪、利培酮、奥氮平等是临床常使用的抗精神病药物，氯丙嗪、硫利达嗪每日用量为200～600 mg，而氟哌啶醇每日用量为6～20 mg，利培酮为每日2～6 mg，奥氮平为每日5～20 mg（表15-1）。用药原则一般为：首次发作疗程1～3年，复发后疗程至少5年以上，部分病情严重、反复发作的患者则需终生服药。给药方法以口服为主，也可酌情肌肉注射或静脉滴注。口服起效时间稍慢，一般在1～4小时，肌肉注射则在15～30分钟内起效。

3. Drug Interactions Because antipsychotic drugs are most commonly metabolized by the liver, other medications that affect the rate of hepatic drug detoxification may have an effect on antipsychotic drug excretion. Drug interactions are often easy to reduce the effect of drug action. For example, cimetidine (Tagamet) may reduce antipsychotic effects and lead to medication failure. Tricyclic antidepressants are also frequently combined with antipsychotics; this combination may increase serum antidepressant level and produce toxicity if levels are not monitored. Fluoxetine and other serotonin reuptake inhibitors may significantly increase antipsychotic drug levels and lead to serious adverse reactions. Some cardiac drugs (particularly quinidine, procainamide and epinephrine, may interact with low-potency antipsychotics; the administration of epinephrine to persons taking medications such as chlorpromazine may result in severe hypotension. In addition, very high levels of caffeine intake may worsen psychosis despite antipsychotic administration. May decrease oral antipsychotic drug absorption and should not be administered within 4 hours of an antipsychotic dose.

3. 药物相互作用 由于抗精神病药物大部分在肝脏代谢，因此凡影响肝脏解毒功能的药物均影响抗精神病药物的排泄。药物间的相互作用会降低药物作用效果，例如：西米替丁可使抗精神病药物的作用减弱，并导致药物失效；三环类抗抑郁药常和抗精神病药混合使用，它会提高抗抑郁药的血药水平，甚至产生毒性反应。氟西汀及其他5-HT再摄取抑制剂会显著增加抗精神病药的血药水平，导致严重的不良反应。一些用于治疗心脏病的药物，如奎尼丁、普鲁卡因酰胺和肾上腺素等，与低效抗精神病药也有相互作用，如使用肾上腺素的患者同时服用氯丙嗪会导致严重的低血压。此外，口服抗精神病药物的患者，摄入过多咖啡会减少药物的吸收，使病情加重，因此在服药4小时内应避免服用咖啡。

4. Use during Pregnancy/Lactation There are no specific known contraindications to the use of antipsychotic medications in pregnancy, although most

4. 孕乳期用药 虽然许多临床医生都会在患者怀孕早期和临近分娩期将用量减至最小或避免给药，但在孕期并不禁止使用抗精

clinicians try to use the minimum possible dose and to avoid administration in early pregnancy and near the time of delivery. Antipsychotic medications are excreted in breast milk so that breastfeeding is contraindicated when these medications must be used following delivery.

神病药。抗精神病药物可经乳液排泄，故服药期间禁止哺乳。

iv. Side Effects and Adverse Effects

（四）药物副作用及不良反应

1. Anticholinergic Effects These side effects include constipation, dry mouth, blurred vision, postural hypotension, urinary hesitancy or retention, weight gain and sedation. These anticholinergic effects may be minimized by choosing drugs with relatively lower anticholinergic action: for example, haloperidol (Haldol), trifluoperazine (Stelazine) and fluphenazine (Prolixin).

1. 抗胆碱能药物的副作用 抗胆碱能药物常见的副作用为便秘、口干、视物模糊、直立性低血压，排尿困难或尿潴留，体重增加和过度镇静。在临床可选择抗胆碱作用弱的药物来减少这些副作用，如氟哌啶醇、三氟拉嗪和氟奋乃静等。

2. Extrapyramidal Side Effects The classical agents such as thioridazine (Mellaril), haloperidol (Haldol), and chlorpromazine (Thorazine) frequently produce a variety of movement disorders, which include akathisia, dystonia, drug-induced parkinsonism and tardive dyskinesia.

2. 锥体外系反应 经典抗精神病药如硫利达嗪、氟哌啶醇、氯丙嗪常引起各种运动障碍，包括以下四种表现：

(1) Akathisia: Akathisia is the most common and consists of a subjective sense of restlessness with a perceived need to pace or otherwise move continuously. It is easy for the nurse to mistake akathisia for anxiety or agitation.

（1）静坐不能：最常见，表现为自主性坐立不安、踱步或不停活动；在临床上，护士常误认为是患者出现焦虑或激惹。

(2) Dystonia: Dystonia consists of sustained, involuntary muscle spasms; these most commonly involve the head and neck but may occasionally occur in other muscle groups. One of the most dramatic dystonia reactions is oculogyric crisis, in which extraocular muscle spasm forces the eyes into a fixed, usually upward gaze.

（2）肌张力障碍：表现为持续性、不随意的肌肉抽搐，常见于头颈部肌肉，偶见于其他肌群，其中最典型的肌张力障碍是动眼危象，表现为眼外肌痉挛，眼球固定，向上凝视。

(3) Parkinsonism: Parkinsonism results in tremor and an unsteady shuffling gait. The features of drug-induced Parkinsonism may closely resemble those of true idiopathic Parkinsonism. The distinction between these two conditions may occasionally be difficult, but idiopathic Parkinsonism most commonly occurs in older individuals who have no history of antipsychotic drug use. In contrast, drug-induced Parkinsonism is common and occurs in up to 30% of individuals who take long-term antipsychotic medications.

（3）类帕金森综合征：表现为震颤和步态不稳。药源性帕金森综合征的特点与特发性帕金森综合征相似，两者有时难以区别。特发性帕金森综合征多见于无抗精神病药物服药史的老年人，而长期服用抗精神病药物的患者有 30% 可发生药源性帕金森综合征。

These three conditions-akathisia, dystonia and Parkinsonism-usually respond rapidly to antipsychotic dosage reduction, anticholinergic drugs or diphenhydramine (Benadryl).

抗胆碱能药物和苯海拉明在药物减量或停用后，可迅速缓解上述三种不良反应。

(4) Tardive Dyskinesia (TD): The fourth movement disorder seen with antipsychotic drugs, tardive dyskinesia, is a more significant adverse effect because it may prove long-lasting despite withdrawal of antipsychotic medication. Tardive dyskinesia is a neurological disorder

（4）迟发性运动障碍：是较严重的不良反应，在停用抗精神病药后可长期存在。迟发性运动障碍是以不随意运动为特征的神经紊乱，常见于舌部和唇部。扮鬼脸、吸吮动作，

characterized by involuntary movements, most commonly of the tongue and lips. Grimacing, sucking movements, and lip smacking are among the most common tardive dyskinesias. When tardive dyskinesia affects the trunk and extremities, the result may be slow and irregular movements that diminish during relaxation and disappear during sleep. On occasion tardive dyskinesia may be so severe as to interfere with walking, eating, or even breathing. Tardive dyskinesia may improve or disappear when medications are stopped and may even improve with continued administration of classical antipsychotics. Anticholinergic drugs are often used to treat medication-related movement disorders, but they have poor effect to treat Tardive dyskinesia.

咋舌也可见于大多数迟发性运动障碍的患者。当迟发性运动障碍影响到躯干、四肢时，患者表现为缓慢而不规则的运动。严重的迟发性运动障碍可影响患者行走、吃饭甚至呼吸。通常停药后，迟发性运动障碍可缓解或消失，抗胆碱能药物常与抗精神病药物同时使用，防止神经症状的发展，但对治疗迟发性运动障碍无效。

3. Neuroleptic Malignant Syndrome (NMS) Neuroleptic malignant syndrome (NMS) is yet another serious complication of antipsychotic medications. This syndrome clinically resembles malignant hypothermia, a condition seen during surgical anesthesia in genetically predisposed individuals. All of the antipsychotic medications, including clozapine, may occasionally result in neuroleptic malignant syndrome. This unusual disorder is associated with sudden fever, rigidity, tachycardia, hypertension, and decreased levels of consciousness. Fever can rise to exceedingly high levels, and death may occur. These individuals are usually thought incorrectly to have an infectious condition, and unnecessary investigations and antibiotic treatment may delay diagnosis. Rapid treatment is required for survival, but this requires a high index of suspicion. Treatment includes discontinuation of antipsychotics and the potential administration of a variety of medications, including anti-parkinsonians, bromocriptine, dantrolene and benzodiazepines.

3. 恶性综合征 恶性综合征是使用抗精神病药物的另一严重并发症，在临床上类似手术麻醉中的恶性低温状态。所有抗精神病药均可引起恶性综合征。这种罕见综合征表现为突发高热、肌强直、心悸、高血压及意识水平降低。发热为高热，可引起死亡，常被误认为感染，及时治疗是存活的关键。治疗方法包括停用抗精神病药，并给予抗帕金森综合征药物、溴隐亭、丹曲林、苯二氮䓬类等药物。

4. Other Side Effects Seizures do occur in some persons with clozapine, and 1% to 2% of persons on clozapine develop bone marrow suppression, which may progress to fatal agranulocytosis. Safe use of clozapine requires weekly monitoring of white blood cell counts with permanent discontinuation if the white cell count goes below $2.0\times10^9/L$.

4. 其他副作用 某些抗精神病药物可导致惊厥，约1%～2%使用氯氮平的患者出现骨髓抑制，并进一步可发展为粒细胞缺乏症。应用氯氮平的患者，需要每周监测白细胞计数，如果白细胞低于$2.0\times10^9/L$应永久性停药。

Antipsychotic medications are frequently used in psychiatric nursing and in general medical practice. Chlorpromazine, long-acting fluphenazine, and haloperidol are included in the World Health Organization list of essential drugs for primary care. The nurse should be familiar with the indications, side effects and adverse effects of both orally administered and parenteral antipsychotics. Table 15-1 presents a summary of selected antipsychotic drugs. Although atypical neuroleptics are more costly on

抗精神病药物常用于临床治疗中，氯氮平、长效氟奋乃静和氟哌啶醇被世界卫生组织列为基本治疗的必需药物，护理工作者应熟悉抗精神病药物的适应证、副作用及不良反应，表15-1概括了抗精神病的代表药物。虽然非典型制剂比氟哌啶醇昂贵，但由于非典型药物副作用少，总的治疗费用可更少，

a per-dose basis than are agents such a haloperidol, the overall cost of treatment with atypical drugs may be less if they lead to fewer visits for the management of side effects. In many psychiatric settings the atypical neuroleptics such as risperidone and olanzapine are preferentially used as initial treatments for clients with previously untreated psychosis.

在大多数情况下，首选非典型抗精神病药如利培酮和奥氮平作为初发精神疾病患者的首选治疗。

II. Drugs for treating mood disorders

二、治疗心境障碍的药物

Drugs for treating mood disorders are used either to treat depressed mood (antidepressants) or to treat mania (mood stabilizers). While these drugs rarely act quickly and are not invariably effective, they can greatly enhance clients' well-being and useful functioning.

治疗心境障碍的药物可治疗抑郁症（抗抑郁剂）和躁狂症（心境稳定剂）。虽然这些药物作用缓慢，疗效不稳定，但可促进患者康复以及功能恢复。

i. Classification

（一）分类

Drugs for treating mood disorders generally fall into four categories: tricyclic (and related) antidepressants, selective serotonin reuptake inhibitors (SSRIs), monoamine oxidase inhibitors (MAOIs) and mood stabilizers. Each one of these categories will be discussed separately in the sections that follow. The tricyclic medications include imipramine (Tofranil), desipramine (Norpramin or Pertofrane), amitriptyline (Elavil), nortriptyline (Pamelor), clomipramine (Anafranil), trimipramine (Surontil), doxepin (Sinequan) and protriptyline (Vivactil), etc. The SSRIs include fluoxetine (Prozae), sertraline (Zoloft), paroxetine (Paxil) and fluvoxamine (Luvox), etc. The MAOIs include pheneizine (Nardil) and tranylcypromine (Parnate). Mood stabilizers include lithium and several anticonvulsants: primarily valaproic acid or divalproex (Depakote) and carbamazepine (Tegretol), etc.

治疗心境障碍药物可分为四类：三环类抗抑郁剂、选择性5-羟色胺再摄取抑制剂（selective serotonin reuptake inhibitors，SSRIs）、单胺氧化酶抑制剂（monoamine oxidase inhibitors，MAOIs）和心境稳定剂。三环类药物包括丙咪嗪、去甲丙咪嗪、多虑平、阿咪替林、马普替林、氯丙咪嗪、三甲丙咪嗪、多塞平、普罗替林等。SSRIs包括氟西汀、舍曲林、帕罗西汀和氟伏沙明等。MAOIs包括苯乙肼和吗氯贝胺。心境稳定剂包括锂盐和抗惊厥药物，如丙戊酸、二丙戊酸盐、卡马西平等。

ii. Drugs Actions

（二）药理作用

A major current theory explaining depression states that depressed individuals have persistent abnormalities in the concentration and distribution of biogenic amines that serve as neurotransmitters within the brain. Most antidepressant medications in common use exert some measurable effect on levels of brain neurotransmitters, most commonly norepinephrine and/or serotonin. The SSRIs typically have negligible effects on norepinephrine systems but are quite specific moderators of brain serotonin levels.

目前认为抑郁症的发生是由于抑郁患者大脑中作为神经递质的生物胺浓度和分布异常。大多数抗抑郁药均可影响大脑神经递质水平，多为去甲肾上腺素和/或5-HT。SSRIs对去甲肾上腺素系统作用微弱，主要是调节机体5-HT水平。

Plasma norepinephrine levels are also linked to mania, but theories about causes of mania are less well developed than those pertaining to depression. Nonetheless, lithium and other mood-stabilizing

躁狂症的发病机制尚不清楚，但认为血浆去甲肾上腺素水平与躁狂症的发生有关。锂盐和其他心境稳定药物治疗双相情感障碍

medications used in the treatment of bipolar disorder act widely in the brain and seem to affect the release of norepinephrine, serotonin and dopamine (another biogenic amine neurotransmitter).

iii. Tricyclic and Related Antidepressants

Tricyclic and related drugs were the first antidepressants to come into clinical use, and these medications still have important roles in treating mood disorders. Although many tricyclic and related antidepressants are available, there are relatively few highly significant differences among them. All of the cyclic antidepressants (tricyclic, tetracyclic,and heterocyclic) have a wide range of biochemical actions in the brain and elsewhere. These actions often result in side effects, and most choices among drugs are made in an effort to minimize such effects. These choices may be somewhat artificial since once in the body the liver modifies many of these drugs. For example, amitriptyline is converted by the liver to nortripyline, and imipramine to desipramine. In general, imipramine or amitriptyline is used when sedation is a desired side of effect, doxepine when both sedation and anxiety reduction are of primary importance, desipramine or nortriptyline when sedation is to be avoided, and protriptyline when some level of psychological stimulation is desired. Trazodone has a very different (and generally milder) spectrum of side effects when compared with tricyclic and heterocyclic antidepressants, but it may be less effective for the management of severe depression.

1. Dose/Administration Antidepressants are only given orally, are typically well absorbed, and reach peak plasma concentrations in 2 to 6 hours. Sedation and side effects of antidepressants are seen within several hours of taking these medications. Clients often report improved sleep patterns from the first night. Antidepressant effect, as with virtually all the antidepressants, is usually significantly delayed, usually for at least 4 to 6 weeks after beginning treatment. Doses are usually begun quite low and increased gradually (typically at intervals of 1 to 4 weeks) until clinical improvement occurs. Cyclic antidepressants generally have half-lives of approximately 24 hours and can usually be given once daily. The half-lives of trazodone, amoxapine, bupropion and venlafaxine are shorter, and these drugs should usually be given in divided doses. Total daily doses must be individualized based on response, side effects, and (occasionally) blood levels. Although assays for therapeutic (and toxic) blood levels are available for most of the tricyclic medications, they are of clear value only for nortriptyline, imipramine and desipramine.

的作用机制主要是影响去甲肾上腺素、5-HT和多巴胺的释放。

（三）三环类及相关抗抑郁药物

三环类及相关药物是投入临床应用的第一类抗抑郁药，这些药物在治疗心境障碍中仍起着非常重要的作用。许多三环类及相关抗抑郁药物在疗效上并无明显差别，所有环类抗抑郁药（三环类、四环类、杂环类）在大脑及其他部位都具有广泛的生物化学功能，这些功能常引起机体不良反应，应尽量选择副作用少的药物。此类药物是人工合成的，一旦进入人体，会经肝脏代谢。如阿咪替林经肝脏代谢为去甲替林，丙咪嗪代谢为去甲丙咪嗪。丙咪嗪镇静嗜睡的副作用较轻，多塞平和阿咪替林镇静抗焦虑作用强，去甲丙咪喹和去甲替林无过度镇静作用。

1. 剂量与用法 抗抑郁药物口服吸收较好，一般 2～6 小时可达到血药高峰。其镇静作用和副作用数小时内出现，患者常从用药第 1 天就可有睡眠改善。抗抑郁的作用起效缓慢，至少需 4～6 周才发挥作用。一般开始时用药剂量低，逐渐加量（1～4 周内）直到临床缓解。环类抗抑郁药半衰期大约为 24 小时，通常每日给药 1 次。阿莫沙平、曲唑酮、安非他酮和万法拉新药物半衰期短，需多次给药。每日总量应根据治疗反应、副作用及血药水平加以调整。如去甲替林每日用量不超过 100 mg，使用时应监测血药浓度，若低于 50 ng/ml 或大于 150 ng/ml 都无抗抑郁作用。其他药物的治疗量大约在 100～200 mg/d，老年人除外。一般用药量每日超过 300～350 mg 时，需监测血药浓度。在临床，需要长期维持治

Nortriptyline dose is generally 100 mg or less daily. The use of nortriptyline often requires careful monitoring of blood levels because antidepressant effects are not seen below 50 ng/ml or above 150 ng/ml. Therapeutic dosage ranges for most other medications are approximately 100 to 200 mg daily. Except in the elderly there is usually no need to measure levels until daily doses of 300 to 350 mg are exceeded. Clients with depression are commonly treated for at least 6 months. For many persons, maintenance treatment should be continued indefinitely. Those for whom long-term treatment should be considered include persons with profound depression, frequently recurring depression(two or more episodes of major depression probably justify long-term treatment), and suicidal ideation or attempts.

疗的精神疾病包括重度抑郁症、反复发作的抑郁症（两次或两次以上的抑郁发作）和有自杀观念或企图者。

2. Drug Actions Tricyclic and related antidepressants are usually, but not invariably, effective in relieving symptoms of depression. Individuals with relatively short duration of symptoms (less than a year) and with unipolar and/or melancholic depression are most likely to benefit from treatment. While some studies have suggested that trazodone is less effective than tricyclics in treating severe depression (usually defined as depression requiring hospitalization), its effectiveness for less severe forms of depression is well established. Trazodone has a significant antianxiety effect in some individuals, and this effect is often seen well before depression improves. The nurse following a client receiving trazodone may observe less reported anxiety or may observe changes in the client's appearance or reaction to stressful situations. When antidepressant effects of trazodone and the cyclic antidepressants become evident after 2 to 4 weeks, the client will report improved mood, better and more restful sleep, and gradual loss of the primary depressive symptoms of anhedonia and dysphoria.

2. 药物作用 三环类药物减轻抑郁症状效果并不稳定，仅对病程短（<1 年）和单相抑郁症患者作用效果较好。研究证明曲唑酮治疗重度抑郁症较三环类差，但对轻度抑郁症效果可靠。临床随访服用曲唑酮的患者，其焦虑症状减少，对应激状态的反应有所改善。曲唑酮和环类抗抑郁制剂服用后 2～4 周产生抗抑郁作用，此时患者常主诉：心境改善、睡眠质量好，并且快感缺乏和烦躁的症状逐渐消失。此外，三环类抗抑郁药物还可用于治疗惊恐障碍（丙咪嗪或去甲替林）、强迫症（氯丙咪嗪）和伴有妄想的抑郁症（阿莫沙平）。

3. Drug Interactions Cyclic antidepressants have a large number of potential interactions with other drugs, but most of these are of doubtful significance. Many of the cyclic drugs have significant anticholinergic side effects, and these may be enhanced to the point of toxicity by other anticholinergic drugs. This interaction is potentially most serious in the elderly and may be produced by antipsychotics, antihistamines, some general anesthetics and premedicating agents, and narcotic pain relievers, particularly meperidine. Norepinephrine may interact with some tricyclics, and even the small amount found in local anesthetics may potentially cause hypertension or arrhythmias if more than about 5 ml is

3. 药物的相互作用 环类抗抑郁剂与其他药物之间有广泛的相互作用。许多三环类药物有抗胆碱的副作用，若同时服用其他抗胆碱药物，可加重其毒性，特别是老年人。抗精神病药物、抗组胺药、麻醉剂、麻醉性镇痛药，特别是哌替啶均可使抗胆碱症状加重。去甲肾上腺素亦可与某些三环类药物相互作用，极少量（5 ml 以上）的去甲肾上腺素即可引起高血压和心律失常。虽然对口服拟交感神经药物和吸入性支气管扩张剂的安全性有质疑，但其与三环类药混用是安全的。SSRIs 和 MAOIs 可导

injected. Whereas the safety of oral sympathomimetics and inhaled bronchodilators is occasionally questioned, the combination of these medications with tricyclics seems to be safe. Tricyclic may interact significantly with SSRIs and MAOIs; these interactions may produce significant elevations of tricyclic dosages and hypertensive crises. Cimetidine, available both by prescription and over the counter, may impair metabolism of tricyclic antidepressants and lead to elevated blood levels with resultant toxicity. In addition, alcohol adds to central nervous system (CNS) depression that is produces by many antidepressant drugs (most cyclics and trazodone), and alcohol-related impairment may occur after fewer drinks in persons taking these medications.

致三环类药物浓度增加，产生高血压危象。丙咪替丁可破坏三环类药物的代谢，导致血药浓度升高引起中毒。此外，酒精可加重抗抑郁药（环类和曲唑酮）引起的中枢神经系统抑制，服用这些药物的患者即使少量饮酒，也会造成酒精性神经损害。

4. Use During Pregnancy/Lactation Cyclic antidepressants should generally not be taken during pregnancy. With the exception of maprotiline (Ludiomil), all of the cyclic drugs are classified in either risk category D (positive evidence of risk) or C (risk cannot be ruled out). The SSRIs are all in category B, though data on safety are limited. When the mother's well-being is judged to require antidepressant treatment, usually an SSRI should be used as there is enough experience with SSRIs in pregnancy to be reasonably experience with SSRIs in pregnancy to be reasonably certain that benefits outweigh risks in almost all persons.

4. **孕乳期用药** 孕期不宜服用环类药物。除马普替林外所有环类药物的危险级别均为D级（危险性确定）和C级（不排除危险性）。SSRIs归为B类。孕期抗抑郁治疗常用SSRIs，试验证明SSRIs在孕期使用利大于弊。

5. Side Effects Cyclic antidepressants act on so many different receptor systems. Many of the actions of antidepressants on receptor systems probably have little or no direct relationship to antidepressant effects, but they are responsible for most drug side effects. While each of the cyclic medications has a different side effects profile, most have some effect on each of the following receptor systems: cholinergic (also called muscarinic), histaminergic, alpha-adrenergic and dopaminergic. Anticholinergic effects include blurred vision, dry mouth, rapid heart rate, constipation, urinary retention and perhaps impaired memory function. Antihistaminic effects include weight gain, sedation, hypotension and interaction with other drugs that cause CNS depression. Alpha-adrenergic effects include postural hypotension, dizziness and potential interaction with some antihypertensive medications. Antidopaminergic effects include movement disorders and endocrine changes. Cyclic medications all have side effects in each of these categories, although desipramine and nortriptyline probably have the best side effects profile of this group of drugs. Trazodone has no anticholinergic effects, moderate alpha-adrenergic effect

5. **副作用** 环类抗抑郁药作用多种不同的受体系统，其中许多作用与抗抑郁无关或无直接关系，却产生副作用。环类药物作用的受体有：胆碱能受体（也为毒蕈碱）、组胺受体，α-肾上腺素能受体和多巴胺受体。抗胆碱作用有视物模糊、口干、心动过速、便秘、尿潴留、记忆损伤。抗组胺作用有体重增加、过度镇静、血压增高、CNS抑制。α-肾上腺素能作用有体位性低血压、头晕、与抗高血压药物有潜在的相互作用。抗多巴胺作用有运动障碍、内分泌改变以及环类药物的各种副作用。其中去甲丙咪嗪和去甲替林副作用最少。曲唑酮无抗胆碱作用，有中度α-肾上腺素能作用（体位性低血压）和极轻的抗多巴胺作用。

(typically manifested by postural hypotension), and very little antidopaminergic effects.

6. Adverse Effects The most significant adverse effects of cyclic antidepressants are seen in accidental or intentional overdose. These drugs typically have a very limited therapeutic margin, and fatal overdose may occur with ingestion of only a few days' supply. Deaths have occurred with only 1 000 mg of amitriptyline. Symptoms of overdose include CNS depression, widening of electrocardiogram (EKG) QRS complexes with associated heart block, shock, seizures and dangerous temperature elevations. Some data suggest that antidepressants may increase the risk of suicide, especially in persons with a history of impulsive or aggressive behavior. Overdose is not necessary for tricyclic-associated fatalities to occur; occasional unexplained, and presumably drug-related, deaths in children taking tricyclics continue be reported.

6. 不良反应 环类抗抑郁药的主要不良反应见于用药过量。这些药物的治疗范围极为有限，仅 1 000 mg 阿咪替林即可致死。过量的表现有 CNS 抑制、心电图 QRS 波宽大伴传导阻滞、休克、惊厥、高热。三环类药物的致死性不一定都由过量引起，有时难以解释，可能与药物有关。儿童服用三环类药物引起死亡多有报道。

Trazodone, along with most other noncyclic antidepressants, is relatively free of direct cardiac side effects and probably safer in overdose than are cyclic medications. Nonetheless, trazodone may produce severe postural hypotension. Trazodone should probably be avoided in geriatric individuals. Trazodone may rarely cause priapism (sustained and painful erection) in men. Tricyclics and occasionally other antidepressants may increase levels of the hormone prolactin. This may result in galactorrhea (leakage of mild from one or both breasts) in women and in loss of libido in both men and women. All of the cyclic antidepressants have a small chance of inducing seizures. Although remarkably free from other adverse effects, bupropion, a noncyclic antidepressant, has had a reputation of being particularly likely to produce seizures.

曲唑酮及其他非环类抗抑郁剂对心脏的副作用较环类药物少，且用药更安全，但曲唑酮可引起严重的直立性低血压，在男性偶还会引起阴茎异常勃起（持续痛性勃起）。三环类和其他抗抑郁药可增加催乳素水平，引起性欲丧失及女性溢乳。安非他酮、非环类抗抑郁药虽然没有其他副作用，也易引起癫痫发作。

iv. Selective Serotonin Reuptake Inhibitors

（四）选择性 5- 羟色胺再摄取抑制剂

In more recent years a senses of selective serotonin reuptake inhibitors (SSRIs) has come into widespread clinical use. Chief among these are fluoxetine (Prozac), sertraline (Zoloft), paroxetine (Paxil), and fluvoxamine (luvox).

选择性 5- 羟色胺再摄取抑制剂（SSRIs）由于抗抑郁效果好，短期与长期副作用都少，被广泛用于临床治疗。常用的 SSRIs 有氟西汀、舍曲林、帕罗西汀和氟伏沙明。

The SSRIs are generally regarded as first-line medications for depressed individuals, particularly outpatients with moderate depression. While studies have clearly established the effectiveness of SSRIs compared with placebo, no study has demonstrated any enhanced effectiveness of SSRIs over cyclic antidepressants. The SSRIs have been shown to be of value in a number of conditions other than depression. For example, SSRIs are clearly effective in treating obsessive-compulsive disorder;

SSRIs 是治疗抑郁的一线药物，特别适用于中度抑郁的门诊患者，安慰剂对照研究证明 SSRIs 疗效确定。除抑郁症外 SSRIs 对其他情况也适用，如氟西汀和氟伏沙明治疗强迫症效果明显。氟西汀和某些 SSRIs 可用于治疗贪食症，并对一些患者的惊恐发作有效。许多经前期综合征患者对 SSRIs 的治疗反应好。

fluoxetine and fluvixamine are well documented to be of value in this condition. Fluoxetine and several other SSRIs have been shown to improve symptoms in bulimia. Data for panic disorder are less extensive but strongly suggest a valuable effect in some individuals. Premenstrual syndrome has been shown to respond. Other data suggest benefit in a variety of other conditions, including migraine, chronic pain, and alcohol dependency/abuse.

此外，SSRIs 还可用于治疗偏头痛、慢性疼痛和酒精依赖 / 滥用。

The SSRIs inhibit the reuptake of serotonin after it is released at the neuronal synapse. This means that serotonin is present for a longer time, and as a consequence its action is augmented. SSRIs increase the effect of an individual's own serotonin release. In most persons, such an increase in serotonergic effect is enough, after a period of time to improve symptoms of depression.

SSRIs 抑制神经突触释放的 5- 羟色胺（5-HT）再摄取，使 5-HT 长期存在，引起 5-HT 作用增强。SSRIs 增加患者自身释放的 5-HT 的作用，从而引起兴奋，5-HT 的作用增强到一定水平，抑郁症状就会得到改善。

Pharmacologically the various SSRIs are strikingly different in the degree to which they inhibit reuptake of both serotonin and several other neurotransmitters. Paroxetine seems to be among the strongest inhibitors of serotonin reuptake, but it also inhibits uptake of norepinephrine and dopamine. Sertraline is a bit less potent in its inhibition of serotonin reuptake but has even more in inhibition of dopamine uptake than paroxetine. In contrast, fluvoxamine differs little from sertraline in its effects on serotonin reuptake, but it is strikingly ineffective in altering dopamine uptake. These differences among the various SSRIs are pharmacologically interesting, but there is as yet no evidence that they have any clinical importance. All of the SSRIs significantly alter serotonin effects at the synapse; the differences in their effects on other neurotransmitters so far seem relatively unimportant.

药理学上，SSRIs 抑制 5-HT 和其他神经递质再摄取的强度不同。帕罗西汀是强效 5-HT 再摄取抑制剂，同时也抑制去甲肾上腺素和多巴胺的摄取。舍曲林抑制 5-HT 再摄取作用稍弱，其抑制多巴胺摄取的作用较帕罗西汀强。氟伏沙明抑制 5-HT 再摄取的作用与舍曲林相近，但明显影响多巴胺的摄取。不同 SSRIs 间的这些差异具有药理学意义，但对临床应用意义并不大，所有 SSRIs 都显著影响突触部位 5-HT 的作用，但对其他递质的影响不大。

1. Dose/Administration The SSRIs are all absorbed after oral administration and are widely distributed throughout the body (including the brain). Dosage of SSRIs must be individualized and differs for each preparation. Compared narrow therapeutic dose "window". Blood levels of SSRIs have not been shown to be of clinical use in assessing nonresponse or toxicity. As with cyclic antidepressants, SSRIs take some time to work, typically at least a month, though some effect on depression may be seen after 10 to 14 days. Doses are rarely altered until after 3 to 4 weeks has elapsed, and there may be no benefit in raising dose for up to 8 weeks.

1. 剂量与用法 口服 SSRIs 吸收好，在全身广泛分布（包括大脑）。SSRIs 用量因人而异，与其他抗抑郁药相比，大多 SSRIs 的治疗范围很窄，临床上不能用 SSRIs 的血药浓度来估计治疗反应或中毒。多数 SSRIs 用药后 1 个月起效，有些 10～14 天即可起效。通常用药 3～4 周无效，才可增加剂量且达 8 周也不见起效。

With the exception of fluoxetine, most SSRIs have elimination half-lives of about 24 hours. Fluoxetine's elimination half-life is somewhat longer, 24 to 72 hours, but unlike other SSRIs, fluoxetine has major metabolites that themselves have half-lives of up to 15 days. This means

大多数 SSRIs 半衰期为 24 小时，氟西汀的半衰期为 24～72 小时。它的主要代谢产物的半衰期可长达 15 天。因此，临床上氟西汀作用时间相当长，停药后多日仍有明显的效果。

that in clinical use fluoxetine is uniquely long acting and has significant effects for many days after discontinuation. This characteristic is useful in preventing emergence of depressive symptoms if one or more doses are missed but may be a problem either when side effects require discontinuation or when it is necessary to switch to another medication (such as a tricyclic or an MAOIs) that may interact with fluoxetine.

这种特性虽可避免因患者漏服而引起的抑郁症状反复，却不利于终止副作用和更换药物，如三环类和 MAOIs，因为这些药物与氟西汀有相互作用。

2. Drug Actions All of the SSRIs effectively relieve symptoms of depression after 2 to 4 weeks. The SSRIs are often useful in management of Obsessive-Compulsive Disorder (though usually at higher dose than for the management of depression). As with depression, improvement of obsessive-compulsive disorder is also delayed for some weeks. Many clients with depression also report significant anxiety, a symptom that generally decreases or disappears as medication brings depression under control. Symptoms of panic disorder also tend to resolve during treatment with SSRIs, although agoraphobia, commonly seen along with Panic Disorder, is less consistently improved.

2. 药物作用 SSRIs 用药 2～4 周可有效减轻抑郁症状。大剂量 SSRIs 也常用于控制强迫症，但起效较慢，常延迟数周。焦虑症状也随抑郁的控制而减轻或消失，惊恐症状亦随治疗而消失，但伴有惊恐发作的广场恐怖症状难以改善。

3. Drug Interactions As noted below, SSRI side and adverse effects are relatively mild: consequently drug interactions are relatively less important than with many of the cyclic antidepressants. Fluvoxamine and paroxetine interact with warfarin (Coumadin). Cimetidine (Tagmet) (available over the counter as well as by prescription) may raise SSRI concentrations by impairing hepatic metabolism. Some clinicians have combined SSRIs and tricyclics in an effort to utilize the latters' sedative qualities, but this practice may not always be safe because SSRI's may raise tricyclic blood levels and increase risk of toxicity. Monoamine oxidase inhibitors may interact significantly with SSRIs, and because of relatively long elimination half-lives, at least 2 weeks should be allowed for drug washout between stopping an SSRI and staring an MAOI (5 weeks for fluoxetine).

3. 药物相互作用 SSRIs 的药物相互作用较少。氟伏沙明和帕罗西汀与华法林可相互作用。西咪替丁通过损害肝脏代谢而使 SSRIs 浓度升高。有些医生将 SSRIs 与三环类药物混用，以消除三环类药物的过度镇静作用，但常不安全，因为 SSRIs 可提高三环类药物的血管水平，增加中毒危险性。单胺氧化酶抑制剂与 SSRIs 作用显著，由于半衰期较长，SSRIs 停药后至少经 2 周（氟西汀 5 周）才可开始使用 MAOIs。

The SSRIs are less likely to increase the sedative or intoxicating potential of alcohol than are cyclic medications. Whereas sertraline absorption is affected when taken with or near meals, other SSRIs are uninfluenced by food.

与三环类药物相比，SSRIs 很少增加酒精镇静和毒性作用。除舍曲林外，进食并不影响 SSRIs 的吸收。

A rare and potentially serious drug interaction (usually with an MAOI) is called the serotonergic syndrome and resembles somewhat symptoms seen in intentional SSRI overdose. Symptoms include agitation, sweating, rigidity, fever, hyperreflexia, tachycardia, and hypotension. On occasion coma and even death may occur. The serotonergic syndrome is most commonly seen following drug interaction between an SSRI and an

5-HT 综合征是一种罕见的，潜在的严重药物相互作用，与 SSRIs 过量引起的症状相似，表现为烦躁、多汗、强直、发热、心动过速、反射亢进和高血压，偶见昏迷甚至死亡。SSRIs 与 MAOIs 间的相互作用常引起此综合征，治疗主要以支持对症为主。

MAOI. As with overdose, treatment is largely supportive.

4. Use during Pregnancy/Lactation The SSRIs are given a category B rating for pregnancy safety. Animal studies do not suggest harm, and there are no human data contraindicating use of the drug in pregnancy. These drugs do appear in breast milk in approximately the same concentration as serum. While no data suggest harm to infants from absorbing SSRIs during breastfeeding, many clinicians counsel caution in combining breast feeding and SSRI administration until long-term studies are available documenting safety for the infant.

4. 孕乳期用药 SSRIs的孕期安全性为B级，动物实验研究未显示其有害，也没有资料证明孕期禁用。药物在乳汁中浓度与血清中相近。虽然没证据表明哺乳期间SSRIs对胎儿有害，但哺乳期间SSRIs应慎用。

5. Side Effects Overall, the SSRIs are among the best-tolerated antidepressants. In short-term trials 10% to 20% of clients have discontinued SSRIs because of side effects, compared with 30% to 35% taking tricyclic medications. Common side effects include anxiety, headache, and gastrointestinal disturbance (nausea, diarrhea). The SSRIs are particularly likely to interfere with sexual functioning (erection in men and orgasm in both men and women). Clients may not volunteer that they are experiencing these side effects, so it is important for the nurse to inquire explicitly about any sexual dysfunction. Since depression is itself associated with decreased libido and sexual functioning, it may occasionally be difficult to the drug or to depression itself. The SSRIs, particularly fluoxetine, can cause akathisia, a symptom of restlessness discussed in this chapter as a side effect of antipsychotic medications.

5. 副作用 SSRIs是最易接受的抗抑郁药，在短期试验中有10%~20%的患者因为副作用而停药，而三环类药物达到30%~35%，常见的副作用有焦虑、头痛、肠胃不适（恶心、腹泻）。SSRIs可影响性功能（勃起和性高潮），患者多不愿提及此副作用，故护理工作者应仔细观察和详细询问。由于抑郁本身也引起性欲、性功能减退，有时难以确定性功能障碍是由药物引起，还是抑郁症本身引起。

6. Adverse Effects The SSRIs are generally free of serious adverse effects, even in intentional overdose. Deaths have occurred following SSRI overdoses, particularly when taken in combination with alcohol. However, death is a rare complication of SSRI overdoses, and most clients recover uneventfully with supportive care. Serotonergic syndrome, discussed earlier under drug interactions, may occasionally occur without known administration of any drug other than SSRIs. As noted earlier, symptoms include agitation, sweating, rigidity, fever, hyperreflexia, tachycardia, and hypotension. Treatment is largely supportive but must be given with vigilance to avoid a potentially fatal outcome.

6. 不良反应 SSRIs不良反应少。SSRIs过量，特别与酒精混用可致死亡，多数用药过量患者经支持治疗可完全恢复。5-HT综合征偶见于SSRIs，患者表现为烦躁、多汗、强直、发热、心动过速、反射亢进、高血压，应给予支持治疗，并警惕死亡发生。

v. Monoamine Oxidase Inhibitors (MAOIs)

Monoamine oxidase inhibitors (MAOIs) are a group of drugs notable for their similar pharmacological actions, their good effectiveness in treatment of depression, and their potentially dangerous interactions with both drugs and foods. The MAOIs are useful "second-line" drugs for treating mood disorders but can only be used safely with careful monitoring in highly motivated clients.

（五）单胺氧化酶抑制剂（MAOIs）

MAOIs能有效治疗抑郁症，是治疗心境障碍的二线药物，因与其他药物和食物间有潜在危险的相互作用，需在严格监测下使用。

1. Indications and Evidence for Effectiveness The

1. 适应证及疗效 MAOIs经证明对抑郁

MAOIs have demonstrated effectiveness in depression, Panic Disorder, some other anxiety disorders (social phobia, obsessive-compulsive disorder, post-traumatic stress disorder), and bulimia. The "classical" nonselective agents isocarboxazid (Marplan), phenelzine (Nardil), and tranylcypromine (Parnate) have generally been regarded as second-or third-line antidepressant medications, to be tried when tricyclics or SSRIs fail. A double-blind crossover study found phenelzine effective in the majority of clients who failed a trial of imipramine. Many of these clients had atypical depression, a condition for which MAOIs and SSRIs are probably more effective than are tricyclic agents. Some data suggest that dysthymia may respond more effectively to MAOIs than to tricyclic agents, but as with atypical depression, most clinicians are likely to utilize SSRIs for these individuals. Elderly clients may respond particularly well to MAOIs.

症、惊恐、焦虑障碍（社交恐惧、强迫症、创伤后应激障碍）和食欲亢进有效。经典的非选择性制剂如异唑肼、苯异肼和反苯环丙胺是公认的二线或三线抗抑郁药，用于三环类和SSRIs无效时。双盲交叉试验发现，苯乙肼对大多数丙咪嗪无效者有疗效。许多非典型抑郁症，使用MAOIs和SSRIs可能比三环类药物更有效。研究证明，MAOIs对恶劣心境的治疗效果好于三环类药物。但对非典型抑郁症，多数临床医生多选用SSRIs，老年患者对MAOIs的治疗反应特别好。

2. Pharmacology The MAOIs act by blocking an enzyme (monoamine oxidase) whose primary purpose is to metabolize three important brain neurotransmitters (norepinephrine, serotonin, dopamine) to biologically inactive forms. Over several weeks, these pharmacologists attribute the clinical usefulness of MAOIs both to this change in receptor levels and to increased amine levels. The MAOIs are commonly categorized by whether or not they fit into the following three groups: those that belong to the chemical family of "hydrazines", and those that inhibit monoamine oxidase reversibly, those that are selective for one of the two forms of monoamine oxidase: MAO-A or MAO-B. The most frequently prescribed MAOI, phenelzine (Nardil) is a hydrazine that is a nonreversible inhibitor and is nonselective. Tranylcypromine (Parnate) is a similar nonhydrazine drug. Moclobemide is both selective for MAO-A affects primarily dopamine and norepinephrine metabolism, whereas MAO-B is relatively selective for serotonin. It seems highly likely that reversible MAO-A inhibitors offer clinical advantages and will soon be available in the United States. Pure MAO-B inhibitors are not in common clinical use, and there is little evidence to suggest that selective inhibitors offer any benefit over nonselective drugs. The MAO-B inhibitor selegiline is widely used in Parkinson's disease but in Parkinsonian doses has not been found useful in treating depression.

2. **药理学** MAOIs通过抑制单胺氧化酶起作用，单胺氧化酶的主要作用是能够将脑中三种重要的神经递质（去甲肾上腺素、5-HT、多巴胺）代谢为具有生物活性的形式。单胺氧化酶通过阻止神经递质的分解，从而增加它们在神经细胞中的浓度，数周后可导致细胞表面神经递质受体数量的改变。MAOIs通常根据以下标准分为三类：① 化学结构属于肼族；② 可逆性抑制单胺氧化酶；③ 选择性抑制单氯氧化酶：MAO-A或MAO-B。常用的MAOI，苯乙肼（Nardil）属于肼族，是非可逆、非选择性抑制剂。反苯环丙胺为非肼族药物。吗氯贝胺可逆的选择性作用于MAO-A。如果存在药物与食物的相互作用时，选用可逆性抑制剂较安全。MAO-A主要影响多巴胺和去甲肾上腺素的代谢，而MAO-B选择作用于5-HT，由此可见，可逆性MAO-A抑制剂对临床应用更有利。单纯MAO-B抑制剂在临床上并不常用，且没有证据证明选择性抑制剂比非选择性抑制剂好。MAO-B抑制剂塞利吉林广泛用于治疗帕金森病，而用于帕金森病的治疗剂量对抑郁症无效。

3. Dose/Administration The MAOIs are all given orally, are well absorbed, and reach peak plasma levels within approximately 1 hour. The half-life is about 12 hours, but because most of these drugs have long-acting metabolites, at least 2 weeks should elapse between

3. **剂量与用法** MAOIs均为口服，吸收好，约1小时可达血药高峰，半衰期为12小时，由于多数药物有长效代谢产物，故更换其他药物时至少应间隔两周。MAOIs应逐渐停

stopping an MAOI and starting a different antidepressant. The MAOIs should be stopped gradually to avoid significant side effects.

药以避免副作用。

4. Drug Actions The MAOIs are used for depression of all degrees of severity. Tranylcypromine is somewhat more commonly employed in very severe depression and may have an effect sooner than other antidepressants, sometimes within 10 days. Tranylcypromine is chemically related to amphetamines (see the next general section on miscellaneous drugs for depression) and like amphetamines produces a stimulant effect that may contribute to drug effectiveness. Otherwise, like other categories of antidepressants, MAOIs take 3 to 4 weeks to improve symptoms of depression. As noted above, monoamine oxidase inhibition occurs quite rapidly, especially with irreversible inhibitors, but antidepressant effect typically takes some time to develop. This delay suggests that enzyme inhibition is only one of the effects that lead to improvement of depressive symptoms.

4. 药物作用 MAOIs用于治疗不同程度的抑郁症。苯环丙胺普遍用于重度抑郁症，起效较快（10天内）。苯环丙胺化学结构与安非他明相似，有类似的兴奋作用。与其他抗抑郁药相似，MAOIs 3～4周可改善抑郁症状。如前所述，MAOIs起效快，特别是不可逆抑制剂，但抗抑郁作用发生较慢，这种延迟说明酶抑制只是改善抑郁症状的作用机制之一。

5. Drug Interactions Significant drug interactions occur with MAOIs and may be quite serious. Since MAOIs inhibit the metabolism and severe stimulation of their analogues may result in prolonged and severe stimulation of nervous system pathways. The major drug interaction risks are other antidepressants (particularly SSRI),narcotic analgesics [especially meperidine (Demerol) and dextromethorphan, a common ingredient in nonprescription cough medications such as Robitussin-DM] , and various preparations containing sympathomimetic drugs. The latter include a variety of decongestants and cold medications. Surgery is particularly dangerous for persons on MAOIs because of the potential inadvertent administration of meperidine to control postoperative pain. The interaction between meperidine and MAOIs may result in coma, fever, and hypertension. Other drug-MAOI interactions may be dangerous and result in very high blood pressure, headache, sweating, and palpitations. Severe interactions may progress to decreased consciousness, extreme fever, intracranial hemorrhage, and death. Inadvertent medication interactions can be treated with a calcium channel blocker, typically nifedipine (Procardia). Usually a single oral dose will rapidly lower blood pressure and block the effects of drug interaction. When nifedipine is ineffective, phentolamine (Regitine) may be given intravenously. Sympathomimetic drugs pose somewhat uncertain and variable risks. In general, "direct" sympathomimetics such as epinephrine, norepinephrine, phenylephrine, isoproterenol, have the least serious interactions. "Indirect" sympathomimetics

5. 药物相互作用 MAOIs的药物相互作用显著且严重。由于MAOIs抑制生物胺的代谢和解毒，摄入胺类及类似物会延长和加重神经系统传导的兴奋性。与其他抗抑郁药（特别是SSRIs）、麻醉镇痛药和各种含有拟交感神经药物成分的制剂之间的相互作用最危险。含拟交感神经成分的药物包括各种解充血药剂和治疗感冒的药物。手术对使用MAOIs的患者特别危险，用于手术后镇痛的哌替啶与MAOIs相互作用会导致昏迷、高热、高血压。其他危险的药物与MAOIs相互作用还可导致患者出现血压过高、头痛、出汗、心悸，严重的可发展为意识不清、极度高热、颅内出血和死亡。意外的药物相互作用可应用钙离子通道阻滞治疗，心痛定口服可迅速降低血压，阻断药物间相互作用。心痛定起效后，可静脉点滴酚妥拉明。直接拟交感神经药物，如肾上腺素、去甲肾上腺素、苯福林、异丙肾上腺素与MAOIs相互作用的危险性较小，间接拟交感神经药物包括安非他明、甲基苯丙胺、麻黄素、伪麻黄碱、苯丙醇胺等，这些药物为兴奋剂或是非处方咳嗽、感冒药的普通成分。其与MAOIs相互作用的危险性较高，共同服用可出现高血压、烦躁、发热、惊厥和昏迷。

include amphetamine, methamphetamine, ephedrine, pseudoephedrine, phenylpropanolamine, and others. Many of these medications are available either as stimulant street drugs or as common ingredients in over-the-counter cough and cold treatments. Individuals on MAOIs must exercise great care to avoid these indirect sympathomimetics. Symptoms are similar to the meperidine interaction and include hypertension, agitation, fever, convulsions and coma.

6. Food and Alcohol Interactions One of the major deterrents to the use of MAOIs is that a number of foods react strongly with these medications to produce serious reactions identical to those that accompany the interaction between MAOIs and sympathomimetics or meperidine.Most offending foods contain significant amounts of the amino acid tyramine, which is an indirect sympathomimetic agent. Individuals taking MAOIs must avoid foods containing more than 6 mg of tyramine. Intake between 6 and 10 mg provokes a moderate reaction: elevated blood pressure, headache, restlessness. Ingestion of 25 mg or tyramine in a single serving, though some "strong" cheeses may have as much as 15 to 17 mg, and fairly high amounts are found in banana peels. Alcoholic beverages may interact with MAOIs, though not all experts agree on the potential seriousness of such interaction. Some imported beers have moderate tyramine concentrations. Clearly, individuals on MAOIs must be carefully instructed on avoiding risk and beverages. Selecting foods that can be safely consumed is not difficult but requires vigilance, especially when eating in restaurants. When MAOIs are prescribed, the nurse will need to assist the client in acquiring the necessary skills to avoid dangerous medication or food interactions.

6. 食物、酒精与MAOIs的相互作用 使用MAOIs的另一危险是许多食物都与MAOIs发生严重的相互作用。许多食物含有大量酪氨酸，它是一种间接拟交感神经成分，服用MAOIs者必须避免含酪氨酸超过6 mg的食物。摄入6～10 mg酪氨酸，即可引起中度反应，表现为血压升高、头痛、坐立不安；摄入量≥25 mg，会导致严重症状，甚至死亡，需急救。服用MAOIs的患者，可因饮食不慎而发生死亡。例如，浓奶酪含有酪氨酸15～17 mg，泡菜中酪氨酸含量也较高，并且发现香蕉皮中含相当多的酪氨酸。此外，含酒精性饮料，也可与MAOIs相互作用，但不是所有专家都认为这种相互作用具有潜在的危险性。因此，服用MAOIs者必须给予严格饮食指导，避免危险性食物及饮料。

7. Use during Pregnancy/Lactation The MAOIs are category C agents in pregnancy. Human data are sparse, and animal data suggest teratogenic potential for some agents. These drugs are usually avoided during pregnancy. Little data exist on use during lactation, and it is probably unwise to use these medications in lactating mothers.

7. 孕乳期用药 MAOIs为孕期C类药物，动物研究证明，有些MAOIs药物有潜在致畸作用，这些药物在孕期和哺乳期应避免使用。

8. Side Effects Common side effects of nonselective MAOIs cause decreased heart rate, hypotension (Which may lead to dizziness or syncope), and a variety of anticholinergic symptoms: dry mouth, blurred vision, and urinary hesitancy. Central nervous system symptoms occur on occasion and include agitation, anxiety, insomnia, and euphoria. Sexual dysfunction, weight gain, peripheral neuropathy, and impaired speech may sometimes occur as side effects. Newer MAOI agents such as moclobemide are remarkably generally free of

8. 副作用 非选择性MAOIs常见副作用有心率减慢、高血压（可引起头晕和晕厥）及各种抗胆碱症状，如口干、视物模糊、排尿困难。偶见中枢神经系统症状，如烦躁、焦虑、失眠、欣快。其他副作用有性功能障碍、体重增加、外周神经病、语言障碍。新型MAOIs制剂如吗氯贝胺没有上述副作用，但偶尔可引起恶心。

these side effects but may occasionally cause nausea.

9. Adverse Effects The most serious adverse effects of nonselective, nonreversible agents include syncope from hypotension, potentially resulting in physical injury and either hepatic abnormality or bone marrow suppression. Routine monitoring of liver functions or blood counts are usually not necessary. On occasion MAOIs can produce hypomania. Clients with a history of mania or hypomania should generally be placed on mood stabilizers rather than antidepressants. When selective MAO-A inhibitors are released, they will probably come into fairly widespread usage because they are generally free of serious adverse effects. Table 15-2 shows a summary of MAOIs as well as the antidepressants.

9. 不良反应 不可逆、非选择性 MAOIs 的严重不良反应包括高血压、晕厥、躯体损害、肝功能异常或骨髓抑制。MAOIs 偶会产生轻度躁狂。有躁狂或轻度躁狂病史的患者通常用心境稳定剂治疗而不用抗抑郁剂。选择性 MAO−A 抑制剂，因其没有严重的不良反应而被广泛使用。表 15−2 概括了 MAOIs 及抗抑郁剂。

Table 15−2 Antidepressant medications

GENERIC NAME	ANTI-CHOLIN-ERGIC	SEDA-TION	NOREPIN-EPHRINE ORTHO-STASIS	SERO-TONIN BLOCKING ACTIVITY	DOSE LIFE/h	RANGE/($mg\cdot d^{-1}$)
Tertiary tricyclics						
Amitriptyline	4+	4+	2+	2+	31-46	25-300
Doxepin	2+	3+	2+	11+0	8-24	25-300
Imipramine	2+	2+	3+	2+	11-25	25-300
Trimipramine	2+	3+	2+	1+	7-30	50-300
Secondary amines						
Amoxapine	3+	2+	1+	3+	8-30	50-600
Desipramine	1+	1+	1+	4+	12-24	25-300
Nortriptyline	2+	2+	1+	2+	18-44	30-100
Protriptyline	3+	1+	1+	4+	67-89	15-600
Phenethylamines						
Venlafaxine	0	0	0	3+	5-11	75-375
Tetracyclic amines						
Maprotiline	2+	2+	1+	3+	21-25	50-225
Mirtazapine	3+	2+	0	4+	20-40	15-450
Phenylpiperazines	1+	3+	3+	3+	2-4	200-600
Nefazodone	1+	3+	2+	0	4-9	150-600
Trazodone						
SSRIs						
Fluoxetine	0	0	0	1+	>72	10-800
Fluvoxamine	0	0	0	1+	16-24	50-300
Paroxetine	0	0	0	1+	10-24	10-500

continued

GENERIC NAME	ANTI-CHOLIN-ERGIC	SEDA-TION	NOREPIN-EPHRINE ORTHO-STASIS	SERO-TONIN BLOCKING ACTIVITY	DOSE LIFE/h	RANGE/($mg \cdot d^{-1}$)
Sertraline	0	0	0	1+	24	50-200
Citalopram	0	0	0	1+	16-24	40
MAOIs						
Phenelzine	0	0	0	0	6-8	45-900
Tranylcypramine	0	0	0	0	6-8	30-600
NASSAs						
Mirtazapine	0	2+	0	3+	20-40	15-45

表 15-2　抗抑郁药

通用名	抗胆碱能效应	镇静作用	去甲肾上腺素静态平衡位	5-羟色胺阻断效能	作用时间/h	剂量范围/($mg \cdot d^{-1}$)
三环抗抑郁剂						
阿咪替林	4+	4+	2+	2+	31～46	25～300
多塞平	2+	3+	2+	11+0	8～24	25～300
丙咪嗪	2+	2+	3+	2+	11～25	25～300
氯咪帕明	2+	3+	2+	1+	7～30	50～300
仲胺						
阿莫沙平	3+	2+	1+	3+	8～30	50～600
地昔帕明	1+	1+	1+	4+	12～24	25～300
去甲替林	2+	2+	1+	2+	18～44	30～100
普罗替林	3+	1+	1+	4+	67～89	15～600
苯乙胺						
文拉法辛	0	0	0	3+	5～11	75～375
四环类						
马普替林	2+	2+	1+	3+	21～25	50～225
米氮平	3+	2+	0	4+	20～40	15～450
苯基哌啶	1+	3+	3+	3+	2～4	200～600
奈法唑酮	1+	3+	2+	0	4～9	150～600
曲唑酮						
选择性 5-羟色胺再吸收抑制剂						
氟西汀	0	0	0	1+	>72	10～800
氟伏沙明	0	0	0	1+	16～24	50～300
帕罗西汀	0	0	0	1+	10～24	10～500
舍曲林	0	0	0	1+	24	50～200

续表

通用名	抗胆碱能效应	镇静作用	去甲肾上腺素静态平衡位	5-羟色胺阻断效能	作用时间/h	剂量范围/（mg·d-1）
西酞普兰	0	0	0	1+	16～24	40
单胺氧化酶抑制剂						
苯乙肼	0	0	0	0	6～8	45～900
反苯环丙胺	0	0	0	0	6～8	30～600
NASSAs						
米氮平	0	2+	0	3+	20～40	15～45

vi. Mood Stabilizers

Mood stabilizers could treat symptoms of mania and, once controlled, to prevent its recurrence. The most commonly utilized antimanic drugs are lithium, carbamazepine (Tegretol), and two very closely related drugs: valproic acid (Depakene)and divalproex (Depakote).

1. Indications and Evidence for Effectiveness Mood stabilizers are indicated for the management of mania. They can be used both to treat acute mania and to prevent the recurrence of mania in individuals who have a history of manic episodes. Antidepressants can provoke manic episodes in bipolar individuals. Prior treatment with mood stabilizers can prevent this somewhat unusual but undesirable outcome.

Numerous studies show that both divalproex and lithium are effective in the control and prevention of mania. About 80% of individuals respond to lithium, though response is typically delayed by at least 1 to 2 weeks.Lithium is generally effective in controlling depressive symptoms in individuals with Bipolar Disorder. Most of these persons do not need other antidepressants. The data for other mood stabilizers are less well established, but antimanic effects have been most convincingly shown for carbamazepine. In general, either lithium or divalproex is used as primary treatment, with the other mood stabilizers employed only if lithium fails or is not tolerated. Divalproex may, however, be particularly effective in managing adolescents with mania or hypomania. In this group of clients it may frequently be the first mood stabilizer utilized.

2. Pharmacology The neurobiology of mania is as yet incompletely understood, and perhaps as a result the precise mechanism of action of the mood stabilizers remains unknown. One of the extraordinary characteristics of lithium is that it has virtually no psychotropic effects in

（六）心境稳定剂

心境稳定剂用于控制躁狂症状及防止复发。常用的抗躁狂药物有锂盐、卡马西平、丙戊酸及二丙戊酸盐。丙戊酸和二丙戊酸盐极其相似，但后者比前者更常用。

1. 适应证及药效 心境稳定剂适用于躁狂，既可治疗躁狂急性发作，也可防止复发。抗抑郁剂可引起双相情感障碍患者的躁狂发作，而心境稳定剂则可防止躁狂发生。

大量研究表明丙戊酸和锂盐均对控制和防止躁狂发作有效。约80%的患者对锂盐有治疗反应，但作用缓慢，通常1～2周后才起效。锂盐可有效控制双相障碍患者的抑郁症状，大多不需再服用其他抗抑郁剂。研究证明，卡马西平抗躁狂效果可靠，可用于治疗特殊类型躁狂。总之，锂盐和二丙戊酸盐是基本治疗药物，只有对锂盐无效或不能耐受时，才选用其他心境稳定剂。二丙戊酸盐特别适用于治疗青少年躁狂或轻度躁狂，为首选药物。

2. 药理学 躁狂症的神经生物学机理还不完全清楚，因此，心境稳定剂的精神药理作用尚不清楚。锂盐最明显的特点是它既不是镇静剂也不是抑制剂，对非躁狂患者不产

nonmanic individuals. Lithium is neither a sedative nor a depressant drug, and it appears not to affect mood in persons who do not have mania.

生精神影响，不影响正常人的心境。

Lithium is well absorbed after an oral dose and is not metabolized in any way after absorption. Peak levels occur within 2 to 4 hours after ingestion of a single dose. Lithium is not bound to protein and is excreted almost completely by the proximal tubules of the kidney. Once in the circulation, lithium has a mean half-life of 18 hours; there is considerable range in this half-life so that lithium levels are often required to establish the appropriate dose. Individuals whose clearance of lithium is more rapid will have lower serum levels at a given dose, whereas those with slower clearance will have higher levels. Since lithium has a narrow therapeutic window (blood levels only a little above the therapeutic range may lead to serious adverse effects), blood levels can allow both effective and safe administration.

锂盐口服吸收效果好，吸收过程中不被代谢。服药后 2～4 小时达血药浓度高峰。锂盐不与蛋白质结合，可在肾脏近曲小管完全排泄。锂盐半衰期为 10～30 mg，平均为 18 小时，由于半衰期范围相当大，测定锂盐血药浓度需知道相应的剂量。清除率高的个体用药后血药水平低，清除率低者血药水平高。锂盐的治疗剂量范围很窄，血药浓度水平稍高于治疗范围即导致严重不良反应。

Carbamazepine (Tegretol) is most commonly used as an anticonvulsant but has become more widely used in the management of mania as well. Like lithium, carbamazepine is absorbed after oral dosage, but unlike lithium, it is metabolized by the liver and circulates in the plasma almost completely bound to protein. The absorption of carbamazepine is also somewhat delayed and is quite variable from individual to individual. Peak levels may not be reached until 24 hours after a dose. The half-life of carbamazepine is also variable and ranges from 10 to 20 hours in individuals who have taken the drug for some weeks. Carbamazepine has the property of inducing increased levels of the enzymes that metabolize it in the liver. As a result, the half-life is much longer in the first few days that the drug is taken of after a single dose.

卡马西平多用于抗惊厥，现在也广泛用于治疗躁狂，口服效果好，在肝脏中代谢，在血液循环中几乎完全与蛋白质结合。卡马西平的吸收稍延迟，且因人而异。用药 24 小时后才达血药浓度高峰。卡马西平半衰期不定，在 10～20 小时之间。卡马西平可增加肝脏中代谢卡马西平酶的水平，因此半衰期在开始用药的几天中较长。

Divalproex more closely resembles lithium in its absorption. Peak concentrations are reached after 1 to 4 hours, and the half-life is about 15 hours. Like carbamazepine, divalproex is strongly bound to plasma proteins and is metabolized in the liver.

二丙戊酸盐的吸收与锂盐相似。1～4 小时达到血药浓度高峰，半衰期约 15 天，与血浆蛋白牢固结合，在肝脏中代谢。

3. Dose/Administration Lithium dosage is typically 1 800 mg for acute mania and 900 to 1 200 mg total daily dose for maintenance, typically in three divided doses. All lithium administration needs to be accompanied by careful monitoring of serum levels, but this is particularly true when high doses are utilized. Lithium levels are most commonly maintained between 0.6 and 1.2 mEq/L, though levels up to 1.5 mEq/L are sometimes required for control of acute symptoms. Levels much above 1.5 mEq/L are often associated with unacceptable symptoms of toxicity such as lethargy and dizziness. Very high levels may produce EKG changes and potentially fatal

3. 剂量与用法 躁狂急性发作，锂盐每日量 1 800 mg，躁狂持续状态每日 900～1 200 mg，分三次服用。使用锂盐要监测血药水平，特别是大剂量使用时。控制急性症状的锂盐血中水平要达到 1.5 mEq/L，但通常维持在 0.6～1.2 mEq/L，高于 1.5 mEq/L 常引起嗜睡、头晕等中毒症状。极高水平可引起心电图改变和潜在致命的心脏毒性反应。卡马西平每日用药总量 400～1 200 mg，分次给药，控制惊厥需要 4～12 μg/ml，二丙戊酸盐每日用量

cardiac toxicity. Carbamazepine is administered in divided doses with a total of 400 to 1 200 mg given daily. Levels are frequently measured, and as in seizure control, the desirable levels are between 4 and 12 μg/ml. Divalproex is similarly given in doses of 500 to 1 500 mg daily to achieve levels of 50 to 100 μg/ml.

500～1 500 mg，血药水平需达到 50～100 μg/ml。

4. Drug Actions Chemically, lithium is a metallic element closely related to sodium and is chemically recognized as sodium in brain pathways. This substitution may affect the way that neurotransmitters react, and it certainly influences many of the aspects of lithium side effects and toxicity to be discussed later. Anticonvulsant drugs such as carbamazepine and divalproex (valproic acid) have effects on brain electrical functions. These effects reduce the brain's susceptibility to disorganized electrical activity, which produces seizure disorders, but their relationship to the control of mania remains incompletely understood.

4. 药物作用 锂盐是与钠相似的金属元素，在大脑通道中与钠的化学性质相同。抗惊厥药物如卡巴西平（丙戊酸盐）可影响大脑，减低大脑易感性，破坏引起惊厥的电活动。它们控制躁狂的机理尚不清楚。

5. Drug Interactions Since lithium interacts with body sodium metabolism, any drug that affects sodium levels may interact with lithium. Similarly since lithium and sodium share the same pathways for renal excretion, a low-salt diet may result in decreased lithium excretion and therefore high lithium levels. Many nonsteroidal anti-inflammatory drugs, including a variety of nonprescription medications, can affect sodium excretion and increase lithium levels. A variety of prescription anti-inflammatory drugs can have similar effects: indomethacin (Indocin), piroxicam (Feldene), and phenylbutazone (Butazolodin). Haloperidol (potentially used to treat psychosis in Bipolar Disorder) may interact to produce a dangerous encephalopathic syndrome potentially leading to permanent NCS damage. Aminophylline, less commonly used for asthma than in past years but still relatively frequently prescribed, can decrease lithium doses and precipitate manic relapse.

5. 药物相互作用 锂盐可影响体内钠的代谢，故任何影响钠水平的药物均与锂盐相互作用。由于锂和钠有相同的肾脏排泄途径，故低盐饮食会降低锂的排泄，从而提高锂的水平。许多非甾体消炎药，可影响锂的排泄，增加锂的水平，如布洛芬、酮洛芬、消炎痛、保泰松等。氟哌啶醇（用于治疗双相障碍）与锂盐相互作用可导致危险的脑病综合征，引起永久性中枢神经系统损伤。氨茶碱可降低锂盐作用，促使躁狂复发。

Carbamazepine is strongly affected by interaction with the large number of drugs that affect the liver cytochrome system. Erythromycin may specifically interact with carbamazepine and raise blood levels, leading to toxicity.

卡马西平与影响肝脏酶系统的药物之间有强烈的相互作用，如红霉素可与卡马西平相互作用，使卡马西平血药水平升高，导致中毒。

Since divalproex and valproic acid are also metabolized by the liver, they have a number of potential interactions that may be of clinical importance. Each prolongs anticoagulant effects in clients treated with Coumadin and increases the effects of MAOIs.

由于二丙戊酸盐和丙戊酸都经肝脏代谢，它们有许多潜在的相互作用在临床上有重要意义。它们均能延长肝素的抗凝效果，并增强 MAOIs 的作用。

6. Use during Pregnancy/Lactation Lithium is potentially cardiotoxic and is usually not advised during pregnancy. Lithium teratogenicity is probably limited to

6. 孕乳期用药 锂盐有潜在心脏毒性，不提倡在孕期服用，锂盐在怀孕前三个月可导致胎儿畸形。卡马西平和二丙戊酸盐在怀孕早期的危险性相对较低，有时用来代替锂

the first trimester. Carbamazepine and divalproex may have less risk during early pregnancy and are sometimes substituted for lithium. The management of mania during pregnancy is a difficult problem that should be undertaken with expert consultation.

盐。但注意治疗孕期躁狂，应在专家指导下进行。

7. Side Effects Lithium has a spectrum of side effects of that are often troubling to clients. Almost everyone who takes this medication develops thirst and polyuria because of the effect of lithium on the kidney. Another very common side effect is tremor, most noticeable in fine motor activities such as writing, buttoning clothes, and sewing. Weight gain is less common but does occur in up to 30% of individuals. A smaller percentage of persons experience chronic diarrhea, which can also be an early sign of toxicity and, when of recent onset, requires that blood levels be measured immediately. The nurse can assist clients to distinguish between nuisance side effects and those that, like diarrhea, can be warning signs for more serious adverse effects. Thyroid enlargement and even frank hypothyroidism may occur in persons taking lithium. Thyroid abnormality is less common than other side effects but does occasionally occur and may require treatment. Most individuals on lithium should have periodic measurements of their thyroid function [usually thyroid-stimulating hormone (TSH)].

7. 副作用 锂盐常见的副作用包括口渴、多尿，以及手抖，特别在精细运动时最明显，如写字、钉纽扣、缝纫。有30%的人体重增加，少部分人还可发生慢性腹泻。此外，服用锂盐还可发生甲状腺肿或明显的甲状腺功能减退。甲状腺异常较其他副作用少见，服用锂盐者应定期测定甲状腺的功能（常用TSH）。

Carbamazepine is generally tolerated than lithium, although occasionally individuals may have dizziness, and drowsiness occurs,at least initially. Unfortunately, carbamazepine may seriously affect bone marrow function and occasionally, liver enzymes. Fatal agranulocytosis (loss of all functioning polymorphonuclear white blood cells) may result if blood counts are not carefully monitored. Agranulocytosis leads to serious infections and may not infrequently prove fatal. Persons beginning carbamazepine treatment generally require frequent (usually weekly) testing of blood counts and often of live enzymes as well. The frequency of testing may decrease if results remain normal over time.

卡马西平比锂盐易于耐受，偶尔会引起头晕，早期常发生嗜睡。卡马西平可严重影响骨髓功能及肝脏酶系统。可引起致死性粒细胞缺乏症（多形棱白细胞功能丧失）。粒细胞缺乏症可导致严重感染，甚至死亡。用卡马西平，要求每周一次检查血细胞数并经常检查肝功能。结果维持正常时，可减少检查次数。

Divalproex is generally very tolerated but has very rarely been associated with fatal liver damage. Individuals on divalproex need careful monitoring of liver functions to help avoid this catastrophic outcome. The nurse can assist clients to remember to get needed blood testing and to be alert for symptoms (loss of appetite, darkened urine, lightened stool, yellow colour to skin, profound fatigue) that may indicate impending liver failure. Lamotrigine has relatively few common side effects, but it is occasionally associated with Steve Johnson Syndrome, a potentially fatal allergic skin condition. Persons taking this medication

二丙戊酸盐易于接受，但可引起致命的肝脏损害。服用二丙戊酸盐需密切监测肝功能以防止发生危险。护理工作者应提醒患者做必要的血液检查，警惕肝脏衰竭的先兆症状（食欲减退、尿黄、柏油便、黄染、疲倦）。

should be instructed to stop it if they have any unusual skin rash or develop sores in their mouth.

8. Adverse Effects Divalproex and carbamazepine are relatively safer in overdose and with inadvertent high blood levels than is lithium. Lithium toxicity may be fatal as a result of cardiac arrhythmias. Individuals on lithium need to be alert for situations in which they may lose excess sodium, as in heavy sweating (such as occurs with vigorous physical exercise). Under such conditions, lithium toxicity may occur without any change in lithium intake. As noted previously, drug interactions (including interactions with drugs commonly available without prescription) may also result in dangerously high lithium levels.

8. **不良反应** 二丙戊酸盐和卡马西平服用过量及血药水平偶然升高的危险性比锂盐低。锂中毒引起的心律失常可导致死亡。服用锂盐者应警惕大量出汗所造成钠盐的大量丧失，因为，在这种情况下，即便没有增加锂盐的摄入量仍会导致锂中毒。

III. Drugs for Treating Anxiety and Sleep Disorders

Symptoms of anxiety and insomnia are most commonly treated with benzodiazepines. Other medications of nonbenzodiazepines useful on occasion include buspirone for generalized anxiety, antidepressants for panic disorder and social phobia, beta blockers for performance anxiety, and a variety of agents for insomnia. Antihistamines, antidepressants, barbiturates, and antipsychotics are sometimes prescribed for anxiety (table 15-3).

三、治疗焦虑和睡眠障碍的药物

苯二氮䓬类是治疗焦虑和失眠的常用药物。有时也使用其他非苯二氮䓬类药物，如丁螺环酮用于治疗广泛性焦虑，抗抑郁剂用于治疗惊恐发作和社交恐怖，β-受体阻滞剂用于治疗表演性焦虑，以及各种治疗失眠的药物。此外，抗组胺药、抗抑郁剂、巴比妥酸盐和抗精神病药有时用于治疗焦虑（表 15-3）。

Table 15-3 Drugs for treating anxiety and sleep disorders

GENERIC NAME	CLINICAL USES	DOSE LIFE/h	RANGE/($mg \cdot d^{-1}$)
Benzodiazepines			
Diazepam	anxiety, insomnia	30-60	5-15
Clordiazepoxide	anxiety, insomnia	30-60	5-30
Fludiazepam	insomnia	50-100	15-30
Clonazepam	anxiety, insomnia, mania	20-40	2-8
Alprazolam	anxiety, insomnia, depression	6-20	0.8-2.4
Estazolam	anxiety, insomnia	10-24	2-6
Lorazepam	anxiety, insomnia	10-20	1-6
Oxazepam	anxiety, insomnia	6-24	30-90
Midazolam	insomnia	2-5	15-30
Nonbenzodiazepines			
Buspirone	anxiety	2.5	15-45
Zolpidem	insomnia	3	5-20
Zopiclone	insomnia	6	7.5-15

表 15-3 抗焦虑及睡眠障碍药物

通用名	临床应用	作用时间 / 小时	剂量范围 / (mg·d⁻¹)
苯二氮䓬类			
地西泮	焦虑，失眠	30～60	5～15
利眠宁	焦虑，失眠	30～60	5～30
氟西泮	失眠	50～100	15～30
氯硝西泮	焦虑，失眠，躁狂	20～40	2～8
阿普唑仑	焦虑，失眠，抑郁	6～20	0.8～2.4
艾司唑仑	焦虑，失眠	10～24	2～6
劳拉西泮	焦虑，失眠	10～20	1～6
奥沙西泮	焦虑，失眠	6～24	30～90
咪达唑仑	失眠	2～5	15～30
非苯二氮䓬类			
丁螺环酮	焦虑	2.5	15～45
唑吡坦	失眠	3	5～20
佐匹克隆	失眠	6	7.5～15

i. Indications and Evidence for Effectiveness

While they have many clinical uses, benzodiazepines have been most distinctly shown to be effective for generalized anxiety, panic disorder and insomnia .Although all benzodiazepines may be equally effective for Panic Disorder, alprazolam (Xanax) was the first benzodiazepine approved for this treatment. There is no evidence that any other similar medication is more effective, but fairly high alprazolam doses are required. Clinicians may use long half-life drugs [diazepam (Valium)] when daily administration is required but may prefer relatively shorter half-lives (i.e., lorazepam [Ativan]) when clients are more likely to benefit from intermittent symptom-driven treatment. The selection of hypnotic medications was discussed above and requires balancing onset of action, morning drowsiness,and rebound insomnia. Triazolam (Halcion) is particularly likely to produce rebound and may result in amnesia.

（一）适应证及疗效

苯二氮䓬类对失眠、广泛性焦虑和惊恐发作特别有效。各种苯二氮䓬类药物对惊恐发作的疗效相同，以阿普唑仑首选，并需大剂量使用。当需要每天用药时医生多选用半衰期长的药物如地西泮，但当间断去除症状治疗对患者有利时，应选用半衰期短的药物如劳拉西泮等。选择安眠药应考虑它的起效时间、嗜睡作用、失眠反跳等因素，如三唑仑容易引起反跳和遗忘。

ii. Pharmacology

The clinical effectiveness of benzodiazepines was first discovered in the mid-1950s. These medications have been in wide use since and remain among the most commonly prescribed drugs. Benzodiazepines are frequently diverted to street sales and are readily available for illicit purchase. Benzodiazepines may produce dependence and are not infrequently chosen as drugs of abuse, particularly in combinations with

（二）药理学

苯二氮䓬类的临床疗效发现于 20 世纪 50 年代中期，是广泛应用的处方药。苯二氮䓬类药物可引起依赖和药物滥用，特别是与其他药物混用时（如酒精）。研究证明，哺乳动物大脑中存在苯二氮䓬受体，这种受体与抑制性神经递质γ-氨基丁酸（GABA）关系密切。苯二氮䓬可增强 GABA 的作用，也可单独

other agents (including alcohol). Subsequent research has shown that there is a benzodiazepine receptor in the mammalian brain and that this receptor is closely tied to the inhibitory neurotransmitter gamma aminobutyric acid (GABA). Benzodiazepines may increase the effectiveness of GABA but may also act separately by affecting brain metabolism of serotonin and norepinephrine. Zolpidem is a nonbenzodiazepine drug that nonetheless binds to benzodiazepine receptors and produces sleep induction with little effect on anxiety.

影响大脑5-HT和去甲肾上腺素的代谢。唑吡坦为非苯二氮䓬类药物，但仍可与苯二氮䓬受体结合，虽可诱导睡眠，但无抗焦虑作用。

Barbiturates, now primarily used for anesthesia induction and seizure control, also augment brain GABA inhibitory effects but through a somewhat different molecular mechanism than that of benzodiazepines. Alcohol probably also exerts its anxiolytic and sedative effects, at least in part through enhancement of GABA transmission.

巴比妥酸盐主要的作用是诱导麻醉和控制惊厥，也增强大脑GABA的抑制作用，但其与苯二氮䓬的分子机理不同。酒精通过增加GABA的传递而产生抗焦虑和镇静作用。

All the benzodiazepines are readily absorbed after oral administration and often reach peak levels within an hour or less. Diazepam (Valium) acts particularly quickly after oral administration. Lorazepam and midazolam (Versed) can be given intramuscularly, and diazepam is frequently given intravenously (most commonly for seizures, but occasionally for anxiety). Nearly a dozen benzodiazepines are available for clinical use, and these vary most significantly in their half-lives. Triazolam, for example, has a half-life of only 6 hours and no clinically significant metabolites. As a result, triazolam is classified as a short-acting benzodiazepine. In contrast, diazepam has both a long half-life (nearly 24 hours)and active metabolites with similar long half-lives. The effect of metabolites can be quite important: flurazepam (Dalmane) itself has quite a short half-life (2 to 3 hours),but its major metabolite has a half-life of more than 2 days. As a result, this commonly used medication may prolong daytime drowsiness when used for treating insomnia.

所有苯二氮䓬类药物口服易吸收，1小时内达药物高峰。地西泮口服起效特别快。劳拉西泮和咪达唑仑可肌肉注射，地西泮多静脉点滴，多用于治疗惊厥，偶用于治疗焦虑。临床上使用的苯二氮䓬类药物约十几种，半衰期各不相同。例如，三唑仑半衰期仅6小时，其代谢产物无临床作用，故归为短效苯二氮䓬药。而地西泮半衰期近24小时，其活性代谢产物也有同样长的半衰期，并且有相当重要的作用。氟西泮本身半衰期很短，仅2～3小时，但主要代谢产物半衰期超过2天，可用于治疗失眠，延长白天睡眠时间。

iii. Dose/Administration

Benzodiazepine doses are quite specific for the individual drugs chosen and vary over a rather wide range. Alprazolam (short to intermediate half-life) and clonazepam (long half-life) are perhaps the two most commonly used benzodiazepine medications for treating anxiety. Alprazolam (Ativan) daily doses range from 0.75 to 8 mg daily, with a common range of 1.5 to 3 mg. Clonazepam (Klonopin) is generally given in a dosage range of 1.5 to 10 mg daily.

（三）剂量与用法

苯二氮䓬类用药剂量范围广，并且因人而异。阿普唑仑（中、短半衰期）和氯硝西泮（长半衰期）是用于治疗焦虑最常用的苯二氮䓬类药物。阿普唑仑每日用量0.75～8 mg，通常为1.5～3 mg，氯硝西泮每日用量为1.5～10 mg。

iv. Drug Actions

Benzodiazepine exerts a significant effect on GABA-ergic CNS pathways and produce both sedation and a

（四）药物作用

苯二氮䓬类主要作用于GABA的中枢神经系统通路，产生镇静，并且能明显减

marked decrease in subjective anxiety. These drugs induce sleep, decrease frequency of awakenings, slightly decrease rapid eye movement (REM) sleep, and moderately decrease slow-wave or deep Stage Ⅲ to Ⅳ sleep. Individuals who take benzodiazepines for sleep generally report an increased subjective sense of sleep quality. Sleep latency (the time to fall asleep) is significantly deceased by short half-life benzodiazepines such as triazolam, but these medications frequently produce rebound insomnia on subsequent nights. Longer half-life benzodiazepines take somewhat longer to produce sleep and cause some hangover the next day. Temazepam (Restoril) is a commonly prescribed hypnotic medication with an intermediate half-life and an onset of action within 2 to 3 hours.

轻主观性焦虑，这些药物引起睡眠，减少觉醒次数，服用苯二氮䓬类者主诉睡眠质量提高。短半衰期苯二氮䓬类如三唑仑可明显缩短睡眠潜伏期（进入睡眠的时间），但常可引起失眠反跳。长半衰期苯二氮䓬起效慢，但作用可延续至第二天。羟基安定是常用的中半衰期安眠药，起效时间为 2～3 小时。

v. Drug and Food Interactions

There are few benzodiazepine drug interactions of clinical significance. Alcohol is additive with the sedative effects of benzodiazepines and will produce increased drowsiness if taken along with these medications. The combination of alcohol and large amounts of benzodiazepines can produce fatal respiratory depression and coma.

（五）药物与食物的相互作用

临床上苯二氮䓬类药物的相互作用不多。酒精增加苯二氮䓬的镇静作用，如果与其同服会加重嗜睡，如与大量苯二氮䓬混用，会导致致命的呼吸衰竭和昏迷。

vi. Use during Pregnancy/Lactation

There is little firm data on which to base recommendations for benzodiazepine use during pregnancy. Alcohol and barbiturates clearly cause fetal damage. Only clonazepam is placed in pregnancy category C: Potential benefits may justify potential risk. Other benzodiazepines are in category D and are contraindicated during pregnancy. Risks during breast feeding are likely smaller, and in contrast to many other psychiatric medications, lower drug concentrations are found in milk than in plasma; consequently benzodiazepines are generally accepted as safe in lactating mothers.

（六）孕乳期用药

孕期不主张使用苯二氮䓬类药物。酒精和苯二氮䓬混用可明显伤害胎儿。只有氯硝西泮归为孕期 C 类药物，其他苯二氮䓬药物均属于 D 类孕期禁用。哺乳期危险性较小，与其他精神药物比较，苯二氮䓬在乳汁中的浓度比血中的低，故哺乳期用药较安全。

vii. Side Effects

Benzodiazepine's side effects are largely limited to sedation, interference with safe driving, and occasional amnesia.

（七）副作用

苯二氮䓬的副作用仅有过度镇静，影响安全驾驶及遗忘。

viii. Adverse Effects

Severe adverse effects are rare, even in intentional overdose. Deaths have occurred in combination with alcohol and other substances but are unusual. The major adverse effects of benzodiazepines involve physical dependence. When given these medications over prolonged periods, many individuals have symptoms of increased anxiety and, rarely, seizures on abrupt withdrawal. Withdrawal should be accomplished slowly over several weeks.

（八）不良反应

严重的不良反应少见，若与酒精和其他物质混用可引起死亡，但不常见。主要的不良反应有躯体依赖，长期服用的患者可出现焦虑加重，以及突然停药诱发惊厥发作。因此，应在几周内逐渐停药。

ix. Nonbenzodiazepine Drugs for Anxiety and Sleep Disorders

While the benzodiazepines are widely used for management of anxiety and insomnia, they are not the only medications of value for treating these conditions. Buspirone (BuSpar) is a unique antianxiety agent that has no effects on the benzodiazepine-GABA receptor. As a consequence, it produces relies of anxiety with virtually no sedation. Zolpidem (Ambien) does act on the benzodiazepine receptor, but it does not have the chemical structure of a benzodiazepine. As a consequence, zolpidem produces only sedation; it does not provide any relief from anxiety. Propranolol(Inderal),a beta blocker, has little demonstrated effect on anxiety, but it has proved useful when performance anxiety produces physical symptoms such as tremor or difficulty speaking. Administration of propranolol prior to activities such as public speaking or playing a musical instrument can sometimes improve performance by reducing tremor or other manifestations of nervousness. There is some limited role for beta blockers in other anxiety disorders. Antidepressants (and very rarely antipsychotics) can sometimes be helpful for control of anxiety or insomnia. As noted previously, trazodone seems particularly anxiolytic and is often used to combat onset insomnia in anxious and/or depressed individuals.

（九）抗焦虑和治疗睡眠障碍的非苯二氮䓬类药物

一些非苯二氮䓬类药物亦可用于治疗焦虑和失眠，例如，丁螺环酮是唯一一种不影响苯二氮䓬—GABA 受体的抗焦虑药，它可减轻焦虑，但不引起镇静嗜睡。唑吡坦虽作用于苯二氮䓬受体，但与苯二氮䓬化学结构不同，只引起镇静嗜睡而不减轻焦虑。普诺奈尔是一种 β 受体阻滞剂，可用于治疗表演性焦虑引起的躯体症状，如手抖或说话困难，但对其他焦虑障碍作用有限。此外，抗抑郁剂也有助于控制焦虑或失眠，如曲唑酮常用于治疗焦虑和 / 或抑郁症的失眠症状。

Section 3 Nursing Care of Clients with Psychiatric Medication

The main purpose of psychiatric drug therapy is to control clients' psychiatric symptoms, so before using medication, nurses should collect client's date, as a criterion to evaluate whether client's symptoms has improved. In the process of psychiatric drug therapy, nurses should also observe the effect of drug, identify side effect immediately and judge client's compliance of the medication, accordingly nurses can take corresponded measurement to insure effectiveness and durability of the drug.

I. Nursing Assessment

1. Drug Compliance Include the client's attitude towards drug therapy, whether understand the relationship between taking medication and illness, whether reject taking medication or hiding medication.

第三节 使用精神药物患者的护理

精神药物治疗的主要作用是控制患者的精神症状，因此在使用药物之前，护理人员应收集患者的相关资料，作为患者用药前后症状是否改善的评判依据。在药物治疗过程中，还应观察患者用药效果，及时识别药物不良反应，判断患者用药的依从性，从而采取相应的护理措施，保证药物治疗的有效性和持久性。

一、护理评估

1. 药物依从性评估 包括患者对药物治疗的态度，是否了解服药与疾病的关系，有无拒绝服药、藏药行为。患者有无影响治疗

Whether have psychiatric symptoms that will affect compliance, such as auditory hallucination, delusion etc. Belief that client and his relevant will take medication continuous.

依从性的精神症状，如幻听、妄想等。患者及家属对坚持服药的信心。

2. Physiological State Include the client's conscious state, nutritional state, eating state, sleeping quality, excretion and activity etc.

2. **生理状况评估** 包括患者的意识状态、营养状况、进食、睡眠、排泄及活动等情况。

3. Mental State Include the client's present psychiatric symptoms, severity, sustained degree, whether have insight, and how the damage degree of insight is.

3. **精神状况评估** 包括患者现存的精神症状、严重程度及持续时间，有无自知力及自知力受损程度。

4. Social Support Include the client's status at home, whether the relationship between families is harmonious, client's economic state, culture background and education level.

4. **社会支持评估** 包括患者在家中的地位及与家庭成员之间的关系是否融洽，患者经济状况、文化背景、受教育程度等。

BOX 15-2 Learning More

Common Manifestations of Poor Medication Compliance in Clients with Mental Illness

The poor medication compliance in psychiatric clients not only delays the condition but also brings difficulty in clinical treatment. Meanwhile, poor compliance is one of the major cause of relapse in psychiatric clients. The common manifestations of poor medication compliance includes the following aspects:

1. Refusing to take medicine on his/her own initiative: Refuse orally or vomit. Clients keep mouth closing after taking medicine or making threats.
2. Refusing to take medicine passively: clients forget or hesitate to take medicine, and do not swallow.
3. Excessive use of drugs. Clients often ask for drugs or take medicine excessively. And they may take medicine without permit or hide side-effect of drugs.

BOX 15-2 知识拓展

精神疾病患者服药依从性不良的常见表现

很多精神疾病患者服药依从性差，不仅延误病情，而且给临床治疗带来较大困难。同时，服药依从性不良也是精神疾病患者病情复发的主要诱因之一。服药依从性不良的常见表现如下：

1. 主动拒绝服药　口头直接拒绝、吐药、服药后闭紧嘴巴或提出恐吓。
2. 被动拒绝服药　忘记服药，服药时磨蹭或将药物含于口中而不咽下。
3. 过度用药　经常要求给予药物，经常服用过量药物，不经询问即服下药物，不诉说药物的不良反应等。

II. Diagnosis/Outcome Identification

二、护理诊断 / 护理目标

i. Nursing diagnosis related to medication includes:

1. Behavior disorder/ noncooperation are related to auditory hallucination, delusion, lacking of self insight, not able to tolerate side effect from psychiatric drug's and fear of side effect.

2. Sanitation/ feeding/ self excretion disorder are related to drug's inhibition of central never system and adverse effect.

3. Change of sleep pattern is related to excess sedative effect or stimulant effect of drug.

1. 护理诊断

（1）遵医行为障碍 / 不合作　与幻听、妄想、自知力缺乏、拒绝服药或不能耐受精神药物不良反应、对药物不良反应产生恐惧等因素有关。

（2）卫生 / 进食 / 如厕自理缺陷　与药物对中枢神经的抑制和药物不良反应有关。

（3）睡眠型态改变　与药物过度镇静或兴奋等作用有关。

4. Risk of injury is related to postural hypotension, instability of gait, stiff limbs, slow action, confusion etc. adverse effect.

ii. Nursing Goal

1.Clients can cooperate with treatment, take proper medication, elevate treatment compliance.

2. Clients retain basic self-care ability.

3. Clients can take medication willingly, improve sleeping pattern and quality.

4. Clients are able to prevent and reduce accident.

（4）有受伤的危险　与直立性低血压、步态不稳、肢体僵硬、行动迟缓、意识混乱等不良反应有关。

2. 护理目标

（1）患者能配合治疗，正确服药，提高治疗依从性。

（2）患者能恢复基本的生活自理能力。

（3）患者能主动服药，改善睡眠型态，提高睡眠质量。

（4）患者能预防和减少意外事故的发生。

III. Nursing Intervention

1. Establishing a good relationship between nurses and clients as well as improving clients' treatment compliance, of which is the safeguard measure has to be taken in the drug treatment process.

2. Strict implementation of medication system need to be used to ensure medications put in plans. Nurse should implement strictly 3-inspections-7-verifications before dispensing, and choose the correct administration route while dispensing. In order to prevent hiding and vomiting behaviors, nurse have to make sure "three arrivals" (hands, mouth, stomach). Reasons and chemical incompatibility for drug using should be known when nurse use multiple drugs. At the same time, nurse should explain destination, ways, and matters needing attention of the drug to clients and family.

3. Careful observation and adverse reaction handling. Watching reaction of clients closely which includes drug effects and side-effect. Assessing symptoms and behaviors of clients objectively, and paying more attention to mental situation as well as body signs of clients. Serious cardiovascular adverse reactions, neuroleptic malignant syndrome, etc should be on alert.

4. Satisfying normal physiological needs of clients in the basic nursing process of strengthening drug treatment. Due to adverse drug reaction in clients with dysphasia should pay attention to choking and not to eat food with bone. If necessary, hand feeding, intravenous nutritional supplement should be given. Clients in urinary retention and constipation should be processed in a timely manner. For orthostatic hypotension and disabled clients, nurse should direct them to exercise slowly or give assistance if necessary.

5. Do a real detailed and objective nursing record.

三、护理措施

1. 建立良好的护患关系，提高患者治疗的依从性　这是药物治疗过程中必须首选采取的保障措施。

2. 严格执行服药制度，保证药物治疗落实到位　发药前严格执行三查七对制度，发药时使用正确给药途径与方法，做到三到（到手、到口、到胃），防止藏药、吐药等行为影响治疗或蓄积顿服。同时使用多种药物时，应了解用药的原因，注意药物间的配伍禁忌。并向家属及患者讲解药物治疗的目的、方法和注意事项。

3. 仔细观察与处理用药后的不良反应　用药后应密切观察患者的反应，包括用药的效果及不良反应。客观评估患者的症状与行为，重视患者的精神症状和躯体症状。对严重心血管系统的不良反应、恶性综合征等应高度警惕，并采取相应的处理措施。

4. 加强药物治疗过程中的基础护理，满足患者正常的生理需要　因药物不良反应吞咽困难的患者应注意噎食，避免进食有骨头的食物，必要时专人喂食、鼻饲或静脉补充营养。对尿潴留及便秘的患者应及时处理。对直立性低血压、运动不能的患者应注意指导患者活动或起床时动作要慢，必要时给予协助，防跌伤。

5. 作好护理记录　真实、详细、客观地

Analyze reasons for poor treatment compliance and give doctors feedback timely, so that doctors can adjust administration according to specific condition of clients.

6. Good guidance for medication and health. Make drug rehabilitation and medication knowledge are understood by clients and their family, which includes drug dosage storage method and general methods of observation as well as treatment of adverse reaction.

作好护理记录，分析患者治疗依从性差的原因，并及时反馈给医生，以便医生针对患者的具体情况调整药物治疗方案。

6. **作好用药与健康指导** 让患者及家属了解药物对疾病康复的作用和用药知识，包括药物服用方法、用量、保管方法以及一般不良反应的观察和处理方法。

IV. Evaluation

Evaluation includes the following aspects:

1. Whether clients are conscious about own health state, and whether can tie in treatment and drugs.

2. Whether clients make progress on ability of daily life and activities of clients.

3. Whether clients occur insomnia, and have a well sleep-wake cycle.

4. Whether clients have accidents, for example, falling.

(Wang Zaichao)

四、护理评价

护理评价包括：

1. 患者自身对健康问题是否有所认识，能否配合治疗，并能按医嘱服药。

2. 患者生活自理能力和日常活动是否有所改善。

3. 患者有无失眠，其睡眠－醒觉周期是否恢复正常，并能正常作息。

4. 患者有无跌倒等意外发生。

（王再超）

Key Points

1. Therapeutic options expanded rapidly beginning in the mid-20th century. While some kinds of drugs now in modern use were discovered or synthesized prior to the mid-20th century, virtually all the studies establishing modern drug effectiveness were carried out after 1950.

2. The potential effects of any drug are a complex balance of each of these factors: absorption, distribution, elimination, and metabolism. Another term for this balance is pharmacokinetics. In most cases, the goal of drug administration is the achievement of a "steady" pharmacokinetic state (often called steady state) in which the amount of drug absorbed is constantly balanced by the competing processes of distribution, elimination, and metabolism.

3. Antipsychotic drugs, also called "major tranquilizers" are administered to control the symptoms of psychosis such as hallucinations and bizarre or paranoid behavior. These drugs tend to produce a calming effect without significantly sedating the client or reducing alertness. A number of antipsychotic medications are considered in this section. There are nearly 20 antipsychotic drugs in clinical use.

内容摘要

1. 20世纪中期，开始了精神药物的研究，精神疾病的治疗方法迅速增多。

2. 当药物的吸收、分布、代谢、清除各因素达到平衡状态时，药物可发挥最大效应，将药物在机体的吸收、分布、代谢及清除过程称为药物动力学。多数情况下，给药的目的在于达到稳定的药物动力学状态，称为稳态，即药物的吸收量在机体的分布、清除和代谢过程中保持恒定。

3. 抗精神病药物也称“强安定剂”，用于控制精神病症状，如幻觉、怪异或偏执行为。这些药物可使患者平静，且不伴有明显的过度镇静或降低警觉的作用。大部分抗精神分裂症药属于此类。

4. Drugs for treating mood disorders are used either to treat depressed mood (antidepressants) or to treat mania (mood stabilizers), which generally fall into four categories: tricyclic (and related) antidepressants, SSRIs, monoamine oxidase inhibitors (MAOIs), and mood stabilizers.

4. 治疗心境障碍的药物可治疗抑郁症（抗抑郁剂）和躁狂（心境稳定剂），可分为四类：三环类抗抑郁剂，选择性5-羟色胺再摄取抑制剂（SSRIs），单胺氧化酶抑制剂（MAOIs）和心境稳定剂。虽然这些药物作用缓慢，疗效不稳定，但可促进患者康复以及功能恢复。

5. Symptoms of anxiety and insomnia are most commonly treated with benzodiazepines. Other medications of nonbenzodiazepines useful on occasion include buspirone, beta blockers et al.

5. 苯二氮䓬类是治疗焦虑和失眠的常用药物，有时也使用其他非苯二氮䓬类药物，如丁螺环酮、β-受体阻滞剂等。

6. Before using medication, nurses should collect client's date, as a criterion to evaluate whether client's symptoms has improved. In the process of psychiatric drug therapy, nurses should also observe the effect of drug, identify side effect immediately and judge client's compliance of the medication, accordingly nurses can take corresponded measurement to insure effectiveness and durability of the drug.

6. 在使用精神药物之前，护理人员应收集患者的相关资料，作为患者用药前后症状是否改善的评判依据。在药物治疗过程中，还应观察患者用药效果，及时识别药物不良反应，判断患者用药的依从性，从而采取相应的护理措施，保证药物治疗的有效性和持久性。

7. In the process of using psychiatric drug，the mainly measures include are following aspects: Establishing a good relationship between nurses and clients; Strict implementation of medication system need to be used to ensure medications put in plans; Careful observation and adverse reaction handling; Satisfying normal physiological needs of clients in the basic nursing process of strengthening drug treatment; Do a real detailed and objective nursing record; Good guidance for medication and health, etc.

7. 应用精神药物的过程中，主要的护理措施包括建立良好的护患关系，提高患者治疗的依从性；严格执行服药制度，保证药物治疗落实到位；仔细观察与处理用药后的不良反应；加强药物治疗过程中的基础护理，满足患者正常的生理需要；作好护理记录，作好用药与健康指导等方面。

Exercises

(Questions 1 to 2 share the same question stem)

A 24-year-old man, who was at acute episode of schizophrenia, had a series of symptoms, such as fever (maximum temperature of 39.4 degrees Celsius), consciousness disorder, with muscle stiffness, breathing difficulties, etc. after 2 days he took Haloperidol.

1. What kind of side effect may the client appear ?
2. What kinds of the measures should be taken by nurses?

(Questions 3 to 4 share the same question stem)

A 45-year-old woman, who suffered from bipolar disorder, is currently in a stage of mania without psychotic symptoms and taking lithium carbonate 0.5 g, 3 times a day for treatment. Having taken 2 months, she appeared nausea, vomiting, diarrhea, blurred vision, two hands tremor and other symptoms.

思考题

（1～2题共用题干）

患者，男，24岁，精神分裂症急性发作，服用氟哌定醇2天后，出现发热（最高体温39.4℃），意识障碍，伴肌肉僵硬、呼吸困难等。

1. 该患者可能出现了副作用？
2. 护士应该采取的护理措施是什么？

（3～4题共用题干）

患者，女，45岁，患有双相情感障碍，目前处于无精神病性症状的躁狂症阶段，正在接受碳酸锂0.5 g，每天3次治疗。服用2个月后，患者出现恶心、呕吐、腹泻、视物模糊、双手震颤等症状。

3. What is the most likely side affect?
4. What is the main and priortizied nursing diagnosis?
(Questions 5 to 6 share the same question stem)
A 16-year-old student in vocational school is a cheerful disposition girl. Latterly, her classmates found that she became more and more lonely, speech less, late for school. Sometimes she muttered, or laughed suddenly at the class. She always puzzled to blame the classmates and said, "why do you scold me?" When the teacher talked with her, she explained, the reason why she didn't want to go to school is that other female classmates envied and cursed her, she even suspected that the classmate put the poison into her cup.
5. What is the main psychiatric symptoms?
6. According to the client's current condition, which kind of the drugs can be considered to use ?

3. 该患者最可能的药物反应是什么？
4. 此时最优先、最主要的护理问题是什么？
（5～6 题共用题干）
患者，女，18 岁，某职校学生，平素性格开朗。近期，同学们发现她变得孤僻，不爱与人讲话和交往，经常迟到，旷课。上课时有时喃喃自语，有时忽然发笑，总是莫名其妙地指责同学说“你为什么骂我？”老师找她谈话，她解释说，班长喜欢她，所以其他女同学嫉妒，在背后议论她，骂她，甚至怀疑同学在她的水杯里放毒，所以不愿去上学。
5. 该患者目前的主要精神症状是什么？
6. 针对患者目前的病情，可以考虑使用的药物是什么？

Chapter 16 Somatic Therapy
第十六章　躯体治疗

Learning Objectives

Memorization

Describe concepts of electroconvulsive therapy (ECT), transcranial magnetic stimulation therapy, light therapy and hypnosis.

Comprehension

1. Analyze the mechanism of action of electroconvulsive therapy (ECT), transcranial magnetic stimulation,light therapy and hypnosis as treatment strategies for psychiatric illness.
2. Detect the adverse effects of electroconvulsive therapy (ECT), transcranial magnetic stimulation,light therapy and hypnosis as treatment strategies for psychiatric illness.
3. Summarize the use, indications of electroconvulsive therapy (ECT), transcranial magnetic stimulation,light therapy and hypnosis as treatment strategies for psychiatric illness.

Application

Discuss the nursing care needs of the patient receiving ECT.

学习目标

识记

能准确描述电抽搐疗法、经颅磁刺激疗法、光感疗法和催眠疗法的概念。

理解

1. 能分析电抽搐疗法、经颅磁刺激疗法、光感疗法以及催眠疗法用来治疗精神疾病时的作用机制等。
2. 能探讨电抽搐疗法、经颅磁刺激疗法、光感疗法以及催眠疗法用来治疗精神疾病时的不良反应等。
3. 能总结电抽搐疗法、经颅磁刺激疗法、光感疗法以及催眠疗法用来治疗精神疾病时的适应证等。

运用

能了解和掌握接受电抽搐疗法的患者的各种需求。

16章

Mandy is a lively, cheerful, and eloquent girl studying in a colleges. She grew up in a superior environment and live a comfortable life. She competed several positions of student union at the first year in college, but all failed. Faced with such "heavy" blow, she fell into the quagmire of self-denial. She was filled with loneliness when she found the people around her playing and laughing together. Furthermore, she was also trapped by some symptoms including nightmares, sleep problems, poor mental state, lack of enthusiasm for life, and even self-closing. She was deeply helpless and even wanted to end her life by asking about painless way to commit suicide.

曼迪，女，某中专院校的学生，是一个活泼开朗、能言善辩的女孩子。从小就在优越的环境中长大，过着衣食无忧的生活。中专第一年时，参加了学校和系上的各类学生干部、干事的竞选，结果都失败了。面对如此"沉重"的打击，一向好胜的她陷入了自我否定的泥潭。每次看到别人高兴地在一起玩或学习时，内心充满了孤独感；晚上常常做噩梦，睡眠出现问题，精神状态不佳，对生活缺乏热情，甚至产生了自闭的状态。她感到空前的绝望和无助，甚至想用一种最不痛苦的方式来结束自己的生命。

Please think about the following questions based on the case:

1. Which somatic therapy is suitable for the patient?
2. What should nurse do before and after the somatic treatment?

请思考：

1. 患者目前可以采取什么躯体治疗方法？
2. 在治疗前后，护士应该为患者提供哪些护理措施？

With the emergence of biological psychiatry and the growing knowledge basis in the neurosciences, interest has increased in somatic therapies for psychiatric illness. The limitations of psychotropic medications, increase in treatment-resistant psychiatric disorders, and refinement in treatment techniques have placed greater emphasis on evaluating the indications for and efficacy of somatic therapeutic interventions.

Psychiatric nurses are involved in caring for patients who are receiving somatic therapy. Thus it is essential that all nurses understand how the way in which these treatment modalities work and the nursing care that enhances their effectiveness. This chapter discusses four contemporary somatic therapies: electroconvulsive therapy, transcranial magnetic stimulation therapy ,light therapy and hypnosis.

随着精神生物学的出现和神经系统科学的发展，躯体疗法在精神疾病的治疗中起到越来越重要的作用。而且由于精神药物治疗的局限性、精神疾病治疗过程中抗药性的增加，以及躯体治疗技术的改进，人们也更加重视评估躯体治疗的适应证和疗效。

躯体治疗过程中的护士需要正确执行治疗方案，全面观察并评价治疗的反应和效果，为患者提供有效的帮助等，这不仅要求护士全面了解躯体治疗的相关知识，而且要掌握治疗过程中的护理技术。本章主要介绍目前四种常用的躯体疗法：电抽搐疗法、经颅磁刺激疗法、光感疗法、催眠疗法。

Section 1 Electroconvulsive Therapy

第一节 电抽搐治疗

Electroconvulsive therapy (ECT) is a treatment in which a grand mal seizure is artificially induced to cause convulsions in an anesthetized patient by passing an electrical current.

电抽搐治疗（electroconvulsive therapy，ECT）是用一定量的电流通过大脑，引起患者意识丧失，引起中枢神经系统癫样放电，产生全身性抽搐发作的一种治疗方法。

Modified electroconvulsive therapy (MECT), modified on the basis of the ECT, makes the seizure significantly reduced or disappeared during electroconvulsive therapy by using intravenous anesthetic and muscle relaxant to selectively block the neuromuscular junction before the electroconvulsive therapy.

无抽搐电痉挛治疗（Modified electroconvulsive therapy，MECT）是在电抽搐治疗的基础上进行的改良，即在ECT治疗前使用静脉麻醉剂和肌肉松弛剂对骨骼肌的神经－肌肉接头进行选择性的阻断，使电抽搐治疗过程中的痉挛明显减轻或消失。

I. Introduction

Electroconvulsive therapy was first described by Cerletti and Bini in 1938 as a treatment for schizophrenia. At that time it was believed that epileptics were rarely schizophrenic. It was hypothesized that convulsions would cure schizophrenia. Later research did not support this hypothesis. Further experience with ECT demonstrated that it is much more effective as a treatment for affective disturbance than it is for schizophrenia. It has also been noted that epilepsy and schizophrenia do sometimes occur concurrently. ECT is now most frequently used as a treatment for severe depression.

一、概　述

Cerletti和Bini在1938年最先使用电抽搐治疗来治疗精神分裂症。当时人们认为癫和精神分裂症不会同时存在，提出了抽搐能治疗精神分裂症的假设。后来的结果表明这是一个错误的假设，但发现电抽搐治疗对情感障碍有较好的治疗效果。目前，电抽搐治疗是治疗重度抑郁最常用的治疗方法。

II. Mechanism of Action

The specific way in which ECT works has been the subject of extensive research, but the precise mechanism of action is still not known. It is believed that the electric current passing through the brain causes a biochemical response. Most theories about the mode of action of ECT focus on its efficacy with depressed patients. The following theories have been proposed:

1. Neurotransmitter theory suggests that ECT acts like tricyclic antidepressants by enhancing deficient neurotransmission in monoaminergic system. Specifically it is thought to improve dopaminergic, serotonergic, and adrenergic neurotransmission.

2. Neuroendocrine theory suggests that ECT releases hypothalamic or pituitary hormones or both, which results in its antidepressant effects. ECT releases prolacting, thyroid-stimulating hormone, adrenocorticotropic hormone, and endorphins, but the specific hormones responsible for the therapeutic effect is not known.

3. Anticonvulsant theory suggests that ECT treatment exerts a profound anticonvulsant effect on the brain that results in an antidepression effect.Some support for this theory is based on the fact that a person's seizure threshold rises and the seizure duration decreases over the

二、作用机制

虽然很多学者对电抽搐治疗的作用机制进行了广泛深入的研究，但其具体的作用机制目前仍不清楚。电流通过大脑引起了生物化学反应。针对电抽搐治疗抑郁患者的作用模式，有以下三种理论解释：

1. **神经递质学说**　认为电抽搐治疗的作用机制与三环类抗抑郁药相似，通过抑制单胺能神经末梢对多巴胺、5-羟色胺和肾上腺素的再摄取，以增加突触间隙单胺类神经递质的浓度。

2. **神经内分泌学说**　认为电抽搐治疗可促使下丘脑和/或垂体释放催乳素、促甲状腺素、促肾上腺皮质激素、内啡肽，从而起到抗抑郁作用。

3. **抗抽搐学说**　认为电抽搐治疗能影响大脑对异常放电的控制能力，起到抗抑郁的作用。在进行电抽搐治疗的过程中，抽搐发作的阈值上升，发作的时间缩短，电抽搐治疗能减少某些癫患者的发作次数。

course of ECT and that some patients with epilepsy have fewer seizures after receiving ECT.

In spite of unanswered questions regarding its mechanism of action, ECT is an effective treatment for many psychiatric disorders and is safe when properly administered.

尽管电抽搐治疗的作用机制仍不清楚，它仍是一种对许多精神障碍非常有效的治疗方法。

III. Indications

The primary indication for ECT is major depression. ECT's response rate of 80% or more is equal to or better than response rates to antidepressant medications. It is particularly useful for people who cannot tolerate or fail to respond to treatment with medication. On occasion, ECT may be used for conditions other than affective disorders. ECT is believed to be quite effective in treating manic episodes,and although controversy surrounds its usefulness for treating schizophrenia, some schizophrenic patients with catatonic stupor or catatonic excitement may respond well to ECT.Finally, ECT should be considered as an initial intervention when its anticipated side effects are less than those associated with drug therapy, such as with the elderly, for patients with heart shock, and during pregnancy.

三、适应证

电抽搐治疗主要用以治疗抑郁症。电抽搐治疗对 80% 的抑郁症患者有治疗作用，其治疗效果与抗抑郁药物相当或更好。电抽搐治疗还可用于不能耐受药物治疗或药物治疗无效的患者。有时，也可用于治疗其他精神障碍：狂躁发作、伴有紧张综合征的精神分裂症。此外，当预期的副作用比药物的副作用小，电抽搐治疗可作为对老人、心脏骤停的患者和孕妇的首选治疗方法。

IV. Contraindications

ECT has no absolute contraindication. Clients with some preexisting encephalic space- occupying lesions and others increasing encephalic pressure, recent encephalic bleeding, recent myocardial infarctions, severe hypertension, retinal detachment and pheochromocytoma are likely to be at increased risk during the course of ECT.

四、禁忌证

电抽搐治疗无绝对禁忌证。尽管如此，有些疾病可增加治疗的危险性，不宜采用电抽搐治疗，如：颅内占位性病变及其他增加颅内压的病变、近期的颅内出血、近期的心肌梗死、严重高血压、视网膜脱落、嗜铬细胞瘤等。

V. Clinical Guidelines

Patients and their families are often apprehensive about ECT; therefore, clinicians must explain the beneficial as well as adverse effects and alternative treatment approaches. Before the ECT treatment is begun, the patient should sign an informed consent form. Clinicians must know local,state,and federal laws about the use of ECT.

i. Pretreatment Evaluation

1. Pretreatment evaluation should include a complete history of the illness, routine examination including physical examination, blood count, urinalysis, serum chemistry profile, electrocardiograph and chest X-rays. An X-ray of the spine is needed if there is other

五、治疗方法

要接受 ECT 治疗的患者及其家属通常都会有担忧和顾虑，因此医护人员必须向患者及家属解释治疗的必要性、治疗的效果及治疗可能出现的不良反应，以取得患者及家属的知情同意。

（一）治疗前准备

1. 详细了解病史，进行系统的体格检查，常规进行血常规、尿常规、生化、心电图、胸片等检查，有其他证据说明患者存在脊柱疾病时，要进行脊柱摄片检查。怀疑患者有

evidence of a spinal illness. Computed tomography (CT) or magnetic resonance imaging (MRI) scan of the head should also be performed if a clinician suspects the presence of a seizure disorder or a space-occupying lesion.

2. Patients' ongoing medications should be assessed for effects, both positive and negative, on the seizure threshold, and for drug interactions with the medications used during ECT. The use of tricyclic and tetracyclic drugs, monoamine oxidase inhibitors, and antipsychotics are generally thought to be acceptable. Benzodiazepines used for anxiety should be withdrawn because of their anticonvulsant activity; lithium should be withdrawn because it can result in increased postictal delirium and can prolong seizure activity; clozapine (Clozaril) and bupropion (wellbutrin) should be withdrawn because they are associated with the development of late-appearing seizures. Lidocaine (Xylocaine) should not be administered during ECT because it markedly increases the seizure threshold; theophylline (Theo-Dur) is contraindicated because it increases the duration of seizures. Reserpine (Serpasil) is also contraindicated because it is associated with further compromise of the respiratory and cardiovascular systems during ECT.

ii. Premedications

1. Muscarinic Anticholinergic Drugs Muscarinic anticholinergic drugs are administered before ECT to minimize oral and respiratory secretions and to block bradycardias, unless the resting heart rate is above 90 beats a minute. The most commonly used drug is atropine, which can be administered 0.3 to 0.6 mg intramuscularly (IM) or subcutaneously (SC) 30 to 60 minutes before the anesthetic or 0.4 to 1.0mg IV 2 or 3 minutes before the anesthetic. An option is to use glycopyrrolate (Robinul) (0.2 to 0.4mg IM, IV or SC), which is less likely to cross the blood-brain barrier and less likely to cause cognitive dysfunction and nausea, although it is thought to have less cardiovascular protective activity than does atropine.

2. General Anesthetics The administration of ECT requires general anesthesia and oxygenation. The depth of anesthesia should be as light as possible, not only to minimize adverse effects but also to avoid elevating the seizure threshold associated with many anesthetics. Methohexital (Brevital) (0.75 to 1.0 mg/kg IV bolus) is the most commonly used anesthetic because of its short duration of action and lower association with postictal arrhythmias than is thiopental (Pentothal) (usual dose 2 to 3 mg/kg IV), although this difference in cardiac effects is not universally accepted.

3. Muscle Relaxants After the onset of the

癫或颅内占位性病变时还需进行CT或磁共振检查。

2. 评估患者目前使用的药物对电抽搐治疗的抽搐阈值的影响，以及与电抽搐治疗中使用的药物之间的相互作用。治疗前应避免使用会影响电抽搐治疗的药物，如苯二氮䓬类药物、锂盐、氯氮平和丁氨苯丙酮、利多卡因、茶碱类药物、利血平等。因为苯二氮䓬类药物具有抗抽搐作用；锂盐可加重治疗后的精神症状及延长抽搐时间；氯氮平和丁氨苯丙酮与迟发性癫的发生有关；利多卡因可显著提高电抽搐的阈值；茶碱类药物可延长抽搐时间；利血平在电抽搐治疗中易诱发呼吸系统、心血管系统严重并发症。而三环类抗抑郁药、四环类抗抑郁药、单胺氧化酶抑制剂及抗精神病药物对治疗影响不大，可继续使用。

（二）治疗前用药

1. 抗胆碱能药物 在接受电抽搐治疗前使用抗胆碱能药物，以减少口腔及气道分泌物，防止治疗中出现窒息和心动过缓。常使用阿托品，在使用麻醉药物前30～60分钟肌肉注射或皮下注射阿托品0.3～0.6mg，或在使用麻醉药物前2～3分钟静脉注射0.4～1.0mg。还可以以肌肉注射、皮下注射或静脉注射的方式使用胃长宁0.2～0.4mg。与阿托品相比，胃长宁不易通过血－脑脊液屏障，可以减轻患者的呕吐症状和认知功能的损害，但对心血管的保护作用较弱。

2. 麻醉药物 电抽搐治疗需进行全身麻醉，麻醉深度应尽可能浅，以减少药物的不良反应，避免麻醉药物引起电抽搐阈值的升高。最常使用的麻醉药物是美索比妥（0.75～1.0mg/kg静脉注射），戊硫代巴比妥（2～3mg/kg静脉注射），相比，美索比妥作用时间短、起效快、较少引起迟发性心律失常。

3. 肌松药 使用麻醉药物，诱导患者发

anesthetic effect, usually within a minute,a muscle relaxant is administered to minimize the risk of bone fractures and other injuries resulting from motor activity during the seizure. The goal is to produce a profound relaxation of the muscles,not necessarily to paralyze them, unless the patient has a history of osteoporosis or spinal injury or has a pacemaker and is, therefore, at risk for injury related to motor activity during the seizure.

生意识状态的改变，达到治疗要求时，开始注射肌松药。目的是使肌肉松弛，防止剧烈抽搐引起骨折和其他损伤。

iii. Stimulus Electrode Placement

ECT can be conducted with either bilaterally or unilaterally placed electrodes. In bilateral placement,which was introduced first, one stimulating electrode is placed bifrontotemporally with the center of each electrode about 2.54 cm above the midpoint of an imaginary line drawn from the tragus to the external canthus.In unilateral ECT, the electrode is placed several centimeters apart over the nondominant hemisphere, almost always the right hemisphere.

（三）电极的放置

电极的放置有双侧和单侧放置两种方法。双侧电极放置是将电抽搐治疗机的两个电极放置在头部两侧外眦和外耳屏连线中点上方垂直距离 2.54 cm 处。单侧放置是将电极均放置在患者的非优势半球一侧，通常是右半球。

The most common approach is to initiate treatment with unilateral ECT because bilateral placement usually results in a more rapid therapeutic response, while unilateral placement results in less marked cognitive adverse effects in the first week or weeks after treatment, although this difference between placements is absent 2 months after treatment.

最常用的是单侧电极放置，因为双侧电极放置虽然起效快，但是单侧电极放置在治疗后的第一个或数个星期内所造成的认知方面的副作用相对较轻，但是二者对患者认知影响的副作用在治疗 2 个月后无明显差异。

If a patient does not improve after four to six unilateral treatments, the technique is switched to the bilateral placement. Initial bilateral placement of the electrodes may be indicated in the following situations: severe depressive symptoms, marked agitation, immediate suicide risk, manic symptoms, catatonic stupor, and treatment-resistant schizophrenia. Some patients are particularly at risk for anesthetic-related adverse effects, and these patients may also be treated with bilateral placement from the beginning to minimize the number of treatments and exposures to anesthetics.

如果患者接受 4～6 次单侧电极放置治疗后，效果不明显，也将改为双侧电极放置。一般双侧电抽搐治疗只用于精神症状严重的患者，如出现严重抑郁、有自杀倾向、躁狂、木僵的患者和其他治疗无效的精神分裂症患者。对容易发生麻醉副作用的患者，也采用双侧电抽搐治疗以缩短治疗的时间，减轻麻醉药物的作用。

iv. Electrical Stimulus

The electrical stimulus must be sufficiently strong to produce a seizure. The electrical stimulus is given in cycles, and each cycle contains a positive and a negative wave. Modern ECT machines use a brief square wave pulse form that administers the electrical stimulus usually in a 1-to-2 ms time period at a rate of 30 to 100 pulses a second. Machines that use an ultra brief pulse (0.5 ms) are not as brief pulse machines.The establishment of a patient's seizure threshold is not straightforward. Generally doses of 3 times the threshold are the most rapidly with the fewest and least and least severe cognitive adverse effects.

（四）治疗电流量

交流电治疗机：电压 80～120 V，通电时间为 0.3～0.6 秒；直流电治疗机：电流量为 80～110 mV，通电时间为 1～3 秒。原则上应取可以引起抽搐发作的最低电量。首先要确定患者的抽搐发作阈值，选择超过抽搐发作阈值 3 倍的电量进行治疗。

v. Induced Seizures

A brief muscular contraction, usually strongest in

（五）抽搐发作

通电后，患者先出现足趾背曲，额面部

a patient's jaw and facial muscles, is seen concurrently with the flow of stimulus current, regardless of whether a seizure occurs. The first behavioral sign of the seizure is often a plantar extension, which lasts 10 to 20 seconds and marks the tonic phase. This phase is followed by rhythmic contractions that decrease in frequency and finally disappear.

肌肉强烈收缩，一般持续 10～20 秒。随后出现全身肌肉的震颤和抽搐，强度逐渐减弱直至消失。

vi. Number and Spacing of ECT Treatments and Maintenance Treatment

ECT treatments are usually administered 2 to 3 times a week; 2-times-weekly treatments are associated with less memory impairment than are 3-times-weekly treatments. In general,the course of treatment of depressive disorder can take 6 to 12 treatments (although up to 20 sessions is possible); the treatment of manic episodes can take 8 to 20 treatments; the treatment of schizophrenia can take more than 15 treatments; and the treatment of catatonia and delirium can take as few as 1 to 4 treatments. Treatment should continue until the patient achieves what is thought to be the maximum therapeutic response. Treatment past that point does not result in any therapeutic benefit but increases the severity and duration of the adverse effects. The point of maximal improvement is usually thought to occur when a patient fails to continue to improve after two consecutive treatments. If a patient is not improving after 6 to 10 sessions, bilateral placement and high-density treatment (3 times the seizure threshold) should be attempted before ECT is abandoned.

A short-term course of ECT induces a remission in symptoms but does not, of itself, prevent a relapse. Post-ECT maintenance treatment should always be considered. Maintenance therapy is generally pharmacological, but maintenance ECT treatments (weekly, biweekly, or monthly) have been reported to be effective relapse prevention treatments,although data from large studies are lacking.Indications for maintenance ECT treatments may include a rapid relapse after initial ECT, severe symptoms,psychotic symptoms, and the inability tolerate medications. If ECT was used because a patient was unresponsive to a specific medication, then, following ECT, the patient either should return to the original medication or should be given a trial of a different medication.

（六）治疗疗程与维持治疗

电抽搐治疗通常每周 2～3 次，每周两次的治疗方法对记忆的损害比较小。一般情况下，抑郁症患者需要接受 6～12 次治疗；躁狂症患者接受 8～20 次治疗；精神分裂症 15 次以上；紧张症和谵妄 1～4 次即可。应坚持持续治疗直到获得最佳疗效。如果 6～10 次治疗效果不佳，应改为双侧电抽搐并增加每周治疗次数和电流量。

短期的电抽搐治疗只能暂时缓解症状，不能预防疾病的复发。因此要在电抽搐治疗后进行维持治疗，每周 1 次，或两周 1 次或每月 1 次的药物维持治疗可有效预防疾病的复发。维持治疗的适用证包括初次治疗后疾病急性发作；症状严重；出现精神症状；不能耐受药物治疗的患者。对某种药物治疗无效的患者，在进行电抽搐治疗的维持治疗时，可以选用原来的药物或试用其他的药物。

vii. Failure of ECT Trial

If a patient fails to improve after a trial of ECT, the patient may again be treated with the pharmacological agents that failed in the past. Although the data are primarily anecdotal, many reports indicate that patients who had previously failed to improve while taking an antidepressant drug do improve while taking the same

（七）ECT 治疗无效

如果患者接受电抽搐治疗后无效，需再次进行药物治疗。有些报道指出，虽然电抽搐治疗失败，对于接受治疗前无效的一些药物治疗，电抽搐治疗后可以增加这些药物的疗效。

drug after receiving a course of ECT treatments, even if the ECT seemed to be a therapeutic failure. Nonetheless,with the increased availability of drugs that act at diverse receptor sites, it is less often necessary to return to a drug that has failed than was formerly true.

VI. Adverse Effects

1. Mortality The mortality rate with ECT is about 0.002 percent per treatment, which is quite equal to that of general anesthesia and childbirth. ECT death is usually from cardiovascular complications and is most likely to occur in patients whose cardiac status is already compromised.

2. Central Nervous System Effects Common side effects associated with ECT are headache, confusion,and delirium shortly after the seizure while the patient is coming out of anesthesia. Marked confusion may occur in up to 10 percent of patients within 30 minutes of the seizure and can be treated with barbiturates and benzodiazepines. Delirium is usually most pronounced after the first few treatments and in patients who receive bilateral ECT or who have coexisting neurological disorders. The delirium characteristically clears within days or a few weeks at the longest.

3. Memory The greatest concern about ECT is the association between ECT and memory loss. About 75 percent of all patients given ECT say that the memory impairment is the worst adverse effect. Although memory impairment during a course of treatment is almost the rule, follow-up data indicate that almost all patients are back to their cognitive baselines after 6 months. Some patients, however, complain of persistent memory difficulties. The degree of cognitive impairment during treatment and the time it takes to return to baseline are related in part to the amount of electrical stimulation used during treatment. In spite of the memory impairment, which usually resolves, there is no evidence of brain damage caused by ECT. This subject has been the focus of several brain-imaging studies, using a variety of modalities; virtually all concluded that permanent brain damage is not an adverse effect of ECT. It is generally agreed by neurologists and epileptologists that seizures that last less than 30 minutes do not cause permanent neuronal damage.

4. Systemic Effects Occasional, usually mild transient cardiac arrhythmias occur during ECT, particularly in patients with existing cardiac disease. The arrhythmias are usually a by-product of the brief postictal bradycardia and, therefore, can often be prevented by

六、治疗的不良反应及并发症

1. 死亡 接受电抽搐治疗的患者病死率0.002%，与麻醉意外和分娩死亡率相当。电抽搐治疗是一种较为安全的治疗手段。引起死亡的原因主要是心血管并发症，常发生于治疗前心功能受损的患者。

2. 中枢神经系统影响 电抽搐治疗后，患者会出现头痛、意识模糊和谵妄。意识模糊发生率为10%，可以使用巴比妥类苯二氮类药物进行治疗。谵妄通常发生于治疗初期，采用双向电抽搐治疗或伴有神经系统病变的患者，症状持续几天或几周后即可消失。

3. 记忆障碍 记忆障碍是人们最关注的问题。接受电抽搐治疗的患者中，大约75%的人认为记忆损害是其最严重的不良反应。接受电抽搐治疗的患者均可出现较为明显的记忆损害，其损害程度与接受电刺激的总量有关。数据表明，治疗结束后6个月，多数患者的认知功能恢复至基线水平。虽然患者记忆有损害，但没有证据表明电抽搐治疗会造成大脑损害，神经学家认为如果电抽搐治疗持续时间不超过30分钟，不会导致永久性的大脑损害。

4. 全身影响 接受电抽搐治疗的患者偶尔会发生心律失常，尤其是心脏病患者。最常见的心律失常是心动过缓，治疗前使用抗胆碱能药物可以预防。心律失常继发于抽搐

increasing the dosage of anticholinergic premedication. Other arrhythmias are secondary to a tachycardia during the seizure and may occur as a patient returns to consciousness. The prophylactic administration of a β-adrenergic receptor antagonist can be useful in such cases. As already mentioned, an apneic state may be prolonged if the metabolism of succinylcholine is impaired. Toxic and allergic reactions to the pharmacological agents used in ECT have rarely been reported. Sore muscles resulting from the seizure motor activity can generally be alleviated by pretreatment with curare or atracurium or by increasing the succinylcholine dose by 10 to 25 percent.

时引起的心动过缓，发生在意识恢复的过程中，可在治疗前使用β-受体阻滞剂进行预防。药物的毒性反应和过敏反应在电抽搐治疗中很少发生。将琥珀酰胆碱的剂量增加10%或25%，可以减轻抽搐发作导致的肌肉酸痛。

BOX 16-1 Learning More

Post-ECT Delirium (PECTD) Related Factors

Individual Factors

According to the reports, age is a risk factor (the older the patients is, the higher the risk is). In addition, suffering from heart disease, the basal ganglia disease, Parkinson's disease and Alzheimer's disease also increases the risk of PECTD; pathological changes of the brain is believed to be a significant factor of PECTD, for instance, Parkinson's disease patients will suffer serious PECTD when receiving ECT.

MECT related variables

PECTD is affected by all kinds of factors, such as the seizure time, the type of narcotic drugs and muscle relaxants and electrode placement.

The occurrence of PECTD is related to bupropion, atenolol, lithium salt, dopaminergic drugs, haloperidol and theophylline and other drugs. Delirium is also a common adverse reaction when the withdrawal of enzodiazepine occurs and combine a variety of antipsychotic drugs.

BOX 16-1 知识拓展

电痉挛治疗后谵妄（Post-ECT delirium, PECTD）的相关因素

个体因素

年龄大是较常报道的危险因素之一；此外共患心脏疾病、基底节病变、帕金森病以及阿尔茨海默病也增加PECTD的风险；脑部的病理改变被认为是发生PECTD的一个重要因素，如帕金森病患者行ECT治疗会出现严重的PECTD。

MECT治疗的相关变量

ECT治疗的抽搐时间、麻醉药物种类及肌肉松弛剂、电极安放位置均对PECTD有一定影响。

PECTD与安非他酮、阿替洛尔、锂盐、多巴胺能药物、氟哌啶醇和茶碱类等药物有关。谵妄也常见于苯二氮䓬类药物戒断及多种抗精神病药联合应用。

BOX 16-2 Learning More

The Safeguard of Unsafety Incidents in MECT

The preparation before the therapy

Before the treatment, visit and introduce the principle, operation method, effect, symptoms and approaches may occur in the process of MECT to eliminate patients' fear. First aid items should be checked again before the treatment.

The observation during the therapy

Observe patients' breathing carefully, and ensure an unobstructed vein tunnel in order to deal with the unsafe

BOX 16-2 知识拓展

无抽搐电痉挛治疗中不安全事件的防范措施

治疗前准备

对拟行MECT者进行访视，向患者介绍治疗的原理、操作方法、效果、治疗过程中可能出现的一些自觉症状以及处理方法，消除其恐惧感。治疗前应再次检查急救物品是否齐全、完好无损。

治疗中观察

仔细观察患者有无呼吸道阻塞或窘迫的迹象，确保静脉通路通畅，以便在发生意外时及时

events timely. Carry out CPR and inject medicines such as adrenaline through the vein tunnel immediately when the patient has no breathing and heartbeat.

The treatment after the therapy

Give the patients who have Post-ECT delirium special care, and prevent them from falling down. The appropriate bed protection should be given for the restless patients.

给药。如出现呼吸、心脏停搏，应立即给予心肺复苏，通过静脉给予肾上腺素等药物。

治疗后处理

对治疗后出现谵妄的患者应派专人守护，防摔伤。对不肯卧床、兴奋躁动的患者可以适当进行床上保护，以防跌伤。

VII. Nursing Care in Electroconvulsive Therapy

七、电抽搐治疗的护理

i. Education and Emotional Support

（一）向患者提供治疗相关的教育及情感支持

Nursing care begins as soon as the patient and family are presented with ECT as a treatment option.Initially, an important role of the nurse is to allow the patient an opportunity to express feelings, including any myths or fantasies about ECT. Patients may describe fear of pain, dying of electrocution, suffering permanent memory loss, or experiencing impaired intellectual functioning. As the patient reveals these fears and concerns, the nurse can clarify misconceptions and emphasize the therapeutic value of the procedure. Supporting the patient and family in their need to discuss, question, and explore feelings and concerns about ECT should be an essential part of nursing care before, during, and after the course of treatment.

患者及家属可能会对电抽搐治疗存有很多顾虑，如：电抽搐治疗会引起疼痛；会导致患者触电死亡；会引起记忆永久丧失或智力受损。护士要鼓励患者及家属说出自己的恐惧和顾虑，澄清他们的误解，强调电抽搐治疗的疗效，帮助患者及家属讨论关于电抽搐治疗的感受和顾虑。

Once the patient has had an opportunity to express feelings, the nurse can begin ECT teaching, taking into consideration the patient's anxiety, readiness to learn, and ability to comprehend. Family teaching should occur at the same time as patient teaching, and the amount of information to be shared should be individualized. The nurse should review with the family and patient the information they have received from the physician regarding the procedure and respond to any questions they might have.

在患者表达了自己对治疗的感受后，护士可根据患者的焦虑情况、学习的愿望和理解能力开始有关电抽搐治疗的教育。同时对患者的家属也进行相关的教育，教育的内容因人而异，并评估患者及家属对相关知识的掌握情况。

During this assessment process, the nurse should also attempt to define specific patient behaviors the family associates with the patient's illness and determine whether the patient or family member has received ECT in the past. Any information about the family's previous experiences with ECT helps the nurse identify familial beliefs about the patient's illness, ECT treatment,and expected prognosis. Both patient and family should also be asked what else they know about ECT such as through friends who have received it or by reading about it or seeing ECT portrayed in movies. Open-ended questions may give the nurse the opportunity to identify and correct misinformation and address specific concerns the patient or family has about

在评估的过程中，护士还应向家属解释其所关心的与疾病相关的行为，了解患者的家属有无看护过接受电抽搐治疗后的患者。有过电抽搐治疗看护经历的家属提供的信息，能帮助护士明确他们对患者的疾病、电抽搐治疗和预后的看法。开放性问题有助于护士判断患者与家属对上述内容是否有正确认识。在治疗过程中，上述护理措施有助于家属对患者提供支持，减轻患者的焦虑。

the procedure. These nursing actions may facilitate the family's ability to provide support to the patient during the treatment course and thus further alleviate the patient's anxiety.

此外，护士可以用相关资料和录像来对患者进行教育。让患者参观治疗的房间，帮助患者了解治疗环境、治疗设备和治疗过程。鼓励患者与接受过有效的电抽搐治疗的其他患者进行交流。护士可以安排家属在治疗前后陪伴患者，可以减轻患者的家属的焦虑和担心。

Various media may also be used to supplement the teaching of the patient and family about ECT, including written materials and videotape presentations. A tour of the treatment suite itself may help familiarize the patient with the area, procedure, and equipment. Encouraging the patient to talk with another patient who has benefited from ECT may be worthwhile. Finally, the nurse should facilitate flexibility in family arrangements, particularly during the patient's first few treatments, allowing for family presence before and after ECT if the patient and family desire. This approach helps allay the family's anxieties and concerns about the treatment while encouraging the family to support the patient.

如果家属不能或不愿陪伴患者，护士要在治疗后向家属提供相关信息及患者的反应，鼓励家属讨论患者的疾病变化。在患者的治疗过程中为患者及其家属提供情感和教育支持是护士角色的重要组成部分。

If the family cannot or does not want to be present, they cannot or does not want to be present during these times, the nurse should contact the family after treatments to provide information and describe the patient's response. The nurse should also encourage the family throughout the course of treatment to discuss changes they observe or questions that arise. Providing emotional support and responding to the educational needs of both patient and family are essential components of the nursing role throughout the patient's treatment.

ii. Informed Consent for Electroconvulsive Therapy

（二）有关患者知情同意的护理

Before ECT treatment begins,the patient should sign an informed consent form. If the patient does not have the capacity to give consent, it can be signed by a legally designated person. This consent acknowledges the patient's rights to obtain or refuse treatment. Although it is the physician's ultimate responsibility to explain the procedure when obtaining consent, the nurse plays an important part in the consent process.

在进行治疗前，患者要签署一份正式的知情同意书，表示自己有权决定接受或拒绝治疗。如果患者自己没有能力，可以由其法定委托人代签。虽然向患者解释治疗的程序，使患者同意接受治疗是医生的责任，但是，护士在此过程中也起着重要的作用。

Informed consent is a dynamic process that is not completed with the signing of a formal document; rather, it continues throughout the course of treatment. As such, it suggests a number of nursing activities. First, it is helpful if a nurse is present when the information for consent is discussed with the patient. The most appropriate nurse is one who has established a trusting and therapeutic relationship with the patient and who is best able to assess whether the patient comprehends the explanation. The presence of a nurse at this time may enable the patient to feel comfortable asking questions, and the nurse may help to simplify the language if necessary. The nurse can also ensure that the patient has been provided with a full

知情同意是一个动态的过程，需要护士为此进行多项护理活动。在患者与医生关于同意治疗进行讨论时，护士应在场。因为护士与患者建立了信任的治疗性关系，可以判断患者是否能理解医生解释的内容，必要时帮助简化患者的问题，保证患者能充分了解治疗的性质、目的和意义，知道自己可以随时退出治疗。在患者签署了知情同意书，还没有开始治疗的过程中，护士应该再次向患者解释有关治疗的信息，坦诚地与患者讨论有

explanation of the treatment, including its nature, purpose, and implications; understands the option to withdraw consent at any time; and has had all questions answered before signing the consent form. After the informed consent is signed, but before the beginning of treatment, the nurse should again thoroughly review this information and discuss the treatment in an open and direct manner, thus communicating that this is an accepted and beneficial form of treatment.

关治疗的情况。

Certain patients pose particular challenges to the nurse when obtaining informed consent.If a patient is unable to make independent judgments and meaningful decisions about care and treatment,the nurse is responsible for acting as a patient advocate. For example, concentration is often impaired in depressed patients, so they are less likely to comprehend and retain new information.For these patients it is essential that the nurse repeat the information at regular intervals because new knowledge is seldom fully absorbed after only one explanation. Then, throughout the patient's treatment course, the nurse should reinforce what the patient already understands, provide reminders of anything that has been forgotten, and be there to answer new questions.

如果患者不能对护理与治疗做出自主决策，护士应该充当患者的代言人。如抑郁患者常伴有注意力障碍，不能理解和保持新的信息，对于此类患者，护士应该间隔一段时间后，重述相关信息。在患者接受治疗期间，护士应该强化患者已经理解的知识，并随时回答患者提出的问题。

iii. Pretreatment Nursing Care

Providing optimal nursing care for the patient undergoing ECT includes evaluating the pretreatment protocol to ensure that it has been followed according to hospital policy. This involves completing appropriate consultations including the patients' medical history, physical illness, the ongoing medications such as antiepileptic drugs and benzodiazepine sedative hypnotics, et al., noting that any abnormalities in laboratory tests have been addressed, measuring the patients' vital signs to see if the therapy should be suspended (body temperature> 38℃, or pulse rate> 130 beats/min, or blood pressure> 160/110 mmHg, suspending the treatment once), measuring weight before the first treatment and checking that equipment and supplies are adequate and functional. The treatment nurse is responsible for ensuring that the treatment suite is properly prepared for the ECT procedure. Although not required to be in the treatment room itself, a crash cart with defibrillator should be readily available for emergency use.

（三）治疗前护理

治疗前准备：仔细核对患者的各项辅助检查结果是否符合治疗要求。了解患者的既往史、用药情况及目前躯体疾病状况。术前是否使用抗癫痫药及苯二氮卓类镇静催眠药。每次治疗前应监测患者的体温、脉搏、呼吸和血压。如有异常及时向医生汇报（如体温 >38 ℃，或脉搏 >130 次 /min，或血压 >160/110 mmHg，暂停治疗一次）。首次治疗前应测量体重。保证治疗设备运转正常，物品充足。

Equipment for Electroconvulsive Therapy: (a) Treatment device and supplies including electrode paste and gel, gauze pads, alcohol preps, saline, and chart paper. (b) Monitoring equipment including ECG and EEG electrodes; blood pressure cuffs (two), peripheral nerve stimulator, and pulse oximeter; stethoscope; reflex hammer. (c) Intravenous and venipuncture supplies.

所需设备：备好治疗设备及物品 导电胶、纱布垫、酒精棉球、生理盐水、脑电图电极和纸、监护设备、听诊器、反射锤、牙垫、注射器、吸氧装置、插管设备和急救药品及其他麻醉医生建议的药品等。

(d) Bite blocks with individual containers. (e) Stretchers with firm mattress and siderails with the capability to elevate the head and feet. (f) Emergency equipments such as suction device; ventilation equipment including tubing, masks, Ambu bags, oral airways; and intubation equipment with an oxygen delivery system capable of providing positive-pressure oxygeng Emergency and other medications are recommended by anesthesia staff.

Patient preparation: Because ECT is similar to a brief surgical procedure, patient preparation is similar. General anesthesia is required, so fluids should be withheld from the patient for 6 to 8 hours before treatment to prevent the potential for aspiration. The exception to this NPO status is in the case of patients who routinely receive cardiac medications, antihypertensive agents, or H_2 blockers. These drugs should be administered several hours before treatment with a small sip of water. The patient should be encouraged to wear comfortable clothing, including street clothes, pajamas, or a hospital gown, provided that it can be opened in the front to facilitate the placement of monitoring equipment. The patient should also be reminded to remove prostheses before coming to the treatment area to prevent loss or damage. This may include dentures, glasses, contact lenses, and hearing aids. The patient's hair should be clean and dry for optimal electrode contact. Hairpins, barrettes, hairnets, and other hair ornaments should also be removed for placement of electrodes. The patient should void immediately before receiving ECT to help prevent incontinence during the procedure and to minimize the potential for bladder distention and damage during treatment.

患者准备：治疗前6～8小时内禁食禁水；如果患者需常规服用心脏药物，降压药或者是H_2受体阻滞剂，则在治疗前几个小时用少量水送服。临近治疗前患者衣着舒适，排空大、小便，取出活动性义齿、发夹及各种装饰物品，解开领扣及腰带。

Environment, supplies and operators preparation: keep quiet and avoid other patients or their families to enter the treatment room. Open the therapy device, monitor and oxygen master switch (open the flow meter when start the treatment), operate the ECG and defibrillator at the same time. Doctors and nurses should keep the coats and hats neat, wash hands before the treatment, and strictly obey the technique procedures when operating the aseptic techniques.

环境、设备及操作员准备：治疗室内保持环境安静，避免其他患者及家属进入。将治疗仪、监护仪打开，心电图、除颤仪处于工作状态，打开氧气总开关（治疗开始时再开流量表）。

医护人员衣帽整齐、清洁，治疗前洗手，无菌技术操作时要严格无菌技术操作规程。

iv. Nursing Care during the Procedure

（四）治疗中护理

The patient should be brought to the treatment suite either ambulatory or by wheelchair, depending on individual need, accompanied by a nurse with whom the patient feels at ease. If possible, the nurse should remain with the patient throughout the treatment to provide support. Because there will be a number of people in the room, including a psychiatrist, the treatment nurse, and the anesthesia staff, the patient should be introduced to each member of the treatment team and given a brief

护士陪同患者进入治疗室，向患者介绍治疗医生、治疗护士、麻醉师及上述人员在治疗过程中的作用。治疗时给予患者心理安慰，减轻患者对治疗的恐惧，请患者仰卧于治疗床上，身体放松。或嘱患者闭眼做深呼吸，以缓解紧张情绪。

explanation of everyone's role in the ECT procedure. In order to reduce patients' fear of treatment and ease the tension, it's necessary to conduct psychological comfort when patients receiving treatments, and put the patient supine on the bed with their body relaxed or guide them close eyes to take deep breaths.

The patient should then be assisted onto a stretcher and asked to remove shoes and socks. This allows for the placement of a blood pressure cuff on an ankle and clear observation of the patient's extremities during the treatment. Once the patient is positioned comfortably on the stretcher, a member of the anesthesia staff inserts a peripheral intravenous line while the treatment nurse and other members of the treatment team place leads for various monitors. One member of the treatment team should explain the procedure while it is occurring. EEG monitoring consists of two electrodes, one on the forehead and one on the left mastoid. A set of three-lead ECGs, connected to the oscilloscope, is placed on the patient's chest. A pulse oximeter is clipped to the patient's finger to monitor oxygen saturation. Blood pressure monitoring throughout the treatment is accomplished by a manual or automatic cuff. A peripheral nerve stimulator, preferably placed on the ankle over the posterior tibial nerve, serves to determine muscle relaxation.

协助患者仰卧治疗台上，四肢自然伸直。脱去鞋袜，便于血压监测和观察末梢循环情况。建立静脉通路，连接脑电监护仪、心电监护仪、血氧饱和度监测仪、血压计和神经刺激仪。

The treating psychiatrist or nurse cleans areas of the patient's head with mild soap at the sites of electrode contact. This cleansing process facilitates optimal stimulus electrode contact during treatment, thus eliminating the potential for skin burns and minimizing the amount of electrical stimulus needed for the treatment.

清洁放置电极部位的头发，以免油污影响通电效果，减少对皮肤的潜在灼伤，最小化治疗所需的电量。

Once the preparation is completed, atropine (0.3 to 0.6 mg) may be administered intravenously to decrease oral secretions and minimize cardiac bradyarrhythmias in response to the electrical stimulus. Next an anesthetic, usually methohexital (usual dose approximately 1 mg/kg), is administered. When the patient is asleep, the blood pressure cuff on the ankle is inflated, allowing it to serve as a tourniquet. A muscle relaxant, succinylcholine (usual dose approximately 0.75 mg/kg), is then administered to minimize the patient's motor response to the ECT treatment. Because the tourniquet is in place on one ankle, the succinylcholine is not effective in that extremity. This is a desired effect because it is used in detecting a motor response of the seizure. Progressive muscle relaxation is monitored by the nerve stimulator, as well as by observing the patient for the cessation of fasciculations. As the muscle relaxant takes effect, the anesthesiologist provides oxygen by mask to the patient through positive pressure ventilation. The changes in blood oxygen saturation of

遵医嘱静脉注射 0.3 ~ 0.6 mg 阿托品以减少口腔及气道分泌物并降低心律失常的发生率。遵医嘱静脉注射美索比妥（1 mg/kg）。遵医嘱注射肌松药如琥珀酰胆碱（0.75 mg/kg），减轻治疗时的抽搐反应。肌肉松弛后，协助麻醉师给予面罩加压给氧，监测患者血氧饱和度的变化，确保血氧饱和度维持在 95% 及以上。尽管使用了肌松药，但通电后患者仍会发生下颌肌肉抽搐，因此，要在患者牙齿间放置牙垫，避免损伤牙齿和舌头。通电过程中，护士要固定患者的下颌和牙垫，防止抽搐过程中牙垫脱落。痉挛发作后，取出患者的牙垫，使患者头后仰，以保持呼吸道通畅。记录抽搐时间。一般抽搐持续 30 ~ 60 秒，超过 2 分钟要给予苯二氮䓬类药物及时终止抽搐。

the patient should be observed carefully when patient's face and limbs and extremities twitch slightly (namely seizures) to ensure that oxygen saturation remains above 95%. Although most muscles become completely relaxed, the patient's jaw muscles are stimulated directly by the ECT, causing the patient's teeth to clench. This creates the need for a protective device, or bite block, to be inserted in the patient's mouth by the treatment nurse before the electrical stimulus. This disposable or autoclavable device prevents tooth damage and tongue or gum laceration during the stimulus. The bite block should be placed between the upper and lower teeth. The nurse should then support the patient's chin firmly against the bite block during delivery of the brief electrical stimulus. After delivery of the stimulus, the bite block may be removed by the nurse to maintain the airway patency. One member of the treatment team records the time elapsed during the seizure. A motor seizure lasting 30 to 60 seconds is generally considered adequate to produce a therapeutic effect, and seizures lasting longer than 2 minutes should be terminated to prevent a prolonged postictal state. The seizure may be terminated by using a benzodiazepine,such as diazepam,thiopental sodium (Pentothal), or additional methohexital, given at half the induction dose. Anesthesia staff continuously ventilates the patient with pure oxygen during the procedures until the patient is able to breathe spontaneously. Vital signs should be monitored by the nurse both before and after the ECT treatment. Once the patient is stabilized,the anesthesiologist clears the patient for transfer to the recovery area.

持续给予纯氧吸入，直到患者恢复自主呼吸。严密监测生命体征。如果病情平稳，协助麻醉师将患者转入恢复室。

v. Posttreatment Nursing Care

The recovery area should be adjacent to the treatment area to provide accessibility for anesthesia staff in case of an emergency. The area should contain oxygen, suction, pulse oximeter, vital sign monitoring, and emergency equipment. The area should be appropriately staffed and provided a minimal amount of sensory stimulation. Once in the recovery area with pulse oximeter in place,the patient should be unobtrusively observed by a staff member in close proximity until the patient awakens. At this time, the staff should be aware of the potential for falls from the stretcher caused by patient restlessness and maintain patient safety. After removing oxyhemoglobin monitor, observe the patient's breathing and awareness until they recover, which generally last 15-30 minutes.

（五）治疗后护理

恢复室应邻近治疗室，一旦发生紧急情况可立即进行抢救。恢复病房内应配备氧气、吸引装置、氧饱和度检测仪、生命体征监测设备和急救设备。应保持病室安静，严密观察病情，注意患者的安全，避免发生坠床意外。保证患者卧床休息，观察患者的呼吸、意识情况，直至呼吸平稳、意识完全恢复后解除血氧监测，一般监护 15 分钟至 30 分钟。

When the patient awakens, a nurse should discuss the treatment and check vital signs. Most patients do not remember receiving the treatment and may be confused and disoriented, similar to patients recovering from anesthesia. The nurse should provide frequent reassurance

患者清醒后，往往出现记忆障碍和定向力障碍，护士应向患者讲解治疗情况，定时检查生命体征。

and reorientation and repeat this information at regular intervals until the patient retains it. Being postictal, the patient may have somewhat concrete thinking. Providing brief, distinct direction is most beneficial.

When the patient is awake and appears ready to return to the hospital room and has maintained a continuous oxygen saturation level of 90% or above, and when vital signs and mental status have returned to an acceptable level, the nurse should help to move the patient from the stretcher to a wheelchair for transport from the recovery area. When a wheelchair is used, the seatbelt should be securely fastened. The patient should be allowed to ambulate if desired. At this time the ECT treatment nurse should convey as much information as possible about the patient's condition to the unit nursing staff. The most beneficial information includes medications given to the patient that may be evidenced in the patient's behavior or vital signs and any change in the procedure or the patient's response to treatment that may affect the patient's behavior on return to the unit.

当患者完全清醒、血氧饱和度在90%以上、生命体征平稳时可送回普通病房。向病房护士交接患者的用药情况、生命体征情况和治疗反应等。

The patient should be observed at least once every 15 minutes; if the patient is agitated, confused, or restless, one-to-one observation may be required until the patient's condition has stabilized. Level of orientation should be assessed every 30 minutes if the patient is awake until mental status returns to baseline. If sleeping, the patient should remain undisturbed unless additional nursing intervention is warranted. Sleeping may help the patient return to baseline values more quickly. The return of the gag reflex should be assessed before administering medication or offering food to the patient. Patients can not eat anything until they regain consciousness, and a small amount of liquid food first until the next meal can they have a normal diet. Avoid a lot and eager eating, especially solid food, since the residual effect used in the treatment of anesthetics and muscle relaxants easily lead to serious unforeseen circumstances,such as choking, etc.

送回病房后，护士应每15分钟观察一次病情，如果患者躁动不安，应进行严密观察直至病情平稳。如果患者清醒，则每30分钟评估一次患者的定向力，通过环境刺激和护理人员的不断提醒，患者可在短期内恢复定向力。如果患者处于睡眠状态，要确保其不受干扰，因为睡眠能促进患者恢复。在给药或进食之前要评估吞咽反射，防止发生呛咳。患者意识完全清醒后方可少量进食进水。切忌大量、急切进食，尤其是固体食物，由于治疗中使用麻醉剂和肌松剂的残余作用易导致噎食等严重意外情况，可先进少量流食，待下顿进餐时间再进食普食。

When fully awake, the patient should be observed when getting out of bed for the first time to ensure full muscle functioning after administration of muscle relaxants. Throughout the posttreatment interval, provision of support and reminders to the patient of having received ECT eliminate patient distress from posttreatment amnesia.

患者完全清醒后第一次下床活动时要进行监护，防止肌肉松弛引起的摔伤。同时，要给予患者精神支持，减轻记忆力障碍给患者带来的痛苦。

Potential side effects immediately after treatment that may be treated symptomatically include headache, muscle soreness, and nausea. Any confusion or disorientation is likely to be of short duration and may respond well to restricted environmental stimulation and frequent nursing contacts to remind the patient of ECT treatment and to

对治疗后潜在不良反应，如头痛、肌肉痛、恶心呕吐等进行相应的对症处理。意识障碍或定向障碍持续的时间一般较短，护理人员可通过减少环境的刺激，经常性的提醒等方式来增强患者的定向能力。

provide reorientation.

vi. Nursing Staff Education

Despite recent increases in the use of ECT and its effectiveness in the treatment of certain psychiatric illnesses, the procedure continues to elicit emotional responses from the public as well as the medical and nursing communities. Some of these responses may be positive. However, many people react negatively to ECT based on outdated ideas and procedures. It is critically important that when a patient is referred for ECT, the patient and family should be presented and unbiased manner. If a nurse has ambivalent or negative feelings about ECT, these feelings will probably be communicated to the patient and render the treatment course less effective. To function as patient advocates,nurses need to examine their attitudes and have as much information about the procedure as possible.

Educational efforts should be directed toward nurses who work on units where ECT is implemented as a treatment strategy. Programs should be developed that address both cognitive and attitudinal content because the more knowledge and clinical experience mental health professionals have with ECT, the more positive their attitude will be toward it.

Such programs might be initiated by asking staff to discuss their beliefs and feelings about ECT, including its potential therapeutic value, perceived risks, nature of the procedure itself, and ethical and legal issues concerning its use. The content can then progress to a discussion of factual material about ECT, including the rationale for the treatment, possible mechanisms of action,its efficacy relative to other treatment options, risks and side effects resulting from ECT, and current research on its indications and benefits. Time should be spent discussing the way in which the procedure has changed over the years, and all nurses should be encouraged to observe the ECT procedure as performed in their institution.

These discussions might be supplemented with written handouts, reference articles, and teaching videotapes about ECT. Finally,this information can be formalized and incorporated into the unit's daily nursing care by the establishment of nursing standards of care for patients receiving ECT and the development of a standardized nursing care plan that identifies appropriate nursing diagnoses, goals, and interventions.

In addition to informing nurses who care for patients undergoing ECT, there is a need to teach the larger nursing community about ECT. Psychiatric nurses who work with ECT can provide in-services to nurses in other clinical

（六）护士培训

尽管电抽搐治疗可以有效治疗某些精神障碍，使用的范围越来越广，但由于受一些观念的影响，公众和某些医护人员仍然不能正确看待电抽搐治疗。如果护士对电抽搐治疗抱有偏见，会给患者及家属带来消极影响，从而影响治疗的效果。作为患者的代言人，护士要端正对电抽搐治疗的态度，掌握相关知识。

因此要对从事电抽搐治疗工作的护士进行培训，着重改变他们对电抽搐治疗的不良认知和态度。关于ECT的知识和临床经验越丰富，对ECT的态度越积极。

首先要求护士讨论对电抽搐治疗的想法和感受，包括电抽搐治疗的意义、危险、治疗的特性和相关的伦理和法律问题。培训的内容包括电抽搐治疗的原理、作用机制、治疗效果及产生的不良反应，以及最新的有关适应证和疗效的研究成果。讨论随着时间推进，ECT实施过程发生了哪些变化，并鼓励护士在其所在机构观察ECT实施的全过程。

通过组织讨论、阅读书面材料和相关文献、观看关于治疗过程的录像，使护士掌握电抽搐治疗护理常规，针对具体患者确定护理诊断、制订护理目标、实施护理计划。

除了对从事电抽搐治疗和护理的精神科护士进行培训以外，还应对其他广大护士进行电抽搐治疗的相关教育，如老年科、神经科、内科等，给他们提供关于ECT最新、最准确的信息，以改变其对ECT的错误观念。

settings, such as geriatrics, neurology, or medicine, to dispel myths, clarify misconceptions, and provide current, accurate information.

VIII. Role of Nurses in Electroconvulsive Therapy

The effectiveness and limitations of ECT have been the subject of considerable debate within the field of psychiatry. Since it is a somatic therapy for psychiatric illness,nurses have participated in both the debate and the implementation of ECT as a treatment opinion for their patients.

Although psychiatric nurses have always had a role in assisting with the ECT procedure, nursing functions have historically been limited to supportive and adjunctive care. With the growing sophistication of nursing science and clinical practice, this role is evolving to include independent and collaborative nursing actions.

八、护士在电抽搐治疗中的角色

目前，电抽搐治疗的作用和局限性成了精神病学的争论主题。虽然精神科护士在治疗过程中担任辅助实施治疗的角色，对治疗提供支持和辅助。

但是随着护理理论和实践的发展，护理成了一门独立的学科，护士在治疗中将进一步发挥作用，特别是精神科高级专科护士如临床护理专家及独立开业者的出现，更使护士在此领域有广阔的发展空间。

Section 2 Other Therapies

I. Transcranial Magnetic Stimulation Therapy

Transcranial magnetic stimulation therapy (TMS) is a noninvasive procedure in which a changing magnetic field is introduced into the brain to influence the brain's activity. The field is generated by passing a large electrical current through a wire stimulation coil over a brief period.

After assessing a patient's resting motor threshold to determine dosing,an insulated coil is placed on or close to a specific area of the patient's head, allowing the magnetic field to pass through the skull and into target areas of the brain.

i. Mechanism of Action

TMS modulates the brain's electrical environment using magnetic fields based on the principle of electromagnetic induction, which pass through the scalp and skull unimpeded. These fields are produced by passing rapidly alternating electrical currents through a coil with a ferromagnetic core. The magnetic field strength produced by TMS varies from 1.5 to 3 T and is comparable to an MRI device. TMS can be administered in a single pulse or as a brief series of pulses, and it can be used for research, diagnostic, and therapeutic purposes. When used clinically, several thousand pulses are usually applied

第二节　其他治疗

一、经颅磁刺激治疗

经颅磁刺激治疗（Transcranial magnetic stimulation therapy，TMS）是一个不断变化的磁场被引入大脑并影响其活动的非侵入性治疗程序。短暂的时期内大量电流通过线圈而产生了磁场。在评估患者的静息运动阈值以确定给药剂量，一种绝缘线圈被放置在或靠近患者头部的特定区域，从而使磁场穿过颅骨并进入脑中的目标区域。

（一）作用机制

基于电磁感应原理，经颅磁刺激疗法利用磁场来调节大脑的电生理环境，穿过头皮和颅骨畅通。这些磁场由交替快速通过线圈和铁磁芯的电流产生。经颅磁刺激疗法所产生的磁场强度在 1.5 到 3 特斯拉之间，与核磁共振磁场强度具有可比性。经颅磁刺激治疗可以以单脉冲或是一个简短的系列脉冲进行，可用于研究、诊断和治疗目的。临床上使用

over a period of minutes to hours. This is called repetitive transcranial magnetic stimulation or "rTMS".

时，通常在几分钟到几小时内达到几千个脉冲，这就是所谓的重复经颅磁刺激治疗。

ii. Indications

（二）适应证

1. Mood Disorders TMS is most widely applied in psychiatric treatment of depression. Researchers propose ideas with TMS treatment of depression based on the fact that prefrontal cortex function changes in patients and transcranial magnetic stimulation can affect people's emotions. Currently the effect of TMS in depression has been proved to be the most positive one.

1. **心境障碍** 目前经颅磁刺激治疗在精神科中应用最多的是治疗抑郁症。研究者根据抑郁症患者存在前额皮层功能的改变，以及经颅磁刺激能影响人的情绪等事实，提出用 TMS 治疗抑郁症的设想。抑郁症的治疗是目前疗效最为肯定的。

2. Anxiety Disorders TMS can be used for a variety of anxiety related disorders for that it can relieve patients' anxiety, such as simple anxiety disorder, stress disorder, adjustment disorder, Depression comorbid anxiety and obsessive compulsive disorder, et al., particularly for refractory obsessive compulsive disorder, which have been proved effective by a number of studies. 12 cases of patients with obsessive compulsive disorder received rTMS with frequency of 20 Hz and intensity of 80% MEp, the outcomes demonstrated that obsessive compulsive symptoms significantly decreased and accompanied by short-term emotional changes within 8 hours after stimulation of the right side of the prefrontal cortex.

2. **焦虑性障碍** 经颅磁刺激治疗可缓解焦虑情绪，故可用于多种焦虑障碍，如单纯性焦虑症、应激障碍、适应障碍、抑郁共病焦虑及强迫症等。特别是对难治性强迫症，已有多项研究证实有效。12 例强迫症的患者采用 rTMS 进行治疗，给予的刺激频率为 20 Hz，刺激强度为 80% MEp，结果显示，在对右侧前额叶刺激后的 8 个小时内，强迫症状明显减弱，并伴有情绪的短期改善。

Futhermore, the results of numerous studies suggested that TMS can be helpful for schizophrenia and posttraumatic stress disorders. TMS has been used for studying motor cortex excitability and inhibition, and schizophrenia patients are considered to have cortical inhibition dysfunction. But it is premature to apply TMS as a diagnostic tool for mental illness. How to combine TMS and functional brain imaging research and select the specific brain areas to stimulate in view of different target symptoms (cognition, positive symptoms and negative symptoms) will be the research direction in the future,which will make it possible to make TMS an effective treatment for schizophrenia.

除此之外，已有研究证实经颅磁刺激治疗还可应用在精神分裂症和创伤后应激障碍的治疗中。经颅磁刺激治疗现已用于运动皮层的兴奋性和抑制性研究，并已发现分裂症患者存在皮层抑制功能障碍。但将经颅磁刺激治疗作为精神疾病的诊断工具，还为时尚早。未来的研究方向是将经颅磁刺激治疗与功能性脑影像研究相结合，针对不同的靶症状（认知、阳性症状和阴性症状），选择特定的脑区进行刺激，将有可能使经颅磁刺激治疗成为治疗分裂症的有效方法。

iii. Adverse Effects

（三）不良反应

TMS is considered quite safe if the safe use guidelines are followed strictly; however, it is unavoidable that some risks may be induced by TMS. Studies have shown that epileptic seizures, syncope, heart rate, blood pressure, hearing loss, pain, headache, malaise, skin Burns and other reactions may be induced after transcranial magnetic stimulation.

若严格遵守安全使用准则，经颅磁刺激治疗是相当安全的；然而，经颅磁刺激治疗也不可避免地会构成一定的风险。有研究表明经颅磁刺激治疗后可能会诱发癫痫发作、晕厥、心率加快、血压升高、听力损害、局部疼痛、头痛、皮肤灼伤等其他反应。

The biggest adverse effect of TMS is the potential for inducing seizures, less than 20 cases of TMS induced seizures have been reported out of tens of thousands of

目前认为其最大的副作用是诱发癫痫发作。据报道，在过去的 25 年里，成千上万的

examined subjects over the past 25 years. Overall the risk of seizure is considered to be <0.01 %. Whether TMS can induce epileptic seizures mainly depends on stimulus intensity, frequency, site of stimulation, et al. The stimulus frequency of inducing epilepsy seizures is usually over 10 Hz, with stimulus intensity above the threshold. Thus, the safety of low-frequency rTMS can be assured.

受试者当中，仅有不到 20 例经颅磁刺激治疗的患者诱发了癫痫发作。因此总体而言，癫痫发作的风险率是低于 0.01 %。经颅磁刺激治疗是否能诱发癫痫发作主要与刺激的强度、频率、刺激部位等因素有关。诱发癫痫发作的刺激频率多在大于 10 Hz，刺激强度均在阈强度以上。因此，低频 rTMS 可以保证其安全性。

In addition, the skin near stimulation point can be burned by rTMS therapy where electrodes recording electroencephalogram (EEG) are placed. The subject and the operator should wear ear muffs to protect hearing, timely arrangements for hearing assessment, cochlear implant patients should not receive TMS. There are no enough studies about long-term effects of TMS, and theoretically no significant side effects will be induced.

此外，rTMS 可引起刺激点附近的脑电图记录电极处的皮肤灼伤。受试者和操作者应戴耳罩以保护听觉，并及时安排听觉评估，耳蜗植人患者不应接受 TMS。目前对 rTMS 的长期效应研究较少，理论上不会有明显副作用。

II. Light Therapy

二、光感治疗

The major indication for light therapy is major depressive disorder with seasonal pattern, characterized by symptoms that appear on a seasonal basis, usually in fall and winter. In light therapy, also called phototherapy, patients are exposed to a bright artificial light source on a daily basis during the treatment. Patients usually sit, with eyes open, about 1 m away from and at eye level with a set of broad spectrum fluorescent bulbs designed to produce the intensity and color composition of outdoor daylight. They then can engage in their usual activities such as reading,writing, or eating. The most recently developed light therapy device is the light visor, a device shaped like a baseball cap and worn on the head, with the light contained in a visor portion suspended above and in front of the eyes. The obvious advantage to such a device is that it allows the person to move about while receiving treatments. However, the results of studies testing the device show great variability in effectiveness.

光感治疗也称光线治疗，主要是利用人工光线治疗季节性抑郁症。这种抑郁症的特点是症状常在特定季节出现，尤其是秋季或冬季。治疗时，患者通常取坐位，光线治疗仪放置在距眼睛约 1 m 远的位置，治疗仪发出类似日光的强烈光线。患者每天接受人工光线照射，治疗的同时患者也可以做其他的事，如：阅读、写作或吃东西。最新研制的光感治疗装置是光疗面罩，光源悬挂在眼前，可以像帽子一样戴在头上。这种装置最大的优点是患者在接受治疗时可以随意走动，缺点是疗效不稳定。

i. Mechanism of Action

（一）作用机制

Mechanism of light therapy still remains unclear. The most accepted theory is that light therapy can change human circadian rhythms. Exposure to light have a differential effect on bodily rhythms (for example, sleep and hormone secretion), depending on the time of day, and hence affect their locations on the phase-response curve. Exposure to light in the morning results in a phase advance, that is, rhythms are shifted to an earlier time; exposure to light in the evening results in a phase delay, that is, rhythms are shifted to a later time. Light therapy can effectively treat the delayed circadian rhythms

光感治疗的机理目前还未完全明确，一般认为是通过影响人的昼夜节律起治疗作用。人有觉醒 / 睡眠的昼夜节律，这种节律受外界白昼 / 黑夜节律的调节，调节部位在下丘脑。通过调整外界昼 / 夜节律，改变下丘脑松果体的激素分泌，能够达到调节觉醒 / 睡眠节律的目的。如早晨接受光照可以使节律变换提前；夜晚接受光照可以使节律变换推迟。季节性抑郁症主要由于季节变换导致觉醒 / 睡眠节律紊乱

associated with major depressive disorder with seasonal pattern. This hypothesis is supported by the observations of several investigators that other depressive disorders do not respond to phototherapy. Light therapy can also influence the secretion of hormone. Melatonin is secreted by the pineal gland during the night. Secretion is stopped by exposure to light during the night but is not stimulated by exposure to darkness during the day. The theory that light exposure works by affecting melatonin secretion has not been supported by subsequent experiments. A high intensity of light was thought to be required for therapeutic effects, but this hypothesis has been disputed by recent studies. Most studies support the idea that 2 hours is more effective than 30 minutes of exposure. Whether light should be administered in the morning or evening or at both times to obtain maximal benefit is undetermined, but most studies support the administration of light in the morning. Full-spectrum light is effective, and some studies have found that narrow-spectrum light is ineffective. Whether an intermediate spectrum of light would be effective is unknown.

造成，因此可以通过人工光线照射调整生理周期来治疗抑郁症状。此外，光感疗法对非季节性抑郁治疗无效也支持上述观点。光感治疗还可以影响激素的分泌，如晚间松果体分泌褪黑素，夜间接受光照可以抑制该激素的分泌，白天避免光照不会诱发激素的分泌。激素水平改变是否与治疗效果有关，目前还没有定论。光照强度和治疗效果之间的关系，目前也还存在争议。多数研究证实光照持续时间 2 小时要比半小时效果好。另外，最佳治疗时间是早上还是晚上，或是早晚均接受治疗，目前还不确定，但多数研究支持早上治疗。光谱的选择一般选用全光谱，窄光谱对治疗无效，中间光谱的疗效还不确定。

ii. Indications

The major indication for light therapy is major depressive disorder with seasonal pattern,which occurs predominantly (80 percent) in women. The mean age of presentation is 40. The symptoms usually appear during winter and remit spontaneously in spring, but sometimes the symptoms appear in summer. The most common symptoms include depression, fatigue, hypersomnia, carbohydrate craving, irritability, and interpersonal difficulties. One third to one half of all patients with the disorder have not previously sought psychiatric help. The remainders have most often been previously classified as having a mood disorder.

（二）适应证

光感治疗的主要适应证是季节性抑郁症，女性居多（80%），平均年龄在 40 岁左右。症状往往冬天出现，而春天自发好转，但少数患者夏季发病。最常见的症状是抑郁、疲劳、嗜睡、多食、易怒、人际交往困难。其中 1/3 至 1/2 患者没有接受正规的精神治疗，其余大部分患者被诊断为心境障碍。

iii. Adverse Effects

The most commonly reported adverse effects are headache, eyestrain. Others include irritability, insomnia, fatigue, nausea, and dryness of eyes. These adverse effects can usually be managed by reducing the length of time that the patient is exposed to the light or increasing the patient's distance from the light. The long-term effects of phototherapy, if any, are currently unknown. Light therapy should be used with caution with specific ophthalmic conditions.

（三）不良反应

光感治疗最常见的不良反应是头疼、眼睛疲劳，另外还有易怒、失眠、疲劳、恶心、眼睛干燥等。这些反应可通过减少光照时间或增大患者与光源的距离得到缓解。光感治疗的远期影响还不清楚。伴有眼部疾患的患者治疗需谨慎。

III. Hypnotherapy

三、催眠疗法

Hypnosis is a natural state of aroused, attentive focal concentration with a relative suspension of peripheral awareness. It involves an intensity of focus that allows the hypnotized person to make maximal use of innate abilities

催眠是一种注意力高度集中，对外界感知暂停，易被唤醒的一种自然状态。接受催眠者在催眠师的引导下注意力高度集中，能

to control perception, memory, and somatic function. Even psychiatrists who make no formal use of hypnosis can enhance their effectiveness by learning to recognize and take advantage of hypnotic mental states.

Alterations in consciousness occur frequently in the course of ordinary life; indeed, such cyclic variation is the norm, not the exception. Certain variations in consciousness may change the relationship between mental and physical states and alter the degree to which concentration is focused. One of these alterations in consciousness is hypnosis, a naturally occurring phenomenon in which focal concentration is intensified at the expense of peripheral awareness. Hypnotic experience involves three main factors absorption, dissociation, and suggestibility. Absorption is an immersion in a central experience at the expense of contextual orientation. When one is intensely involved in a central object of consciousness, one tends to ignore perceptions, thoughts, memories, or motor activities at the periphery. In a hypnotic age regression, subjects act as though they were younger, suspending awareness that they really are decades older than the assumed age. The incongruity is available to them, yet they easily ignore it. Dissociated information is temporarily and reversibly unavailable to consciousness, but may nonetheless influence conscious(or other unconscious) experience. A rape victim may have no conscious memory of the crime,yet become anxious when exposed to stimuli reminiscent of the event. Suggestibility is enhanced in hypnosis. Because of their intense absorption in the trance experience, hypnotized individuals usually accept instructions relatively uncritically. They are also less prone to distinguish an instruction as coming from another rather than themselves and so will tend to act on another person's ideas as though they were their own.

(Yang Min)

够最大限度地调动机体的潜能来控制感知、记忆和躯体功能，因此，催眠可以作为治疗或辅助治疗精神疾病的方法。精神疾病医师掌握一定的催眠技术有助于提高治疗效果。

在日常生活中，意识的改变经常发生，属于正常情况。某些意识的变化可以改变精神状态与生理状态的关系，并可改变注意力集中的强度。催眠就是一种意识状态的改变，是一种注意力高度集中的自然发生的现象。引发催眠有三个关键因素：全神贯注、分离和暗示。全神贯注是把注意力集中在某个事物上，而忽略了其他。如催眠状态下老年人举动可以如同年轻人，忽略了自己的实际年龄要比假定年龄大几十岁。分离是指暂时地、可逆地失去意识，如受到强暴的受害者失去对犯罪过程的记忆。暗示是人类最简单、最典型的条件反射。在催眠状态下，难以判断指令是别人发出的还是自己的意愿，因此容易接受暗示。

（杨　敏）

Key Points

1. Electroconvulsive therapy (ECT) is a treatment in which a grand mal seizure is artificially induced to cause convulsions in an anesthetized patient by passing an electrical current.

2. Nursing care in electroconvulsive therapy includes: education and emotional support, informed consent for electroconvulsive therapy; pretreatment nursing care,nursing care during the process, posttreatment nursing care and nursing staff education.

内容摘要

1. 电抽搐治疗是用一定量的电流通过大脑，引起患者意识丧失，引起中枢神经系统癫样放电，产生全身性抽搐发作的一种治疗方法。

2. 电抽搐治疗的护理包括向患者提供治疗相关的教育及情感支持；有关患者知情同意的护理；进行治疗前、治疗中和治疗后的护理；护士培训。

3. Transcranial magnetic stimulation therapy (TMS) is a non-invasive brain stimulation procedure that can alter neuronal activity through administration of various pulse sequences and frequencies.

4. The major indication for light therapy is major depressive disorder with seasonal pattern, characterized by symptoms that appear on a seasonal basis, usually in fall and winter.In light therapy,also called phototherapy, patients are exposed to a bright artificial light source on a daily basis during the treatment.

5. Hypnosis is a natural state of aroused,attentive focal concentration with a relative suspension of peripheral awareness.Hypnosis has been shown to be an effective adjunct to the treatment of a variety of psychiatric symptoms and problems.

3. 经颅磁刺激是一种非侵入性的脑刺激治疗程序，可以通过不同的脉冲序列和频率管理改变神经元的活动。

4. 光感治疗也称光线治疗，主要是利用人工光线治疗季节性抑郁症。

5. 催眠是一种注意力高度集中，对外界感知暂停，易被唤醒的一种自然状态。催眠可以作为多种精神症状和精神疾病的辅助治疗方法。

Exercises

(Questions 1 to 2 share the same question stem)

Xiaoqian, 23 years old, is a college student. She lived with her grandmother because her parents divorced when she was young. Unfortunately she has been thinking herself as a bad girl and loathed by people around her after being raped. She is of extremely low self-esteem, is troubled by insomnia, and felt lonely and alienated in her university life. She felt so hopeless and helpless that she wanted to commit a suicide recently. She visited a psychiatrist accompanied by her roommate yesterday.

1. what somatic treatments doctors can take for the patient's condition?
2. what adverse effects will the patients have after somatic treatment?

(Questions 3 to 4 share the same question stem)

A 62-year-old woman with diagnosis of severe depression was suggested to have ECT tomorrow morning. Her daughter came to her primary nurse and asked if her mother would feel painful during the therapy?

3. how should the primary nurse response to the patient's daughter?
4. What should the patient and her family expect for the therapy?

思考题

（1～2题共用题干）

王小倩，女，23岁，某大学学生。童年时，因父母离异被寄养在外婆家，不幸遭流氓强暴后，始终认为自己不是个好女孩，所有人都讨厌自己。大学4年中，从来没有快乐过，极度自卑，失眠，注意力不集中，孤独不合群，有自杀意念。昨日由室友陪伴前往当地某医院精神科门诊咨询医生，医生对其进行了抑郁自评量表测试，标准分65分，属重度抑郁。结合症状，被诊断为抑郁性神经症。

1. 针对患者的病情，医生可采取哪种躯体治疗方法?
2. 患者在接受治疗后，可能出现哪些不良反应?

（3～4题共用题干）

一名重度抑郁症的62岁女性患者被安排在第二天早上做电休克治疗。她的女儿问护士：“我母亲做治疗时会很痛苦吗？”

3. 该责任护士该如何回答患者女儿的问题?
4. 关于ECT治疗，患者或家属的合理预期是什么?

Chapter 17 Psychotherapy and Nursing Care

第十七章 心理治疗与护理

Learning Objectives

Memorization

1. Describe concepts of psychotherapy, psychoanalysis, behavioral therapy, cognitive therapy, and client-centered therapy.
2. Describe classification of psychotherapy, indicators and techniques of each main psychotherapy approach.

Comprehension

1. Explain and distinguish mechanism of each main psychotherapy approach.
2. Expound correct psychotherapy approach and techniques in different psychiatric nursing settings.

Application

Apply psychotherapy in the practice of psychiatric nursing settings.

学习目标

识记

1. 能准确描述心理治疗、精神分析法、行为疗法、认知疗法、患者中心疗法的概念。
2. 能正确阐述心理治疗的分类以及主要心理治疗的适应证和主要技术。

理解

1. 能解释和区分每种主要心理治疗的作用机制。
2. 能针对不同的精神科护理病例选择正确的心理治疗方法和技术。

运用

能将心理治疗运用到精神科护理实践中。

Grandpa Li, 66 years old, married, was hospitalized one day ago because of severe cough, sputum, and dyspnea, and was diagnosed as chronic obstructive pulmonary disease (COPD). He has suffered COPD for 10 years. When the disease got severe, his activities of daily living need to depend on his families. Due to the recurrent disease and gradually increased and there is no cure for, he considered himself "someone else's burden", resulting in depression and even suicidal thoughts.

Please think about the following questions based on the case:

1. What might be the potential nursing diagnoses for the client?
2. What kind of psychotherapy approach is appropriate for helping the client?

李爷爷，今年66岁，已婚，住院前一天因剧烈咳嗽、咳痰、呼吸困难，并被诊断为慢性阻塞性肺疾病。他遭受了慢性阻塞性肺病10年，发病时更加严重，他的日常活动需要依赖于他的家庭。由于病情反复发作且逐渐加重，也没有特效药，他认为自己是"别人的负担"，导致抑郁，甚至自杀的念头。

请思考：

1. 该患者可能的护理诊断是什么？
2. 哪种心理治疗方法适合于帮助该患者？

Psychotherapy can inform, illuminate and improve the everyday practice of psychiatry and psychiatric nursing. Many clients are helped through processes that allow them to gain insight, to examine their thoughts and behaviors, and to try out new ways of relating to others. While each therapy has its strong proponents and clearly unique benefits. Nurses in virtually any area of practice may often need to give their opinions regarding the value of specific therapeutic approaches to clients. Some nurses in advanced practice roles function as therapists, offering direct psychotherapies to clients. To offer service better to clients, and to improve the quality of nursing, nurses must study the theory and technique of psychotherapy and apply them in nursing practice. This chapter provides the main psychotherapy approaches for various mental disorders.

心理治疗为精神障碍治疗和护理提供了广阔的前景，极大地丰富和改进了帮助和治疗精神障碍患者的思路和方法。很多精神障碍患者通过心理治疗进行内省、重审自己的观念和行为、尝试以新的方式与他人相处而获得帮助。然而，每一种治疗方法都有其独特的适用范围和用途。在临床实践中，护士常常要为患者选择特殊的治疗方法进行咨询，有的护士还作为治疗者直接为患者做心理治疗。为更好地为患者服务，提高护理质量，护士必须学习和研究有关心理治疗的理论和技术，并将之应用于护理实践中。本章提供了各种精神障碍的主要心理治疗方法。

Section 1 Introduction

第一节 概 述

Psychotherapy is the treatment of mental or emotional disorders through psychological rather than physical methods, although it is often done in conjunction with somatic therapy, especially medications.

尽管心理治疗常常与躯体治疗，特别是药物治疗联合使用，但心理治疗不是通过生理手段来处理患者的问题，而是通过应用有关心理学理论及其方法来治疗患者的精神或情感障碍。

I. Definition and Classification of Psychotherapy

i. Definition of Psychotherapy

Psychotherapy has many definitions based on the variety of approaches' theories. An overall definition of psychotherapy encompasses the great variety of approaches: psychotherapy is a form of treatment based on the systematic use of a relationship between therapist and client – as opposed to pharmacological or social methods – to produce changes in cognition, feelings and behavior.

The advantage of this definition is that it emphasizes the essentially interpersonal nature of the psychotherapeutic relationship, from which much of its power derives; technique, although of no less importance, can only be effective if a good therapeutic alliance is established. This definition is also wide-ranging enough to include most of the varieties of psychotherapy currently practiced.

ii. Classification of Psychotherapy

The psychotherapies can be classified according to theory, technique, setting, mode and length.

psychotherapy encompasses a large number of treatment methods, each developed from different theories about the causes of psychological problems and mental illnesses. The main approaches are analytic, behavioral, cognitive, and experiential-humanistic approaches. Analytic approaches derive from the primarily lengthy, intensive psychoanalysis and rely on helping individuals gain insight into feelings and behaviors. Behavioral approaches help individuals to gain tools that allow them to change behavior (and often feelings). Cognitive approaches aim to modify maladaptive thoughts, self-statements, or beliefs.

Experiential-humanistic approaches attempt to create an experience that will facilitate growth and personal development. There are many specific types of therapy within each category. Currently, many therapists describe their approach as eclectic or integrative, meaning that they combine ideas and techniques from a variety of therapies and often tailor their treatment to the particular psychological problem of a client. But no matter what kind of psychotherapy approach is used, to establish rapport with the client is very important.

一、心理治疗的概念及分类

（一）心理治疗的概念

心理学家们从各自的理论观点出发，提出了很多关于心理治疗的定义。从广义上讲，心理治疗也称精神治疗，是指以治疗者与患者之间建立良好协调关系为基础，由经过训练的专业人员运用心理学专业知识和技巧，影响改变患者的认知、情绪和行为等心理活动，从而改善患者的心理状态和行为以及与此相关的痛苦与症状。

上述概念强调了心理治疗中的治疗性关系，它对治疗进程和疗效的取得起着举足轻重的影响。尽管心理治疗的技术也同样重要，只有在治疗者与患者之间建立了良好的协调关系时，心理治疗的技术才能发挥更好的疗效。该概念也涵盖了当前所应用的大多数心理治疗方法。

（二）心理治疗的分类

心理治疗种类繁多，具体可根据其各自的理论观点、技术方法、应用场所、治疗模式及时间长短进行分类。

根据心理学派理论主要分为分析法、行为疗法、认知疗法和人本主义心理治疗。分析法源自原本耗时的经典精神分析法，旨在帮助个体对自己不良的情感和行为获得内省；行为疗法是帮助患者改变不适应的行为和情感；认知疗法的目的是修正适应不良的思想，自我陈述或信仰。

人本主义心理治疗则努力为患者创造一个有利于个体成长和个人发展的心理感受。以上每一流派又可细分为多种心理治疗方法。目前，很多心理治疗工作者已不再固守于某一流派和坚持某种单一的心理治疗方法，而是根据患者的具体心理问题采取折中疗法。但无论采用哪种心理治疗方法，与患者建立融洽的关系非常重要。

Therapists' intervention techniques can be divided into those that are directive, interpretive, supportive, challenging and expressive; most therapies contain a combination of techniques, although the proportions vary greatly. Psychotherapeutic settings also vary widely from in-client units to mental health centers and day hospitals, from psychotherapy departments to general practitioners' surgeries. Therapy can be in individual, group or family mode. The length of psychotherapeutic treatment varies from one or two sessions to several years, although the average therapy takes probably no more than a few months.

根据治疗技术可分为指导法、解释法、支持疗法、挑战法和宣泄法；大多数治疗者已联合采用多种方法，只是每种方法所占比例不同而已。根据应用场所，心理治疗又可分为住院治疗、心理卫生中心治疗、心理治疗专门科室治疗、一般诊疗室治疗。根据治疗模式可分为个体心理治疗和集体心理治疗或家庭心理治疗；而根据治疗时间长短则分为短程和长程心理 治疗，尽管心理治疗持续时间平均不超过几个月，短程心理治疗只需进行 1～2 次就可达到目的，长程心理治疗可能要持续数年之久。

II. The Role of Nurses in Psychotherapy

二、护士在心理治疗中的角色

Registered nurses may provide counseling and client education related to crisis, stress, and mental health and may also provide referral to community sources for both therapy and counseling. In addition, experienced psychiatric nurses may provide support and carry out interventions based on any of the psychotherapeutic approaches. Nurses with MSN and/or Ph.D. provide both counseling and psychotherapy in some settings.

护士在心理治疗中充当着不可轻视的角色。注册护士可以为患者提供心理咨询和有关危机、应激以及心理卫生方面的宣教，也可以针对社区资源就心理治疗和心理咨询提供参考意见。另外，有经验的精神科护士可以应用心理治疗的技术为患者提供支持，并采取相应的措施进行干预。具有护理硕士和 / 或哲学博士学位的护士在某些场所可以直接为患者提供心理咨询和心理治疗。

Section 2 Psychoanalysis

第二节 精神分析法

Psychoanalysis is the oldest and best known of the insight-oriented therapies. It is derived from the Freudian view of psychosexual development and focuses on the uncovering of unconscious memories and processes.

精神分析法是最早、最著名的内省治疗。精神分析法起源于弗洛伊德的性心理发展理论，着重揭示患者的潜意识记忆和潜意识过程。

I. Mechanism of Action

一、作用机制

In Freud's view, much of an individual's personality develops before the age of six. Freud proposed that children pass through a series of psychosexual stages, during which they express sexual energy in different ways. The innate sexual and aggressive drives cause feelings

弗洛伊德认为，大多数人的个性在六岁前就开始显现。他提出，儿童经历了一系列的性心理阶段，在不同的阶段他们通过不同的方式来表达他们的性冲动。这种天生的性

and thoughts that the person regards as unacceptable. In response, the individual represses these feelings, driving them into the unconscious mind. In the process, three basic personality structures are formed: the id, the ego, and the superego. The id represents unchecked, instinctual drives; the superego is the voice of social conscience; and the ego is the rational thinking that mediates between the id and superego and deals with reality. These three systems function as a whole, not separately. Id forces are unconscious and often emerge without an individual's awareness, causing fear, anxiety, depression, or other distressing symptoms.

冲动产生的情感和想法往往使人在现实生活中难以接受。于是，人们将这种不为社会道德规范所接受的情感压抑在潜意识中。在这一过程中，就形成了人格的三个基本组成部分：本我、自我、超我。本我表现本能的冲动，其活动遵循“快乐原则”；超我反映社会的道德的要求和行为准则，遵守“至善原则”；自我是理性的思考，在本我与超我之间，遵循“现实原则”活动，对上按超我要求控制本我，对下通过调节满足本我中本能的释放。这三者构成一个整体，相互作用，不可分割。如果三者间到达动态平衡，则保持身心健康；平衡失调则导致身心障碍的发生。如本能冲动过强，超过自我的控制力，这些被压抑的本能冲动平时虽不被意识，但并非消失，遇有机会常会浮现出来，如触景生情，从而引起恐惧、焦虑、压抑或其他不适症状。

Treatment should involve helping the client become aware of, and gain insight into, his or her unconscious conflicts and repressed thoughts to eliminate these symptoms. Psychoanalysis places particular emphasis on helping clients uncover memories about early childhood trauma and conflict, which as the source of emotional problems in adults.

治疗上应该帮助患者认识到自己的潜意识的心理冲突和被压抑的情感，获得内省来消除症状。心理分析尤其强调帮助患者发掘有关孩童时期的损伤和冲突的记忆，而正是这些记忆导致成年后的情感障碍。

II. Indication

二、适应证

Psychoanalysis may be used with the following clinical conditions: primarily oedipal conflict, experiences internal conflict, obtains symptom relief through understanding, psychologically minded, able to experience and observe strong affects without acting out, supportive relationships available in both the present and the past.

精神分析法主要用于各种神经症患者以及某些心身障碍的某些症状，如原发性恋母情结冲突、内部冲突困扰等。用精神分析法治疗的患者要有领悟能力并通过领悟可获得症状减轻，而且该患者过去和现在都可获得有效的支持。

III. Techniques of Psychoanalysis

三、精神分析法的基本技术

Some psychoanalysis techniques used to treat clients are free association, dream interpretation, transference, and resistance.

Free association is a method in which clients say whatever thoughts come to their minds about dreams, fantasies, and memories. The analyst's interpretations of

精神分析治疗采用的技术有自由联想、释梦、移情和阻抗分析。

自由联想是让患者把自己心理想到的浮现在脑子里的一切包括梦境、幻想和记忆都诉说出来。治疗者通过对患者所讲的内容加

this material could provide clients with insight into their unconscious—insight that would help them become less anxious, less depressed, or better in other ways.

以分析和解释，使患者认识到自己的潜意识，达到内省——这种内省可以帮助他们减轻焦虑和压抑，或减轻其他不适。

Dream interpretation is a psychoanalytic technique based on the assumption that dreams contain underlying, hidden meanings and symbols that provides clues to unconscious thoughts and desires. The psychoanalyst's task is to look behind the dream's often bizarre disguises and symbols and decipher clues to unconscious, repressed memories, thoughts, feelings, and conflicts.

释梦这种精神分析法的原理是基于梦的内容包含隐藏的含义和征象，以此提供线索帮助患者发掘自己潜意识里的想法和欲望。治疗者的任务就是揭开梦的伪装，洞察梦所隐藏的含义和征象，寻求潜意识里被压抑的记忆、思想、感觉和心理冲突。

Transference is the client's emotional response to the therapist. During therapy, clients transfer repressed feelings toward their family members to their relationship with the therapist. Transference exposes these repressed feelings and allows the client to work through them.

移情是患者将自己的情感活动转移到治疗者身上。在治疗过程中，患者将他们被压抑的对家人的情感转移到治疗者身上。通过移情分析可以揭示这些被压抑的情感，从而帮助患者深入认识自身情感和内心活动，推动治疗。

For most clients, working out transference and achieving insight into their problem are long and difficult processes for the client has so many defenses against admitting repressed thoughts and feelings into consciousness. These defenses lead to resistance. Resistance is the client's reluctance to work through or deal with feelings or to recognize unconscious conflicts. It may show up in many ways: clients may come late or cancel sessions, argue continually, criticize the analyst, or develop physical problems. The analyst must use tact and patience in getting the client to accept threatening interpretations and overcome resistance.

对于多数患者而言，要让他们产生移情、对自己的心理问题达到内省是一段漫长而困难的过程。因为，在这过程中，要使潜意识里被压抑的心理冲突重新进入到意识中来，患者常会产生很多防御心理，这些防御心理便导致了阻抗。所谓阻抗，就是患者不愿意挖掘，或涉及情感问题，或不愿意承认自己潜意识里的心理冲突。阻抗可表现为以下几种方式：患者可能迟到或取消约定；反复就某一事情与治疗者进行争论；对治疗者无端指责或出现身体不适。治疗者在治疗过程中必须应用技巧，耐心帮助患者接受治疗，克服阻抗。

The practice of Freud's classical psychoanalysis has declined in recent years, driven there by its high costs and long time, the restrictive reimbursement policies of health plans, and the development of briefer and equally effective therapies that called the psychodynamic approach. Modern psychoanalysts tend to focus more on current functioning and make less use of free association techniques but share many of the features of psychoanalysis—such as discussing the client's feelings and breaking down the client's defenses and resistances.

近年来经典的弗洛伊德精神分析治疗法应用有下降趋势，原因有该法耗时长，费用昂贵；健康保险补偿制度的限制；更简便但等效的精神动力治疗的发展。现代心理分析学者更注重时效，他们较少应用自由联想技术，但仍采用了心理分析的许多特征如讨论患者的感觉，降低患者的防御和阻抗心理。

IV. The Role of Nurses in Psychoanalysis

四、精神分析疗法中护士角色

Psychoanalysis is most consistent with nursing theories that emphasize human development and the

精神分析疗法大部分理论与护理理论相一致，他们都关注人类的发展和过去的经历

influence of the past experiences on present behaviors. A nurse should explicitly evaluate in the context of a client's past history and use the psychoanalysis technique of interpretation to help the client gain insight into, his or her unconscious conflicts and repressed thoughts and let the client understand how the historical factors influence present needs, frustrations, conflict, and anxiety.

对当前行为的影响。护士应当正确评价患者以往的经历与当前状况的关系，通过运用解释这一精神分析疗法的技术帮助患者了解自己内在的心理活动，将被压抑的潜意识活动的内容疏导出来，并让他明白是以往的经历影响他现在的生活，产生挫折感、心理冲突和焦虑。

Section 3 Behavioral Therapy

第三节　行为疗法

Behavioral therapy is defined as interventions that reinforce or promote desirable behaviors or alter undesirable ones. As psychoanalysis reached its peak of popularity in the 1950s, there was a great increase in the popularity of learning principles that came from Pavlov's work on classical conditioning, Skinner's work on operant conditioning and Bandura's model. Researchers and clinicians began to apply these learning principles to change human behavior with methods based on a strong experimental foundation. Thus, behavior therapy developed by providing more effective methods of changing human behavior out of dissatisfaction with psychoanalysis.

行为疗法是采取措施强化促进适应的行为、改变不适应行为的心理治疗方法。当精神分析疗法在19世纪50年代被广泛应用时，以巴甫洛夫的经典的条件反射、斯金纳的操作条件反射和班都拉的模仿学习为理论基础的行为疗法也迅速发展。研究者们开始应用这些以实验确立的有关学习的原则和方式来矫正人们的非适应性行为。这样，行为疗法通过更多有效的方法弥补了精神分析疗法的不足并逐渐发展。

I. Mechanism of Action

一、作用机制

Behavioral therapies differ dramatically from psychodynamic and humanistic therapies. Behavioral therapists do not explore an individual's thoughts, feelings, dreams, or past experiences. Rather, they focus on the behavior that is causing distress for their clients. They believe that behavior of all kinds, both normal and abnormal, is the product of learning. By applying the principles of learning, they help individuals replace distressing behaviors with more appropriate ones.

行为疗法完全不同于精神动力疗法和来访者中心疗法。行为疗法并不探究个人的思想、情感、梦或过去的经历，而是关注那些导致患者不适应的行为。行为主义治疗者认为，人的一切行为，包括适应性行为和非适应性行为，都可以通过学习获得。行为疗法可以帮助人们通过学习消除一些不适应的行为，获得适应的行为。

II. Indication

二、适应证

Typical problems treated with behavioral therapy include alcohol or drug addiction, phobias (such as a fear of heights), and anxiety. Modern behavioral therapists work with other problems, such as depression, by having

行为疗法主要治疗酒精或药物成瘾、恐惧症（如恐高症）和焦虑。现代行为疗法还用于其他的方面的治疗，如针对抑郁症，治

clients develop specific behavioral goals—such as returning to work, talking with others, or cooking a meal. Because behavioral therapy can work through nonverbal means, it can also help people who would not respond to other forms of therapy. For example, behavioral therapists can teach social and self-care skills to children with severe learning disabilities and to individuals with schizophrenia who are out of touch with reality.

疗者通过让患者完成特定的目标任务——如重新工作，和他人交谈，或做一顿美餐等，达到治疗目的。因为行为疗法可以用非言语手段进行治疗，所以它还可应用于对其他治疗方式无效的患者。例如，行为治疗学家能够帮助那些学习功能严重障碍的孩子和脱离现实的精神分裂症患者学习社会适应能力和自我照顾技能。

III. Techniques of Behavioral Therapy

Behavioral therapists begin treatment by finding out as much as they can about the client's problem and the circumstances surrounding it. They do not infer causes or look for hidden meanings, but rather focus on observable and measurable behaviors. Therapists may use a number of specific techniques to alter behavior. These techniques include relaxation training, biofeedback, systematic desensitization, graded exposure, flooding, positive reinforcement, modeling, aversion therapy, and social skills training.

三、行为疗法常用技术

行为治疗家开始治疗时尽可能多收集一些有关患者不良行为及其周围环境的资料。治疗者并不去探究原因或挖掘隐藏的含义，而是关注可观察到和可测量的行为活动。治疗者常用一些特定的技术来矫正患者的不良行为。这些技术包括放松训练、生物反馈技术、系统脱敏技术、等级暴露疗法、满灌疗法、正强化技术、示范法、厌恶疗法、社交技能训练。

i. Relaxation Training

Relaxation is defined as a psychophysiological state characterized by parasympathetic dominance involving multiple visceral and somatic symptoms including the absence of physical, mental, and emotional tension. Herbert Benson first used the term relaxation response when referring to the psychophysiological state in which muscles are relaxed; tension is released; blood pressure, heart rate, and respiratory rate are decreased; and the parasympathetic nervous system is activated. As a therapeutic tool, relaxation training effectively decreases tension and anxiety. The basic premise is that muscle tension is related to anxiety. If tense muscles can be made to relax, anxiety will be reduced.

Several relaxation techniques are used in nursing practice to evoke the relaxation response. Progressive muscle relaxation (PMR) is a technique of alternately tensing and relaxing muscle groups throughout the body to become aware of tension and the contrast between muscle tension and relaxation.

1. Before Beginning the Exercise The relaxation procedure should be described; the client should be in a quiet and relaxed area, take a comfortable position, and concentrate on quiet and calm.

（一）放松训练

放松是一种以副交感神经系统兴奋占优势为特征的心身状态，包括多种内脏和躯体症状，表现为身体无紧张感、精神宁静和情绪紧张消失。

Herbert Benson 第一个使用放松反应这一术语来描述肌肉放松，不紧张，血压、心率、呼吸频率下降，副交感神经被激活的心身状态。作为一种治疗手段，放松训练能有效地减轻紧张和焦虑。放松训练技术的基本前提是肌肉紧张与焦虑有关；如果紧张的肌肉被放松，那么焦虑将减轻。

在护理实践中，几种放松技术常被用来激发放松反应。渐进式肌肉放松是一种交替紧张和放松全身肌肉群、让患者学会体验肌肉紧张和肌肉放松之间个人感觉上的差别的技术。放松训练可按以下程序进行：

1. 准备工作 向患者讲解放松程序，选择一个安静、轻松的环境，让患者处于舒适的位置，且集中精力，保持安静和平静。

2. Instruction to Relax The client begins by taking a deep breath and exhaling slowly. He or she is then advised to tense each muscle group for approximately 10 seconds while the therapist describes how tense and uncomfortable this body part feels. Next the client is asked to relax the same muscle group for 20 to 30 seconds and notice how it feels—warm, soft, and calm. This technique services to focus attention on body parts, one by one, and to make the client very aware of what it feels like when that part is tense, and how it feels to relax that same part. The sequence of PMR is listed in table 17-1.

2. 指导患者如何放松 先深吸气再缓慢呼气。然后，依次紧张全身的每一组肌群并保持约10秒，同时训练者描述该肌群所在部位紧张和不适的感觉。接下来，放松同一组肌群约20～30秒并注意体验放松后的感觉——温暖、柔软和沉着。放松训练技术帮助患者学会体验身体每一部分肌肉依次紧张和放松时的感觉。渐进式肌肉放松训练具体步骤见表17-1。

The final exercise asks the client to become completely relaxed, beginning with the toes and moving up through the body to the eyes and forehead.

最后，全身完全放松，从下至上，从脚趾向上到躯干、眼睛、前额全部处于放松状态。

There are some points for attention. The order of progressive muscle relaxation should be determined beforehand. Once implemented, it should not be arbitrarily disrupted. Relaxation training can be taught by demonstration to the patient by the therapist at first. And the therapist gives instructions and the patient follows them for the second time. After having learned, the patient can practice on his/her own, but can also follow the guidance training tapes provided by the therapist, usually 1-2 times a day, 15 minutes each time.

注意事项：全身肌群放松的顺序要事先确定，一旦执行，不宜任意打乱。放松训练可由治疗者先教患者做一遍，边示范边带患者做。第二遍由治疗者发指令，患者跟随执行，学会后由患者去自行练习，也可由治疗者提供指导训练的录音带，通常每天练习1～2次，每次15分钟。

Once learned the procedure, the client can perform these exercises only for the muscles that usually become tense. Clients may also eliminate the tensing exercises and perform only the relaxation ones.

一旦学会了这一放松训练程序，患者可以针对经常受累的肌群进行紧张和放松的练习，也可以不做肌肉紧张训练而只做放松练习。

Other relaxation techniques include meditation (such as Chinese Qigong, Indian yoga) and "countdown". In meditation, people try to relax both the mind and the body. In many forms of meditation, people begin by sitting comfortably on a cushion or chair. Then they gradually relax their body, begin to breathe slowly, and concentrate on a sensation—such as the inhaling and exhaling of breath—or on an image or object. All these techniques have been found to promote relaxation, enhance sleep, reduce pain, and increase creativity.

其他放松技术包括冥想（如中国的气功，印度的瑜伽）和倒数数字。在冥想过程中，人们尽力去放松自己的精神和身体。在形式多样的冥想中，人们开始通常舒服地坐在软垫或椅子上，然后逐渐地放松他们的身体，慢慢地呼吸，全神贯注于吸气和呼气，或全神贯注于某一想象或物体上。所有放松技术都被证明能促进放松，促进睡眠，减轻疼痛，增加创造力。

The purpose of using relaxation technique in nursing practice is to help the client first acknowledge the degree to which the person feels tension and anxiety, to provide a contrast to the daily experience of tension by teaching relaxation, and to give the client the ability to use relaxation therapy as a self-help intervention.

在护理实践中使用放松技术的目的是通过教会患者放松训练的方法帮助患者首先了解自己的紧张和焦虑感觉的程度，并通过做放松训练对比每天紧张程度的体验；其次让患者学会放松治疗法，作为一种自我帮助的手段。

Table 17-1 Sequence of progressive muscle relaxation

Muscle group	Tension-relaxation exercise
Hands	The fists are tensed and relaxed, and then the fingers are extended and relaxed
Biceps and triceps	They are tensed and relaxed
Forehead	The forehead is tensed and relaxed
Eyes	They are opened as wide as possible and relaxed, then closed as hard as possible and relaxed
Mouth	The mouth is opened as wide as possible and relaxed. The lips form a pout and relaxed. The tongue is extended out as far as possible and relaxed, then retracted into the throat and then relaxed; pressed hard into the roof of the mouth and relaxed, then pressed hard into the floor of the mouth and relaxed
Neck	The head is turned slowly as far to the right as possible and relaxed, then turned to the left and relaxed. It is then brought forward until the chin touches the chest and relaxed
Shoulders	They are pulled back and relaxed and then pushed forward and relaxed
Back	The trunk of the body is pushed forward so that the entire back is arched, then relaxed
Stomach	It is pulled in as much as possible and relaxed, then extended and relaxed
Buttocks	The buttocks muscles are tensed and then relaxed
Toes	The toes are pressed into the bottom of the shoes and relaxed. They are then bent to touch the top inside of the shoes and relaxed
Feet	With legs supported, the feet are bent with the toes pointing toward the head and then relaxed. Feet are then bent in the opposite direction and relaxed
Thighs	The legs are extended and raised approximately 6 inches off the floor and then relaxed. The backs of the feet are pressed into the floor and relaxed

表 17-1 渐进式肌肉放松训练

肌肉群	紧张—放松练习
双手	伸出前臂，握紧拳头，然后放松
肱二头肌和肱三头肌	用力弯曲双臂，绷紧双臂肌肉，然后放松
前额	绷紧额头的肌肉，皱额，然后放松
眼睛	尽可能地睁大眼睛，然后放松；再尽可能地闭紧眼睛，然后放松
嘴	尽量张大嘴巴后放松；用力撅嘴再放松；用力把舌头往外伸后放松；尽可能地将舌头向咽喉部回缩后放松；用舌头用力抵住上颚再放松；再用舌头用力抵住下颚再放松
颈部	将头尽可能地转向左边，放松；再将头尽可能地转向右边，放松；然后低头，尽可能地让下颌贴到胸部再放松
肩部	先向后用力扩展双肩，放松；再向前用力合紧双肩，放松
背部	躯干尽可能向前倾，使背部成弓形
腹部	用力收腹，放松；再用力将腹部鼓起，放松
臀部	尽可能地紧张臀部肌肉，上提会阴，放松
脚趾	脚趾用力抓紧鞋底，放松；再翘起脚趾，用力顶住鞋面，放松
脚	以小腿配合，先将脚尖用劲向头的方向翘，放松；然后再指向相反的方向，放松
大腿	将腿伸直并抬高，放松；再将腿伸直并用脚跟向前向下压紧地面，放松

ii. Biofeedback

Biofeedback is a special type of feedback that refers to information provided externally by a machine to a person about normal subthreshold biological or physiological processes. Small electrodes connected to the biofeedback equipment are attached to the client's forehead. Brain waves, muscle tension, body temperature, heart rate, and blood pressure, which the movement mediated by involuntary autonomic nervous system, can then be monitored for small changes. These changes are communicated to the client by auditory and visual means. The more relaxed the client becomes, the more pleasant the sounds or sights that are presented. These pleasant sights and sounds stop when the client stops relaxing, and they resume when the client achieves the relaxed state again. The client is encouraged to apply the technique in stressful situations after developing the ability to relax. A wide variety of biofeedback modalities have been used to treat numerous conditions, such as migraine headaches, palpitations, asthma, and neuromuscular rehabilitation.

（二）生物反馈技术

生物反馈技术是一种特殊类型的反馈，它是指通过现代电子仪器，将人体内不能被感知的生理信息描记，并转换成能被人们理解的反馈信号。将与生物反馈装置相连接的小电极接在人的前额上，可以监测由神经系统自动调节的脑电波、肌肉紧张度、体温、心率、血压的微小的变化。患者通过听觉、视觉了解这些变化。患者越放松，就会呈现出令人越愉快的声音和视觉图像。当患者停止放松，令人愉快的声音和视觉图像也会停止，而患者重新恢复放松状态时，愉快的声音和视觉图像就又恢复。生物反馈技术疗法是让患者学会放松技术和利用脑的意识来调节自身的生理功能，主要靠自我训练，仪器监测反馈只是初期帮助自我训练的手段，此后大部分靠自我练习。患者掌握了放松技术和自我调控生理功能的能力后，当他们陷入应激情境时就可应用这一技术来应对应激。各种各样的生物反馈技术已被广泛地应用于多种情况的处理，如偏头痛、心悸、哮喘、神经肌肉的康复。

iii. Systematic Desensitization

Systematic desensitization is a procedure that gradually teaches people to be relaxed in a situation that would otherwise frighten them. It is often used to treat phobias and other anxiety disorders. The word desensitization refers to making people less sensitive to or frightened of certain situations.

（三）系统脱敏疗法

系统脱敏疗法是一种教人们处于恐惧情境中学会如何逐步放松的治疗程序。系统脱敏疗法又称为交互抑制，认为放松状态与焦虑是两个对抗过程，两者相互抑制，即交互抑制。这一技术通常用来治疗恐怖症和焦虑性障碍。脱敏即指使人们对某些情形不再敏感或减轻恐惧。

Systematic desensitization is divided into the following three steps:

1. Establishment of an Anxiety Hierarchy The therapist and client establish an anxiety hierarchy—a list of fear-provoking situations arranged in order of how much fear they provoke in the client. For a woman afraid of cats, for example, holding a cat may rank at the top of her anxiety hierarchy, whereas seeing a small picture of a cat may rank at the bottom.

2. Relaxation Training The therapist has the client relax using one of the relaxation techniques described above.

3. Desensitization Desensitization generally includes imaginal desensitization and vivo exposure two stages.

系统脱敏分为以下三个步骤：

1. 针对问题建立焦虑或恐惧事件等级 根据引起患者恐惧的程度，治疗者和患者一起建立焦虑或恐惧事件等级。例如女人怕猫，抱着猫可能是恐怖程度的最高等，而看到猫的图片是恐怖程度的最低级。

2. 进行放松训练 治疗者用以上提到的放松技术使患者放松。

3. 脱敏 一般分想象脱敏和现实脱敏两个阶段。

Imaginal desensitization: Then the therapist asks the client to imagine each situation on the anxiety hierarchy, beginning with the least-feared situation and moving upward. For example, the woman may first imagine seeing a picture of a cat, and then imagine seeing a real cat from far away, then from a short distance, and so forth. If the client feels anxiety at any stage, he or she is instructed to stop thinking about the situation and to return to a state of deep relaxation. The relaxation and the imagined scene are paired until the client feels no further anxiety. Eventually the client can remain free of anxiety while imagining the most-feared situation.

想象脱敏：治疗者要求患者从低级到高级去想象每一事件等级的状况。先想象低强度的刺激，产生焦虑，然后放松，对抗和抑制焦虑；再想象，出现焦虑，再放松，直至不再焦虑。之后进入下一强度等级的刺激想象，又产生焦虑，又用放松对抗。如此反复进行。仍是女人和猫的例子，先让女人想象猫的图片，然后想象从远处看猫，接着从近处看猫，如此类推。如果患者在任一级别感到焦虑时，则应停止往引起更高的焦虑或恐惧情境级别想象，回到深度放松状态。放松和想象画面相互配合直到患者不再感到恐惧。最终患者可在想象恐怖情景的最高级别时也不再害怕了即可转入现实脱敏或模拟现实脱敏。

Vivo exposure: Asking a client to encounter the feared situation is a technique called in vivo exposure. For the woman who is afraid of cats, a therapist might arrange to the place where there are many cats. The therapist would model for the client how to approach a cat and how to touch it. The therapist may also encourage the women to walk gradually closer to the cat, reinforcing her progress with praise and reassurance as she does so. The goal for the therapist and client would be for the woman to touch the cat.

现实脱敏：要求患者去面对能令他产生恐惧的现实情景并进行逐级脱敏称为现实脱敏。对于女人害怕猫，通过想象脱敏后，治疗者可能会把她安排在一个有很多猫的环境里，并示范如何去接近、触摸猫。治疗者可能也会通过鼓励她逐渐靠近猫，当她按照治疗者要求的做的话，治疗者可用肯定、赞扬话语来加强她的遵医行为。治疗者和患者的目的都是为了消除患者对猫的恐惧，直至敢触摸猫。

iv. Graded Exposure

Graded exposure is similar to systematic desensitization except that relaxation training is not involved and treatment is usually carried out in a real-life context.

（四）逐级暴露疗法

逐级暴露疗法与系统脱敏疗法相似，但它不包含放松训练，且治疗通常是在现实情境中进行的。

v. Flooding

There is a premise that escaping from an anxiety-provoking experience reinforces the anxiety through conditioning. Based on it, flooding is a behavioral technique to extinguish anxiety and prevent the conditioned avoidance behavior by not allowing the client to escape but encouraging the client to actually confront the feared situation. In the technique, with no relaxation exercises, the client experience fear, which gradually subsides after a time. The success of the procedure depends on the client's remaining in the fear-generating situation until he or she is calm and feeling a sense of mastery. The technique is used for special phobias. Because of the psychological discomfort involved, flooding is contraindicated in clients for whom intense anxiety would be hazardous (e.g., clients with heart disease or fragile

（五）满灌疗法

满灌疗法的前提条件是患者逃离令他感到焦虑的情境的经历通过条件作用强化了他的焦虑程度。在此条件下，满灌疗法通过不让患者逃离，鼓励患者勇敢地去面对令其害怕的情境，进而阻止了该条件反射的产生，达到消除焦虑恐惧的目的。此疗法中，不用放松训练，让患者面对害怕的情境，这种害怕的感觉经历一段时间后就会逐渐减弱。该疗法的成功有赖于患者一直处于害怕的情境中，直到他平静下来并感到自己可以控制局势。满灌疗法用于特别的恐怖症。由于可产生心理上的不适，对于那些严重焦虑可引起

psychological adaptation).

危险后果的患者，满灌疗法是不适宜的（如有心脏病或心理适应能力差的患者）。

vi. Positive Reinforcement

If a behavioral response is followed by a generally rewarding event, such as food, avoidance of pain, or praise, it tends to be strengthened and to occur more frequently. Positive reinforcement has been used in a variety of situations.

（六）正强化技术

如果某种行为通过食物、免于疼痛或称赞的形式受到鼓励，这种行为就会被强化，且会更频繁的发生。正强化被应用于各种各样的情况。如在实际生活中，儿童表现好的给予奖励小红花、小礼品，成人工作学习好可获得奖学金、评为先进等。应用强化技术应注意适宜、及时、灵活等原则。

vii. Modeling

Modeling refers to having a client learn a new behavior by observation, without having to perform the behavior until the client feels ready. Just as irrational fears may be acquired by learning, they can be unlearned by observing a fearless model confront the feared object. With phobic children, it is very useful that a therapist places them with other children of their own age and sex who approach the feared object or situation, such as having injection. With adults, a therapist may describe the feared activity in a calm manner with which the client can identify, or the therapist may act out with the client the process of mastering the feared activity. The modeling technique has been used successful with agoraphobia, job interview, and shyness by having a therapist accompany the client into the feared situation.

（七）示范法

示范法指的是让患者通过观看实例介绍、电视录像、现身示范等方式去学习新的行为。就像某些后天习得的非理性的恐惧一样，通过观看勇敢面对该种恐惧的大无畏行为，这种恐惧心理同样可以被消除。示范法的最典型的应用见于恐怖症治疗。对于有恐惧症的儿童，治疗者将他们和其他同年龄、同性别儿童放在一起，让他们观看其他儿童勇敢面对会让他们感到恐惧的事物和情境。例如其他儿童勇敢接受注射的情境。对有恐怖症的儿童消除恐怖是十分有用的。对于成年人，治疗者可以用一种平静的方式向患者讲述令患者感到恐惧的活动，或者向患者演示在进行该活动中如何消除恐惧的过程，也可以利用其他人现身说法证实该活动并非想象中那样痛苦和危险，则可消除患者的恐惧。示范法通过治疗者的言传身教让患者去面对令其感到恐惧的情境已经成功治疗了陌生环境恐惧症、面试恐惧症和胆怯症。

viii. Aversion Therapy

When an unpleasant stimulus (punishment) is presented immediately after a special behavior response, the response is eventually inhibited and extinguished. There are many kinds of unpleasant stimuli: electric shocks, substances that induce vomiting, corporal punishment, or social disapproval. In this method, clients receive an unpleasant stimulus whenever they perform an undesirable behavior. For example, therapists treating clients with alcoholism may have them ingest the drug disulfiram (Antabuse). The drug makes the patients violently sick if they drink alcohol. The undesirable

（八）厌恶疗法

一种不良行为出现时立即给予一定的厌恶刺激（惩罚），则该不良行为会逐渐减弱或消退。厌恶刺激的种类很多，如电击、致呕物、体罚、或社会谴责。在这种疗法过程中，一旦患者有不良行为将给予厌恶刺激。例如，对于酗酒患者，治疗者给他们服用一种药物（戒酒硫，安塔布司）后，患者一旦再喝酒就会使患者剧烈呕吐。经过反复的处罚过程，不良行为通常会消失。厌恶疗法也用于治疗性变态或其他反常行为和强迫症。

behavior usually disappears after a series of such sequences. Aversion therapy has also been used for paraphilias and other behaviors with impulsive or compulsive qualities.

ix. Social Skills Training

Social skills training is a method of helping people who have problems interacting with others. Clients learn basic social skills such as initiating conversations, making eye contact, standing at the appropriate distance, controlling voice volume and pitch, and responding to questions. The therapist first describes and models the behavior. Then the client practices the behavior in skits or role-playing exercises. The therapist watches the exercises and provides constructive criticism and further modeling. Therapists often conduct this kind of training with groups of people with similar problems. Social skills training often can help people with schizophrenia function more easily in public situations and reduce their risk of relapse or rehospitalization.

One popular form of social skills training is assertiveness training, another technique pioneered by Joseph Wolpe. The technique teaches people, often those who are shy, to make appropriate responses when someone does something to them that seems inappropriate or offensive or violates their rights. For example, if a woman has trouble saying no to a coworker who inappropriately asks her to handle some of her job responsibilities, she may benefit from learning how to become more assertive. In the example, the therapist would model assertive behavior for the client, who would then role-play and rehearse appropriate responses to her coworker.

（九）社交技能训练

社交技能训练是帮助那些与他人交往有障碍者的一种方法，可以通过学习一些基本的社交技能来提高社交能力：学会如何进入交谈，怎样保持眼神接触，保持合适的距离，如何控制音量和音调以及如何回答问题等。治疗者首先解释并示范这些行为。然后患者反复练习这些行为或进行角色扮演。治疗者观看患者的练习，提出建设性的意见并进一步示范。治疗者通常对有相同问题的一群患者同时进行训练。社交技能训练常能帮助那些精神分裂症的患者更好地适应社会，减少复发和再入院。

非常流行的一种社交技能训练方式是自信训练，其倡导者是Joseph Wolpe。该技能通常训练那些当别人侵犯了他的权利或冒犯了他的时候羞于反击的人。例如，当一个女人面对一个经常要她办一些超过她职责范围的事情的同事很难说“不”时，她可能会从此训练中受益，学会如何更果断的拒绝她的同事。在这个例子中，治疗者将为该患者示范果断的行为，她将反复练习以回应她的同事。

IV. Role of Nurses in Behavioral Therapy

Nurses are important members of the treatment team in the implementation of behavior therapy. Because nurses are the only members of the team who manage client behavior on a 24-hour basis, it is essential that they have input into the treatment plan. They are the group called on most often to carry out selective reinforcement, modeling, skills training, and role playing. Because of their direct client contact, nurses are best able to observe clients, assess problem areas, and recommend targets for behavioral intervention. The nursing process provides a systematic method of directing care for clients who need assistance with modification of maladaptive behavior. It is a dynamic process that allows each plan of care to be individualized for the personal requirements of each client.

As nurses play an indispensable role in behavioral therapy, behavioral therapy can be widely used in nursing

四、护士在行为疗法中的角色

在实施行为治疗中，护士是治疗组中重要的角色。因为护士是唯一24小时和患者接触的人员，毫无疑问她们已经融入了治疗计划中。护士常常是进行选择性的强化治疗、示范治疗、技能训练和角色扮演的人选。因为护士和患者直接接触，她们是观察患者、对患者的问题进行评估和推荐行为干预目标的最佳人员。对于那些需要帮助来改变不良行为的患者，护理程序提供了一个直接照顾患者的系统方法。护理程序是一个动态的过程，可针对每一个患者的需求制订相应的护理计划。

由于护士在行为治疗中承担着不可或缺的角色，行为疗法可广泛运用于护理实践中。

practice. Positive reinforcement such as affirmation, praise and encouragement can be applied to strengthen patients'compliance and fight against disease. For example, in the course of medical treatment, some patients do not know much about certain examinations, have fear, can not accept or cooperate with certain examinations or operations. If nurses organize patients to watch videos beforehand, or ask other patients to present their views, so that patients can understand that the actual situation is not as painful and dangerous as they imagine, they can eliminate their concerns and receive examination and treatment. Relaxation techniques can help both patients and nurses alleviate their tension and anxiety.

Section 4 Cognitive Therapy

Cognitive therapy can be defined as interventions that reinforce and promote desirable or alter undesirable cognitive functioning. Cognitive therapies are similar to behavioral therapies in that they focus on specific problems. However, they emphasize changing beliefs and thoughts, rather than observable behaviors. Cognitive therapists believe that irrational beliefs or distorted thinking patterns can cause a variety of serious problems, including depression and chronic anxiety. They try to teach people to think in more rational, constructive ways.

I. Mechanism of Action

Men are disturbed not by events, but by the views which they take of them. The model for cognitive therapy is based on cognition, and more specifically, the personal cognitive appraisal of an event, and the emotions or behaviors that result from that appraisal. The goals of cognitive therapy are to make clients aware of their cognitive distortions and to effect change through correction of these distortions.

The distorted cognitions, which are called cognitive distortions or cognitive errors, usually present by automatic thoughts. Common cognitive distortions or cognitive errors are as following:

1. Arbitrary Inference An individual automatically comes to a conclusion about an incident

如运用肯定、赞扬和鼓励等正强化来加强患者的遵医行为和与疾病斗争的行为。又如在医疗过程中，有些患者对某些检查不甚了解，有恐惧心理，不能接受或配合某些检查或手术，若护士事先组织患者看录像，或者请其他患者现身说法，使患者了解到实际情况并非像想象中那样痛苦和危险，则可消除顾虑，接受检查治疗。运用放松技术既可帮助患者也可帮助护士自身减轻紧张情绪和焦虑。

第四节　认知疗法

认知疗法可定义为强化或促进期望的认知功能或改变不期望的认知功能的干预措施。认知疗法与行为疗法都同样关注一些特殊的问题。但认知疗法着重改变信念和想法，而不是着重改变可观察到的行为。认知疗法治疗者认为不合理的信念或歪曲的思维方式能导致一系列严重的问题，包括抑郁和慢性焦虑。认知疗法治疗者们试图教会人们用更理性、更有建设性的方式去思考。

一、作用机制

人们的行为、情感不是由事物本身所影响和决定的，而是由人们对事物的认知所影响和决定的。认知疗法模式是根据认知，特别是根据个体对激发事件的认知评价以及由此所产生的情感或行为来进行治疗的。认知疗法的目的是改变人们对某一事件或情境的歪曲的认知，从而产生持久的情感和行为的改变。歪曲的认知称为认知歪曲或认知错误，通常表现为自动思维。常见的认知歪曲或认知错误有如下几种：

1. 主观臆断　在证据缺乏的情况下，对某一事件就机械地做出推断，有时甚至用自

without the facts to support it, even sometimes despite contradictory evidence to support it.

2. Overgeneralization An individual makes conclusions on the basis of a single incident.

3. Dichotomous Thinking An individual views situations in all-or-nothing, black-or-white, good-or-bad terms.

4. Selective Abstraction It is a conclusion that is based on only a selected portion of the evidence. The selected portion is usually the negative evidence or what the individual views as a failure, rather than any successes that have occurred.

5. Magnification or Minimization It is to exaggerate the negative significance of an event or to undervalue the positive significance of an event.

6. Catastrophic Thinking It refers to always thinking that the worst will occur without considering the possibility of more likely, positive outcomes.

7. Personalization The person takes complete responsibility for situations without considering that other circumstances may have contributed to the outcome.

Cognitive therapy focuses on correcting patients'cognitive distortions.

相矛盾的证据来支持推断。

2. 过度引申 在单个具体事件的基础上做出普遍性的结论。

3. 非此即彼的绝对思想 看问题走极端，认为凡事不好即坏，非白即黑。

4. 选择性概括 仅仅以选择的一小部分证据为基础就得出结论。被选择的部分通常是反面的证据或是失败的例子，而不是成功的例子。

5. 夸大和缩小 过分夸大某一事情（事件）的消极意义，低估它的积极意义。

6. 悲观思维 总是把事情往坏的方面想，而不去想可能的好的结果。

7. 牵连个人 倾向将与己无关之事联系到自己身上，引咎自责；或认为自己应对事件负全责，而不考虑环境和其他因素对结果的影响。

认知疗法重点在于矫正患者的认知歪曲。

II. Indication

Cognitive therapy is used for a broad range of emotional disorders. In addition to the original use with depression, cognitive therapy may be used with the following clinical conditions: panic disorder, generalized anxiety disorder, social phobias, obsessive-compulsive disorder, posttraumatic stress disorder, eating disorder, substance abuse, personality disorder, schizophrenia, couples' problems, bipolar disorder, hypochondriasis, and somatoform disorder. The emphasis of therapy must be varied and individualized for clients according to their specific diagnosis, symptoms, and level of functioning.

二、适应证

认知疗法被广泛用于情感障碍的治疗。除了最初用于治疗抑郁，认知疗法还可用于以下临床情况：惊恐症，广泛性焦虑障碍，社交恐怖症，强迫症，损伤后应激功能障碍，饮食失调，药物滥用，人格障碍，精神分裂症，婚姻危机，两极倒错，疑病症，身心障碍。这一疗法强调必须根据患者各自具体的诊断、症状、功能水平制订不同的个体化治疗计划。

III. Techniques of Cognitive Therapy

i. Main Approaches of Cognitive Therapy

1. Rational-emotive Therapy Albert Ellis's rational-emotive therapy is also called ABCDE therapy (figure 17-1). In this therapy, irrational beliefs and illogical thinking are regarded as the major cause of most emotional disturbances. In her view, negative

三、认知疗法常用技术

（一）主要认知疗法

1. 理性情感治疗 Albert Ellis 的理性情感治疗法也称为 ABCDE 理论（图 17-1）。该理论指出，多数的情感障碍是由非理性的信念和不合理的思维造成的。Ellis 认为，消极的事件本身（事件，A）如失业、爱情破裂并不会

events (event, A) such as losing a job or breaking up with a lover do not by themselves cause depression or anxiety (consequence, C). Rather, emotional disorders result when a person perceives the events in an irrational way (belief, B), such as by thinking, "I'm a worthless human being."

直接导致抑郁或焦虑（后果，C），而是当一个人用非理性的方式（信念，B）去认知该事件时，如认为"我是一个没用的人"，才会导致情感障碍。

Although many techniques, the most common technique used by rational-emotive therapists is that of disputing irrational thoughts (disputation, D). First the therapist identifies irrational beliefs by talking with the client about his or her problems. Examples of irrational beliefs, according to Ellis, include the idea that unhappiness is caused by external events, the idea that one must be accepted and loved by everyone, and the idea that one must always be competent and successful to be a worthwhile person.

尽管有许多方法，然而理性情感治疗者最常用的方法仍是驳斥非理性的思维（驳斥，D）。首先，治疗者通过与患者针对问题进行交谈鉴别出哪些是非理性思维。Ellis 认为非理性信念包括不幸是由外部事件导致的；一个人必须被所有人接受和喜爱；一个人必须总是有能力和凡事成功才有价值。

To dispute the client's irrational beliefs and longstanding assumptions, rational-emotive therapists often use confrontational techniques. For example, if a student tells the therapist, "I must get an A on the test or I will be a failure in life," the therapist might say, "Why must you? Do you think your entire career as a student will be through if you get a B?" The therapist helps the client replace irrational thoughts with more reasonable ones (effective consequence, E), such as "I would like to get an A on the test, but if I don't, I have strategies I can use to do better next time."

为了驳斥患者非理性的信念和长时间以来形成的错误观点，理性情感治疗者经常使用针锋相对的技巧。例如，如果一个学生告诉治疗者，"我必须在测验中得 A，否则我将是一个失败者。"治疗者则应说，"为什么你必须得 A？难道如果你得了 B 的话你作为学生的全部生涯就此彻底结束了么？"治疗者应该帮助患者用更理性的思维来取代非理性的思维（有效的结局，E），如"我希望在测验中得 A，但是如果我没有，我有办法在下一次做得更好。"

2. Beck's Cognitive Therapy In Beck's view, depressed people tend to have negative views of themselves, interpret their experiences negatively, and feel hopeless about their future. He sees these tendencies as a problem of faulty thinking. Practitioners of Beck's technique challenge the client's absolute, extreme

2. Beck 的认知疗法 Beck 认为，抑郁的人总是对他们自己持消极的态度，消极地看待他们的经历，对未来感到无望。这些想法就是非理性思维的问题所在。Beck 认知疗法的实践者们向患者这种绝对的、极端的思维发

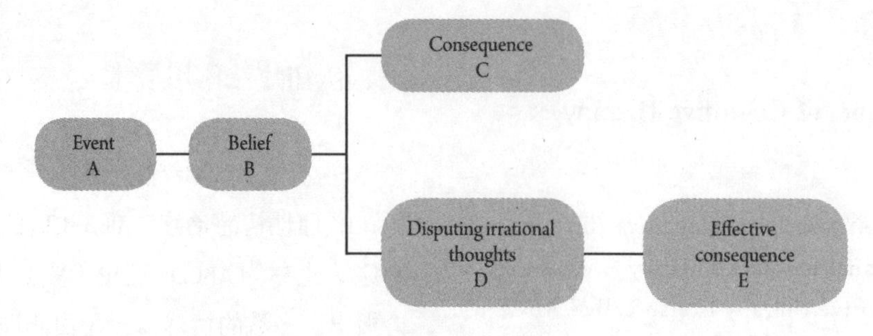

Figure 17-1 Albert Ellis's rational-emotive therapy

statements. They try to help the client identify distorted thinking, such as thinking about negative events in catastrophic terms, and then suggest ways to change the thinking.

Cognitive therapists often give their clients homework assignments designed to help them identify their own irrational patterns of thinking and to reinforce what they learn in therapy. For example, clients often keep a daily log in which they write down distressing emotions, the situation that caused the emotions, their thoughts at the time, whether the thoughts were distorted or not, and alternative ways of thinking about the situation.

起了挑战。他们尽力帮助患者明确什么是歪曲的思维，如用悲观的词语去思考消极事件，并为改变歪曲的思维提出建设性意见。

认知疗法治疗学家们经常给他们的患者布置家庭作业，其目的是帮助他们明确自己那些非理性的思维模式和强化他们在治疗中所学到的内容。例如，患者经常随身携带日记本，记下痛苦的情感，导致该情感的状况，他们在此时的想法，不管这种想法是否是歪曲的，和针对此状况可供选择的其他思维方式。

ii. Common Cognitive Techniques

1. Recognizing Automatic Thoughts Automatic thoughts are cognitions that intervene between external events and the person's emotional reaction to the event. These thoughts occur almost without notice and they are often negative and based on erroneous logic. An example of an automatic thought is the thinking "I'm a failure" after doing poorly on one test. Another example is a person's thought that "He doesn't like me" if someone passes the person in the hall without saying hello.

In cognitive therapy, clients must firstly recognize the automatic thoughts, especially those thoughts occur before angry, anxiety, and depression. A therapist may help the client elicit and recognize automatic thoughts by questions, imagery, and role-play, or by asking the client to write down all of the negative thoughts he experiences; and then, through analyzing each thought and explaining why it is irrational or exaggerated, the therapist may help the client recognize existing and affect of the automatic thoughts.

2. Generating Alternative To help the client see a broader range of possibilities than had originally been considered for an event, the therapist guides the client in generating alternatives to undermine inaccurate and distorted automatic thoughts.

3. Examining the Evidence The client and therapist set forth the automatic thought as the hypothesis, and they test the evidence both for and against the hypothesis.

4. Reattribution It is believed that depressed clients attribute life events in a negatively distorted manner; that is, they have a tendency to blame themselves for adverse life events and believe that the negative situation will last indefinitely. Through reattribution, the client is asked to substitute a nondepressed, positive thought in place of the negative one.

（二）常用认知干预技术

1. 识别自动思想 自动思想是介于外部事件与个体对此事件不良情绪反应之间的认知。这些思维常在不知不觉中产生，其内容常是消极的，并基于错误的逻辑。例如，某人在考试成绩不好时就认为“我是一个失败者”；某人在走廊和他人相遇时，对方没跟其打招呼就认为“他不喜欢我”等。

在认知疗法中，患者必须首先认识到什么是自动思想，尤其是在恼怒、焦虑和抑郁发生之前。治疗者可以通过提问、形象比喻和角色扮演，或要求患者写下他体验到的所有的消极思想来帮助患者认识自动思想。接着，通过分析每种自动思维和解释它为什么是非理性的或言过其实的来帮助患者认识到自动思想的存在和影响。

2. 改变极端的信念 帮助患者从更广的角度去看待思考一个事件，用现实的或理性的信念替代极端或错误的信念。

3. 检验假设 把患者的上述自动思维变成假设形式，然后检验支持和不支持此错误假设的证据，以事实来证明患者认知的错误和歪曲。

4. 重归因技术 抑郁的患者总是以消极、歪曲的方式看待生活中的事件。在遭遇挫折后，他们总是责备自己并认为不利的情况会一直持续。通过重新归因，要求患者用非抑郁的、积极的心态取代消极的心态对待生活。

5. Daily Record of Dysfunctional Thoughts The tool of three-column, or more column recording is used as homework for clients outside of therapy to modify automatic thoughts. In three-column recording, clients are asked to keep a written record of situations that occur, the automatic thoughts that elicited by the situation, and rational thoughts; in four or more column recording, clients are asked to add analysis of cognitive distortions or emotional response. Table 17-2 presents an example of a four-column recording.

5. 记录每天的不适应思维 除了治疗以外，作为家庭作业的三栏笔记法和多栏笔记法也是改变患者的自动思想的工具。三栏笔记法要求患者记录每天发生的事件，由此事件产生的自动思想和理智的思维；四栏或多栏笔记法还要求患者记录对歪曲认知的分析或情感反应。表 17–2 为四栏笔记法的例子。

There are almost no pure cognitive or behavioral therapists. Usually therapists combine cognitive and behavioral techniques in an approach known as cognitive-behavioral therapy, one of the most influential eclectic approaches. For example, to treat a woman with depression, a therapist may help her identify irrational thinking patterns that cause the distressing feelings and to replace these irrational thoughts with new ways of thinking. The therapist may also train her in relaxation techniques and have her try new behaviors that help her become more active and less depressed. Thus the outcomes of therapy are more effective.

目前几乎没有纯粹的认知疗法治疗学家或行为治疗学家。治疗者通常将认知疗法技术与行为疗法技术结合在一起进行治疗，这就是所谓的认知行为疗法。它是目前最有影响力的折衷治疗方法之一。例如，治疗一位患有抑郁症的女患者，治疗者可能帮助她明确是非理性的思考方式引起了她痛苦的感觉，并代以新的理性的思考方式去看待问题；同时，治疗者也可能教给她放松技术并让她尝试能够让她变得更积极向上的行为。这样，治疗的结果会更有效。

Table 17–2 Daily record of dysfunctional thoughts

situation	automatic thought	analysis	rational thought
I did poorly on the test	I'm a failure	Overgeneralization	I'm not a failure. I have done lot of things very well. Failed on one test doesn't mean I will fail forever
My son failed on the terminal examination	I'm not a good mother	Personalization	There are many things may contribute to the failing of son's test. As a mother, my responsibility is mainly to help my son to analyze the causes of failing and promote him to make progress in his study. I have no need to blame myself by taking complete responsibility for the situation

表 17–2 每天的不适应思维记录表

事件	自动思维	分析	理智的思维
我这次考试没考好	我是一个失败者	过度引申	我不是一个失败者，很多事都做得很好，这一次失败不表示我永远都失败
我儿子这次期末考试考砸了	我不是一个好妈妈	牵连个人	有很多原因导致我儿子考试失败。作为一个母亲，我的主要任务是帮助儿子分析失败的原因，促使他在学习中进步，而不是将所有的责任归咎于自己，责备自己

IV. Role of Nurses in Cognitive Therapy

Many of the cognitive therapy techniques are within the scope of nursing practice. Nurses may elicit clients' basic beliefs about a situation, and then the clients' beliefs are gently challenged. In nursing practice, we often encounter some patients with anxiety, depression and even suicide due to cognitive distortions. For example, some patients with chronic obstructive pulmonary disease (COPD) may suffer from repeated attacks and aggravation of the disease, but there is no radical cure yet, they think that they are "the end of everything, the burden of others", which leads to depression and even suicidal thoughts. Nurses should help patients realize that they have exaggerated the importance of the disease and belittled the value of their lives; as long as patients can timely treat and control the disease, adhere to breathing exercise, pay attention to nutrition and posture energy saving, actively prevent and treat cold and appropriate body exercise, they can stabilize the condition and achieve a higher quality of life. At the same time, encouraging patients to try to do something within their abilities can also reduce negative cognition. As the role of the psychiatric nurse continues to expand, the knowledge and skills associated with a variety of therapies will become more involved.

四、护士在认知疗法中的角色

许多认知疗法技术包含在护理实践的范围之内。护士在护理实践中如能启发患者了解是自己对某一状况所持的歪曲的认知和信念导致了目前的情感行为障碍，在治疗过程中患者的不合理的信念就会逐渐消除。在护理实践中，我们常会遇到一些患者因认知歪曲而出现焦虑、抑郁、甚至自杀的情况。如有的慢性阻塞性肺疾病患者因疾病反复发作并逐渐加重而目前尚无根治办法，便认为自己“一切完了，是别人的包袱”，从而产生抑郁甚至产生自杀念头。护士应帮助患者认识到是他自己夸大了疾病的重要性，贬低了自己生活的价值；只要患者能及时治疗控制病情，坚持呼吸锻炼，注意营养和体位节能，积极防治感冒和适当全身锻炼，是可以稳定病情、获得较高的生活质量的。同时鼓励患者尝试做一些力所能及的事情，可减少负性认知。随着精神科护士角色的扩展，更多的各种治疗的知识和技能将会融入护理实践中。

BOX 17-1 Learning More

Cognitive-Behavioral Therapy(CBT)

I. Three fundamental propositions

1. Cognitive activity affects behavior.
2. Cognitive activity may be monitored and altered.
3. Desired behavior change may be effected through cognitive change.

II. Major cognitive-behavioral therapies

1. Cognitive Restructuring They assume that emotional distress is the consequence of maladaptive thoughts. The goal is to examine and challenge maladaptive thought patterns, and to establish more adaptive thought patterns.
2. Coping Skills Therapies They focus on the development of a repertoire of skills designed to assist the client in coping with a variety of stressful situations.
3. Problem-solving Therapies They may be characterized as a combination of cognitive restructuring techniques and coping skills training procedures. Problem-solving therapies emphasize the development of general strategies for dealing with a broad range of personal problems, and stress the importance of an active collaboration between client and therapist in the planning of the treatment program.

BOX 17-1 知识扩展

认知行为疗法

一、三个基本假设

1. 认知活动影响行为。
2. 认知活动可以监测和改变。
3. 期望行为的改变可能会通过认知改变来实现。

二、主要认知行为疗法

1. 认知重建 认为情绪困扰是适应不良思想的后果。我们的目标是研究和挑战适应不良的思维模式，并建立更具适应性思维模式。
2. 应对技巧疗法 旨在协助患者发掘针对各种应激情境的应对技巧。
3. 问题解决疗法 问题解决疗法被认为是认知重建技术和应对技能培训程序的结合。该疗法强调总体发展策略，处理范围广泛的个人问题，并强调在治疗过程中患者和治疗师之间有效合作的重要性。

Section 5 Client-centered Therapy

第五节　来访者中心疗法

Client-centered therapy, also called person-centered therapy, based on experiential- humanistic theories, is founded by Carl Rogers. Client-centered therapy has helped to make therapists aware of the need to develop a positive working relationship with their clients.

来访者中心疗法，又称以人为中心的疗法，是以人本主义理论为基础，由 Carl Rogers 创立的。来访者中心疗法是让治疗者意识到要与来访者之间发展积极的人际工作关系的必要性。

I. Mechanism of Action

一、作用机制

Client-centered therapy assumes that each person has an actualizing tendency to develop one's full potential and the client, not the therapist, is responsible for change. The task of the therapist is to show empathy and positive regard in helping the client reach her or her potential.

来访者中心疗法假设每一个人都有要发挥自己的潜能和自我实现的倾向，并且是来访者本人而不是治疗者对改变现状负有主要责任。治疗者的任务是给予来访者通情，设身处地的理解其内心世界，而且无条件关注其情感，以帮助来访者充分发挥其潜能。

II. Indication

二、适应证

Many therapists, not just those of humanistic orientation, have adopted elements of Rogers's approach to resolve a wide variety of personal problems.

许多治疗者，不仅仅是那些人本主义治疗者，也包括其他学派的治疗家，都已经采用了 Rogers 的方法来解决各种各样的人格问题。

III. Techniques of Client-Centered Therapy

三、来访者中心疗法基本技术

Person-centered therapy emphasizes understanding and caring rather than diagnosis, advice, and persuasion. Rogers strongly believed that the quality of the therapist-client relationship influences the success of therapy. Three personal characteristics of the therapist—empathy, unconditional positive regard, and genuineness—would bring about the client's change and grow.

来访者中心疗法强调理解和关爱多于诊断、建议和说服。Rogers 特别强调治疗者和来访者的关系的好坏直接影响治疗的成功与否。治疗者的三种重要态度或基本条件——通情、无条件的积极关注和坦诚将使来访者改变不适应的行为和促进自我发展。

Empathy is the ability to understand what the client is saying and feeling with open and nonjudgmental ways. An empathic therapist demonstrates a deep understanding of the client's thoughts, ideas, experiences, and feelings and communicates with empathic understanding to the client.

通情就是去体验来访者的情感和感受，与来访者的体验同步，但又不对此进行判断或受到它们的感染。治疗者与患者交流时能够做到通情，则能对来访者的思想、情感和体验达到深入理解和领悟。

Unconditional positive regard is the ability to communicate caring, respect, and regard for the client. An accepting therapist cares for the client

无条件的积极关注是治疗者对来访者表示他的无条件的关心，接受和尊重。即使治

unconditionally, even if the therapist does not always agree with him or her.

疗者不是一直都赞同来访者的看法，仍给予来访者无条件的关心。

Genuineness is the ability to be real and nondefensive in interactions with the client. A genuine therapist expresses true interest in the client and is open and honest.

坦诚就是真实的、毫无掩饰的对待来访者。一个坦诚的治疗者在来访者面前不加任何修饰，以自己本来面目出现，真诚、真实、真情。

Rogers believed that when clients feel Unconditional positive regard from a genuine therapist and feel empathically understood, they will be less anxious and more willing to reveal themselves and their weaknesses. By doing so, clients gain a better understanding of their own lives, move toward self-acceptance, and can make progress in resolving a wide variety of personal problems.

Rogers 认为，当来访者感觉到治疗者的坦诚、无条件的积极关注和通情时，会减少他的焦虑并更愿意把他心灵深处的一切感觉和想法全部倾诉出来。这样，来访者就能更好地了解自己的生活，接受自我，并在不断的解决各种各样个人问题的过程中取得进步。

The therapist does not interpret client behaviors; rather the therapist attempts only to understand the client's inner feelings. In client-centered therapy, the client's autonomy is respected and protected; the client is viewed as the expert about himself, the therapist is a supportive facilitator to answer questions, give explanations, and shape experiments for the client to try. The therapy ideally results in the client's ability to see self differently and to promote self-growth and maturation.

治疗者不对来访者的行为做出解释，而仅仅是试图去理解和体验来访者的内心感受。在来访者中心疗法的治疗过程中，来访者的自我实现的能力受到尊重和保护。来访者被认为是他自己的专家，治疗者则是一个协助者，回答来访者提出的问题，给出解释和说明，为来访者营造一个有利于自我发展的环境，让来访者去改变自己不适应的行为和发展自我。理想的治疗结果是来访者能看到自己的改变、成长和成熟。

IV. Role of Nurses in Client-Centered Therapy

四、以人为中心疗法中的护士角色

There is a very strong philosophical similarity between the nursing concept of human care and the client-centered psychotherapy. In nursing, caring is a unique philosophy that emphasizes the nurse-client relationship and places value on positive regard, acceptance, human care, and nurturance. These qualities are an implicit part of the client-centered therapy. Thus, principles of client-centered therapy, with emphasis on a caring, humanistic relationship, fit well in practice directed by nursing theory in which the goal is to provide a safe psychological environment for the client to explore the meaning of his/her life, work, illness, or current circumstance.

护理工作和来访者中心疗法在理论方面有很多的相似处。在护理工作中，关怀是唯一的护理原则，它强调建立良好的护患关系的重要性，强调对患者的积极的关注、接受、人文关怀和扶持。而这些特点正是来访者中心疗法中不可或缺的部分。这样，强调关怀和人际关系的来访者中心疗法的原理在指导实践上与护理原理完全吻合，他们的共同目标就是为患者提供一个安全的心理环境，让患者自己去探索其生活、工作、疾病以及目前环境对其自我发展成熟的意义。

Section 6 Complementary Therapies

第六节　补充治疗

Besides the above main kinds of psychotherapy, there are many complementary therapies that are beneficial to reduce symptoms and to promote client's well-being.

除了上述主要的心理治疗外，还有很多补充治疗，这些补充治疗对减轻患者的症状和促进身心健康都大有益处。

I. Introduction

一、概　述

Complementary therapies, belonging to complementary medicine, are those interventions being used as an adjunct to medical care and psychiatric treatment that are thought to have effects on stress, sleep disturbance, anxiety, and/or other emotions. Complementary therapies have many benefits, which may outweigh the barriers that are often associated with conventional therapies, such as less cost, more convenience, fewer side effects, more individualized care, and more contact with practitioners. So they often seem to available, accessible, and therefore more appealing to the health-care consumer. Few complementary therapies claim to cure diseases; rather they propose to have therapeutic benefits on the reduction or relief of symptoms and the promotion of well-being. Complementary therapies assist the practitioner to view the client in a holistic manner. Most complementary therapies consider the mind and body connection and strive to enhance the body's own natural healing powers. Terms such as harmony and balance are often associated with complementary care. In fact, restoring harmony and balance between body and mind is often the goal of complementary health care approaches.

补充治疗，或称辅助疗法，是指那些属于辅助医学范畴，对应激、睡眠障碍、焦虑和其他情绪障碍有效的医疗和精神治疗的辅助治疗方法。补充疗法弥补了传统疗法的不足之处，具有花费少、副作用小、更方便采用和实施、更富个性化等优点，因此，常被卫生保健服务对象视为有效和易于接受的治疗方法，受到人们的欢迎。补充疗法旨在减轻或解除症状和促进健康，而不是治疗疾病。该疗法将个体视为一个身心统一的整体，致力于提高个体身体本身的自然愈合能力，强调个体的协调和平衡，治疗目标是恢复身心的协调一致和平衡。

II. Types of Complementary Therapies

二、补充疗法的种类

There are several types of complementary therapies used in psychiatric mental health care including guided imagery, massage, therapeutic touch, and music therapy.

精神神经疾病治疗的补充疗法有很多种，常用的有想象力放松、按摩、治疗性触摸和音乐疗法等。

i. Guided Imagery

（一）想象力放松

Guided imagery is a technique that builds on the relaxation response and adds visual or other sensory images to enhance the relaxation and/or to present an image for the client that is one of healing.

想象力放松是一种建立于松弛反应基础上，配合视觉或其他感觉想象以加强放松效果和为患者呈现轻松映象的康复技术。

"Pleasant memory technique" is one of a simple guided imagery technique in which a client comfortable and relaxed is told to close her eyes and is given the

"愉快记忆技术"是一种简单的想象力放松技术，应用该技术放松时，患者处于舒适体位，心神宁静，在治疗者的指导下，闭

suggestion to think back to an enjoyable event. Thinking of a pleasant event can bring many positive sensations to the client, as he will remember sights, sounds, and smells of a joyful time. A nurse can extend the technique by asking the client to think of a "special place" or a "safe place" where he has positive memories when the client is undergoing medical procedures that are uncomfortable and/or scary. The nurse can suggest that the client go back to the pleasant place brought up in her memory and think about being there rather than in hospital or other similarly negative situation. Such questions will assist the client in developing the scene: "How does it look?" "What does it smell like?" "What does it feel like?" The client will be encouraged to express thoughts and feelings about the experience to whatever degree the client is comfortable disclosing her personal experiences.

上双眼，回忆起过去某件快乐的事情。想起愉快的事情可给患者带来积极的感受，因为愉快的往事可让患者记起当时那段快乐时光里所看到的美好情景、所听到的愉悦的声音、所闻到的温馨的气味，让人心情舒畅，回味无穷。护士可将愉快记忆技术扩展应用到临床实践中，如当患者正在进行不舒适或可引起恐慌的医疗检查或治疗时，护士可让患者回想起一个有着美好记忆的特殊地方或安全的地方，并想象着自己回到了那里，而不是处在医院或其他类似的不舒适的环境中，从而在轻松的气氛中减轻医疗处置带来的不适。护士还可通过询问这样一些问题来引导患者忆起当时愉快的场景："那地方看起来怎样？闻起来如何？给人好到什么程度的感觉？"并鼓励患者尽情回味当时的舒适程度，充分表达自己当时的所想所感，以促进放松。

Relaxation and guided imagery techniques have great use in nursing practice such as in preparing clients to go through procedures, maternity care for preparation for and management of labor and childbirth.

放松技术和想象力放松技术在护理实践中应用较多，如用于患者的特殊检查、治疗和手术准备，产妇分娩的准备和分娩过程，通过放松，大大减少了患者的痛苦和不适。

ii. Massage

（二）按摩

Massage is the stimulation of the skin and underlying tissues for the purposes of increasing circulation and inducing a relaxation response. Massage has been used in China for the treatment of diseases more than 5 000 years ago. The Eastern style of massage focuses on balancing the body's vital energy (chi) as it flows through pathways, while the western style of massage affects muscles, connective tissues, such as tendons and ligaments, and the cardiovascular system.

按摩是一种通过刺激皮肤和皮下组织以达到加快血液循环和引发松弛反应的技术。按摩术在中国已有五千多年的历史，常用于治病。东方按摩术着重于使体内的气在经脉中穿流通畅，保持平衡；西方按摩术侧重于影响肌肉、肌腱和韧带等结缔组织和心血管系统。

The back rub is one of massage techniques and a very traditional part of care, frequently given to clients on bedrest, confined to wheelchairs, and before the hours of sleep. And stimulating the skin to increase circulation during bathing is also a basic massage technique. It has been shown to be beneficial by using massage in the following conditions: anxiety, chronic back and neck pain, arthritis, sciatica, migraine headaches, muscle spasms, insomnia, pain of labor and delivery, stress-related disorders, and whiplash, as well as high blood pressure, acute infection, osteoporosis, phlebitis, skin conditions, varicose veins, or over the site of a recent injury, bruise, or burn.

背部按摩是按摩技术之一，也是一个传统按摩的部位，常常用于卧床患者、坐轮椅的患者和睡前。淋浴时按摩皮肤以促进血液循环也是一种基本的按摩技术。事实证明，运用按摩有益于下列情况的好转：焦虑、慢性颈背痛疼、关节炎、坐骨神经痛、偏头痛、肌肉痉挛、失眠、分娩阵痛、应激相关障碍、抽搐、高血压、急性感染、骨质疏松症、静脉炎、压疮、静脉曲张，或最近损伤、擦伤或烧伤部位的上方肌体的保护。

BOX 17-2 Experience Sharing

Effects of Acupressure Training on Older Adults' Sleep Quality and Cognitive Function

We explored the effects of acupressure training on older adults' sleep quality and cognitive function. Ninety older adults with impaired sleep quality were randomly divided into equal control and experimental groups; 82 completed the 1-year follow-up. Participants in the control group were given instructions on sleep health, while those in the experimental group received sleep health instructions plus individual and small group acupressure training sessions and support to practice the intervention on their own each day. All participants were assessed by trained assistants blind to study group allocation using Chinese versions of the Pittsburgh sleep quality index, the Epworth Sleepiness Scale, the Mini-Mental State Examination, and four subscales from the revised Chinese version of the Wechsler memory scale, at baseline and at 3, 6, and 12 months. Repeated measures analysis of variance showed that acupressure training improved older adults' sleep quality and cognitive function, but the mediating effect of sleep on the relationship between acupressure training and cognitive function was not supported.

BOX 17-2 经验分享

穴位按摩对老年人的睡眠质量和认知功能的影响

该研究旨在探讨穴位按摩对老年人的睡眠质量和认知功能的影响。将90位睡眠质量受损的老年人随机分为对照组和实验组，每组45人，其中82位完成了1年的随访。对照组给予睡眠知识健康宣教，在此基础上，穴位按摩组还给予穴位按摩训练。分别于干预前、干预3个月、6个月、12个月末运用匹兹堡睡眠质量指数、爱波沃斯嗜睡量表、简易精神状态量表、韦氏记忆量表中国修订版中背数、图片记忆、联想记忆、理解记忆四个分量表测量两组研究对象的睡眠质量及认知功能。重复测量方差分析显示，穴位按摩能提高老年人的睡眠质量和认知功能，但中介效应分析结果还不足以验证穴位按摩是通过改善睡眠质量来提高认知功能的。

iii. Therapeutic Touch

Therapeutic touch (TT) is a specific technique developed in the 1970s by a nurse named Dolores Krieger at New York University. TT is based on the philosophy that the human body projects a field of energy around it. Pain or illness occurs while the energy field becomes blocked. TT involves the intentional exchange of energy between the practitioner and client by the practitioner's hands to correct the blockages, thereby relieving the discomfort and improving health.

The goal of TT is to repattern the energy field. Based on the premise that the energy field extends beyond the surface of the body, the practitioner need not actually touch the client's skin. TT is done by performing slow, rhythmic, sweeping hand motions over the client's entire body with hands remaining two to four inches from the skin. Heat should be felt where the energy is blocked. The therapist "massages" the energy field in that area, smoothing it out, and thus correcting the obstruction.

TT has been embraced by nursing in all areas of practice and is probably one of the most widely researched

（三）治疗性触摸

治疗性触摸是20世纪70年代由美国纽约大学一名叫Krieger的护士创立的一种特殊的治疗技术。治疗性触摸基于以下原理：人身体周围存在能量场，当能量场发生阻滞时便出现痛疼和疾病。治疗性触摸被认为是能量场的互动，由操作者的手引起操作者与患者之间能量场的互动来纠正患者能量场的阻塞，从而减轻不适和促进健康。

治疗性触摸的目的是使能量场畅通。基于能量场向体表外扩展的前提，操作者的手无须直接接触患者的皮肤，而是与患者身体保持9～15m的距离。操作者以冥想的意识程度进入治疗状态，以集中注意力帮助作为独特整体的患者，并用手从患者身体从头到脚进行缓慢的、有节律的、清扫式的移动。手在移动过程中，一旦遇到能量阻滞的部位就会感觉发热。治疗者用手在阻滞的能量场区域移动以疏通能量场，消除阻塞。

治疗性触摸已被广泛的运用于护理实践和护理研究中。最近更多研究表明，治疗性

interventions in the nursing literature. More recent studies have demonstrated TT to have a positive and consistent effect in producing a relaxation response, controlling headache pain, reducing anxiety and stress, promoting accelerated wound healing, and in treatment of alcohol and drug abuse, as well as promoting health maintenance. TT has been useful in the treatment of chronic health conditions.

触摸对引发松弛反应、控制头痛、减轻焦虑和应激、促进加速伤口愈合、治疗酗酒和药物成瘾以及促进健康保持都有积极的一致性效果。治疗性触摸对治疗慢性疾病非常有用。

iv. Music Therapy

（四）音乐治疗

When a client is unable or unwilling to express emotion through words, the visual and expressive arts provide the nurse with an opportunity to communicate with the client in avenues that need not verbal expression or the rational, cognitive processes. Arts permit the client and nurse to interact on emotional and intuitive levels.

当患者不能或不愿用言语来表达情感时，可视艺术和表现艺术给护士提供了一个与患者之间不必用言语表达或用理性认知过程分析进行交流的机会，而是凭借情感和直觉进行互动。

Music therapy is concerned with the use of specific kinds of music and its capability to effect changes in behavior, emotions, and physiology. The goal of music therapy is the reduction of psychophysiological stress, pain, anxiety, or isolation. The healing abilities of music are intimately bound to the personal experience of inner relaxation. Soothing music can produce a hypometabolic response characteristic of relaxation in which autonomic, immune, endocrine, and neuropeptide systems are altered. Likewise, music therapy activates a psychological response in that there is a reduction of tension, anxiety, and fear. Music therapy has been applied in birthing rooms, in operating rooms, during massage therapy sessions, during counseling sessions, on psychiatric inpatient units, and during addictions treatment. Many researches have shown that playing music has a desired effect in reducing anxiety in surgical clients and in assisting clients having sleep disturbances to sleep.

音乐治疗注重音乐的选择和该音乐对改变行为、情感和生理功能效果的能力。音乐治疗的目的是减轻心身应激、痛疼、焦虑、或孤独感。音乐治疗的效果与个体对内部放松的体验能力有关。轻音乐可引发新陈代谢降低，从而导致自主神经系统、免疫系统、内分泌系统和神经肽系统发生改变而出现松弛状态。同样，音乐治疗可激发心理反应而减轻紧张、焦虑和恐惧。音乐治疗被应用于产房、手术室、按摩治疗过程中、心理咨询进程中、精神科住院病房和成瘾治疗中。很多研究表明，音乐治疗对减轻外科患者的焦虑和促进睡眠障碍患者的睡眠起到理想的效果。

III. The Role of Nurses in Complementary Therapies

三、补充治疗中护士的角色

Complementary therapies can have an important impact on psychiatric nursing practice. More and more clients seek out the healing properties of these complementary care strategies. Complementary therapies are beneficial, safe, cost-effective, and easily implemented throughout psychiatric settings. Most complementary therapies can be prescribed and implemented by nurses. With holistic framework, nursing is in an ideal position to gain ownership of many complementary therapies for the management of symptoms experienced by psychiatric clients. Therefore, nurses must be familiar with these therapies and implement them to reduce or relief discomfort of psychiatric clients and enhance their well-

补充治疗在精神科护理实践中影响重大。这些治疗安全有效、花费少，又易于实施，越来越多的服务对象受益于补充治疗并选择补充治疗以增加疗效。大多数补充治疗可凭护嘱由护士实施。因此，护士必须熟悉这些治疗并将其应用到护理实践中去以减轻或消除精神障碍患者的不适，促进其健康；同时，应该进行更深入的科学研究以进一步证明补

being. At the same time, nurses should continue to follow the research literature to track more evidences regarding the effectiveness of these therapies.

(Zeng Hui)

充治疗的有效性，挖掘其潜能，使服务对象受益更多。

（曾 慧）

Key Points

1. Psychoanalysis focuses on helping clients become aware of, and get insight into their unconscious conflicts and repressed thoughts, which are the causes of their problems, by free association, dream interpretation, transference analysis, and assistance overcome.
2. Behavioral therapy emphasizes to change disruptive behaviors based on principles of learning by relaxation training, biofeedback, systematic desensitization, graded exposure, flooding, positive reinforcement, modeling, aversion therapy, and social skills training
3. Cognitive therapy is to help clients recognize their automatic, negative, irrational thoughts and replace them with positive ones.
4. Client-centered therapy produces a warm and supportive atmosphere by a therapist with empathy, unconditional positive regard, and genuineness to let the clients feel comfortable and could deal with their problems better.
5. Complementary therapies include guided imagery, massage, therapeutic touch, music therapy, etc.
6. Nurses in psychotherapy may provide counseling, education, support, or direct psychotherapies to clients.

内容摘要

1. 精神分析法通过运用自由联想、梦的解析、移情分析和克服阻抗着重帮助患者达到内省，意识到其潜意识的冲突和压抑的思维是导致他们问题的症结。
2. 行为疗法强调在学习理论基础上通过放松训练、生物反馈技术、系统脱敏技术、等级暴露疗法、满灌疗法、正强化技术、示范法、厌恶疗法和社交技能训练来改变不良行为。
3. 认知疗法是帮助患者认识他们的自动的、消极的、非理性的思维，并代之以积极思维来改变歪曲认知。
4. 来访者中心疗法则由具备通情、无条件积极关注和真诚品质的治疗者为患者提供一个温暖、支持性环境，让患者感觉舒适，使患者能更好地处理解决自己的问题。
5. 补充疗法包括想象力放松、按摩、治疗性触摸和音乐治疗等。
6. 在心理治疗中，护士可为患者提供咨询、健康宣教、心理支持或直接心理治疗。

Exercises

(Questions 1 to 2 share the same question stem)

A 36-year-old woman had a minor traffic accident. She refuses to drive and says, "I shouldn't be allowed to be a driver." When asked why, she answers, "I could have killed someone!"

1. What kind of cognitive distortion does the client have?
2. What psychotherapy approach is more appropriate for helping this client?

(Questions 3 to 4 share the same question stem)

A 5-year-old boy is crying and trying to escape from the setting of vaccination. When asked why, he says, "It should be painful, someone is crying."

3. What is the most appropriate clinical diagnosis for the little boy?

思考题

（1～2题共用题干）

一位36岁的女性曾开车发生过小的交通事故。她拒绝开车，并说，“我不应该成为一名司机。”当问及为什么时，她回答说，“我差点成了马路杀手！”

1. 此患者存在何种认知歪曲？
2. 哪种心理治疗方法更适合于帮助该患者？

（3～4题共用题干）

一个5岁的男孩在哭，并试图逃离疫苗接种现场。当问及为什么时，他说，“这应该很痛，有人在哭呢。”

3. 该男孩最合适的临床诊断是什么？

4. What technique of psychotherapy should be applied for helping the little boy at this situation?

(Questions 5 to 6 share the same question stem)
A 50 years old man usually feels tension, worries about the safety of his families and his own health status, companying with physical symptoms such as sweating, trembling, dizziness or a rapid heartbeat. Several times of physical examination showed negative outcome.
5. What is the main problem for the client?
6. What psychotherapy approach is more appropriate for helping this client?

4. 在这种情况下，护士可采用何种心理治疗技术帮助这位小男孩接受疫苗接种？
（5～6题共用题干）
一名50岁的男性常常感到紧张，总担心他家人的安全和他自己的健康状况，并伴有躯体症状，如出汗、颤抖、头晕或心跳加速。但几次体检结果都是阴性。
5. 该患者的主要健康问题是什么？
6. 哪种心理治疗方法更适合于帮助该患者？

Chapter 18 Continuity of Mental Health Nursing Care

第十八章　精神卫生连续性护理

Learning Objectives

Memorization

1. Describe the concepts of continuity of mental health nursing care, psychiatric rehabilitation, community mental health nursing care, psychiatric case management and psychiatric family care.
2. Summarize the characteristics of a collaborative model of the interdisciplinary team and the roles of mental health nurses as members of this team.
3. Describe the principles of psychiatric rehabilitation, community mental health nursing care and psychiatric family care.

Comprehension

1. Analyze methods to promote referred mental health clients along the continuum of care.
2. Discuss the models of case management in community mental health nursing care.
3. Explore approaches to provide family therapy for people living with mental health problems.

Application

1. Develop appropriate plans of care for mental health clients across the continuum of care.
2. Develop psychiatric rehabilitation programs for clients living with mental health problems.
3. Provide effective education during psychiatric family care.

学习目标

识记

1. 能准确描述精神卫生连续性护理、精神康复、社区精神卫生护理、精神卫生个案管理和精神卫生家庭护理的概念。
2. 能准确概述精神卫生多学科团队合作式模型中护士的角色。
3. 能识别精神康复、社区精神卫生护理以及精神卫生家庭护理的原则。

理解

1. 能准确分析精神卫生连续性护理中如何实施转介。
2. 能讨论社区精神卫生护理中个案管理的相关模型。
3. 能探讨精神卫生连续性护理过程中恰当的家庭治疗方法。

运用

1. 在精神卫生连续性护理过程中制订恰当的护理计划。
2. 为精神障碍患者设计精神康复项目。
3. 在精神卫生家庭护理中提供有效心理健康教育措施。

Mrs Chen, aged 76, has been living alone in her small apartment for 6 months since the death of her husband, to whom she had been married for 51 years and had no children. Mrs Chen was an elementary school teacher for 40 years, retiring at age 65 with an adequate pension. A niece remains in regular contact with Mrs Chen and contacted her physician when she observed that Mrs Chen was not eating properly, was losing weight, and seemed to be isolating herself more often. She had not left her apartment in weeks. Her physician referred her to psychiatric home health care. Carol, a community psychiatric nurse, completed a preliminary home visit with Mrs Chen, conducted an assessment and found that her mood was dysphoric and tearful at times, but she was cooperative, and denied thoughts of self-harm. Mrs Chen stated, "I feel so alone; so useless." There is a subjective report of occasional dizziness and loss of 9.07 kg since the death of her husband.

Please think about the following questions based on the case:

1. What might be potential nursing diagnoses for Mrs Chen?

2. What should the community psychiatric health nurse include in a referral letter about Mrs Chen to the psychiatric home health care unit?

陈太太，76岁，自丈夫去世后已独居在一个小公寓中六个月。她和她丈夫结婚51年，无子，在一所小学教学40年，65岁时退休，退休金充裕。她的侄女会定期看望或联系她。当她发现陈太太进食欠佳，体重下降，与周围环境的隔绝与时俱增，并且已经几个星期没有离开过公寓后，她联系了陈太太的医生。医生将其转诊至一家精神科照护中心。在陈太太转诊前，一位社区精神科护士卡罗尔对她进行了一次家访，并做了初步评估，发现陈太太烦躁不安，时常落泪。但是陈太太很配合，否认有自伤的想法，她透露感觉自己很孤独，没有什么价值。陈太太还报告自己偶尔有眩晕感，自从丈夫去世后体重下降了9.07 kg。

请思考：

1. 陈太太目前及潜在的护理诊断是什么？

2. 将陈太太转诊至精神科照护中心时，应当如何撰写转诊信？

"*Mental Health Action Plan 2013-2020*" of World Health Organization and "*Chinese National Mental Health Work Plan (2015-2020)*" recognizes that one of the major objectives of mental health work is the provision of comprehensive, integrated mental health and social care services in community-based settings, and the improvement of the collaborations of hospitals, communities and rehabilitation institutes. The priority work is to provide seamless connection mental health services of prevention, treatment and rehabilitation, which based on the continuity of nursing care and the development of tertiary prevention system. "Chinese National Mental Health Work Plan (2015-2020)" also indicated that one of the major goals of mental health is the "people in 70% of Chinese cities have access to community mental health nursing and rehabilitation care by 2020, and 50% of people can have home-based care". This Chapter explores the basic concepts, elements and interventions of the continuity of mental health nursing care. Psychiatric rehabilitation, community mental health nursing and psychiatric family care are the focus.

世界卫生组织《2013—2020年精神卫生综合行动计划》及《全国精神卫生工作规划（2015—2020年）》明确提出当前精神卫生工作的主要目标之一是建设综合型、一体化的精神卫生和社会保障服务，强调精神卫生领域医院、社区及其他康复场所的多机构合作。通过落实精神卫生连续性护理，促进精神障碍三级预防体系的建立，从而实现精神障碍预防、治疗和康复的无缝衔接是当前精神卫生主要工作内容之一。《全国精神卫生工作规划（2015—2020年）》还指出，到2020年，我国70%以上的县（市、区）应设有精神障碍康复机构，50%以上的居家患者能接受康复服务。本章主要探讨精神卫生连续性护理的基本概念、主要内容以及干预方法，其中精神康复、社区精神卫生护理以及精神卫生家庭护理是重点讨论内容。

Section 1 Introduction

第一节 概 述

Continuity of nursing care is based on the individual's needs and provides the client with a wide range of treatment modalities to help an individual in achieving his or her optimal level of functioning. People living with mental health problems should be able to access care from hospital to community. Continuity of mental health nursing care services must ensure an orderly transition from one service to the next appropriate service and uninterrupted movement as the individual transitions along diverse elements of the service delivery system. Continuity of mental health nursing care is considered by clients and clinicians as an essential feature of good quality care of long-term disorders, yet there is general agreement that it is a complex concept and lacks clarity in conceptualization and operationalization.

连续性护理是基于个体的需要，为护理对象提供一系列的护理措施来帮助个体达到他/她的理想功能水平。尽管连续性护理是一个复杂的概念，将其概念化和操作化的工作还尚待完成，但是社区、家庭和康复是这一概念的核心部分。存在精神健康问题的人可以寻求从医院层面至社区层面的帮助。精神卫生连续性护理服务的主要目标包括：① 确保两次精神卫生服务之间有序的过渡；② 当精神障碍患者在多个机构中辗转寻求多样化的服务时能够顺利交接。虽然连续性护理的概念并未有统一的定论，目前，精神障碍患者和精神科医务人员都将精神卫生连续性护理视为提高护理质量和患者生活质量的关键要素。

Continuity of mental health nursing care requires the collaboration of clinics, clients' families, their communities and rehabilitation centers. Nurses are the essential members of this collaborative team approach which involves promotion of mental health, treatment, rehabilitation and coordination.

精神卫生连续性护理涉及医院、家庭、社区和各类康复机构的协同合作，因而多学科团队成员间的紧密合作尤为重要。护士作为团队的一员，在精神卫生健康促进、治疗和康复领域开展工作，负责机构间的协调。

I. Interdisciplinary Team and the Role of Nurses

一、精神卫生连续性护理的多学科团队和护士角色

1. Interdisciplinary Team Regardless of the treatment setting, rehabilitation program, or population, an interdisciplinary team approach is the most useful in dealing with the multifaceted problems of clients with mental illness. Interdisciplinary teamwork has been shown to be the main mechanism to ensure truly holistic care, because it helps provide clients with seamless service throughout their disease trajectory and across the boundaries of primary, secondary, and tertiary care. The health care team has already changed from a medical model to a collaborative model (figure 18-1).

Collaborative interdisciplinary teams are characterized by: (a)different members of the team have expertise in specific areas as well as a set of common skills across all professions; they can meet the client's needs more effectively in collaboration; (b)inclusion

1. 精神卫生多学科团队 无论治疗环境如何，采取何种康复计划，或是针对何种人群，多学科团队都是处理精神障碍患者多方面问题的最有效方法。跨学科的团队工作已被证明是确保实现整体护理的主要机制，因为它有助于在整个疾病的程中为患者提供无缝服务，还可以跨越一级、二级和三级预防的界限。多学科团队已经由以医疗团队为主导的模型转向合作式模型（图 18-1）。

合作式模型的特点：① 团队成员拥有特定领域的专业知识，但也掌握一套结合了多学科特点的通用技能；② 将精神障碍患者及家庭纳入多学科团队，并且平等对待；③ 所

of family and client as equal partners alongside paid professionals;(c)shared decision making;(d)extremely strong and functional communication mechanisms.

有团队成员共同决策；④ 沟通机制顺畅，通过合作，能够更有效地满足护理对象的需求。

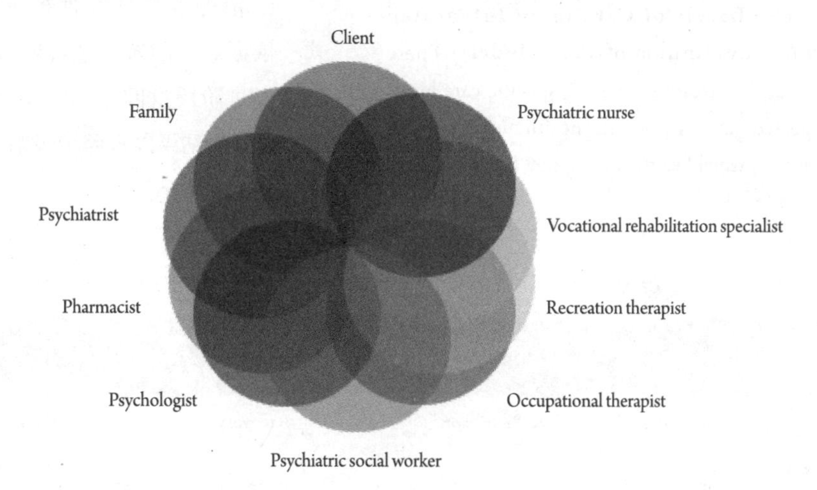

Figure 18-1 Collaborative model

2. Role of Nurses

(1) The role of nurses is to assess the individual's current level of functioning comprehensively and thus direct the person to appropriate resources to enhance quality of life and decrease fragmentation of care.

(2) Nurses are the only members of the multidisciplinary team who provide 24-hour care during the hospital stay.

(3) Nurses coordinate a number of community services which are involved in the continuum of care. The community services include housing, medicine clinic, dental service, outclient counseling, and self-help groups for the family.

(4) Nurses should include the individual and the family or significant other(s) in multidisciplinary conferences as much as possible. This is very important.

(5) Nurses can deliver direct care to help reintegrate people with mental illness into community living, as well as assist the individual in linking with other community resources.

(6) Because the variability of nursing activity based on service setting and geographic location is diverse, psychiatric nurses might assume multiple roles, such as nurse practitioner, case manager, evaluation and triage nurse, utilization review nurse, client educator, risk manager, quality improvement officer, marketing and development specialist and corporate managers and executives.

2. 精神卫生护士的角色

（1）全面评估患者当前的功能水平，从而指导其寻找合适的资源以提高生活质量，减少碎片化护理。

（2）在住院期间提供 24 小时服务，护士也是团队中唯一提供 24 小时服务的成员。

（3）协调连续性护理中的多种社区服务项目，其中包括住房，医疗诊所，牙科服务，门诊咨询和家庭自助小组等。

（4）推动精神障碍患者及家庭或其他相关人员参与到多学科团队会议中来，这一点尤为重要。

（5）护士可以通过直接的护理帮助精神障碍患者重新融入社区生活，还可以为其联系其他社区资源。

（6）因为服务环境和地理位置的变化所导致的护理活动的不同，精神科护士可能承担多种角色，如精神科开业护士，个案管理者，评估和分诊护士，采纳评审护士，健康教育者，风险管理者，质量改善官员，营销和开发专家以及企业管理者和执行者。

II. Components of Continuity of Mental Health Nursing Care

i. Models of Continuity of Nursing Care

1. The Levels of Care in an Integrated Behavioral Continuum of Care Model There are four stages of treatment having specific care levels with expected outcomes. Mental health nurses provide continuity in mental health nursing care based on these levels (table 18-1).

二、精神卫生连续性护理的内容

（一）精神卫生连续性护理的模型

1. 精神卫生连续性护理的综合行为模式 依据危急阶段、急性阶段、保持阶段和健康促进阶段这四个治疗阶段，设定对应的目标、预期结果以及照护级别（表 18-1）。

Table 18-1 Levels of care for each stage of treatment in an integrated behavioral continuum of care model

Stages of treatment	Crisis	Acute	Maintenance	Health Promotion
Goal	Stabilization	Remission	Recovery	Optimal level of wellness
Expected outcome	No harm to self or others	Symptom relief	Improved functioning	Attain optimal quality of life
Level of care	--Outpatient hospitalization --24-hour mobile emergency intervention --Crisis stabilization unit and beds --23-hour observation beds --Outpatient detoxification --Telephone access and triage	--Partial hospitalization --Intensive remission-oriented Outpatient treatment --Assertive community treatment --Intensive in-home intervention --23-hour respite beds* --Telepsychiatry	--Rehabilitative day treatment --Multimodal recovery-oriented outpatient --Relapse prevention --Rehabilitation-oriented residential --Supported independent living	--Education --Respite care --Drop-in centers --Peer support --Social activities --School --Employment --Housing

*They are for people that do not need a long admission. e.g. by a traumatic event and distressed but not mentally ill or someone drunk and suicidal.

表 18-1 精神卫生连续性护理综合行为模式中的护理阶段

治疗阶段	危急阶段	急性阶段	保持阶段	健康促进阶段
目标	稳定	缓解	恢复	达到最佳的健康水平
预期结果	不伤害自己或他人	缓解症状	改进功能	达到最优生活质量
照护级别	-- 住院治疗 --24 小时的机动紧急干预 -- 在特定科室住院稳定危机状态 --23 小时观察床 -- 门诊脱毒治疗 -- 电话随访、分诊	-- 日间治疗项目 -- 重症缓解型门诊 -- 主动式社区治疗 -- 密集型居家干预 --23 小时观察床（临时）* -- 远程精神专科干预	-- 日间康复治疗 -- 综合性的恢复导向型门诊 -- 预防复发 -- 康复导向型的居家护理 -- 支持独立生活	-- 健康教育 -- 临时照护 -- 提供教育、咨询或娱乐服务）的青少年活动中心 -- 同伴支持 -- 社交或从 -- 学校 -- 就业 -- 住房

*23 小时观察床（临时）：是指为需要短暂入院的存在精神健康问题的人群提供的一种服务，如经历急性应激和创伤但不足以诊断为精神障碍的人群，或存在酗酒、自杀问题的人群等。

2. Treatment Focused and Rehabilitation Focused Services　Treatment focused services for clients living with mental health problems must take into consideration those clients with impairments, as opposed to clients with mental health problems requiring rehabilitation focused services due to activity limitations and participation restrictions (box 18-1).

2. 以治疗为中心和以康复为中心的服务模式　在精神卫生连续性护理的过程中，护理对象身体功能发生明显损害时需要提供以治疗为中心的服务，而活动受限或参与受限的护理对象则提供以康复为中心的服务（box 18−1）。

BOX 18-1　Learning More

Aspects of Continuity of Mental Health Care and the Impact of Mental Illness

Components	Treatment Focused Services	Rehabilitation Focused Services	
	The impact of a severe mental illness		
	Impairment: Problems in body function or structure such as a significant deviation or loss, such as: hallucinations, delusions or depression	Activity Limitation: Difficulties a person may have in executing activities, such as lack of work adjustment skills, social skills or Activities of Daily Life (ADL) skills.	Participation Restriction: Problems a person may experience in involvement in life situations, such as: discrimination, poverty, unemployment or homelessness.
Medication	x		
Crises Intervention	x		
Case Management	x	x	x
Specialist Clinical Interventions	x	x	
Recovery and Wellbeing		x	x
Skill Development		x	x
Access to Community			x
Services			

BOX 18−1　知识拓展

精神卫生连续性护理的几个方面和对精神障碍的影响

项目	以治疗为中心的服务	以康复为中心的服务	
	对重性精神病的影响		
	损害 身体功能的明显改变，包括歪曲的信念或功能丧失。比如：幻觉、妄想或抑郁	活动受限 进行活动时遇到困难。比如工作适应能力不强，社交能力和日常生活能力的缺乏	参与受限 生活中遇到问题。如：遭遇歧视、生活贫困、失业或无家可归
药物治疗	x		
危机干预	x		
个案管理	x	x	x
临床护理专家干预	x	x	
恢复健康		x	x
发展技能		x	x
获得社区服务			x

ii. Services Patterns of Continuity Mental Health Nursing Care

Except for in-hospital nursing care during the acute stage, programs of continuity mental health nursing care are provided in rehabilitation facilities, the community and in homes. Psychiatric rehabilitation, community mental health nursing care and psychiatric family care are the primary services. Understanding and clarifying the principles and nursing interventions used in these services are essential for nursing students. Providing referrals based on the needs of the clients is one of the most important components in continuity mental health nursing care.

1. Psychiatric Rehabilitation Psychiatric rehabilitation, also termed psychosocial rehabilitation, is defined as the formal principles and active specialized strategies within a comprehensive mental health service system, and external to the system, that supports people with a mental illness to address difficulties in their life roles and participation restriction in society. Psychiatric rehabilitation has two essential features. Firstly, there is identification and minimization of the cause of disability. Secondly, at the same time help must be given if individuals are to develop and use their talents, through which they will acquire confidence and self-esteem from success in social roles. Psychiatric rehabilitation program is conducted in a variety of settings, such as in-patient units, outpatient settings, day hospitals, half-way house, patient's home and the community.

Goals of psychiatric rehabilitation include: (a) enhancing and supporting the person's journey towards recovery and wellbeing. (b) Identification of the person's needs and life goals. (c) Providing relationship and environment supports. (d) Assisting in the development of skills critical for effective life management. (e) Increasing a person's capacity for independence and interdependence. (f) Successful access to community resources and opportunities. (g) Participation in community life without the experience of discrimination and prejudice.

2. Community Mental Health Nursing Care Community mental health nursing care represents the responsibility to a population rather than simply to a geographically defined catchment area. It is a multi-faceted and multidisciplinary approach involving not only those responsible for providing statutory health and social services but also the family, non-government organizations, and, the community itself. The majority of Community Psychiatric Nursing Services (CPNS) are based either in a psychiatric hospital itself, or a day hospital/center.

Four important elements are involved in community

（二）精神卫生连续性护理的服务类型

除了急性期的住院护理，精神卫生连续性护理的院外项目主要在康复机构、社区及家庭中实施，因此，精神康复、社区精神卫生护理以及精神卫生家庭护理是主要的院外护理服务类型。明确这三大类型的护理原则及护理干预措施非常重要。此外，根据护理对象的需求，合理实施转诊，也是精神卫生连续性护理的工作内容之一。

1. **精神康复** 也称为心理社会康复，指在综合的精神服务系统或相关系统中，依据相应的原则主动采取专业策略，帮助患者解决生活角色适应障碍和社交障碍，促进其融入社会。精神康复过程主要有两个特点：① 明确及减少患者残障的原因及诱因；② 帮助其发挥、运用个人的能力与潜能，使他们能够自信自尊的生活在社区。精神康复项目可以在不同的环境中实施，如医院病房、门诊部、日间医院、中途宿舍、患者家中或社区。

精神康复的目标包括：① 鼓励和支持患者的康复过程；② 帮助患者识别需求，明确生活目标；③ 提供人际关系和环境方面的支持；④ 协助发展有效管理生活的重要技能；⑤ 增强患者的独立能力和人际交往的能力；⑥ 帮助患者成功获取社会资源和机会；⑦ 帮助患者参与社区生活，免于遭受歧视和偏见。

2. **社区精神卫生护理** 是针对整个社区人群的护理，它包括多层面的工作并需要多种精神科专业人员的团队合作，它不仅包括政府所提供的医疗社区服务，还包括家庭、私营机构及整个社区提供的照顾。社区精神卫生护理的服务主要由精神障碍专科医院或日间医院 / 中心提供。

社区精神卫生护理主要包括下列四方

care:(a)The care outside of large institutions.(b)The delivery of various professional services outside of hospitals or similar institutions.(c)The reliance on the "whole community itself" to provide care.(d)The provision of care as close to a normal environment as possible.

面的内容：① 在大型医院以外提供的护理；② 在医院外提供各类专业照顾；③ 依赖整个社区为患者提供照顾；④ 尽量在患者生活的日常环境中提供照顾。

3. Psychiatric Family Care Psychiatric family care focuses on supporting the biopsychosocial integrity and functioning of the family of clients with mental disorders as defined by its members. This includes family assessment, education, health teaching, support, counseling and family therapy. Having a family member with mental health problems affect the wellbeing of other family members, even if they are not the primary caregivers. Many family members report that they are unprepared for their responsibilities. In surveys, more than one third of family members were found to be depressed. Close family members are almost twice as likely to experience chronic pain. Families become the major source of support and rehabilitation. Of clients discharged from acute care, 65% to 70% return to their families. Even when clients do not live at home, their families are often the only source of support. Families need access to information, education, training and family advocacy.

3. 精神卫生家庭护理 主要目的是维持精神障碍患者家庭的完整性及良好的家庭功能，措施包括家庭评估、健康教育、支持、辅导及家庭治疗等。一名患有精神障碍的家庭成员会影响到其他家庭成员的健康，即便这些家庭成员并不是主要照顾者。许多家庭成员反映他们对于所要承担的责任还没有做好充分准备。在一些调查中发现，精神障碍患者所在的家庭，超过三分之一的家庭成员感到压抑，而亲密家人发生过慢性疼痛的比率是其他家庭的两倍。65%～70% 的精神障碍患者在脱离疾病的急性期后会返回到家庭，家庭常常成为精神障碍患者重要的支持系统。尽管有些患者不在家中居住，但家庭通常是他们的唯一支柱。家庭成员需要在获取信息、教育、培训以及家庭权利保护等方面获得支持。

III. Referrals along the Continuum of Mental Health Care

三、精神连续性护理过程中的转介机制

Referral is sending an individual from one clinician to another or from one service setting to another for either care or consultation. The processes of referral are based on the individual's assessed needs and the organization's ability to provide care. The nurse may initiate a referral and transfer a client to other services that provide the required care. A decision tree can be used to match the needs of the individual with appropriate services based on safety needs and intensity of supervision needed, severity of symptoms, level of functioning, and the type of treatment needed.

转介是将某个护理对象从一所医疗服务机构转向另一个机构寻求治疗或咨询的过程。转介是精神卫生连续性护理的核心内容，顺利、安全的转介才能保证连续性护理落实到位。转介服务必须基于护理对象的需求和转介机构能为护理对象提供照护的能力。在多学科团队中，护士可以根据护理对象的需求发起转介，将其转介至其他机构。护士可以根据决策树做出更匹配护理对象需求的转介，在此过程中应当依据护理对象的安全需求、需要巡视的频率、症状严重程度、功能水平和需要的治疗类型等。

A good referral enables an agency to prioritize and assess potential admissions, allows the agency to assess urgency, and enables the agency to plan care. A good referral depends on knowledge of facilities, skill in selection, objectivity, timing (e.g. do an early referrals and do referrals while the relationship is good), and follow up.

一个好的转介能够确保医疗机构按照轻重缓急评估潜在的入院需求，允许医疗机构评估紧迫性，保证医疗机构能够尽早制订照护计划。转介是否恰当取决于护士对各类医疗机构的了解、选择机构的技巧、客观性、

It requires a nurse to:

1. Communicate Clearly with Patients (a) Provide name, phone number, address, directions of the receiving institute to the client. (b) Do they need to organize transportation? (c) Discuss their expectations. (d) Discuss the nature, purpose and value of a referral. (e) Verify the best method to contact the client and family in the interim. (f) Offer written material about the referral source. (g) Alert the institute to expect the client and agree to confirm arrival.

2. Write a Letter of Referral A letter of referral is necessary and it should be clearly articulated and include: (a) Reasons for referral. (b) Issues discussed with client. (c) Client's understanding of reason for referral. (d) Any agreements made with client and family. (e) Avenues for communicating outcomes of referral.

3. Implement Risk Assessment It is imperative that risk assessment is fully completed and examples provided, such as "has continuous thoughts of suicide" "when angry voices tell him to kill his mother" "impulsive when angry" "with a history of medication noncompliance" "has acute detoxification ".

4. Clarify Goals of Admission to Hospital Determining the admission goals is essential for referral. Admission goals could be included to focus on the following: for further assessment and observation, close monitoring, stabilization of medication, secure place for treatment because of unpredictable behavior, 24-hour observation to diagnose and assess, medication review when there is a history of failed medication trials, review of diurnal mood variation, development of long term strategies to deal with illness comorbidity of physical and mental illness making treatment in any other facility problematic, treatment outside the family environment and why, diagnostic dilemma, assessment of psychometric testing, ascertain appropriate management, difficult to engage in long term therapy, community treatment does not appear to have been effective, to assess whether behavior is a result of environmental influences, requires specific unit.

5. Take a Referral According to Procedure It is appropriate to use case formulation when doing a

及时性（比如，早期转介，在建立良好关系时进行转介）和后续服务。它要求护士：

1. 保持与患者的清晰、顺畅沟通 ①向患者提供接诊方联络人的姓名、电话号码、地址、方位。②明确患者是否需要安排交通？③明确患者及家庭成员对转介的期待。④向患者介绍转介的性质、目的和价值。⑤明确在转介其间联系患者的方式。⑥向患者及家庭成员提供关于转介机构情况的书面材料。⑦确保患者愿意转介并顺利到达转介机构。

2. 写一封转介信 一封符合要求的转介信对于转介尤为重要，转介信应清楚地表达写明：①转介原因；②患者存在的问题；③患者对转介原因的理解；④与患者及家庭成员一起确定的方便继续进行治疗的任何安排；⑤沟通转介结果的渠道。

3. 实施风险评估 全面风险评估是转介的重要内容，在描述风险的时候应当举出具体的例子，如转介对象"持续存在自杀的想法""有愤怒的声音告诉他要杀死自己的母亲""生气的时候易激惹""药物服用过程中存在不遵医行为""存在物质滥用的戒断反应"。

4. 明确住院治疗的目标 确定住院治疗的目标是转介必不可少的内容。住院目标可以归纳为解决以下问题：进一步评估和观察，密切监测，确保药物的稳定使用，由于存在不可预测的行为需要提供一个安全的地方进行治疗，需要24小时的全面观察以供诊断和充分评估，曾有药物治疗失败需进行药物再次审查，回顾每日的情绪变化，形成长期策略以应对疾病带来的挑战，同时患有躯体和精神障碍，其他机构的治疗无法满足需求，必须在家庭以外的环境中进行治疗，存在诊断困境，心理测验的评估，确定适当的管理方式，难以进行长期治疗，社区治疗效果不显著，评估行为是否是环境因素影响的结果，需要专家团会诊。

5. 按程序实施转介 在转介过程中，恰当的方法包括运用案例陈述患者存在的问题；概

referral: outline how an admission fits into long term plan, complete all requested information, ensure information is current and legible, discuss referral with agency, and notify appropriate agency coordinator. It is inappropriate to merely send photocopied notes instead of completing a specific referral form, leave goals of admission blank, and give the client/parents the form to complete or provide additional information. Table 18-2 shows how to take a referral.

述出院后的长期计划；完成转诊信中所有要求的信息；确保提供的信息是最新的；与接收机构讨论转介的问题；通知转介过程中各方的协调人员；确保相关机构的充分参与。

不恰当的方法包括仅仅只发送病例的影印文件而不给出总结了重点的转介信；转介接收机构的入院目标空白；让服务对象或家属自己填写表格；使用戏剧化的方式描述而非实事求是。表 18–2 展示了如何实施转介的要点。

Table 18-2 Taking a referral

Key points	Details
i. What is the problem?	As opposed to the diagnosis
ii. For whom is it a problem?	Is it a problem for the school, the parents the partner? Is it an administrative/management problem for the treating agency?
iii. Precipitants.	Describe why now?
iv. People involved	Who is already involved? Who is actually currently involved? Who is mistakenly involved? Who has been involved in the past?
v. Perceived Urgency	Clarify timeframes: “urgent” may not mean the same to the referrer as to yourself
vi. Expectations	Is this a referral or a recommendation? The former will be accompanied by assessment but in the latter case an assessment may not have come from the contacting agency. The expectations of the referrer are assessed at the time of referral and readdressed when the family is seen. Clarify whether the referrer is asking for a second opinion or wants to hand over management. Who will monitor safety, take responsibility for coordinating care, or medical assessment?
vii. Preparation	What are the referrers going to tell the family about service to be provided? What are children going to be told?
viii. Responsibility	Who is responsible for what? (Child protection/monitoring/medication etc.)
ix. Discharge	What is the discharge plan?

表 18-2 如何实施转介

要点	描述
1. 描述当前的问题是什么？	基于服务对象的诊断，描述当前存在的问题
2. 当前的情况对哪些人或机构造成了困扰	对于学校或工作单位而言，对于其父母亲或侣而言是否造成了困扰？对治疗机构而言会导致是行政 / 管理问题吗？
3. 转介的紧迫性	描述为什么现在必须转介？
4. 转介涉及哪些人或机构	当前谁正参与其中？之前哪些人或机构参与了进来？之前哪些人或机构不应当参与？还需要哪些人或机构参与？
5. 具体描述导致当前转介紧迫性的原因	不能宽泛描述“非常紧急”，因为对于紧急的定义不同的人和机构有不同的解读，因此必须描述当前的具体事件
6. 明确目的，阐明当前的行为是转介还是建议	明确描述这是转介还是建议，转介需要接收机构的评估，但建议可能并不需要接收机构的评估；在转介时，转介者必须评估这次转介的目的，并对患者和家属做出明确说明；明确说明转介者是否需要征求他人的补充意见或者希望将当前的案例移交。明确由谁负责监控安全，谁负责协调照护，谁负责医疗评估

续表

要点	描述
7. 做好准备工作	转介者应当做好准备向患者及家属解释为何需要转介？思考如何对儿童解释？
8. 明确的责任分工	明确分工，各司其职，如确定儿童保护、监控、用药等各方面的负责人员
9. 明确何时终止计划	制订出院计划

Section 2 Psychiatric Rehabilitation

I. Fundamental Principles of Psychiatric Rehabilitation

1. Normalizing Roles and Relationships Psychiatric rehabilitation asserts that people with serious mental illness need not be separated from the rest of society, treated within an especially controlling environment, or relegated to only a limited range of living circumstances, work opportunities, or social relationships. Rather it is assumed that a full range of life experiences is within their grasp.

2. Acknowledging the Potential for Growth There is the belief that people with serious mental illness, despite the disabling aspects of their conditions, have a unique potential to develop skills, make personal choices, manage their illness, and achieve many goals that may have once seemed unattainable.

3. Focusing on Here-and-now Services Psychiatric rehabilitation services often begin pragmatically (for example, by focusing on housing needs, vocational needs, social isolation and financial crises) and work with clients to address their most urgent concerns. Rehabilitation programs also aim to strengthen the client's ability to accept and meet the responsibilities of day-to-day life.

4. Learning-by-doing To address problem areas, health care practitioners provide opportunities for problem solving within a real world environment. The program encourages more actual engagement in the problem itself and an emphasis on working with people in their homes, at their jobs, and in their communities.

5. Approaching Community Life Holistically Psychiatric rehabilitation programs recognize the interrelatedness of the various domains of community life. Consequently, although rehabilitation programs often begin with a single social, vocational, or residential focus, they soon add other elements of rehabilitation programs,

第二节　精神康复

一、精神康复的基本原则

1. 角色和关系正常化　精神康复主张患严重精神障碍患者不需与社会隔离，也不需要在特定的环境中接受治疗或被限制于某些居住环境、工作机构或社交圈子。患者有权利在社区中自由的生活。

2. 相信患者有发展的潜能　严重精神障碍患者除了在某些方面有残障之外，在其他方面有潜能去发展其技能、做出个人选择、控制自己的病情，而且可能实现先前认为无法企及的目标。

3. 着重于实质的服务　精神康复注重解决患者的实际问题（例如帮助患者解决住房需要、工作需求、社交隔离和财物的困难）。精神康复工作者与缓和共同找出最迫切要解决的问题，康复项目也旨在增强病患者的能力，以面对和适应日常生活。

4. 边做边学　在找出最迫切需要解决的问题之后，精神康复工作者会帮助患者在实际生活环境中接受训练，寻找解决问题的方法，并强调与家属、同事和朋友合作以共同解决困难。

5. 全面投入社区生活　精神康复项目与社区生活息息相关。虽然康复项目通常始于社交、就业、住房中的一个重点，但项目会很快增加其他康复的元素，例如教育、技能训练等。因此，成功的社区生活取决于康复项目中

recognizing that successful community living depends on simultaneously addressing needs in many arenas.

是否包含照顾患者生活细节所需的服务。

II. Role of the Nurse in Psychiatric Rehabilitation

Psychiatric nurses play an important role in psychiatric rehabilitation. The traditional inpatient nurse role moves into diverse out-patient, rehabilitative, and community-based settings. Most rehabilitation programs have a full-time nurse who functions as part of the multidisciplinary team. Psychiatric nurses will encounter mentally ill individuals at varying phases in recovery and will practice in many different treatment settings across the continuum of care.

1. Assessment Regardless of the situation or setting, the nurse must perform a comprehensive assessment at the point of first contact with an individual on the five dimensions of a person-physical, emotional, intellectual, social, spiritual-with the focus toward developing a psychiatric rehabilitation emphasis.

2. Provide Psychiatric Rehabilitation Programs to Match Individual's Needs When choosing appropriate psychiatric rehabilitation programs, initial assessments should be considered. This includes a focus on the client's financial issues, the type of treatment being sought, their current physical condition, and their ability to agree to or consent to treatment. It must be determined if the organization has the ability to provide direct care or if referral to another service should be considered.

3. Prevent Relapse in Several Different Ways Nurses act as a referral source for the programs, trainer or leader of the programs, or an after-care source for patients when the program is completed. Additionally, psychiatric nurses can help the patient and family by promoting optimism, sticking to goals and aspirations, and focusing on the person's strengths. They must have knowledge on the latest trends in effective treatment and available community resources. They must appreciate the stigmas that may hinder psychiatric rehabilitation. Above all, psychiatric nurses demonstrate patient advocacy by networking with community agencies and vocational specialists to ensure that the patient has available resources in the community to lessen the chances of symptom relapse.

二、护士在精神康复中的角色

精神科护士在精神康复中承担重要的角色，传统的精神专科医院护士的角色在门诊部、康复中心或社区服务中心等机构中大大得到扩展及提高。多数精神康复项目都有护士的参与，是精神康复团队中的重要成员。精神科护士需要为不同康复阶段的精神障碍患者提供护理，在社区中也需要在不同的环境中为患者提供连续性护理。

1. 评估 精神康复注重准确诊断及运用恰当的治疗与康复计划。不论在任何环境及情况下，护士必须在首次会见患者时，对患者进行仔细及全面的评估。评估内容主要包括五个方面：身体、情绪、智力、社交及精神状态。

2. 选择及提供恰当的康复活动 在选择康复机构及项目时，护士应充分考虑初次评估的结果，患者可以利用的资源，患者的类型，患者对选择和接受服务的能力，以及服务机构能否提供适当的服务等。护士可让患者参与进行康复项目的选择，或将患者转诊到其他服务机构以满足患者的需要。

3. 采用多种方式协助预防疾病复发 精神科护士可采用不同的方式协助患者预防疾病的复发，包括介绍患者参与康复项目，作为康复项目的训练者、领导者，在项目结束后继续提供连续性护理等。同时，护士应鼓励患者对前景保持乐观，坚持达到目标，并积极发掘患者的优点以帮助其克服困难。护士应该掌握最新的治疗知识及可供患者使用的社区资源，并应认识到歧视对精神障碍患者康复的负面影响，积极为患者争取应有的权益。通过与社区机构的联系，确保患者有足够的社区资源，以减少疾病的复发。

III. Program Elements in Psychiatric Rehabilitation

Psychiatric rehabilitation can be divided into acute or chronic stage as well as hospital-based and community-based. The following programs are discussed in this same order:

i. Discharge Planning

Discharge planning is an integral part of psychiatric nursing care and should be considered a part of the psychiatric rehabilitation process. The goal of discharge planning is to provide the client with the resources he or she needs to function as independently as possible in the least restrictive environment and to avoid rehospitalization.

1. Implement Discharge Assessment Based On Checklist It includes medications, activity of daily livings, mental health after-care, residence, follow-up in physical health care, special education, financial, or other needs.

2. Record Discharge Planning Activities (a) The client's response to proposed after-care treatment. (b) Follow-up for psychiatric and physical health problems. (c) Discharge instructions. (d) Medication education, food-drug interactions, drug-drug interactions, and special diet instructions. (e) Discharge assessment results.

3. Explain after-care plans and instruction to the client and family in details. Because clients with mental illnesses may have limited cognitive abilities and residual motivational and anxiety problems, it is helpful to make after-care appointments before the client leaves the facility. The nurse should than provide written instructions about where and when to go for the appointment and a contact person's name and telephone number at an after-care placement. Finally, the nurse should review emergency telephone numbers and contacts and medication instructions.

ii. Relapse Prevention Programs

1. Causes of Relapse Relapse of mental illness symptoms is the major reason for rehospitalization in many countries. The term relapse refers to the recurrence or marked increase in severity of the symptoms of

三、精神康复项目的内容

精神康复根据时期可以分为急性期和慢性期精神康复，根据地点可以分为医院精神康复、社区精神康复等，不同时间、不同地点康复内容不同。下列精神康复项目的内容按照由急性至慢性，由医院至社区的顺序列出：

（一）制订出院计划

出院计划是精神科护理、精神康复的重要组成部分，目的是为患者提供所有可以利用的资源，使其尽快自立，避免再次入院。

1. 实施出院前评估 精神科护士应对即将出院的精神障碍患者进行评估以方便医护人员更好地实施连续性护理和制订出院计划，主要包括：① 药物治疗；② 日常生活活动能力；③ 精神健康连续性护理状况；④ 住所；⑤ 躯体健康护理进展状况；⑥ 特殊的教育经历、经济状况或其他需要。

2. 制订出院计划并记录 ① 评估患者对护理措施的反应，治疗的反应及进展；② 精神卫生和躯体健康问题的后续跟进；③ 出院指导；④ 对患者所进行的用药方面的教育，食物及药物的相互作用，药物之间的相互作用和特别的饮食指导等内容；⑤ 出院前评估的结果。

3. 向患者及家属详细介绍出院计划 护士应向患者及家属详细解释所有连续性护理计划和指导，在患者出院前，约好所有复诊时间，为患者提供书面的指导，详细告知复诊的时间和地点，紧急时候可拨的电话号码和药物服用的指导等，以保证患者出院后的连续治疗。

（二）预防复发

1. 复发的原因 疾病复发是精神科患者再入院的主要原因。“复发”一词是指在病情好转或稳定后，患者再次患病或原有疾病的

a disease, especially following a period of apparent improvement or stability. The primary reasons for relapse include stopping medications or reducing dosages without medical supervision. Clients should be supervised and educated to take medications in a correct and timely manner during regular outpatient visits and long-term follow-up. Homelessness and unemployment create threats to a client's identity and state of wellness and can also affect relapse.

2. Relapse Prevention Much effort has been directed at the creation of relapse prevention programs for the major mental illnesses and addiction disorders. Relapse prevention programs generally seek to: (a) Provide an understanding of the illness for clients and families. (b) Enable clients and families to come to terms with the chronic nature of the illness. (c) Promote recognition of early warning signs of relapse. (d) Educate clients and families about prescribed medication and the importance of compliance. (e) Educate clients and families about side effects of medication and ways to deal with them. (f) Provide information about other disease management strategies (e.g., stress management, exercise) in the prevention of relapse.

Research has shown that nurses conducting highly structured health education programs from admission through the immediate post-discharge period are effective in preventing relapse in clients having schizophrenia. These programs include didactic courses, with audiovisual and written materials, and pretests and posttests.

iii. Activities of Daily Living

One of the problems of clients with serious mental illness is the impact of the mental disorders on clients' instrumental functioning; many clients have deterioration in their abilities of self-care and life skills. Fundamentals of personal hygiene, appropriate clothing, proper nutrition and meal preparation, budgeting, and public transportation are skills that some clients may have lost during long period of institutional care, or may be too unmotivated or distracted by their illness to address. Health care practitioners help in a variety of ways. Special classes in day hospitals, working on immediate issues within the residential program, field trips, and community events are ways in which skills are taught, rehearsed, practiced, and learned.

iv. Social Programs

Clients with severe mental illness often face problems of social isolation and loneliness. Many of

症状加重。自行停药、减药是精神障碍复发的主要原因，因此通过定期门诊和长期随访，督促患者服药，并通过教育健康，提高患者对服药的依从性是减少复发的首要措施。其次无家可归和失业会使患者感到很大的威胁，并影响其情绪，因此提供相应社会支持也很重要。

2. 预防复发的措施 为有效预防和避免复发，可采取以下措施：① 患者和家属充分理解疾病的症状；② 指导患者和家属适应疾病带来的长期问题；③ 指导患者和家属认识疾病复发的早期症状；④ 指导患者和家属认识到药物治疗的作用及服从药物治疗的重要性；⑤ 教育患者和家属识别药物副作用并及时处理；⑥ 提供有关处理疾病方法的信息，如压力应对的方法等，以预防复发。

有研究证明，在患者入院时开始采取健康教育措施，包括教育讲座、视听教材及讲义、教育前后的测验评价，随后同患者及家属一起在住院时或出院后继续完善预防复发的计划并实施，可以有效预防了精神分裂症患者疾病的复发。

（三）日常活动能力训练

精神障碍患者的日常活动功能通常会受到影响。患者因长期住院，或因患病后受疾病症状的困扰，保持个人卫生、衣着、饮食、财物管理及运用公共交通工具等能力受到限制。慢性退缩型的患者往往失去自我照顾能力，生活技能退化。医护人员应采用行为矫正的方法，训练患者养成规律生活习惯，培养生活自理能力和使用工具的能力，例如在日间医院提供特殊的技能课程，帮助患者学习处理日常活动，安排外出训练和社区活动等，使患者有机会在社区实践中学会各种生活技能。

（四）社交技能训练

隔离和孤独是严重精神障碍患者经常出现的问题。针对精神障碍的患者，采用授课、讨

those discharged do not have the necessary social skills to live independently. Classroom programs, discussion, demonstration, repetitive exercises and social activities can provide opportunities to form friendships, practice social interactions and conversational techniques. Social activities such as clubs, educational and current events classes, psychoeducational programs, health maintenance programs, recreational services, and evening gatherings for movies, dancing, and barbecuing are ways to decrease stigma and provide peer support.

论、示范、角色扮演和重复练习的方法，也可组织娱乐服务活动，训练基本的社交礼仪、倾听、语言表达和解决问题的能力，以增进社交技能、改善人际关系和争取社会支持。

v. Mental Rehabilitation Training

Individual and group based activities can be designed to improve coping strategies, by using cognitive remediation therapy and mood adjustment interventions. Patients who lack confidence or are unable to cope with stressors can benefit extensively from these programs.

（五）心理康复训练

针对自信心缺乏、难以应对压力的患者，采用个体和小组治疗相结合的方法，进行认知矫正，调整情绪，提高应对挫折的能力。

vi. Recreation Therapy

Nurses can design interactive or competitive activities to assist patients to increase interests and cultivate hobbies, such as games, chess, cards, music, painting and sports. Client participation can promote enjoyment of life instead of withdrawal or isolation.

（六）文娱治疗

通过多种参与性、学习性和竞技性的活动，比如游戏、棋牌、音乐、绘画、体育比赛等，增加患者的生活情趣，培养爱好，陶冶情操，享受生活。

vii. Residential Programs

One of the most urgent needs for many clients is a safe, affordable, decent place to live and call their own. Early in the history of psychiatric rehabilitation, some service providers started establishing group homes, such as half-way houses, for clients who had no homes or chose to live independently from their families. Half-way houses provide accommodations to clients during the transitional period from hospital to community. Their focus is to improve clients' independent daily activity living skills and help them reintegrate into society.

（七）居住环境的安排

安全、舒适并且可以负担得起的住所对精神障碍患者来说极其重要。在精神康复发展的初期，有一些机构为那些无家可归，或决定不与家属同住的患者提供住所，如中途宿舍等。中途宿舍是为从医院踏入社区的精神障碍患者所提供的短暂住宿，帮助他们提升独立生活的能力并重新融入社会。

viii. Occupational Programs

Work is an important element of a person's life. Many psychiatric rehabilitation programs attach considerable importance to work. There are four levels of vocational training programs.

（八）就业安排及工作能力训练

工作是一个人生活中重要的组成部分，许多精神康复项目都注重为患者创造和提供工作的机会，以增强患者的能力，使其获得满足感。

1. Sheltered workshops provide training and employment where allowance is made for a person's disability and the person is protected from full competition. They also offer permanent employment to persons with specified disabilities as well as temporary employment to retrain skills. The work training helps clients to appreciate their work capabilities and capacity for further growth.

1. 职业康复训练的第一步是在庇护工场中从事低压力、非竞争性的工作，从而学习工作技能。

2. Transitional employment programs offer the same support as supported employment programs,

2. 第二步是过渡性就业，由社区或康复机构与企业签订协议，担保完成某项初级的工作。

but the employment is temporary. This type of work has a time frame and is agreed on by the employer and the participant. The person works at the temporary position until he or she can find permanent, competitive employment.

3. Supported employment programs provide on-site support and job-coaching services on a one-to-one basis. They occur in real work settings and are used for clients with severe mental illnesses. The primary focus is to maintain attachment between the mentally ill person and the workforce.

4. Independent employment, providers assist clients with mental disorders to obtain independent employment. Clients need assessment, coordination and support from mental health professionals until they can work in a competitive environment.

Practitioners working in this arena may be job developers (working with employers to open job opportunities for clients); job coaches (helping clients locate jobs and prepare for interviews and working alongside clients on the job until they can gradually minimize the intensity and visibility of their support); or long-term support workers (providing ongoing counseling, problem solving, and occasionally on-site interventions to sustain the client's long-term involvement in the labor market).

ix. Educational Programs

A growing emphasis is on helping clients return to school. Such programs are important because many clients have their onset of mental illness in their late teens or early twenties which cuts them off from educational advancement. Many service providers offer basic education and high school equivalency programs, and a few offer "vocational training" programs. These educational programs enhance clients' future work opportunities but also encourage them to pursue higher education.

3. 第三步是辅助性就业，患者在康复机构安排下以正常雇员的身份工作并获得相应薪水，但需要精神卫生服务者的评估、协调和支持。

4. 最后是独立就业，同正常人一样从事竞争性的工作岗位。

医护人员可以作为工作的寻找者（与雇主合作，寻找更多的就业职位），辅导者（帮助患者找到工作及准备工作面试，协助患者工作直至他们适应了工作环境）或长期的支持者（提供长期辅导、解决问题和在工作期间的帮助，以支持患者长期工作）。

（九）教育培训

鼓励患者重返学校是目前所大力提倡的康复计划，对患严重精神障碍患者尤其重要。由于大部分患者多在青少年时期发病，导致他们未能完成学业。因此，应根据患者的实际情况，为患者提供基础教育或高中程度的教育课程，或职业训练课程。不仅可以帮助患者提高其工作能力，且能激励他们重返学校接受更高的教育。

Section 3 Community Mental Health Care

I. Principles of Community Mental Health Care

1. Coordinated Service It should be noted that an effective community mental health care service is coordinated and involves a clinical team (medical and

第三节　社区精神卫生护理

一、社区精神卫生护理的原则

1. **多部门协作**　社区精神服务需要卫生、教育、民政、公安、残联和劳动等部门密切配合，还要动员患者家属、邻居、单位、街

nursing staff, social workers and occupational therapists) which liaises with other service providers, e.g., non-government organizations which provide residential and recreational facilities, special education departments, labor offices and vocational training centers, etc.

道以及基层保健组织，福利机构，人民团体如妇联、康复中心等的热心参与，形成一个完整的服务网络，才能使优先的人力和资源发挥最大的效益。社区精神卫生护理是在精神障碍急性期得到控制后，在这个时期患者可以接受由医疗或社会福利专业人员负责的机构、中途宿舍、活动中心或庇护工场等的照顾，或由亲友、邻居、朋友和志愿者在社区照顾。

2. Ongoing Process Services begin from the point where management of acute psychiatric illness is completed, whether in a hospital or an outpatient clinic and are an ongoing long-term process. These can be provided by hostels, half-way houses, activity centers, sheltered workshops, and other mental health centers. They are supervised by professional workers in the medical and social setting; or through care and support by relatives, neighbors, friends and volunteers in the community. Occasionally, the neighborhood or the entire social community is involved.

2. 连续性 应努力建立一个“患者可以在各组成部分之间自由流动的服务体系”，避免患者在多种服务项目之间陷入无人照顾的裂缝之中。比如发病初期患者可以寻求门诊治疗；疾病严重时可住院或行日间治疗；出院时有社区服务交接的机制；在社区症状加重时能够及时向专科医院转诊；病情缓解后可进行职业康复，还可以接受居委会监护网络的照顾。

3. Comprehensive Services Community mental health services vary in intensity from outreach to outpatient and, from day care to inpatient care. They also involve psychotherapy (individual, family, and community) and rehabilitation activities.

3. 综合性 以不同强度提供形式多样的服务，从外展服务到门诊服务，从日间治疗到住院治疗，还包括心理治疗（个人、家庭和团体）和康复训练。

4. Assertive or Directive Care Psychiatric community care has to be “assertive” or directive, as psychiatric clients often lack the initiative to seek assistance. It usually involves the development of a strong psychosocial support system between the clients and their relatives and friends, social skills training for the clients and an effective psychoeducation program for the family members.

4. 自主性 精神障碍患者在社区通常不会主动寻求协助。因此，社区精神卫生护理必须有“自主性”或“直接性”，即护理人员必须在专业判断的基础上主动为患者提供服务。

5. Developing a Caring Community Community mental health care has to be conducive in developing a genuine “caring community” for clients. Instead of assuming the community is caring and supportive for the clients, the health professionals should be responsible for developing and building a supportive rehabilitation environment for community integration of clients. Members of the general community must be encouraged to interact with clients to enhance their understanding and acceptance towards these clients and their illnesses. On the other hand, clients must be encouraged to serve the community and become responsible and contributing members of society. Joint volunteer service projects with social welfare agencies and psychiatric rehabilitation organizations can be a good

5. 以关怀为核心 社区精神卫生护理必须为患者建立一个真正的“关怀社区”。专业医护人员必须为重新融入社区生活的患者建立一个支持性的康复环境。一方面，应鼓励社区居民与精神障碍患者多接触，以提高社区居民对精神障碍患者的了解和接纳。另一方面，应鼓励患者参与社区服务，积极为社区做贡献。如鼓励患者参加由社会福利机构和精神障碍康复组织举办的义工计划，使患者有机会正常地接触社会及社区居民。

starting point for the clients to serve the community, which could allow "normal" interaction with "normal" members of society.

II. Roles of Nurses in Community Mental Health Nursing

Community Psychiatric Nurses (CPNs) follow up clients who require services once they are discharged. The main objective of the service is to minimize the chance of relapse of thus reducing the utilization of hospital beds. CPNS also provide a service to clients not previously admitted to hospitals aimed at strengthening their coping capabilities and preventing further deterioration due to inadequate and inappropriate management at the primary stage of their illness. CPNS has become an increasingly important component of a comprehensive community service (table 18-3).

二、护士在社区精神卫生中的角色

社区精神科护士跟踪随访在出院后需要社区服务的患者。随着社区精神科护士的服务需求逐渐增加，社区精神科护士的角色亦逐渐扩展。例如，在社区中工作的社区精神科团队均有社区精神科护士参与，有些社区精神科护士也参与初级预防工作，以提高社区居民的精神健康。一些精神科专科医院拥有社区精神科护士团队，例如老年、儿童精神科专科社区护士。这些角色的扩展配合和满足了在社区中照顾患者的需要（表 18-3）。

Table 18-3 Roles and work areas of CPNs

Institutes	Roles	Work areas of tertiary prevention
Hospital-based	Residential nurse	Tertiary
	Discharge preparation service team	Secondary to tertiary
	Day care nurse	Tertiary
	Disease manager or file manager in community mental health clinic	Secondary to tertiary
	Team member of outpatient or mental health care, assist in managing suicide, family violence and rape victims	Primary to secondary
Community-based	Nurse in community mental health clinic	Primary to tertiary
	Case manager or file manager in community mental health clinic	Primary focused, could cover secondary to tertiary
	Case manager, nurse-in charge, or responsible nurse of community rehabilitation center, rehabilitation home and mental health nursing home	Tertiary

表 18-3 社区精神卫生护理人员的专业角色与三阶段预防的工作范围

机构	社区精神卫生护理人员的角色	所属三阶段预防的工作范围
以医院为基础	居家护理人员	三段预防
	出院准备服务小组	二、三段预防
	日间留院护理人员	三段预防
	社区精神科或心理卫生科的档案管理员或疾病管理师	二、三段预防
	参与门诊或心理卫生医疗团队，协助自杀、家暴及强暴受害个案的处置	一、二段预防

续表

机构	社区精神卫生护理人员的角色	所属三阶段预防的工作范围
以社区为基础	社区卫生服务中心公共卫生科护士	一至三段预防
	社区精神卫生中心的个案管理员或社工	以一段预防为主，也可涵盖二、三段预防
	社区康复中心、康复之家以及精神科护理之家的机构负责人（管理者）或个案管理护士或主护护士	三段预防

III. Program Elements in Community Mental Health Nursing

i. Mental Health Medical Services

1. Inpatient Services Some beds are provided in community mental health clinics to admit individuals who are incapable of living independently or are a risk to themselves or others. The services are on a short-term basis for clients experiencing complications, having poor treatment effects or needing diagnosis clarification and referral to mental health hospitals.

2. Outpatient Services Community outpatient services aim to provide dynamic assessment, counseling, prescription drugs for stable clients, and screening and referral for community residents who have mental health problems. Outreach services, such as telephone follow-up, community or home visits, should also be provided to patients who are unwilling or unable to be seen in a clinic.

3. Day Care Services Day care is a form of partial hospitalization, between outpatient and inpatient services. Clients receive adequate treatment and rehabilitation services, without leaving their community life. Day care can be done at dedicated centers or in patients' homes, similar to home-based beds in China. In addition to medications, psychological treatment which includes a variety of skills training is provided.

ii. Mental Health Prevention and Rehabilitation Services

Mental health care services are provided for all residents of the community, such as health education to improve knowledge of mental health, create a healthy living environment, improve individual mental health status, and develop good social adaptability. This also permits early identification and early intervention for residents in high-risk groups. In addition, mental health rehabilitation services are available for those already affected with mental disorders.

iii. Mental Health Social Services

Programs focus on providing care and management of people with mental disorders in the community,

三、社区精神卫生的服务内容

（一）精神卫生医疗服务

1. 住院服务 当患者不能照顾自己或由于精神病性症状对自己或他人构成威胁时，社区精神卫生中心需要中设置少量住院床位，供患者短期住院。对诊断不明、治疗困难或伴有严重并发症的患者应及时向专科医院转诊。

2. 门诊服务 社区门诊的任务是为病情稳定的患者进行动态评估、解答咨询、提供处方药物，并为社区居民的心理健康问题提供筛查和转诊。此外，还应向不愿或不能来诊的患者提供外展服务，如电话随访，社区或家庭访视。

3. 日间治疗 日间治疗是部分住院的一种形式，介于门诊和住院服务之间。患者既可以接受充分的治疗和康复服务，也能不脱离社区生活。日间治疗可以在专设中心，也可以在患者家中，类似于我国的家庭病床。治疗内容除了药物治疗、心理治疗，也包括各种技能训练。

（二）精神卫生保健和康复服务

精神卫生保健服务针对社区所有居民，普及精神卫生知识、创造健康生活环境、提高个体心理健康水平，培养良好社会适应能力。同时，针对高危人群进行早期识别和早期干预。此外，针对已经患病的人群，提供精神卫生康复服务。

（三）精神卫生社会服务

提供社区精神障碍患者的监护和管理，在住房、交通设施、信息获得、文娱设施、

public services in housing, transport facilities, access to information, recreational facilities, legal protection, political activities, education and employment opportunities and reducing barriers for people with mental disorders. Mental health services also provide psychological support for families, information consultation, advocacy to reduce public discrimination and prejudice against people with mental disorders.

法律保障、政治活动、受教育及就业的机会方面提供公共服务，为精神障碍患者生活减少阻碍。为患者的家庭提供心理支持、信息咨询，倡导公众减少对精神障碍患者的歧视与偏见。

iv. Case Management

（四）个案管理

Mitchell and Reaghard (1996) maintained that the purpose of case management is to serve as a client advocate by means of increased coordination of services. Case management comprises the activities aimed at linking the service system to the client and coordinating the various service components to achieve a successful outcome.

个案管理的目标是增加各服务之间合作，以保护患者的权利，最大限度地为患者联系及协调多项不同的服务，以确保他们之间能互相合作而达到所需效果。工作包括确保提供连续性照顾，克服系统的僵化、服务的片面、资源运用的不足、不能充分使用服务设施等问题。个案管理中，每位患者均有一位管理者，负责评估患者的需要，提出方案及进行护理计划等工作。

Mental health case management is almost exclusively a tertiary (rehabilitative) preventive effort aimed at clients who have a history of serious mental illness. Like all preventive efforts, priority is given to people most in need of case management services.

精神健康个案管理主要是为患有严重精神障碍的患者提供三级预防保健服务。与其他预防工作一样，此项工作需要有轻重缓急，最需要的患者获得优先服务，包括经常需要住院服务、社区精神卫生服务、急诊服务及危机处理服务的患者。

1. Goals of Case Management The goal of case management services is to decrease a client's use of services and thus make more services available to people not in a high-priority group. Specific outcome goals for heavy user groups include the following: (a) increased community tenure, measured by a reduction in the number of admissions to psychiatric hospitals and number of days of hospitalization and reduced use of emergency services; (b) decreased frequency of crisis situations; (c) increased independence in living arrangements; (d) increased involvement in vocational activities; (e) enhanced social support networks including families, peers, and support systems in the community; (f) achievement of client-initiated goals.

1. 个案管理目标 个案管理的目标是了解患者经常使用各种医疗服务的原因，以减少这些患者经常使用住院服务，从而节省资源，使这些资源可以运用于其他方面。因此，为大量使用各种服务的患者提供个案管理可以达到以下目标：① 有效使用社区资源，可以从不同的方面度量目标是否达到，如住院次数是否减少，使用日间医院及急诊服务是否减少等；② 减少危机的出现；③ 加强日常生活的独立性；④ 增强工作能力；⑤ 加强社交网络，包括家庭、朋友及其他支持体系；⑥ 达到患者制订的目标。

In principle, every member of the health care team could be a case manager. However, it is argued that CPNs are in a better position to be case managers. CPNs provide direct client care in their homes, and are in the best position to actively assess clients' level of functioning in the community and persistently see that client's needs are met. Gibbs, et al (1995) believed that nurses acting as

理论上，所有在医疗系统工作的专业人员均可作为个案管理的负责人。但是，社区精神科护士最适合担当此角色。社区精神科护士在患者家中直接提供护理，评估患者在社区的功能，了解患者的需求是否得到满足。Gibbs等（1995）认为护士担当个案管理者可

the case manager can promote consistency and lead to a strong nurse-client relationship that optimizes assessment and care-giving work in a way that cannot be achieved by a team of people as case manager.

以为患者提供专业的照顾，同时，社区精神科护士与患者所建立的良好护患关系是对患者进行有效的评估和护理的基础。因此，护士是最佳的个案管理者。

2. Key Functions of Case Management Although no definition of case management is universally accepted, most case management literature includes the following five functions:

(1) Identification and outreach: A comprehensive delivery system must have strategies to locate potential clients, inform them of available services, and ensure access to these services. Establishing and maintaining close working relationships with potential referral sources such as hospitals, community mental health centers, and social service agencies, is essential to meeting these goals.

2. 个案管理的核心活动 尽管目前对个案管理没有统一的定义，但护理界普遍认为个案管理主要应包括以下几方面的内容。

（1）发现个案，主动帮助：一个完善的医疗系统应能够及时发现有潜在问题的患者，及时告知其可获取服务的方法，确保患者能及时得到所需服务，以减少病情复发及需要住院机会。要达到上述目标，个案管理者需要与转介的组织或机构，如医院、社区精神卫生中心及社区服务机构等维持密切的合作关系。

(2) Assessment: Thorough assessment of a client's strengths and deficits is required for an effective service plan. Assessments should consider all aspects of a person's life, including psychological, emotional, financial, medical, educational, vocational, social, and residential needs. The knowledge and skills needed for comprehensive assessment are generally beyond the ability of one case manager and require a multidisciplinary approach. This assessment strategy facilitates an important goal of case management--the client's active involvement in the process.

（2）评估：全面评估患者各方面的需要，包括心理、情绪、经济、医疗、教育、工作、社交及居住等，在评估的基础上，根据患者的需要制订一套行之有效的服务计划。必须明确，对患者进行有效综合评估需要各医务人员合作，并需要患者自愿而主动参与，而非某个人的能力所能完全达到。

(3) Service planning and linkage with needed services: A comprehensive service plan guides all case management activities with a client. Therefore, nurses must formulate service plans carefully with extensive client and family involvement. The overall goal of the service plan is to assist people with mental illness to live in the community. It is developed based on needs identified during the assessment process and requires the participation of the client, the client's social network, and professional care resources. It should clearly state treatment objectives and specific actions that will be taken to meet them. The major components of the plan include the following (Worley, 1997): (a) specification of problem areas to be addressed; (b) identification of goals; (c) identification of the service and supports needed to achieve goals; (d) identification of the people or agencies who will undertake specific activities to achieve the objectives of the plan. (e) specification of a timeline for the completion of each objective; (f) identification of changes expected to result from the completion of each objective.

（3）制订服务计划，提供相关服务：综合性服务计划指导所有个案管理的活动。服务计划的目标是帮助精神障碍患者成功地投入社区生活，这需要能够对患者准确地进行评估，并需要患者及其家属参与计划的制订与实施。此外，需要与患者的社交网络、各专业的服务机构及各医疗康复资源连结，明确患者治疗的目的及活动。Worley（1997）认为个案管理服务计划主要包括：① 明确患者需要解决的问题；② 制订目标；③ 找出达到目标所需的服务及支持；④ 明确实施计划所需的专业人士或机构；⑤ 制订达到目标的时限；⑥ 制订计划预期的结果。

(4) Monitoring of service delivery: The monitoring function of case management serves two basic purposes. It ensures that the objectives of the service plan are being met and provides the information necessary for ongoing plan evaluation. The case manager assists the client in obtaining the services specified in the service plan. Because the needs of people with chronic mental illness are usually complex and require the services of many agencies, the case manager must be a coordinator and facilitator. Periodic review of the client's progress with each service provider is one of the case manager's duties. The case manager uses information gained from these contacts in periodic reviews of the entire service plan.

(5) Advocacy: Helping people receive all available services and influencing providers to improve existing services and develop new ones also are important case manager functions. A case manager has to help clients overcome barriers that keep them from getting the services or attain entitlements they need to live successfully in the community.

3. Critical Pathways of Care Critical pathways of care (CPCs) have emerged as the tools for provision of care in a case management system. A critical pathway is a type of abbreviated plan of care that provides outcome-based guidelines for goal achievement within a designated length of stay. Only one nursing diagnosis is used in this sample. A CPC may have nursing diagnoses for several individual problems.

CPCs are meant to be used by the entire interdisciplinary team, which may include nurse case manager, clinical nurse specialist, social worker, psychiatrist, psychologist, dietitian, occupational therapist, recreational therapist, chaplain, and others. The team decides what categories of care are to be performed, by what date, and by whom. Each member of the team is then expected to carry out his or her function according to the time line designated on the CPC. The nurse, as case manager, is ultimately responsible for ensuring that each of the assignments is carried out. If variations occur at any time in any of the categories of care, the rationales must be documented in the progress notes.

v. Assertive Community Treatment (ACT)

The ACT model emphasizes a multidisciplinary team approach that provides a comprehensive range of

（4）监督并评价服务系统：个案管理的监督及评价有两个功能：① 确保计划是否达到目标；② 提供有用的信息不断评价服务计划。长期慢性精神障碍患者的需求复杂，常需要不同机构的人员为其提供各项服务，个案管理者因而担当了统筹及协调的角色，以帮助患者获得所需的各项服务。管理者定期随访以了解各服务机构对患者服务的进展，接触各机构以获得各种有效的资料，从而全面地监督服务计划的实施情况。

（5）权利保护：个案管理者的重要角色是帮助患者获得各项服务，并尽可能最大限度的利用及完善各种现有服务，发展新的服务项目，使服务更加完善有效。管理者应帮助患者克服接受服务时所遇到的各种困难，并协助保障其获得社区生活的各项基本权益。

3. **护理路径** 护理路径是为照顾一组同类型患者（例如精神分裂症）的需要而制订的标准护理计划，护理路径可作为个案管理的工具，以有效的组织、安排及布置各项服务工作。护理路径这种标准护理计划将医疗团队给予患者的所有护理措施组织协调成一体，详述医疗团队中每个成员在照顾患者时的责任、护理措施、服务时限和护理措施的预期效果，指导护士为患者实施护理措施。护理路径也为护理的规范化、标准化提供了方法及途径。

收集临床护理路径的资料后，将所有主要的临界事件列出，包括主要的治疗护理措施，各医疗团队期望达到的目标等，制订新的临床护理路径，然后将新制订的临床护理路径和同类诊断患者以往的病历记录相比较，并需在医疗团队中传阅及评价（包括精神科护士、精神科医生、医疗社工、临床心理专家、职业治疗师等）。评价后作出修订，最后定稿。

（五）主动式社区治疗

主动式社区治疗是目前研究最为广泛、效果也最被推崇的社区服务模式。ACT 强调

treatment, rehabilitation and supportive services to help clients meet the requirement for community living, thus preventing rehospitalization. This model combines the best features of service brokerage and clinical case management and emphasizes outreach to clients in their natural settings. Primary features of this model include high staff-to-client ratios with caseloads no larger than 10 to 15 clients for each case manager, 24-hour responsibility for clients, and assertive outreach and treatment in the community. Because this case management model is labor intensive and thus more costly than traditional models, it is usually reserved for clients who have great difficulty in adjusting to their illnesses, a poor record of poor compliance, complex needs, and a record of frequent admissions..

通过多专业团队合作，为患者提供综合性的治疗、康复及支持服务，使患者得到恰当的社区照顾，从而减少再入院的机会。此模式强调患者在正常的环境中治疗及康复，其特点是专业人员与患者的人数比例较高（即每个工作人员负责的患者人数少）。在患者的原生环境（家中、邻舍或工作场所）中提供每天 24 小时不间断服务。因为此模式需要的工作人员较多，所需资源相对较多。一般只适合一些病情比较复杂且难处理的患者，比如那些不愿意接受治疗及经常入院的患者。

Section 4 Family Care

I. Family assessment

1. Family Function The level of family functioning can be determined by assessing such areas as the family's ability to negotiate and change when appropriate, respect for individual's choices, and the absence of intimidation. High-functioning families have open and clear communication and members are able to be both independent from and connected to their families.

2. Assessment of Vulnerability to Relapse Families are very concerned with their mentally ill member's vulnerability to relapse. Although families are not to be blamed for mental disorders, their interactions may influence the course of the disorder. Relapse is less common in families who see the client as ill (rather than lazy or manipulative) and provide support to one another. Relapse is more common in families who are highly critical, highly anxious, and preoccupied with their problems. Researchers have studied two family patterns, family expressed emotion (EE) and family affective style (AS). Families rated as high EE tend to be hostile, critical, and emotionally over involved with the client. Families rated as high AS are intrusive and make guilt-inducing remarks during emotionally charged family discussions. Both high EE and AS families are predictors of relapse for people who are psychiatrically disabled. Families are more

第四节　家庭护理

一、家庭评估

1. 家庭功能　应通过一系列的评估，了解家庭功能。评估内容包括家庭中的磋商能力，应对变化的能力，尊重家属选择的能力，以及是否强迫他人接受自己意见等情况。良好的家庭功能体现为明确而开放的沟通，家属既保持自己的独立性，同时也与家庭保持紧密的联系。

2. 复发的评估　疾病的复发往往是家庭最担心的问题，虽然家庭不会因某一成员罹患精神障碍而受责，但家庭关系确实会影响患者的病情进展及病程。在相互支持的家庭中，疾病较少复发。相反，过度焦虑紧张的家庭，患者疾病的复发较为常见。家庭模式相关研究证明，有两种家庭模式容易复发：过度表达情感的家庭和感性的家庭。过度表达情感的家庭倾向于敌对、批评及对患者投入太多情感。感性的家庭对成员过分干预，在家庭讨论时互相攻击对方，家属容易产生内疚。

likely to be excessively critical or over-involved when they lack information about the disorder and when they believe the symptoms are under the client's control. Family members who do not understand the nature of psychiatric disability may mistake the negative symptoms as laziness.

Medication noncompliance is another factor related to relapse. Medication noncompliance is linked to lack of insight into the disorder, medication side effects, cost of medication, missed outpatient appointments, and negative client/family attitudes toward medication.

药物治疗依从性差是精神障碍复发的原因。药物治疗依从性差是由于患者对自身疾病认识不足，或药物治疗的副作用、药物治疗的费用，以及患者和家庭对药物治疗的消极态度有关。滥用药物、酗酒及其他非遵医行为等会进一步损害患者的精神健康。

3. Family Burden Family burden affects the quality of life of the patients with mental disorders and their family members, and it is one of the key elements of family assessment (table 18-4).

3. **家庭负担** 家庭负担严重影响精神障碍患者及家庭成员的生活质量，是家庭评估的重要内容（表 18-4）。

Table 18-4 Family subjective burden and objective burden

Subjective Burden	Objective Burden
● Level of worry for the future	● Time helping client with daily living
● Distress due to family member's illness	● Time supervising the client
● Resentment of providing care for ill family member	● The actual tangible work of caring
● Extent of feeling of burden	● Effects on household, e.g. financial loss effects on health, children and family routine
● How much the client is seen as demanding, unreasonable or manipulating	● Tasks required to care for ill family member
● Emotional impact: relationship pressure with client, tension in family life	● Disruption to caregiver's life: time for, own work and chores
● Feeling of depression and anxiety	
● Level of hopelessness	
● Fear for safety of family members	

表 18-4 家庭的主观及客观负担

主观负担	客观负担
一对未来的担心程度	一帮助患者处理日常生活需要的时间
一因为家庭成员的生病导致的忧虑	一监护患者需要的时间
一对要为生病的家庭成员提供照顾不满	一照顾患者的实际工作强度
一感觉到的负担的程度	一对家庭的影响，如经济损失、对健康、孩子和家庭日常生活的影响
一家庭成员感受到的患者下列行为的程度：苛求、不可理喻、操纵	一照顾生病的家庭成员的任务
一情感影响：和患者的关系压力、家庭生活紧张程度	一照顾者生活被打乱：时间、自己的工作、家庭琐事
一感到抑郁或焦虑	

续表

主观负担	客观负担
—无望的程度	
—担心家庭成员的安全	

4. Home Visit Wheeler (1998) identifies the following components of the comprehensive assessment that must be completed during an initial visit or a second visit with the client: (a) client's perception of the problem and need for assistance. (b) Information regarding client's strengths and personal habits. (c) Health history, recent changes, support systems, vital signs, current medications, client's understanding and compliance with medications, nutritional and elimination assessment. (d) Activities of daily living (ADLs) assessment.(e) Substance use assessment. (f) Neurological assessment. (g) Mental status examination. (h) Comprehension of proverbs. (i) Global Assessment of Functioning (GAF) scale rating.

Other important assessments include information about acute or chronic medical conditions, patterns of sleep and rest, solitude and social interaction, use of leisure time, education and work history, issues related to religion or spirituality, and adequacy of the home environment. Box 18-2 presents some tips for home visit practice.

4. 家庭访视 Wheeler（1998）确定了家庭访视综合评估中应包含的部分，一般必须在前两次家访时完成：① 家访对象对自身问题的看法以及需要哪些协助。② 家访对象的优势和个人习惯的信息。③ 健康史，最近的变化，支持系统，生命体征，目前的药物，家访对象对药物的理解和药物治疗依从性，营养和排泄评估。④ 日常生活活动能力（ADL）的评估。⑤ 物质滥用情况评估。⑥ 神经系统评价。⑦ 精神状态检查。⑧ 对谚语（箴言）的理解。⑨ 功能大体评定（GAF）量表评分。其他重要的评估包括急性或慢性疾病的信息，睡眠和休息，孤独感和社会交往情况，如果时间充裕，还可以评估教育和工作经历，宗教和信仰，以及家庭环境是否良好。Box 18–2 列出了家访实践的一些技巧。

BOX 18-2 Learning More

Safety Tips for Home-Care Practice

S—Stay alert

Be alert and observant of the surroundings. When driving up to the client's home, pay attention to who is on the street around or near the client's residence; observe the condition of the neighborhood. Are there any thriving businesses in the area or are the streets deserted? Is litter present on the streets or are they clean and well kept? Pay attention to unusual noises or movement.

A—Announce your arrival in advance

If the client knows when to expect the nurse, he or she will be watchful for the arrival. Entrance into the residence will be immediate. Home-health nurses are generally viewed as friends of the neighborhood. Neighbors become aware of the schedule and often become protective. Sometimes the informal neighborhood leaders will alert the nurse when something is wrong, such as the presence of drug activity or an increase in crime.

BOX 18–2 知识拓展

家庭护理实践的安全技巧

S- 保持警惕

对周围的环境保持警觉和敏锐的观察。当驱车前往患者家中时，要注意谁在街边或谁正靠近患者的家。关注附近的情况。该地区经济是否景气？街道是否整洁？注意不寻常的噪音或活动。

A- 提前告知家访时间

患者若提前得知家访时间，家访过程会更加顺利。由于家访护士通常被患者视为邻里朋友，因而提前列出家访时间表会成为一种保护性因素。当周围出现一些危险因素，比如有人在吸毒或出现犯罪事件时，会有人善意提醒护士。

F—Follow your "gut"

Intuition is an excellent warning system. Any situations that create a feeling of discomfort should be taken seriously. If the nurse observes a group of individuals in the distance who instill a feeling of threat of fear, he or she should cross the street, enter the safety of a business, or return to the automobile and drive away. Likewise, when in the client's home, if the nurse feels threatened by family dynamics or a tense situation, he or she should leave immediately. If help is required with the situation, a phone call can be made once the nurse is safely away from danger.

E—Expect the unexpected

When the nurse expects the unexpected, he or she will be ready for any eventuality. Being mentally prepared to handle an unsafe situation will help the nurse avoid being caught "off guard." With experience and increased confidence, fear usually diminishes; however, the prudent home healthcare nurse is always cautious.

F- 相信你的"直觉"

"直觉"是躯体灵敏的警告系统。任何产生不适感的情况都应受到重视。如果护士看到在远处的一群人给你带来一种恐惧和威胁的感觉，应立即前往安全的地方寻求保护或驱车返回。在患者家中的时候，如果护士因为家庭关系或紧张局势而感受到威胁，也应立即离开。如果需要帮助，可在脱离危险之后立即拨打求助电话。

E- 预则立，不预则废

尽量分析各种可能发生的情形并做好充分准备。为处理危险情况做好心理准备将有助于护士避免突然袭击。随着经验的积累和信心的增加，恐惧通常会减少，但是小心驶得万年船。

II. Family Interventions

1. Principles of Family Care Family interventions focus on supporting the biopsychosocial integrity and functioning of the family as defined by its members. Include: (a) family intervention should be developed within a collaborative framework and be tailored to the needs of each family. (b) The aim is to empower the family to cope and adjust to the crisis of mental disorder. (c) The approach to pre-existing problems within the family should be guided by general crisis intervention principles. (d) It is important to determine the wishes of the person with the mental disorder regarding the involvement of the family. In some instances, people do not want their families involved, and the basis for this feeling should always be carefully explored. A young person's need for confidentiality and the importance of establishing a therapeutic relationship should be balanced against the needs of the family for support.

2. Psychoeducation Psychoeducation has many purposes and functions. The most important function is the transfer of information and the development of skills. Other functions include:

(1) Emotional catharsis and support: Newly diagnosed clients need to come to terms with their illness, and families need to work through feelings related to the illness. A new diagnosis of major psychiatric illness presents a crisis for the family and the client. Typically, the families may engage in a variety of normalizing behaviors to rationalize and explain their ill family member's

二、家庭干预

1. 家庭护理的原则 家庭护理措施的主要目的是维持家庭的完整性及良好的家庭功能，措施包括健康教育、支持、辅导及家庭治疗等。指导家庭护理措施的原则：① 家庭护理措施应针对家庭的特定需要，由家属与医护人员协调制订；② 其主要目标是协助家庭处理及适应精神障碍带来的危机及问题；③ 根据一般的危机措施原则处理已存在的家庭问题；④ 应考虑精神障碍患者是否希望其家属参与治疗与护理。有些患者不希望其家属参与，比如年轻患者常要求保护隐私，因此，护士应在与患者建立治疗性信任关系或邀请家属参与之间进行适当的平衡。

2. 心理健康教育 心理健康教育有多种目的和功能，其中最重要的功能是传达信息、发展技能，其他功能包括：

（1）情感的宣泄和支持：新近被诊断为精神障碍的患者需要时间接受疾病，而家属亦需要处理自己的情绪，这对家庭和患者都是生活的巨大变化及危机。一般家属会以合理化的方式将患者的异常行为解释为正常，并出现否认、情绪困扰、责备行为、忧伤、负罪感等反

behavior. Denial, emotional turmoil, blaming behavior, grief, and feelings of guilt are some typical responses. Psychoeducational programs need to allow time for the expression of these feelings without forgetting their educational purpose and moving to a therapy model.

应。心理健康教育为患者及家属提供了情感宣泄的机会，并及时提供教育及治疗。

(2) Development of support network: Family psychoeducation is often offered on a group basis in which several families meet together. These programs thus provide the nucleus of a new support network. Sometimes families of people with mental illness have withdrawn from social connections as they attempt to cope with their family members. Meeting and listening to other families allow them to begin to realize that they are not alone, to share solutions to problems, and to develop bonds with a new network of people who share their problems. People who receive their psychoeducational programs in a multiple family group format do better than those who participate in an individual family program. Psychoeducation also provides opportunities for sharing in a group, but in this case an assessment must be made of the client's readiness.

（2）发展支持性网络体系：家庭心理健康教育经常由不同的家庭共同参与。此方法提供了一个新的支持网络体系和分享经验的机会。有精神障碍患者的家庭有时会拒绝与外界接触，以应对家人患病所带来的问题。通过与同类疾病的患者和家属进行讨论，家属可以听到其他类似家庭的情况，同样的经历及感受可消除其孤独感，而共同讨论他们所面临的具体问题及解决方式，可增加彼此的了解及信任，以发展成一个同病相怜的支持网络体系。

(3) Information sharing: Psychoeducation involves considerable sharing of information about the illness and its management. Families who have lived with and struggled to manage their family members at home provide information about the client's functioning in the community, activities that do and do not help, and the client's response to medication and other treatment. Families have often resented mental health professionals for their lack of respect for the family, its interest, and its potential contribution. Family psychoeducation recognizes families as important allies in the treatment of the client and requires that the professional form a different relationship with the family than the traditional one. The program typically includes information about the disease process to give the client and family a conceptual framework with which to understand it. The information shared may vary according to the professional's background or psychoeducational approach.

（3）分享信息：在心理健康教育中，小组成员可相互讨论疾病的知识及其处理方法。可以相互分享患者在社区的功能状态，有效或无效的应对方法，患者对药物或其他治疗的反应等信息。家庭是帮助患者的一个重要元素，专业人员必须认识到家庭在患者康复中具有重要的作用，需要家属与专业人员建立新的合作伙伴关系，并向家属提供有关疾病及治疗的信息，使家属对疾病有进一步的了解。

(4) Skill development: A variety of skills are taught within psychoeducational models. Specific skills dealt with in each program vary with the target population, goals and conceptual framework, and needs of the group. Nevertheless, common skills include assertiveness training, problem solving skills, activities of daily living, cognitive training, communication skills, and stress management techniques. Techniques for teaching these skills are widely reported in the nursing literature and can be assimilated within a psychoeducational program.

（4）技能训练：心理健康教育需教授各种各样的生活技巧，常用的技巧包括自我表达训练、解决问题的技巧、日常生活的技巧、认知训练、沟通技巧、压力应对技巧。一般应根据不同的课程、对象、目的和理论架构而选择不同的技能培训。

(5) Linking with community and other resources:

（5）加强与社区的联系及资源的应用：有

Families of people with mental illness have often become alienated from their communities and friends. Preoccupation with the problem in the family, feelings that others will not understand, worry about stigmatization, and feelings of guilt and shame interact to support and sustain this isolation. Psychoeducational programs provide opportunities to renew community linkages. Multiple family groups and workshops provide a forum for the exchange of information and ideas with other families, which can reduce the sense of isolation and reinforce the understanding that problems are shared.

精神障碍患者的家庭常感到被他人歧视而产生烦恼、内疚及羞耻感。这些感觉使他们与社区和朋友疏远，倍感孤立。心理健康教育可加强家庭与社区的联系。家庭小组及工作培训场所可向家庭提供交流心得的机会，以减少家庭的隔离感，并帮助解决家庭遇到的实际问题。

(6) Symptom monitoring and self-management: In psychoeducational programs, clients and families can learn to understand the illness, identify early or prodromal symptoms, and act to prevent exacerbation of symptoms. This can help a client to develop early insight, to be able to self-monitor and self-control. A problem with many clients who are frequently readmitted (and with some families of these clients) is that they can identify symptoms requiring hospitalization but tend to overlook earlier signs of increasing tension. One goal of psychoeducation is to encourage clients to notice symptoms at an earlier stage when less radical intervention is needed.

（6）疾病症状的监测和自我照顾：在心理健康教育计划中，患者和家庭学习如何认识精神障碍的病征，以便识别早期或先兆期的症状，以采取行动，防止病情恶化。这可帮助患者及时产生洞察力，发展自我监测及控制的能力。因为多次入院的患者及其家属常忽略发病的早期症状，心理健康教育的目的之一是鼓励患者注意到早期阶段症状，以便及早发现及早治疗并控制疾病的进一步发展。

(7) General health promotion: Good general health is critical to mental health; clients should understand the need to maintain regular patterns of rest, nutrition, exercise, and general health care because these are important to them and also because they leave the body in optimal condition to withstand stress.

（7）一般性健康教育：有效的健康教育是维持健康的关键，患者应意识到适当休息、饮食、运动及维持健康等方法的重要。因为这些知识可帮助他们维持正常的身体状况，减轻压力。

(8) Home visits: Home visits by nurses have been reported intermittently in the treatment of patients with mental illness for many years. With the advent of community care and the continuing search for cost effectiveness, home visits to people with psychiatric illness are again becoming common. Psychoeducational models can be incorporated into intensive case management approaches by nurses and others.

（8）家庭访视：心理健康教育中常采用家庭访视的形式，随着社区护理的出现，护士对精神障碍患者进行家庭访视将更为深入。护士和其他医护人员可将心理健康教育结合到个案管理中，例如社区精神卫生护士可为精神障碍患者及其家属提供心理健康教育。

3. Family Therapy In the U.S., a clinical nurse specialist or nurse practitioner with a graduate degree in psychiatric nursing has received supervised clinical experience and has extensive knowledge and skills in psychiatric and mental health nursing. They can serve as a family therapist. The three main stages of family therapy are the initial interview, the intervention or working phase, and the termination phase.

3. 家庭治疗 在美国，具备研究生学位的临床护理专家或开业护士在获得足够的受督导的临床经验，并且在精神和心理健康护理方面拥有广泛的知识和技能后，可以成为家庭治疗师。家庭治疗主要包括三个阶段，即最初接触、治疗阶段和终止阶段。精神科护士通常也承担家庭治疗师的职责。

(1) Initial interview: During the initial interview, the therapist must be able to assess and synthesize the information the family has given and formulate ideas or interventions for bringing about positive changes to resolve the identified problems. There are specific stages

（1）最初接触：在初始的会面期间，治疗师必须评估及综合所有家属提供的信息，从而确立目标并制订计划及措施。最初的接触阶段可能包含以下过程：① 约会，初次与家庭

during an initial interview in which the therapist facilitates the process of determining which problems the family has identified as needing attention. These stages include: (a) engagement stage, the family is met and put at ease, all family members should involve. (b) Assessment stage: Problem(s) that concern the family are and family function identified. (c) Exploration stage: The therapist and family explore additional problems that may have a bearing on present family concerns. (d) Goal-setting stage: The therapist synthesizes information, and the family members state what they would like to see changed. (e) Termination stage: The initial interview ends, an appointment is set for the next session, and it is determined which family members need to attend.

会见，所有家庭成员均需参加；② 评估，家庭成员所提出的问题以及家庭功能；③ 调查分析，治疗师和家属分析其他被忽视的问题；④ 确立目标，治疗师综合所有资料，家庭成员说明其所期待的改变；⑤ 终止，即以接触评估为主的阶段初步结束，为下一阶段作出准备，并决定哪些家属需要继续参加治疗。

(2) Intervention or working phase: The goal of the working phase is to help the family accept and adjust to change. During this second phase families do a lot of work, and the therapist participates in the therapeutic process. Usually family sessions occur once a week for approximately one hour. During this phase, the therapist identifies strengths and problems of the family. Twelve family strengths were identified. The therapist should determine which of these strengths are present in the family seeking help. Identified strengths are useful in helping the family remain stable when other relationships seem threatened by change.

（2）治疗阶段：治疗阶段的目标是帮助家庭接受并适应家庭的变故。在此阶段，治疗师、患者和家属共同参与，一般每周 1 次，每次约 1 小时。治疗师的角色是协助家庭建立开放而诚恳的沟通方式，并及时向家庭提出建议，引导家庭面对问题，解决问题。家庭成员需明确家庭的优势；学习适当表达情绪的方法，尤其是有暴力问题、沟通不足的家庭；学会处理冲突。随着治疗的继续，家庭成员开始明白角色并非固定不变，而是随时变化及调整。每个人都会成长，可以变得更加具有独立、自主性。随着治疗的发展，家庭成员不但会增加彼此之间的了解，也可惊喜地看到成员行为的改变。

(3) Termination phase: Sometimes families want to terminate the sessions prematurely. This desire may be indicated by behavior. Family members begin to be late or do not show up for scheduled appointments, or not all members continue to participate, as agreed upon at the initial interview. Such behavior may occur if the family perceives that a certain type of change is threatening to the family's present functioning. At this point, it is important for the therapist to review the identified problems with the family and renegotiate the contract and number of family sessions. This review is helpful in recognizing which problems remain and which goals have been met. If the family has achieved the goals and the identified specific problems have been resolved, then it is time to initiate the termination phase.

（3）终止阶段：如果家属已完成目标，并解决了存在的问题，便可适当地进入终止阶段。然而，若家庭仍有未解决地问题，治疗师则不应该终止疗程。若家庭已经学会怎样有效地处理问题，发展了相应的支持系统，并学会了如何进行开放、诚恳、直接地沟通，家庭权力及角色经过了适当地分散及重组，家属能够独立地解决问题，原来存在的问题或患者的症状已减轻，可以终止家庭治疗。

However, the therapist should remember that no family terminates therapy without experiencing some problems. Also, some family members may be somewhat reluctant to terminate the sessions. Nevertheless,

但是家庭成员有时会提前终止疗程，表现为开始迟到或者不出席家庭治疗，或者并非所有成员都继续遵守之前的承诺参与疗程。

termination should take place. By now, the family has learned how to solve its own problems in a healthy manner, has developed its own internal support system, and has learned to communicate in an open, honest, and direct manner. Power has been appropriately assigned and redistributed, and family members are able to work out and resolve problems at home without the therapist's help or intervention. The original problems or symptoms have been alleviated, and it is time for termination of family therapy sessions.

(Yang Bingxiang)

如果成员觉得家庭的转变带来负面影响或威胁时，就会出现上述行为。这时，治疗师需要回顾及重新评估家庭的问题，且继续与家庭成员沟通有关问题。回顾及评估可帮助治疗师明确家庭还存在哪些问题，以及哪些目标已经达成或尚未达到。

（杨冰香）

Key Points

1. The continuity of mental health nursing care is a comprehensive system of services and programs designed to match the needs of the individual with the appropriate treatment in a setting that varies according to levels of service, structure, and intensity of care.
2. Interdisciplinary team changed from a medical team model to a collaborative model, which emphasizes shared decision making and includes family as a member of the team providing a service to meet the needs of the client.
3. The nurse may initiate a referral and transfer a client to other services that provide the care required by the individual. A good referral depends on knowledge of facilities, skill in selection, objectivity, timing, and follow up.
4. Psychiatric rehabilitation program is conducted in a variety of settings, such as in-patient units, outpatient settings, day hospitals, half-way house, patient's home and the community. psychiatric rehabilitation including social programs, residential programs, vocational programs, educational programs, discharge planning and relapse prevention programs.
5. Community mental health care is an ongoing long-term management process; it is a comprehensive and coordinated service and provides assertive care.
6. Case management comprises all activities aimed at linking the service system to the client and coordinating the various service components to achieve a successful outcome. Service broker model, clinical model/extended brokerage model, assertive outreach model/assertive community treatment are the three commonly used theoretical models.
7. Critical pathways of care (CPCs) have emerged as the tools for provision of care in a case management system.

内容摘要

1. 精神卫生连续性护理综合了各种服务和项目，为护理对象提供一系列的护理措施来帮助个体达到他/她的理想功能水平，所提供的服务层级、结构以及服务强度都有所不同。
2. 多学科团队已经由以医疗团队为主导的模型转向合作式模型，强调包括家属在内的团队成员共同决策以满足护理对象的需求。
3. 在多学科团队中，护士可以根据护理对象的需求发起转介，将其转介至其他机构。转介恰当与否取决于护士对各类医疗机构的了解，选择机构的技巧，客观性，及时性和后续服务。
4. 精神康复项目可以在不同的地方进行，例如医院病房、门诊部、日间医院、中途宿舍、患者家中或社区；康复项目通过工作、教育和社交训练，以及满足患者对医疗及住房的需求，帮助精神障碍患者重新融入社会。
5. 社区精神卫生护理是一个持续的过程，旨在提供综合性、自主性服务，以建立关怀社区。它涵盖医疗服务、保健康复服务、社会服务、个案管理及社区主动治疗。
6. 个案管理是在社区为精神障碍患者提供服务的一个主要方法，精神科护士在个案管理中担任重要的角色。在个案管理中，管理者需要评估患者的需要，提出方案，和团队合作制订及实施护理计划，以及监督服务和评价资源的使用情况，以确保服务符合患者的需要。
7. 护理路径是为照顾一组同类型患者（例如精神分裂症）的需要而制订的标准护理计

Each member of the team is then expected to carry out his or her function according to the time line designated on the CPC. The nurse, as case manager, is ultimately responsible for ensuring that each of the assignments is carried out.

划，可以有效地组织、安排及布置各项服务工作。

8. Family function, vulnerability to relapse, and family burden are the major elements that should be assessed during psychiatric family care. Home visit is one of the effective ways to do a comprehensive assessment.

8. 家庭功能、复发的可能性、家庭负担是家庭评估的主要内容，家庭访视是实施综合评估的一种有效的方法。

9. Family interventions focus on supporting the biopsychosocial integrity and functioning of the family as defined by its members. The most important psychoeducation function is the transfer of information and the development of skills.

9. 家庭护理侧重于向家庭提供生理及心理支持，维持健康的家庭功能。心理健康教育可帮助家属更加了解精神障碍、家庭系统并应对各种挑战。

10. Family therapy can be implemented by a psychiatric clinical nurse specialist or nurse practitioner. The three main stages of family therapy are the initial interview, the intervention or working phase, and the termination phase.

10. 家庭治疗包括最初接触、治疗和终止三个阶段。它可以帮助家庭培养开放的沟通模式，使家属发挥理想的功能。

Exercises

(Questions 1 to 2 share the same question stem)

Ann is a psychiatric home nurse. She has received an order to begin regular visits to Mrs. W., a 78-year-old widow who lives alone. Mrs. W's primary-care physician has diagnosed her as depressed. Ann found out that Mrs. W. is physically too weak to travel without risk of injury.

1. What might be a priority nursing diagnosis for Mrs. W?
2. Mrs. W. says to Ann, "What's the use? I don't have anything to live for anymore." What type of information should be obtained in an assessment?

(Questions 3 to 4 share the same question stem)

Jane is single, 33 years old, and has a history of multiple psychiatric admissions. She was referred to the community mental health center case management unit upon discharge from a 6-month stay at the state hospital. She had a diagnosis of undifferentiated schizophrenia in remission and was discharged to the care of her family on resperidone 4 mg daily. Jane has occasional auditory hallucinations, is somewhat suspicious, and has a long history of disruptive family relationships and noncompliance with medications. Lisa, the psychiatric nurse case manager, volunteered to take the case and made an appointment with the family for a home visit.

3. Lisa feels fearful when she arrives at Jane's home, what should Lisa do first?
4. What might be a priority nursing diagnosis for Jane?

思考题

（1～2 题共用题干）

Ann 是精神科护理中心的护士，她遵医嘱需要对 W 太太，一位独居的 78 岁丧偶老年妇女进行常规家访。W 太太被她的社区医生诊断为抑郁症，在家访中 Ann 发现 W 太太过于虚弱以至于存在跌倒受伤的风险

1. W 太太目前首要的护理诊断是什么？
2. W 太太对 Ann 说，“这有什么用呢，我已经没有值得活下去的理由了。”Ann 应该进一步评估哪一方面的信息？

（3～4 题共用题干）

Jane 是一名 33 岁的单身女性，曾经反复多次入住精神专科医院。在州立精神专科医院住了长达六个月后，Jane 被转介至社区精神卫生中心个案管理科。被诊断为“精神分裂症：未定型，缓解期”，出院医嘱：利培酮，4 mg，每日一次。Jane 存在偶发性幻听，有时敏感多疑，长期制造紧张的家庭关系，服药依从性差。Lisa 是一名精神科个案管理师，自愿接手 Jane 的个案管理，并同 Jane 的家庭约定了一次家庭访视。

3. Lisa 在到达 Jane 的家里时，有一种恐惧的感觉，Lisa 此时优先采取的措施什么？
4. Jane 当前首要的护理诊断是什么？

(Questions 5 to 6 share the same question stem)

When Lisa arrived, the family was visibly upset and related that in the week since Jane had been home, she slept much of the day and roamed around the house during the night, taking long showers, slamming kitchen cabinet doors, and playing loud rock music. When she was awake during the day, she should disappear for hours at a time, causing great anxiety for the family. The mother was tearful and wringing her hands in an agitated manner while the father sat on the sofa with his head bowed. Jane sprawled in a chair and intermittently swore at her mother as the mother described these events.

5. What might be the major family concern with Jane residing in the home?

6. Lisa recognizes that Jane's illness dominates the household. What type of interventions should be done first?

（5～6题共用题干）

当Lisa到达Jane的家里时，发现她的家人自从上周Jane出院回家后就一直焦虑不安，Jane的睡眠昼夜颠倒，彻夜不眠，白天酣睡。在夜间洗很长时间的洗澡，把厨房的柜门搞得砰砰响，把摇滚乐的声音调得很大。在白天很短的醒着的时间里，Jane总是会突然消失几个小时，导致家里人非常担心。她的母亲暗自垂泪，不停绞双手，焦虑不安，她的父亲低头窝在沙发上，在她母亲讲述这些事情的时候，Jane躺卧在椅子上不时朝她母亲吼两句。

5. Jane给家庭带来的最主要的负担是什么?

6. Lisa意识到Jane的疾病彻底支配着这个家庭的日常生活，她应当优先采取的护理措施是什么?

英文索引

A

a generic approach	274
abuse	340
action control	141
active phase	165
addiction	340
adventitious crises	269
affective response	249
agoraphobia	300
akathisia	474
Albert Ellis's rational-emotive therapy	543
alcohol intoxication	346
alprazolam	494
Alzheimer's disease	376
amphetamine-type stimulants (ATS)	352
anankastic personality disorder	234
anatomical abnormalities	163
anorexia nervosa	440
anticholinergic effects	479
antihistaminic effects	479
antimanic drugs	489
antipsychotic drugs	469
antisocial personality disorder	232
anxiety disorders	284
anxious personality disorder	234
assertive Community Treatment (ACT)	579
attention deficit and hyperactivity disorder (ADHD)	409
autistic disorder	402
autonomy	137

aversion	540
avoidant personality disorder	234

B

behavioral responses	250
behavioral therapy	534
beneficence	138
benzodiazepines	493
biofeedback	538
bipolar disorder	208
block D_2 and serotonin (5-HT_2) receptors	472
blockers of dopamine D_2 receptors	472
bulimia nervosa	444
buspirone	497

C

case management	577
choke	122
chronic motor or vocal tic disorder	425
circadian rhythm sleep disorder	451
client-centered therapy	548
clonazepam	495
cognitive appraisal	248
cognitive rehabilitation	178
cognitive therapy	542
collaborative model	560
community mental health nursing care	564
completed suicide	104
compulsions	308
concreteness	068
conduct disorders	415
confidentiality	138
continuity of nursing care	560
contract for safety	113
conversion symptoms	324
coping mechanisms	251
coping resources	251
counter-transference	074
critical pathways of care	579

D

D_2 dopamine receptors	472
day care	576
delirious mania	206
delirium	370
dementia	372
dependence	340
dependent personality disorder	235
depressive episode	207
dissocial conduct disorder	417
dissocial personality disorder	232
drug compliance	497
dystonia	474

E

eating different objects	124
electric convulsive therapy (ECT)	103
electroconvulsive therapy	210
electroconvulsive therapy (ECT)	505
emotional disorder	428
emotional stability disorder	035
emotionally unstable personality disorder	233
environmental manipulation	274
environmental supports	178
ethics	132
evidence-based nursing practice	053

F

family-oriented therapies are	177
flooding	539

G

general support	274
generalized anxiety disorder	289
genuineness	549
graded exposure	539
group therapy	177
guided imagery	550

H

half-way houses	572
hallucination	167
haloperidol	098
high potency	470
histrionic personality disorder	234
hypnosis	524
hypochondriasis	319
hypomania	206

I

3-inspections-7-verifications	499
independent employment	573
individual Approach	274
informed Consent	138
insight	043
insomnia	447
intelligence	042
interdisciplinary team	560
intoxication	341
intrusion symptoms	257
involuntary admission	147

J

justice	139

K

Korsakoff's Psychosis	349

L

light therapy	523
long-acting preparations	470
low-potency	470

M

major tranquilizers	469
manic episode	205
massage	551
maturational crises	268

mental health	004
mental illness	008
mental retardation	392
mental Status Examination	033
modeling	540
modified electroconvulsive therapy (MECT)	506
monoamine oxidase inhibitors	476
mood	201
mood disorders	202
mood stabilizers	476
music therapy	553

N

negative symptoms	473
neuroleptic malignant syndrome (NMS)	475
neurosis	283
neurotransmitters	091
nonmaleficence	139
nurse-client relationship	063
nursing assessment	031
nursing diagnosis	045
nursing ethnics	132
nursing evaluation	055
nursing implementation	054
nursing interventions	049
nursing process	029

O

obsessions	042
obsessive-compulsive disorder	305
opioids	350
oppositional Defiant Disorder	418
oral assaults	090
other medications of nonbenzodiazepines	493

P

panic	286
paranoid personality disorder	230
Parkinsonism	474
persistent mood disorder	209

personality change	228
personality disorders	228
personality traits	227
phenothiazines	470
phobic anxiety disorder of children	430
phobic anxiety disorders	297
phototherapy	523
physical attacks	090
physiological responses	250
positive reinforcement	540
positive symptoms	473
primary appraisal	249
primary hypersomnia	450
problem-oriented recording	056
prodromal phase	165
progressive muscle relaxation	535
protein-drug complexes	468
psychiatric contingency	089
psychiatric family care	565
psychiatric nursing	011
psychiatric rehabilitation	564
psychoactive substances	340
psychoanalysis	531
psychotherapy	530
psychotropic drugs	466

R

rapport	066
referral	565
relapse	570
relaxation	535
residual phase	169
respect	137
restraint	101
reward system	343
risperidone	470

S

schizoid personality disorder	231
schizoid Personality Phase	165

schizophrenia	160
Seclusion	101
secondary appraisal	249
selective serotonin reuptake inhibitors (SSRIs)	098, 476
self-determinism	141
self-disclosure	068
self-harming	117
separation anxiety disorder of children	429
sheltered workshops	572
short-acting preparations	472
situational crises	269
social anxiety disorder of children	430
social phobia	300
social responses	250
social skill training	177
social skills training	541
somatization disorder	316
specific phobia	299
spontaneous leave	118
steady state	468
stress	248
substance-related disorders	340
suicidal attempt	104
suicidal gesture	104
suicidal ideation	104
suicidal threat	104
suicide	103
suicide prevention center or crisis management of America	115
supported employment	573
sustained avoidance	256
sustained hypervigilance	257
systematic desensitization	538

T

tardive dyskinesia	474
the "atypical" antipsychotic drugs	470
the "typical" antipsychotic drugs	470
the code of ethics	140
the dissociative symptoms	324
the distance of communication	099

the frontal lobes	091
the half-life	468
the hypothalamus	091
the limbic system	091
the newest drugs (atypical agents)	470
the side effect of extrapyramidal symptoms (ESP)	122
therapeutic touch (TT)	552
therapy	540
tic disorders	424
tobacco use disorder	355
tolerance	341
Tourette's syndrome	425
transcranial magnetic stimulation therapy (TMS)	521
transference	073
transient tic disorder	425
transitional employment	572
trauma and stressor-related disorder	252
tricyclic and related drugs	477

U

unconditional positive regard	549

V

vascular dementia (VaD)	379
verbal persuasion	100
violence	090
voluntary admission	146

W

Wernicke's encephalopathy	349
withdrawal	341

中文索引

A

阿尔茨海默病 376
阿片类物质 350
Albert Ellis 的理性情感治疗法 543
安全契约 113
按摩 551

B

半衰期 468
保密原则 138
暴力行为 090
Beck 的认知疗法 544
苯丙胺类兴奋剂 352
苯二氮䓬类 493
庇护工场 572
边缘系统 091
表演型人格障碍 234

C

残留期 169
操纵 276
成瘾 340
澄清 276
痴呆 372
迟发性运动障碍 175

持续性心境障碍 209
抽动秽语综合征 425
出走 118
闯入性症状 256
创伤后应激障碍 253
创伤与应激相关障碍 252
催眠 524
错觉 167

D

蛋白质 - 药物复合物 468
电抽搐治疗 103
电抽搐治疗 505
丁螺环酮 497
独立就业 573
短暂性抽动障碍 425
多巴胺功能亢进假说 162
多学科团队 560

E

额叶 091
恶性综合征 474
儿童抽动症 424
儿童孤独症 402
儿童恐惧症 430
儿童情绪障碍 428
儿童社交恐惧症 430

F

发泄 275
发展性危机 268
反社会型人格障碍 232
反向移情 074

防御性支持	277
放松	535
非苯二氮䓬类药物	493
非经典抗精神病药物	470
非自愿入院	147
分离性焦虑障碍	429
分离症状	324
分裂样人格障碍	231
酚噻嗪类	470
氟哌啶醇	098
辅助性就业	573

G

隔离	101
个案管理	577
个别化方法	274
公正原则	139
光感治疗	523
光线治疗	523
过渡性就业	572

H

《护士伦理守则》	140
合作式模型	560
和谐关系	066
护患关系	063
护理程序	029
护理措施	049
护理路径	579
护理伦理学	132
护理评估	031
护理评价	055
护理实施	054
护理诊断	045

环境干预	274
环境支持	178
幻觉	167
回避型人格障碍	234
回避症状	256
活跃期	165

J

肌张力障碍	474
即时沟通	068
急性肌张力障碍	174
急性应激障碍	252
继发性评价	249
家庭导向治疗	177
建议	276
渐进式肌肉放松	535
交往距离	099
焦虑性人格障碍	234
焦虑障碍	284
戒断	341
经典抗精神病药物	470
经颅磁刺激治疗	521
精神发育迟滞	392
精神分裂症	159
精神分裂症人格期	165
精神分析法	531
精神活性物质	340
精神疾病	008
精神健康	004
精神康复	564
精神科护理学	011
精神科意外事件	089
精神卫生家庭护理	565
精神药物	466

精神状况检查 033
警觉性增高症状 257
静坐不能 175
酒精中毒 346
具体化 068

K

抗精神病药物 469
抗躁狂药物 489
科萨科夫综合征 349
恐惧性焦虑障碍 297

L

来访者中心疗法 548
滥用 340
类帕金森综合征 474
利培酮 470
连续性护理 560
惊恐 286
伦理 132
氯硝西泮 495

M

满灌疗法 539
慢性抽动障碍 425
美国的自杀预防中心或危机干预中心 115

N

耐受性 341
脑结构异常 163

O

偶然性危机	269

P

偏执型人格障碍	230
品行障碍	415

Q

5- 羟色胺受体假说	162
前驱期	165
强安定剂	469
强迫观念	042
强迫行为	308
强迫型人格障碍	234
强迫障碍	305
轻躁狂	206
情感淡漠	169
情感稳定性障碍	035
情绪不稳型人格障碍	233
情绪反应	249
情绪取向机制	252
躯体化障碍	316
全面支持	274

R

人格	227
人格改变	228
人格障碍	228
认知康复	178
认知疗法	542
认知评价	248
日间治疗	576

S

社会反应	250
社会技能训练	177
社交技能训练	541
社交恐惧障碍	300
社交紊乱型人格障碍	232
社区精神卫生护理	564
神经递质	091
神经性贪食症	444
神经性厌食症	440
神经症	283
生理反应	250
生物反馈技术	538
失眠症	447
失认	375
失用	375
失语	375
示范法	540
事故性危机	269
适应性障碍	253
嗜睡症	450
双相障碍	208
思维贫乏	170
思维形式障碍	169

T

坦诚	549
探索解决问题的方法	277
特殊恐惧障碍	299
提升自尊	277
通情	548
同理心	066
吞食异物	124

W

妄想	169
危机	268
韦尼克脑病	349
稳态	468
问题取向机制	252
无抽搐电痉挛治疗	210
无抽搐电痉挛治疗	506
无害原则	139
无条件的积极关注	549
舞蹈症状	175
物质相关障碍	340

X

系统脱敏疗法	538
下丘脑	091
想象力放松	550
小组治疗	177
血管性痴呆	379
心境	201
心境障碍	202
心理治疗	530
新型药物	470
兴趣缺失	170
行为反应	250
行为控制	141
行为疗法	534
行为强化	276
选择性 5- 羟色胺再摄取抑制剂	098
循证护理实践	053

Y

烟草使用障碍	355
言语劝诱	100
广场恐惧障碍	300
广泛性焦虑障碍	289
厌恶疗法	540
阳性症状	471
药物依从性	497
噎食	122
一般性方法	274
依赖	340
依赖型人格障碍	235
移情	073
疑病障碍	319
以问题为中心的记录	056
抑郁发作	207
意志缺乏	170
音乐治疗	553
应对机制	251
应对资源	251
应激	248
有利原则	138
原发性评价	249
约束	101
运动不能	175
运动困难	175

Z

躁狂发作	205
谵妄	370
谵妄型躁狂	206
帕金森综合征	175
正强化	540

知情同意原则	138
治疗性触摸	552
智能	042
中毒	341
中途宿舍	572
昼夜节律障碍	451
逐级暴露疗法	539
主动式社区治疗	579
注意缺陷与多动障碍	409
专业技术职务	135
转换症状	324
转介	565
锥体外系不良反应	122
自杀	103
自杀死亡	104
自杀威胁	104
自杀未遂	104
自杀意念	104
自杀姿态	104
自伤	117
自我暴露	068
自我认定障碍	168
自愿入院	146
自知力	043
自主决策	141
自主原则	137
尊重原则	137

参考文献

1……• 陈瑞全，吴建贤．经颅磁刺激在脑卒中康复治疗中的应用 [J]. 世界最新医学信息文摘：连续型电子期刊，2015，64:45-47.

2……• 邓荆云．精神疾病护理 [M]. 北京：人民卫生出版社，2014.

3……• 范青，梅力，肖泽萍．焦虑障碍的流行病学研究进展 [J]. 中华精神科杂志，2010，43（3）：183-186.

4……• 方贻儒，刘铁榜，杨甫德，等．双相障碍抑郁发作药物治疗专家建议 [J]. 中国神经精神疾病杂志，2013，39（7）：385-390.

5……• 郝香，徐瑞雪．精神科病房强制性护理干预潜在的法律问题及管理对策 [J]. 中国社区医师，2015（11）：158-160.

6……• 胡强，万玉美，苏亮，等．中国普通人群焦虑障碍患病率的荟萃分析 [J]. 中国精神科杂志，2013，46（4）：204-211.

7……• 郝伟，于欣．精神病学 [M]. 7 版．北京：人民卫生出版社，2013.

8……• 刘哲宁．精神科护理学 [M]. 3 版．北京：人民卫生出版社，2013.

9……• 雷慧．精神科护理学 [M]. 3 版．北京：人民卫生出版社，2014：107-119.

10……• 李小妹，王文茹．精神科护理学 [M]. 北京：人民卫生出版社，2006.

11……• 祁革，朱宏日，王宁，等．无抽搐电痉挛治疗中不安全事件原因分析及防范措施 [J]. 解放军医药杂志，2013，25（1）：70-71.

12……• 王艳芳，李家凤．精神科护理中相关的法律问题探讨 [J]. 中国误诊学杂志，2010，10（26）：6379-6380.

13……• 许晓丽，赵丽云，房红芸，等．2010—2012 年中国 15 岁及以上居民饮酒状况 [J]. 卫生研究，2016，45（4）：534-537.

14……• 杨雪，任艳萍，姜玮，等．电痉挛治疗后谵妄的表现、评估及处理．精神医学杂志，2015（3）：228-231.

15……• 余雨枫．精神科护理学 [M]. 2 版．北京：人民卫生出版社，2016.

16……• 尤春景．经颅磁刺激技术在神经康域的应用 [J]. 中国医疗器械信息，2010，16（2）：9-11.

17……• 张焱，孙岚，田伟．重复经颅穴位磁刺激对偏瘫患者康复的影响 [J]. 中国康复理论与实践，2010，16（8）：781-782.

18……• 郑亚琦．精神科护理工作常见的法律问题与对策 [J]. 当代医学，2011, 17（34）：30-31.

彩 插

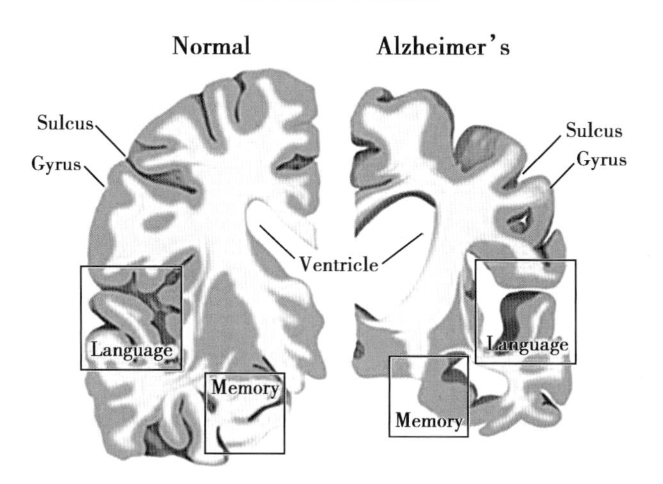

Figure 12-1　Brain with Alzheimer's disease

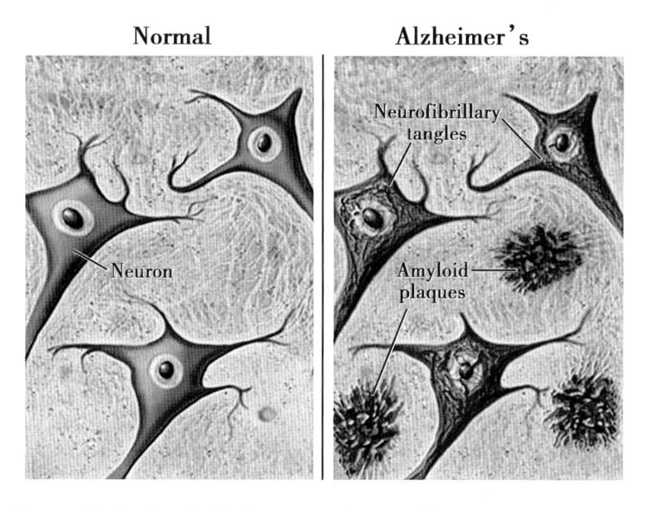

Figure 12-2　Amyloid plaques and neurofibrillary tangles